EVIDENCE-BASED PRACTICE

for NURSING and HEALTHCARE
QUALITY IMPROVEMENT

EVIDENCE-BASED PRACTICE

for NURSING and HEALTHCARE QUALITY IMPROVEMENT

Geri LoBiondo-Wood, PhD, RN, FAAN
Professor and Coordinator, PhD in Nursing Program
University of Texas Health Science Center at Houston—Cizik School of Nursing
Houston, Texas

Judith Haber, PhD, RN, FAAN
The Ursula Springer Leadership Professor in Nursing
New York University
Rory Meyers College of Nursing
New York, New York

Marita G. Titler, PhD, RN, FAAN
Professor and Dumas Endowed Chair
University of Michigan School of Nursing
Ann Arbor, Michigan

ELSEVIER

ELSEVIER

3251 Riverport Lane
St. Louis, Missouri 63043

Executive Content Strategist: Lee Henderson
Content Development Manager: Lisa Newton/Ellen Wurm-Cutter
Content Development Specialist: Melissa Rawe/Sarah Vora
Publishing Services Manager: Julie Eddy
Senior Project Manager: Tracey Schriefer
Design Direction: Patrick Ferguson

Printed in China

Last digit is the print number: 9 8 7 6 5 4 3 2 1

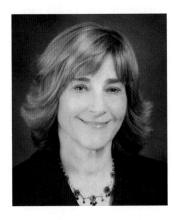

Geri LoBiondo-Wood, PhD, RN, FAAN, is Professor and Coordinator of the PhD in Nursing Program at the University of Texas Health Science Center at Houston, Cizik School of Nursing (UTHSC-Houston) and former Director of Research and Evidence-Based Practice Planning and Development at the MD Anderson Cancer Center, Houston, Texas. She received her diploma in nursing at St. Mary's Hospital School of Nursing in Rochester, New York; bachelor's and master's degrees from the University of Rochester; and a PhD in Nursing Theory and Research from New York University. Her research and publications focus on families, chronic illness, symptom management in children, and oncology nursing. Dr. LoBiondo-Wood is an editor of the award-winning textbook, *Nursing Research: Methods and Critical Appraisal for Evidence-Based Practice,* now in its 9th edition and translated into six languages. Dr. LoBiondo-Wood teaches and mentors doctoral students in research and works extensively with health care organizations on how to promote evidence-based practice (EBP) and conduct research. At MD Anderson Cancer Center, she developed and implemented the Evidence-Based Resource Unit Nurse (EB-RUN) Program, a hospital-wide program that involved all levels of nurses in the application of research evidence to practice. She has extensive national and international experience guiding nurses and other health care professionals in the development and utilization of research. Dr. LoBiondo-Wood is on the editorial board of *Progress in Transplantation* and is a reviewer for *Nursing Research, Oncology Nursing Forum, Oncology Nursing,* and *Journal of Professional Nursing.* For the fourth consecutive year in 2017, she received a Future of Nursing Scholars Program grant from the Robert Wood Johnson Foundation to fund full-time doctoral students.

Dr. LoBiondo-Wood has been active locally and nationally in many professional organizations including the Oncology Nursing Society, Southern Nursing Research Society, Midwest Nursing Research Society, and North American Transplant Coordinators Organization. She has served as Grant Review Chairperson for the American Nurses Foundation and has received local and national awards for teaching and contributions to nursing. In 1997 she received the Distinguished Alumnus Award from the New York University Division of Nursing Alumni Association. In 2001 she was inducted as a Fellow of the American Academy of Nursing and in 2007 became a Fellow of the University of Texas Academy of Health Science Education. In 2012 she was appointed a Distinguished Teaching Professor in the University of Texas system, and in 2016 she received the John P. McGovern Outstanding Teacher Award for Graduate Education from the University of Texas Health Science Center at Houston.

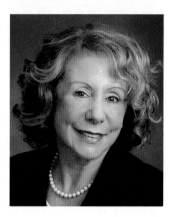

Judith Haber, PhD, RN, FAAN, is the Ursula Springer Leadership Professor in Nursing at the Rory Meyers College of Nursing at New York University. She received her undergraduate nursing education at Adelphi University in New York and holds a master's degree in Adult Psychiatric-Mental Health Nursing and a PhD in Nursing Theory and Research from New York University. Dr. Haber is internationally recognized as a clinician and educator in psychiatric–mental health nursing. She has extensive clinical experience in psychiatric nursing, having been an advanced practice psychiatric nurse in private practice for more than 30 years, specializing in treatment of families coping with the psychosocial sequelae of acute and chronic catastrophic illness. She was the editor of the award-winning classic textbook, *Comprehensive Psychiatric Nursing,* published in eight editions and translated into five languages. Her NIH-funded program of research addressed physical and psychosocial adjustment to illness, focusing specifically on women with breast cancer and their partners and, more recently, breast cancer survivorship. Dr. Haber is also an editor of the award-winning textbook, *Nursing Research: Methods and Critical Appraisal for Evidence-Based Practice,* now in its 9th edition and translated into six languages. She teaches and mentors master's, DNP, and PhD students in EBP and has worked extensively with health care organizations and their nursing staffs on promoting evidence-based culture in acute care settings. Dr. Haber also is committed to an interprofessional program of clinical scholarship related to population health by improving oral-systemic health outcomes. She leads the *Oral Health Nursing Education and Practice (OHNEP)* program funded through the National Interprofessional Initiative on Oral Health (NIIOH) by the DentaQuest and Arcora Foundations, and the HRSA-funded *Teaching Oral Systemic Health (TOSH)* program. Dr. Haber has been active locally and nationally in many professional organizations including the American Nurses Association, the American Psychiatric Nurses Association, and the American Academy of Nursing. She has received numerous local, state, and national awards for public policy, clinical practice, and research, including the APNA Psychiatric Nurse of the Year Award in 1998 and 2005 and the APNA Outstanding Research Award in 2005. She received the 2007 NYU College of Nursing Distinguished Alumnus Award, the 2011 NYU Distinguished Teaching Award, and the 2013 NYU Alumni Meritorious Service Award. In 2015 Dr. Haber received the Sigma Theta Tau Marie Hippensteel Award for Excellence in Nursing Practice; in 2017 she was a recipient of the DentaQuest Health Equity Hero Award. She is a Fellow of the American Academy of Nursing and the New York Academy of Medicine. She has consulted, presented, and published widely on evidence-based practice, interprofessional education and practice, and oral-systemic health issues.

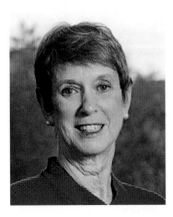

Marita G. Titler, PhD, RN, FAAN is the Rhetaugh G. Dumas Endowed Professor and Chair of the Department of Systems, Population, and Leadership at the University of Michigan School of Nursing. She is the former Director of Research and Quality at the University of Iowa Hospital and Clinics and the inventor of the Iowa Model of EBP to Improve Quality of Care. She received her bachelor's degree in nursing from Mount Mercy College in Cedar Rapids, Iowa, and her master's and PhD from the University of Iowa College of Nursing in Iowa City, Iowa. Dr. Titler is an internationally recognized expert in EBP and translation science. She teaches and mentors graduate students in EBP and implementation science and has authored more than 150 publications in referred journals including *Medical Care*, *Health Services Research*, and *Implementation Science*. Dr. Titler has been an important contributor to all nine editions of *Nursing Research: Methods and Critical Appraisal for Evidence-Based Practice*. Her program of research is in outcome effectiveness and implementation science supported by federal (NIH, AHRQ, CDC) and foundation funding (RWJF). She has been PI on five translation and outcome effectiveness studies funded by AHRQ (R01), NINR (R01) NCI (R01), and RWJF and co-investigator on numerous others funded by NIH, AHRQ, VA, and the CDC. Dr. Titler is the PI of the T32 institutional training grant *Complexity: Innovations in Promoting Health and Safety* (T32 NR016914). She has served on study sections for NIH, AHRQ, the Canadian Foundation for Innovation, and the Canadian Institute for Health Research. She has been a member of several national committees including the National Advisory Council for AHRQ and the Committee on Standards for Developing Trustworthy Clinical Practice Guidelines for the Institute of Medicine. Dr. Titler is active nationally in several professional organizations including the American Academy of Nursing, National Academy of Medicine, Council for the Advancement of Nursing Science, and Academy Health. She is currently a member of the NCI Symptom Management and Health-Related Quality of Life Steering Committee (SxQoL SC). She has received numerous awards for her work including the American Organization of Nurse Executives National Researcher Award, Sigma Theta Tau International Elizabeth McWilliams Miller Award for Excellence in Research, the Friends of NINR President's Award for Translation Science, and the Distinguished Alumni Award from the University of Iowa. She was inducted into the American Academy of Nursing in 1994 and the National Academy of Medicine and New York Academy of Medicine in 2016.

CONTRIBUTORS

Christine Ann Anderson, PhD
Clinical Assistant Professor
School of Nursing
University of Michigan
Ann Arbor, Michigan

Carol Bova, PhD, RN, ANP
Professor
Director of PhD Program
Graduate School of Nursing
University of Massachusetts Medical School
Worcester, Massachusetts

Maja Djukic, PhD, RN
Assistant Professor
Rory Meyers College of Nursing
New York University
New York, New York

Sheila Maria Gephart, PhD, RN
Assistant Professor
College of Nursing
The University of Arizona
Tucson, Arizona

Mattia J. Gilmartin, PhD, RN
Executive Director
NICHE Nurses Improving Care for
    Health System Elders
Rory Meyers College of Nursing
New York University
New York, New York

Susan Kaplan Jacobs, MA, MLS, BSN
Health Sciences Librarian
Elmer Holmes Bobst Library
New York University
New York, New York

Carl Kirton, DNP, RN, MBA
Chief Nursing Officer
Patient Care Services
University Hospital
Newark, New Jersey;
Adjunct Clinical Associate Professor
Rory Meyers College of Nursing
New York University
New York, New York;
Lecturer
Business Administration
St. Peter's University
Jersey City, New Jersey

Barbara Krainovich-Miller, EdD, RN, PMHCNS-BC, ANEF, FAAN
Consultant
New York, New York;
Adjunct Clinical Professor
Rory Meyers College of Nursing
New York University
New York, New York

Barbara R. Medvec, DNP, RN, NEA-BC
Clinical Assistant Professor
School of Nursing
Department of Systems, Populations and Leadership
University of Michigan
Ann Arbor, Michigan

Amy Lynn Msowoya, DNP, FNP-C
Family Nurse Practitioner
Stetson Hills Family Medicine-Anthem
Stetson Hills Family Medicine
Glendale, Arizona

Dona Rinaldi, EdD
Professor and Chair
Department of Nursing
The University of Scranton
Scranton, Pennsylvania

Leah Shever, PhD
Director of Nursing Research, Quality, and
    Innovation
Department of Nursing
The University of Michigan Health System
Ann Arbor, Michigan

Susan Sullivan-Bolyai, DNSc, CNS, RN, FAAN
Professor
Associate Dean for Research and Innovation
Graduate School of Nursing
University of Massachusetts Medical School
Worcester, Massachusetts

REVIEWERS

Karen E. Alexander, PhD, RN, CNOR
Program Director, RN-BSN
Assistant Professor
Department of Nursing
University of Houston Clear Lake-Pearland
Houston, Texas

Shirley M. Newberry, PhD, RN, PHN
Professor Emeritus
Department of Nursing
Winona State University
Winona, Minnesota

TO THE FACULTY

The foundation of this first edition of **Evidence-Based Practice for Nursing and Healthcare Quality Improvement** is the belief that evidence-based practice is integral to preparing the next generation of clinical, educational, and administrative leaders. As the health care system transforms and new health care models, payment systems, and treatment modalities are introduced, evidence-based decision making, in collaboration with patients, their families and the health care team, becomes ever more important.

The translation of research into practice is linked with all aspects of patient care. Clinical research provides findings that require evaluation before implementation. A key recommendation from the National Academy of Medicine (NAM) and multiple national and global health care organizations is a compelling call to base practice on evidence. Achieving a practice that provides high quality and cost-effective care and satisfying patient experiences requires practitioners in all clinical areas and specialties to gather, critically appraise, recommend and deliver practices based on evidence.

As editors, we believe that all health care practitioners need to be competent to use research evidence wisely. As individual studies are reviewed and assessed, it is essential that they also be synthesized as a body of evidence to identify the overall risks and benefits of advocating for a change in policy and/or practice. We realize that critically appraising the findings of research studies and determining the applicability of findings to practice is a challenge. Possessing the knowledge necessary to accept this challenge is a key to preparing students for future roles as clinical, educational, and administrative leaders.

The primary audiences for this textbook are master's and doctoral students and practicing clinicians changing the landscape of advanced clinical practice by building their knowledge base about the principles and methods of EBP and their applicability to practice.

The purpose of this innovative textbook is to provide a user-friendly road map for master's and doctoral students and clinicians that underscores the importance of evidence as a significant foundation for their practices, including the hows and whys of the EBP and quality improvement processes. This textbook features an implementation science approach to EBP that includes implementation and dissemination strategies. It prepares clinicians to become knowledgeable research consumers and practitioners by providing the following:

- Overview of EBP using the Iowa Model
- Overview of EBP and quality improvement models
- Model for developing compelling clinical questions
- Pragmatic road map for the searching the literature using an information literacy framework associated with developing clinical questions
- Five robust chapters on critical appraisal of quantitative and qualitative research designs
- Unique chapter on Quality Improvement models and application to practice
- Five exciting chapters on implementation strategies for EBP, quality improvement, and patient engagement
- Two unique concluding chapters on evaluation and dissemination of EBP projects
- Six appendices featuring published articles including a meta-analysis, randomized controlled study, quality improvement project, and two EBP projects, all of which are integrated as exemplars throughout the text
- Interprofessional Professional Education Collaborative (IPEC) competencies that provide an important collaborative framework to guide interprofessional teams working on evidence-based initiatives
- Numerous pedagogical chapter features including **Learning Outcomes, Key Terms, Evidence-Based Practice Tips, QI Checkpoints, IPE Tips, IT Resources, Decision-Making Algorithms, and Key Points** plus numerous clinical examples, tables, boxes, and figures

In this first edition of *Evidence-Based Practice for Nursing and Healthcare Quality Improvement*, the text is organized into three parts.

PART I – INTRODUCTION contains two chapters. Chapter 1, "Overview of Evidence-Based Practice," provides a compelling overview and historical roots of EBP. It presents the exciting steps of evidence-based practice based on the Iowa Model, which is a thread throughout this textbook. It also introduces the importance of the clinical leader's role as a member of an interprofessional EBP team. Chapter 2, "Models and Evidence," provides in-depth information about the Iowa Model and its principles; it also features other EBP models. This chapter also provides a concise overview of types of clinical questions, evidence retrieval, and grading and synthesizing of evidence, all of which are addressed in detail in subsequent chapters. The chapter introduces an evidence hierarchy model that is used throughout the text. This chapter also includes tips for building clinical questions and a summary of the GRADE Working Group criteria for assessment of study quality. It provides an example of a Table of Evidence (TOE) for organizing retrieved and critically appraised studies. The engaging style and content of this chapter are designed to make subsequent chapters more user-friendly for students.

PART II – PROCESSES OF DEVELOPING EBP AND QUESTIONS IN VARIOUS CLINICAL SETTINGS. The next eight chapters address and explicate processes essential for developing clinical questions, searching the literature, and assessing identified study methods and analyses. Chapter 3, "Developing Compelling Clinical Questions," focuses on important strategies for developing and operationalizing clinical questions in EBP. Chapter 4, "Search and Critical Appraisal of the Literature," provides a user-friendly guide for students conducting focused or comprehensive searches. Innovative strategies are presented for synthesizing the evidence for a body of evidence. Chapter 5, "Principles of Assessing Research Quality," offers a powerful presentation of the key principles for assessment of quantitative designs. It helps develop students' knowledge about sources of bias that affect how a study's design impacts evaluation, interpretation, and application of findings. Chapters 6 through 9 address quantitative and qualitative designs, illustrate the importance of critical appraisal issues for specific designs, and develop competencies related to synthesizing the overall strength and quality of evidence provided by a group of studies. Chapter 10, "Understanding Statistics for Evidence-Based Practice," presents a pragmatic overview of statistical processes used in research studies and EBP. The aim of this chapter is to increase student competence in understanding, interpreting, and critically appraising statistics used for data analysis in published research studies to enhance clinical decision making about the applicability of findings to practice.

PART III – IMPLEMENTATION. This unique section of the text is designed to teach methods for successful implementation of EBPs in a variety of settings such as communities, health care organizations, and ambulatory care. The five chapters in this section provide a compelling, in-depth presentation of EBP and quality improvement processes for planning, launching, and implementing successful EBP and quality improvement initiatives. Chapter 11, "Evidence-Based Approaches for Improving Healthcare Quality," presents major quality improvement models used in health care and promotes the clinical leader's role in advancing quality improvement initiatives and selecting quality measures that are most appropriate for specific practice settings. The chapter emphasizes the importance of applying and evaluating quality improvement interventions that align with national quality aims, priorities, and initiatives. Chapter 12, "Planning for Success," provides an exciting overview of the Translating Research into Practice (TRIP) model to guide selection of implementation strategies that promote adoption of EBPs. This chapter also emphasizes the importance of quality improvement as a foundation for EBP, principles of implementation, an action plan, and ethical considerations in EBP. Chapter 13, "Launching Implementation," focuses on innovative implementation strategies to address two of the four components of the TRIP model: the characteristics of the EBP clinical topic and communication. The research base and exemplars for each of the implementation strategies are discussed. Examples of implementation strategies to address the characteristics of the EBP topic include quick reference guides and clinical decision support tools. Examples regarding communication include opinion leadership, education, and academic detailing.

Chapter 14, "Implementation Strategies for Stakeholders," focuses on more important implementation strategies to address the remaining two components of the TRIP model: the users of the EBP and the social system. The research base and innovative exemplars for each of the implementation strategies are discussed. Transformative examples of implementation strategies that target users of the EBPs, also called members of a social system (e.g., nurses, physicians, and clerical staff), include performance gap assessment and audit and feedback. Examples of implementation strategies to address the social system, also known as the context of care delivery, include environmental scanning and engagement with key leaders in the practice setting.

Chapter 15, "Patient-Centered Evidence-Based Practices," provides a unique perspective on using innovative evidence-based strategies to engage individuals, families, and communities as partners. The goal is to advance a self-care agenda using consumer activation, health literacy, shared decision-making aids, and virtual health modalities.

PART IV – EVALUATION AND DISSEMINATION. The two chapters in this section offer students engaging approaches and tools to evaluate the impact of EBPs and methods for disseminating their work to colleagues and external audiences in the form of presentations, publications, and social media. Dissemination is the final and most important step in 9 EBP.

Chapter 16, "Evaluation of Evidence-Based Practice," outlines the key steps and methods for evaluating the impact of implementing EBPs. Emphasis is placed on the use of QI principles, selection of process and outcome indicators and data sources, analysis and display of evaluative data, considerations for addressing fiscal outcomes, and production of an evaluation summary for key stakeholders.

Chapter 17, "Dissemination," challenges clinical leaders to identify innovative virtual and face-to-face dissemination strategies that creatively communicate, educate, market, and present the findings of EBP initiatives to internal and external stakeholders.

Advancing an evidence-based foundation for clinical leaders is an essential priority for the future of the nursing profession. The first edition of *Evidence-Based Practice for Nursing and Healthcare Quality Improvement* provides an outstanding call to action. It guides graduate students to develop significant competence in understanding, interpreting, critically appraising, synthesizing, and engaging in clinical decision making about the applicability of evidence to improve health care and patient and population outcomes. To the extent that this objective is accomplished, the next generation of nursing leaders will have a cadre of colleagues who strive to provide evidence-based, high-quality, cost-effective, and satisfying health care experiences for individuals, families, and communities.

Geri LoBiondo-Wood
Geri.L.Wood@uth.tmc.edu
Judith Haber
jh33@nyu.edu
Marita Titler
mtitler@med.umich.edu

TO THE STUDENT

We invite you to join us on an exciting journey into the realm of evidence-based practice (EBP) to improve quality of care. Both EBP and quality improvement (QI) are terms often heard in health care. Our contributions to EBP at the national and local levels places the nursing profession at the forefront of change and supports care that is high quality, safe, and cost-effective. Use of evidence to improve quality of care requires not only knowledge of the EBP and QI processes but also knowledge of the collaborative interprofessional and intraprofessional processes involved in effective team membership and/or leadership.

Your EBP journey begins as you turn the first page of *Evidence-Based Practice for Nursing and Healthcare Quality Improvement*. You will discover that using evidence and quality data is essential to improving health care, which positions you, as a nursing leader, at the center of change. You will discover that EBP is integral to meeting the challenge of quality whole-person care in partnership with patients and their families and significant others, and with the communities in which they live. Finally, you will discover the richness of developing a foundation of advanced knowledge and skills to prepare you for the central role you will play as a clinical leader making a significant contribution to your organization or practice's patient outcomes!

We think you will enjoy reading this text. Your graduate courses that address EBP and QI will be filled with new and challenging learning experiences that will advance your EBP and quality improvement knowledge and skills. The first edition of *Evidence-Based Practice for Nursing and Healthcare Quality Improvement* is an exciting dialogue about cutting-edge trends for enhancing your evidence-based leadership role, whether it is in a clinical, educational, or administrative setting.

The four-part organization and special features of this text are designed to help you develop your critical thinking, information literacy, and evidence-based clinical decision-making skills while providing a user-friendly approach to learning that expands your competence in dealing with these new and challenging experiences.

EBP skills are needed in all clinical, education, and administration settings and can be applied to every patient population, clinical practice or system issue. Whether your clinical practice involves primary or specialty care and provides inpatient or outpatient treatment in a hospital, clinic, or home setting, you will be challenged to apply your evidence-based practice skills and use research as the foundation for your EBP. *Evidence-Based Practice for Nursing and Healthcare Quality Improvement* will guide you through this exciting adventure as you discover your vital leadership role in building a professional, evidence-based practice.

ACKNOWLEDGMENTS

No major undertaking is accomplished alone. Many individuals and groups contribute directly or indirectly to the success of a project. With deep appreciation and gratitude, we acknowledge the help and support of the following people:

- Our faculty and students, particularly those at the University of Texas Health Science Center at Houston Cizik School of Nursing, the Rory Meyers College of Nursing at New York University, and the University of Michigan School of Nursing. Their interest, lively curiosity, and challenging questions sparked ideas for this innovative new text.
- Our colleagues in community and practice settings that inform our vision and critical thinking for translating research into practice.
- Our chapter contributors, whose passion for research, EBP expertise, cooperation, commitment, and punctuality made them a joy to have as colleagues.
- Our colleagues, who have taken time out of their busy professional lives to offer feedback and constructive criticism that helped us prepare this first edition.
- Susan Mellott, for her generous help with Chapter 11.
- Our administrative support staff, who helped us with version control of chapters and facilitated communication among us.
- Our editors, Lee Henderson, Melissa Rawe, Tracey Schriefer, and Sarah Vora, for their patience and willingness to listen to yet another creative idea about teaching EBP in a meaningful way, and for their expert help with manuscript preparation and production.
- Our families: Rich Scharchburg; Brian Wood; Lenny, Andrew, Abbe, Brett, and Meredith Haber; Laurie, Bob, Mikey, Benjy, and Noah Goldberg; Sarah Titler, Eric Chamberlin, and Sloan; Nate and Robin Titler; and Grace, Madison, and Wyatt for their unending love, faith, understanding, and support throughout what is inevitably a consuming but exciting experience.

Geri LoBiondo-Wood
Judith Haber
Marita Titler

CONTENTS

1

Overview of Evidence-Based Practice

Marita Titler, Geri LoBiondo-Wood, Judith Haber

LEARNING OUTCOMES

After reading this chapter, you should be able to do the following:

- Describe the historical perspective of evidence-based practice (EBP).
- Compare and contrast conduct of research, EBP, translation science, and quality improvement.
- Describe Donabedian's Framework for Quality Improvement.
- Describe strategies and work of agencies that demonstrate the national agenda for EBP.
- Describe the steps of EBP.
- Identify rationale for including consumers on EBP teams.
- Describe actions that can be used to promote EBPs in the clinical setting.

KEY TERMS

Conduct of research
Evidence-based practice
Implementation science

Outcomes
Processes of care
Quality improvement

Translation science

Since the early 2000s, the advancement of knowledge about effective interventions to achieve improved outcomes has exploded. As nursing leaders prepared at the master's and doctoral levels, you will assume responsibility for ensuring that evidence from nursing science and the science of other disciplines is used in practice. Whether as faculty or as clinical leaders in health care organizations, you will be preparing the nursing workforce to be members of interprofessional and intraprofessional health care teams that use the best available evidence to achieve optimal outcomes across health care settings and populations. Among

the greatest challenges you will face as nursing leaders is engaging your colleagues in committing to using an evidence-based approach to guide practice. In your role, you will lead or be interprofessional and intraprofessional team members, asking relevant clinical questions, accessing and assessing the best information, implementing evidence-based practice (EBP), and evaluating the effect on expected outcomes. Meeting this challenge is integral to improving the health of populations, reducing the per capita cost of health care, and enhancing the experience of care (Berwick et al., 2008). Whittington and colleagues (2015) have demonstrated that three components are important to meeting this challenge:

1. development of a foundation for population management,
2. management of services at scale for a population, and
3. building a learning system to support the work.

The application of evidence to improve quality of care and patient outcomes is central to health care improvement. The United States faces the triple threat of explosive growth in chronic illness incidence, persistent challenges to improve population health and safety, and rising health care expenditures (IOM, 2012b; Ward, Schiller, & Goodman, 2014). Although US spending in health exceeds that of all other developed nations, key measures of health lag behind, particularly for preventable chronic conditions and associated functional decline (Squires & Anderson, 2015). Several reports of the IOM (now called the National Academy of Medicine) describe multiple opportunities for implementation of evidence in health care to improve population health and health care delivery (IOM, 2009, 2011, 2012, 2013, 2015). Despite the availability of evidence-based recommendations for practice, the 2014 National Healthcare Quality and Disparities Report demonstrated that evidence-based care is delivered only 70% of the time, an improvement of just 4% since 2005 (AHRQ, 2015). This problem demonstrates the gap between the availability of evidence-based recommendations and application to improve patient care and population health. This gap is linked to poor health outcomes such as obesity, poor nutrition, health care–acquired infections, injurious falls, and pressure ulcers (Conway, Pogorzelska, Larson, & Stone, 2012; Shever, Titler, Mackin, & Kueny, 2010; Sving, Gunningberg, Högman, & Mamhidir, 2012; CDC, 2016). This chapter provides an overview of EBP to lay the groundwork for you to actualize EBP in health care.

IPE TIP

Evidence-based practice is a team activity! The IPEC Competencies in Appendix G provide a framework for you to use when thinking about how successful EBP teams operate. The IPEC Competencies suggest that understanding the roles and responsibilities of team members from different professions, valuing, and respecting what each team member has to offer, and communicating effectively contribute to teams that function as a strong unit.

HISTORICAL OVERVIEW

Nursing has a rich history of using research in practice, pioneered by Florence Nightingale, who used data to change practices that contributed to high mortality rates in hospitals and communities (Nightingale, 1858, 1859, 1863a, 1863b). Beginning in the 1970s, nursing science has grown, and findings have become available to guide practice. EBP (called *research utilization*) was advanced by demonstration projects and programs such as the following:

- Conduct and Utilization of Research in Nursing (CURN) project (Horsley et al., 1983),
- Western Interstate Commission for Higher Education in Nursing (WICHEN) regional program on nursing research development (Kreuger, 1978; Kreuger, Nelson, & Wolanin, 1978; Lindeman & Krueger, 1977),
- Nursing Child Assessment Satellite Training project (NCAST; King, Barnard, and Hoehn, 1981),
- Moving New Knowledge Into Practice Project (Cronenwett, 1995; Funk, Tornquist, & Champagne, 1989), and
- Orange County Research Utilization in Nursing Project (Rutledge & Donaldson, 1995).

These seminal projects laid the groundwork for application of research findings in practice to improve patient care, known today as *evidence-based practice*. More recently, the nursing profession has provided major leadership for improving care through EBP (Kirchhoff, 2004), and today nurses are leading the way in translation science (Brooks et al., 2009; Estabrooks et al., 2008; Newhouse et al., 2013; Titler et al., 2009, 2016; Wilson et al., 2016), and EBP (Dickinson & Shever, 2012; Dockham et al., 2016; Kelly & Titler, 2010; Kueny et al., 2015; Madsen et al., 2005; Mark, Titler, & Lattimer, 2014; Shever & Dickinson, 2013; Titler & Moore, 2010; Titler, 2010, 2011, 2014). As a result, the scientific body of knowledge translation and the application of evidence in health care are growing. Advancements in implementation science can expedite and sustain the successful integration of evidence in practice to improve care delivery, population health, and health outcomes (Henly et al., 2015).

EBP TIP

The knowledge advanced from implementation science, coupled with health care environments that promote the use of evidence-based practices, will help close the evidence practice gap (NINR Strategic Plan, 2016).

DEFINITION OF TERMS

Various terms are used in the field of EBP (Table 1.1). It is essential that you start or advance your involvement in EBP by crystalizing your understanding of the differences between conduct of research and EBP. As detailed in Table 1.2, you will note that EBP and conduct of research have distinct purposes, questions, approaches, and evaluation methods. Conduct of research is the systematic investigation of a phenomenon to answer research questions or hypotheses that generate new knowledge and advance the state of the science. For example, as an investigator, you may be testing the efficacy of a mobile e-application designed to improve self-care of individuals with heart failure (HF) because the state of the science is questionable and prior studies are nonrandomized with small sample sizes. As a randomized controlled trial, your study aims to advance science by using a more rigorous design in which subjects in your study will meet specific inclusion criteria, and be randomized to the experimental or comparison arm (see Chapter 6). Measures of self-care management with demonstrated reliability and validity will be collected at baseline, after the completion of the intervention, and for specified follow-up time points. Upon study completion, you will disseminate your research at scientific conferences and in scientific journals.

Evidence-based practice is the conscientious and judicious use of current best evidence in conjunction with clinical expertise, patient values, and circumstances to guide health care decisions (Straus, Glasziou, Richardson, & Haynes, 2011; Titler, 2014). Best evidence includes findings from randomized controlled trials, evidence from other scientific designs such as descriptive and qualitative research, and information from case reports and scientific principles. When enough reliable research evidence is available, practice should be guided by research findings in conjunction with clinical expertise and patient values. In some cases, however, a sufficient research base may not be available, and health care decision making is derived principally from other evidence sources such as scientific principles, case reports, and outcomes of quality improvement (QI) projects. For example, there is a strong evidence base for a psychoeducational intervention for dyads of adult cancer patients and caregivers that provides them with information and support for improving coping and quality of life, and decreasing distress (Dockham et al., 2016; Northouse et al., 2005, 2007, 2010, 2013).

When thinking about use of this intervention in your practice, you will need to consider the following:
- the components of the intervention,
- whether you or other staff have the expertise to deliver this intervention,
- the perceptions of the populations of cancer patients you care for, and
- in what circumstances you will offer this intervention (e.g., newly diagnosed cancer patients vs. those at end of life).

In making these decisions, you will need to carefully weigh the research regarding the following:
- multiple components of the psychoeducational intervention tested,
- setting and format in which it has been tested (group format of three or four dyads in a cancer support community agency; individual dyads in the home),
- qualifications and specialized training of the interventionist (e.g., master's-prepared nurse, licensed master's-prepared social worker), and
- inclusion and exclusion criteria of the dyads (patients and caregivers) included in the studies.

EBP TIP

When planning for implementation of EBPs, remember that it is not just the importance or value of the EBP topic as perceived by users and stakeholders (e.g., ease of use, valued part of practice) that will influence their adoption. It is the interaction among the characteristics of the EBP topic, the intended users, and a particular context of practice that determines the rate and extent of adoption.

Quality improvement is both a philosophy of organizational functioning and a set of analysis tools and change techniques to reduce variations in the quality of care provided by health care organizations (Nelson et al., 2007). QI emphasizes customer satisfaction, teams and teamwork, and the continuous improvement of work processes. Other defining features include setting organizational performance goals and expectations, use of data to make decisions, and standardization of work processes to reduce variation across providers and service encounters (Nelson et al., 2007) (see Chapter 11). For example, members of your health care organization's QI council are concerned about an increase in fall rates over the past 6 months that are higher than those of peer organizations in NDNQI reports. You are charged with

TABLE 1.1   Terms Used in EBP and Implementation Science

Term	Description
Translational research	A dynamic continuum from basic research through application of research findings in practice, communities, and public health settings to improve health and health outcomes; progresses across five phases: preclinical and animal studies (T0/basic science research); proof of concept/Phase 1 clinical trials (T1/testing efficacy and safety with small group of humans); Phase 2 and Phase 3 clinical trials (T3/testing the efficacy and safety with larger group of humans; compare to common treatments); Phase 4 clinical trials and clinical outcomes research (T4/translation to practice); Phase 5 population-level outcomes research (T5/translation to community)
	The translational phases along this continuum are sometimes referred to as "bench-to-bedside" and "bedside-to-community" (Institute of Medicine [IOM], 2013).
Conduct of research	Systematic investigation of a phenomenon to answer research questions or hypotheses that advances the state of the science
Implementation science (also called translation science)	Field of science that focuses on testing implementation interventions to improve uptake and use of evidence to improve patient outcomes and population health, and explicate what implementation strategies work for whom, in what settings, and why (Eccles & Mittman, 2006; Titler, 2010, 2014)
Dissemination research	Targeted distribution of information and intervention materials to a specific public health or clinical practice audience with the intent to spread, scale up, and sustain knowledge use and evidence-based interventions (National Institutes of Health, 2013a)
Comparative effectiveness research	Generation and synthesis of evidence that compares benefits and harms of alternative methods to prevent, diagnose, treat, and monitor a clinical condition, or to improve the delivery of care
	Purpose: to assist consumers, clinicians, purchasers, and policy makers to make informed decisions that will improve health care at both the individual and population levels
	This definition implies the direct comparison of two or more effective interventions in patients who are typical of day-to-day clinical care (IOM, 2009).
Knowledge translation	A term primarily used in Canadian implementation research and defined by the Canadian Institute for Health Research (www.cihr-irsc.ca/e/) as "a dynamic and iterative process that includes synthesis, dissemination, exchange, and ethically sound application of knowledge to improve the health of Canadians, provide more effective health services and products, and strengthen the health care system"
Knowledge transfer	"The process of getting knowledge from producers to potential users" (Graham et al., 2006)
	Knowledge transfer has been criticized for its "unidirectional notion and its lack of concern with the implementation of transferred knowledge" (Graham et al., 2006).
Evidence-based practice	Conscientious and judicious use of current best evidence in conjunction with clinical expertise and patient values to guide health care decisions (Straus et al., 2011; Titler, 2014)
Quality improvement	A set of statistical analysis tools and change techniques used to reduce variations in the quality of care provided by health care organizations (Nelson et al., 2007)
Evidence-based policy	Policy developed through a continuous process that uses the best available quantitative and qualitative evidence to improve public health outcomes (Browson, Chriqui, & Stamatakis, 2009)
Evidence-informed decision making (EIDM)	Process of combining a range of sources of evidence to inform a decision
	In practice, this occurs within a political context that requires consideration of a range of other factors including research evidence, community views, budget constraints, and expert opinion (Armstrong et al., 2013).
Policy dissemination and implementation research	Research focused on generating knowledge to effectively spread research evidence among policy makers and integrate evidence-based interventions into policy designs (Purtel, Peters, & Brownson, 2016).

TABLE 1.2   Comparison of EBP and Conduct of Research

Components	Conduct of Research[a]	EBP[b]
Purpose	Knowledge/science generation Example: Test an intervention to improve cognitive performance of older adults with HF.	Application of research findings and/or other evidence in local practice and/or communities Example: Implement evidence-based fall prevention interventions targeted to patient-specific fall risk factors for hospitalized older adults.
Synthesis of the science/ knowledge	Identify gaps in the science Example: Despite high prevalence and severe consequences of memory loss in HF, there are no research-based therapies to improve memory in HF patients. Few studies have tested interventions to improve cognition in HF. Prior studies have been small sample sizes, and lacked control groups.	Synthesize the evidence and set forth EBP recommendations. Example: Because falls are complex and risks for falls are multifactorial, beneficial effects of fall reduction interventions increase when interventions target patient-specific fall risk factors. Fall prevention interventions should be customized to the individual's identified fall risk factors. Example: For those with mobility risk factors (e.g., gait instability, lower limb weakness, required assistance getting out of bed), the following EBPs are recommended: • Ambulate 3–4 times per day with assistance as needed unless contraindicated. • Refer to physical therapy for assessment and gait and strength training. • Minimize use of immobilizing equipment (e.g., indwelling urinary catheters, restraints). • Ensure proper assist equipment (e.g., walker, cane) is readily available and in proper working condition.
Question	Research questions or hypotheses that advance the state of the science Example: Compared with active control and usual-care control groups, do HF patients who receive BrainHQ have greater improvement in delayed recall memory, instrumental activities of daily living, and health-related quality of life?	Clinical question or purpose of the EBP project derived from the PICO Example: Does implementing EB fall prevention interventions that target patient-specific risk factors decrease falls and fall injuries of hospitalized older adults? The purpose of this EBP project is to implement EB fall prevention interventions targeted to hospitalized older adults' fall-specific risk factors for those cared for in noncritical care settings to decrease falls and fall injuries.
Approach	Research design that is aligned with the research questions/hypotheses (e.g., observational; RCT; step-wedge design) Example: A three-arm RCT comparing BrainHQ with computerized general cognitive stimulation with crossword puzzles (active control) and usual care with no computerized cognitive stimulation (usual care).	Nonresearch design: Track measures (see Evaluation in this table) for a specified period of time preimplementation, during implementation, and postimplementation. Example: Falls and types of fall injuries for 6 months before implementation, midway through implementation (3 months), and after implementation (6 months)

Continued

TABLE 1.2	**Comparison of EBP and Conduct of Research—cont'd**	
Components	**Conduct of Research**[a]	**EBP**[b]
Evaluation	Standardized dependent measures with known reliability and validity Example: Hopkins Verbal Learning Test—Revised delayed recall measure; instrumental activities of daily living; Everyday Problems Test; Minnesota Living with Heart Failure Questionnaire	QI metrics that address both processes of care and patient outcomes. Use standardized QI measures when available. Example: *Outcome indicator*—fall rates defined as an unplanned descent to the floor, calculated, at the unit level, by the number of inpatient falls multiplied by 1000 and divided by the total number of inpatient days *Process indicator*—If a specific fall risk factor was present, was an EB fall prevention intervention implemented that targeted the patient-specific fall risk factor? Number of patient days a specific risk factor is present, such as gait instability (1285 patient days); number of times an EB fall prevention intervention was implemented that targeted the patient-specific fall risk factor per 100 patient days; rates of correct intervention per 100 patient days (e.g., 31/100 patient days; 88/100 patient days)

[a]Examples from National Institute of Nursing Research–funded R01 (NR016116), "Cognitive Intervention to Improve Memory in Heart Failure Patients" principal investigator: S. Pressler.

[b]Examples from Titler, M.G., Conlon, P., Reynolds, M.A., Ripley, R., Tsodikov, A., Wilson, D.S. et al. (2016). The effect of a translating research into practice intervention to promote use of evidence-based fall prevention interventions in hospitalized adults: a prospective pre-post implementation study in the U.S. *Applied Nursing Research, 31,* 52–59.

BrainHQ, A computerized cognitive training program; *EB,* evidence-based; *EBP,* evidence-based practice; *HF,* heart failure; *PICO,* problem/patients/populations, intervention, comparison, outcome; *QI,* quality improvement; *RCT,* randomized controlled trial.

addressing this concern. How might you use principles of QI and organizational quality data in conjunction with evidence to guide your approach?

QI CHECKPOINT

W. Edwards Deming is the father of modern QI, which started in the 1940s. Deming's QI approach is centered on process management—that is, managing processes of care (Best & Neuhauser, 2005).

The principles for QI set forth by Deming include the following: (1) QI must be data driven; (2) improving pro-cesses of care is necessary to improve **outcomes**; (3) about 20% of the health care processes account for nearly 80% of the inefficiencies and wide variations in process of care (Pareto principle); and (4) managing processes of care means engaging clinicians who understand the care delivery process and are equipped to figure out improving processes of care over time (Haughom, 2016). A common QI framework used with EBP is *Structure-Process-Outcome* (Donabedian, 1966). *Structure* includes the physical and organizational components of care delivery such as facilities, equipment, and staffing. *Process* of care is the services

and treatments patients receive (e.g., early removal of Foley catheters). *Outcomes* are the effect that the processes of care have on patients and populations, such as catheter-associated urinary tract infection (CAUTI) rates. This framework will be helpful as you plan for EBP implementation (see Chapter 12) and evaluation (see Chapter 16).

QI and EBP have similarities and differences. As depicted in Fig. 1.1, EBP is a type of QI that focuses on implementing evidence-based processes of care to improve patient outcomes and population health. Not all QI, however, is based on scientific findings; it may use organization-specific data to guide actions for improving care processes. For example, if QI data in your organization shows a wide variation in clinic wait times, organizational QI data about care processes (e.g., number of scheduled patients in specific time blocks) may be used to determine actions to decrease variation across clinics and shorten clinic wait times. This is a QI project, but not an EBP project. Both are important for quality of care. In comparison, your QI data may reveal high rates of CAUTI. Review of the evidence reveals a set of EBP recommendations that can be implemented to lower CAUTI rates in the identified patient population. The process of care in this example is guided by the most current evidence from

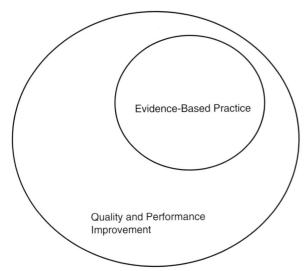

Fig. 1.1 Relationship Between EBP and Quality Improvement.

research and other evidence sources (e.g., early removal of Foley catheters) to decrease CAUTI. QI data (e.g., CAUTI rates) are tracked over time with expectations that your rates will decline. The Donabedian framework of QI is useful in considering the types of metrics to use in evaluating the impact of EBPs (Donabedian, 1966).

Translation science, also more recently known as implementation science, is a type of research conduct. This field of science focuses on testing implementation of interventions to improve uptake and use of evidence to improve patient outcomes and population health, as well as, to clarify what implementation strategies work for whom, in what settings, and why (NIH, 2017;Titler, 2014). An emerging body of knowledge in translation science provides a scientific base for guiding the selection of implementation strategies to promote adoption of EBPs in real-world settings (Dobbins et al., 2009; Titler, 2010; Titler et al., 2016). Thus EBP and translation science, although related, are not interchangeable terms. EBP is the actual application of evidence in practice (the "doing of" EBP), whereas translation science is the study of implementation interventions, factors, and contextual variables that effect knowledge uptake and use in practices and communities. Translation science is research; various research designs and methods are used to address research hypotheses. For example, a translation science study used a clustered randomized trial design to test the effectiveness of a multifaceted implementation intervention designed to improve use of EBPS for acute pain management of older adults hospitalized with a hip fracture (Brooks et al., 2009; Titler et al., 2009)

EBP TIP

EBP is the actual application of evidence in practice (the "doing of" EBP), whereas translation science is the study of implementation interventions, factors, and contextual variables that effect knowledge uptake and use in practices and communities.

THE NATIONAL AGENDA FOR EVIDENCE-BASED PRACTICE

As current and future leaders, it is important for you to recognize that the national agenda for EBP is clearly in the forefront of health care. Multiple federal and national agencies are dedicated to promoting quality, safety, and population health through the application of evidence. EBP is now a national standard, as demonstrated by the agendas of several agencies including the following:

- Agency for Healthcare Quality and Research (AHRQ),
- Centers for Medicare and Medicaid Services (CMS),
- Joint Commission for Accreditation of Healthcare Organizations (JCAHO),
- Centers for Disease Control and Prevention (CDC),
- U.S. Preventive Services Task Force (USPSTF),
- National Quality Forum (NQF), and
- Institute for Healthcare Improvement (IHI).

Table 1.3 provides a general description of each agency's evidence-based initiatives and examples of evidence-based standards, recommendations, or programs.

IT RESOURCES

Agency websites noted in Table 1.3 are rich resources for locating evidence-based information on a variety of health care topics.

As systems-level change agents, you will need to be knowledgeable about the CMS's Value-Based Programs (VBPs), which illustrate the national importance of evidence-based health care. These VBPs reward health care systems with incentive payments for the quality of care provided to people with Medicare coverage and support the three-part aim of better care for individuals, better health for populations, and lower cost. The VBPs include items such as (1) using incentives to improve care, (2) tying payment to value through new payment models, (3) changing how care is delivered through better coordination across health care settings, and (4) more attention to population health (CMS, 2016).

TABLE 1.3   National Agency EBP Initiatives

Agency	General Description: Evidence-Based Initiatives	Examples of Evidence-Based Standards or Recommendations
Centers for Medicare and Medicaid Services (http://www.CMS.gov)	Value-based programs: incentive payments for the quality of care provided to people with Medicare coverage • Hospital Value-Based Purchasing • Hospital Readmission Reduction • Value Modifier (Physician Value-Based Modifier) • Hospital-Acquired Conditions	HF: discharge instructions inclusive of activity, diet, provider follow-up, monitoring/addressing signs and symptoms for worsening HF, weight monitoring; these are important evidence-based components for self-care management of HF after hospital discharge. Prevention of CAUTI: Research demonstrates that the proper insertion and early removal of urinary catheters can reduce CAUTIs. Unplanned hospital readmission for those with HF: based on research demonstrating that effective coordination of care can lower the risk of readmission for patients with HF. Care coordination, home-based interventions, and exercise-based rehabilitation therapy among patients with HF all contribute to reducing the risk of hospitalization.
Joint Commission for Accreditation of Healthcare Organizations (https://www.jointcommission.org)	Sets standards of care for accreditation of health care organizations Standards informed by scientific literature and expert consensus and reviewed by the Board of Commissioners	Fall prevention Patient/family education Prevention of CAUTI Prevention of medication errors
Centers for Disease Control and Prevention (https://www.cdc.gov)	Works to protect the United States from health, safety, and security threats, both foreign and in the United States Fights disease and supports communities and citizens in doing the same As the nation's health protection agency, the CDC saves lives and protects people from health threats. To accomplish the mission, the CDC conducts critical science and provides health information that protects our nation against expensive and dangerous health threats, and responds when these arise.	Fall prevention in communities Medication adherence evidence-based behavioral interventions Evidence-based interventions for HIV prevention Prevention of CAUTI Promoting heart-healthy and stroke-free communities Immunizations Diabetes (Types 1 and 2)

TABLE 1.3   National Agency EBP Initiatives—cont'd

Agency for Healthcare Quality and Research (https://www.AHRQ.gov)	Lead federal agency charged with improving the safety and quality of America's health care system Ensures that the evidence is understood and used in an effort to achieve the goals of better care, smarter spending of health care dollars, and healthier people Funds health services research	EPCs: develop EBP reports that provide comprehensive, science-based information on common, costly conditions, and new health care technologies and strategies. EPCs review all relevant scientific literature on a wide spectrum of clinical and health services topics. EPCs also produce technical reports on methodological topics and other types of evidence. National Guideline Clearinghouse (NGC): publicly available database of evidence-based clinical practice guidelines and related documents. Updated weekly with new content, NGC provides an accessible mechanism for obtaining objective, detailed information on clinical practice guidelines to further dissemination, and implementation. Certified Healthcare Safety Professional initiative: funds three Centers of Excellence and a coordinating center to study how health care delivery systems promote EBPs in delivering care, and to understand the relationships among the successful dissemination of patient-centered outcomes research, patient outcomes, and effective use of resources Funds dissemination and implementation research (e.g., Developing New Clinical Decision Support to Disseminate and Implement Patient-Centered Outcomes Research Findings (R18); Utilizing Health Information Technology to Scale and Spread Successful Practice Models Using Patient-reported Outcomes (R18); Advancing Patient Safety Implementation through Safe Medication Use Research (R18)
U.S. Preventive Services Task Force (https://www.uspreventiveservicestaskforce.org)	Independent, volunteer panel of national experts in prevention and evidence-based health care The Task Force works to improve the health of all Americans by making evidence-based recommendations about clinical preventive services such as screenings, counseling services, and preventive medications. Task Force members come from the fields of preventive medicine and primary care, including internal medicine, family medicine, pediatrics, behavioral health, obstetrics and gynecology, and nursing. Their recommendations are based on a rigorous review of existing peer-reviewed evidence and are intended to help clinicians and patients decide together whether a preventive service is right for a patient's needs.	Task Force: assigns each recommendation a letter grade (an A, B, C, or D grade or an I statement) based on strength of the evidence and balance of benefits and harms of a preventive service. The Task Force does not consider costs of a preventive service when determining a recommendation grade. Recommendations apply only to people who have no signs or symptoms of a specific disease or condition under evaluation, and recommendations address only services offered in the primary care setting or services referred by a primary care clinician. Recommendations that are A (high certainty of substantial net benefit) and B (high certainty that net benefit is moderate or moderate certainty the net benefit is moderate to substantial) are linked to coverage in the ACA and form the basis for decisions of others about how to implement coverage consistent with the task force grade and ACA (Siu et al., 2015). Recommendations are published on Task Force's website and/or in a peer-reviewed journal.

Continued

TABLE 1.3 National Agency EBP Initiatives—cont'd

National Quality Forum (http://www.qualityforum.org)	The NQF is a not-for-profit, nonpartisan, membership-based organization that works to catalyze health care improvements. NQF measures and standards serve as a critically important foundation for initiatives to enhance health care value, make patient care safer, and achieve better outcomes. NQF-defined measures or health care practices are evidence-based approaches to improving care. The federal government, states, and private-sector organizations use NQF's endorsed measures, which must meet rigorous criteria, to evaluate performance and share information with patients and families.	Falls prevalence Falls with injury Restraint prevalence (vest and limb only) Ventilator-associated pneumonia Central line catheter-associated bloodstream infection rate Smoking cessation Skill mix Nursing care hours per patient day Counseling on physical activity in older adults Influenza immunization Pneumonia vaccination for older adults Colorectal cancer screening
Institute for Healthcare Improvement (http://www.IHI.org)	The IHI takes a unique approach to working with health systems, countries, and organizations on improving quality, safety, and value in health care. IHI focuses on the science of improvement, an applied science that emphasizes innovation, rapid-cycle testing in the field, and spread to generate learning about what changes, in which contexts, produce improvements. It is characterized by the combination of expert subject knowledge with improvement methods and tools. It is multidisciplinary — drawing on clinical science, systems theory, psychology, statistics, and other fields.	Developing a patient and family-centered intensive care unit Communication about end-of-life care The opioid crisis Building systems of safety

ACA, Affordable Care Act; *CAUTI,* catheter associated urinary tract infection; *CDC,* Centers for Disease Control and Prevention; *EBP,* evidence-based practice; *EPC,* evidence-based practice center; *HF,* heart failure; *IHI,* Institute for Healthcare Improvement; *NGC,* National Guideline Clearinghouse; *NQF,* National Quality Forum.

The four original value-based programs are the following:
1. Hospital Value-Based Purchasing (HVBP) Program,
2. Hospital Readmission Reduction (HRR) Program,
3. Value Modifier (VM) Program (also called the Physician Value-Based Modifier or PVBM), and
4. Hospital Acquired Conditions (HAC) Program.

Driven by the CMS's VBPs, hospitals are paid for acute care services based on the quality of care rather than quantity of the services provided. *Quality measures are based on evidence.* For example, the inpatient quality measures for those with HF include discharge instructions to include weight monitoring, activity, diet, provider follow-up, and monitoring and addressing signs and symptoms for worsening HF. These are important evidence-based components for self-care management of HF after hospital discharge. A second example, CAUTI, is a quality measure because research demonstrates that proper insertion and early removal of urinary catheters can reduce CAUTIs. Similarly, unplanned hospital readmission for those with HF is based on research demonstrating that effective coordination of care can lower the risk of readmission for patients with HF. Care coordination, home-based interventions, and exercise-based rehabilitation therapy among patients with HF all contribute to reducing the risk of hospitalization (CMS, 2016; see Chapter 15).

The National Institutes of Health funds research in translation and implementation science. For example, the funding announcement, PAR-13-055 Dissemination and Implementation Research in Health, is a call for grant applications that investigate innovative approaches to identifying, understanding, and overcoming barriers to the adoption, adaptation, integration, scale-up, and sustainability of evidence-based interventions, tools, policies, and guidelines (Purtle, Peters, & Brownson, 2016; Tinkle et al., 2013). An example is testing the effect of three dissemination strategies to address weight management among US military veterans: tailored print communication (TPC), tailored motivation interviews (TMI) via telephone, and TPC and TMI combined (principal investigator: M. K. Campbell; R01CA124400; Tinkle et al., 2013).

STEPS OF EVIDENCE-BASED PRACTICE

Multiple models of EBP and translation science are available for you to use as an organizing framework for your agency's EBP initiatives (see Chapter 2). The Iowa Model of Evidence-Based Practice, illustrated in Fig. 1.2, is as an example of an EBP model that serves as a guide for clinicians (Titler et al., 2001). This model has been widely disseminated and used in academic and practice settings. Using the Iowa Model of EBP as a guide, the steps of EBP are overviewed in Table 1.4 with linkages to other chapters that provide detailed information about completing each step.

EBP TIP

Adoption of EBPs is influenced by the nature of the clinical topic (e.g., the type and strength of evidence, complexity) and the manner in which it is communicated to members (nurses) of a social system (organization, setting).

THE EVIDENCE-BASED PRACTICE TEAM

The composition of your EBP team will vary depending on the question being asked, the patient population, and the anticipated resources needed. You want to think about potential EBP teams comprising a broad array of health professionals including, but not limited to, nurses, nurse practitioners and midwives, physicians, physician assistants, social workers, pharmacists, and occupational and physical therapists. You might broaden your thinking about other potential members who have important contributions to make, such as QI specialists, staff from infection control or finance, health science librarians, or IT support staff. Depending on your patient population and practice setting, point-of-care providers such as care coordinators, patient navigators, and community health workers also may offer important contributions to your EBP team.

ENGAGING CONSUMERS IN EVIDENCE-BASED PRACTICE

Although not traditionally included as part of the EBP team, engaging patients, family members, and consumers as team members is receiving more attention (Moore, Kane-Low, Titler, Dalton, & Sampselle, 2014; Moore, Titler, Kane-Low, Dalton, & Sampselle, 2015; Shuman et al., 2016). Consideration should be given to including a layperson on your EBP team who has experience with the topic. For example, a team focusing on prevention of necrotizing enterocolitis (NEC) in premature neonates may invite a parent to participate on the team because feeding breast milk (instead of formula) is one strategy to prevent NEC.

There are several rationales for including consumers in EBP teams. First, they can lend their expertise as recipients of health care and provide input into practices important to them. Second, involving consumers may increase their understanding of why certain EBPs are used in what circumstances and why they are important. Third, consumers may be helpful in championing the use of EBPs. Fourth, consumers may provide insights into evaluation components of EBPs such as specific health outcomes and satisfaction (see Chapter 16).

CALL TO ACTION

Application of evidence in practice is now a national health care agenda. Each of us are called to act within our practice organizations to lead EBP

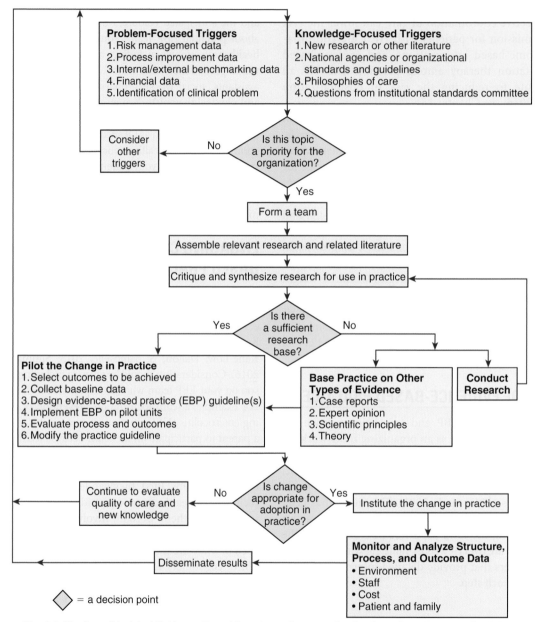

Fig. 1.2 The Iowa Model of Evidence-Based Practice to Promote Quality Care (From Titler, M. G., Kleiber, C., Steelman, V., Rakel, B., Budreau, G., Everett, L. Q., et al. (2001). The Iowa model of evidence-based practice to promote quality care. *Critical Care Nursing Clinical of North America, 13*(4), 497–509.)

TABLE 1.4 Overview of EBP Steps and Chapter Linkages

EBP Step	Description	Factors to consider	Book chapter(s)
Select an EBP Topic			
Topic selection is often driven by problem-and/or knowledge-focused triggers. Example: increasing early mobility in the critical care unit	Problem-focused: QI and risk surveillance data, financial data, recurrent clinical problems. Knowledge-focused: research publications, scientific papers at research conferences, EBP guidelines	Be sure to include clinicians who will implement the potential practice changes in selecting the topic. Do clinicians view the topic as contributing significantly to the quality of care? Consider QI data in topic selection.	Chapter 3: Developing Compelling Clinical Questions Chapter 11: Evidence-Based Approaches for Improving Healthcare Quality Chapter 12: Planning for Success
Form a Team			
Example: physical therapists, staff nurses, advanced practice nurses, physicians	The composition of the team is directed by the topic selected and should include those in the delivery of the EBPs. Consider other key stakeholders who may not be team members but can facilitate the work of the team (see Box 1.1).	An important early task for the team is to use PICO in formulation of the clinical question. This helps set boundaries for the project and assists in evidence retrieval.	Chapter 3: Developing Compelling Clinical Questions Chapter 12: Planning for Success
Evidence Retrieval			
Search for evidence sources on your topic	Use search engines. Retrieve relevant research and related literature, including clinical studies, meta-analyses, systematic reviews, and EBP guidelines.	Keep track of your search strategies. Include websites such as AHRQ, CDC, etc.	Chapter 4: Search and Critical Appraisal of the Literature.
Critical Appraisal of the Evidence			
Requires critique of all types of evidence (e.g., research, systematic reviews, EBP guidelines)	Should be a shared responsibility with one individual providing the leadership (e.g., advance practice nurse). A group approach distributes the workload, helps those responsible for implementing the EBPs to understand the scientific base, arms nurses with citations and research-based language to use in advocating for practice changes with and across disciplines, and provides novices an environment to learn critique and application of research findings.	Critical appraisal tools are available for specific research designs, EBP guidelines, systematic reviews, etc. Understanding statistical methods is important to determining whether study findings are congruent with research design and study aims.	Chapter 2: Models and Evidence Chapter 4: Search and Critical Appraisal of the Literature. Chapter 5: Principles of Assessing Research Quality Chapter 6: Intervention Studies Chapter 7: Observational Studies Chapter 8: Systematic Reviews and Clinical Practice Guidelines Chapter 9: Qualitative Studies Chapter 10: Understanding Statistics for Evidence-Based Practice

Continued

TABLE 1.4   Overview of EBP Steps and Chapter Linkages—cont'd

EBP Step	Description	Factors to consider	Book chapter(s)
Evidence Synthesis			
Synthesis is integrating and linking different types and sources of evidence into a comprehensive whole, thereby providing a foundation for making EBP recommendations.	Evidence synthesis uses tools and techniques to combine multiple sources of evidence. In general, there are two types of synthesis: narrative synthesis (e.g., systematic reviews) and quantitative synthesis (e.g., meta-analysis).	Various tools and strategies are helpful in synthesizing the evidence. Considerations for inclusion of evidence in a synthesis are overall scientific merit, similarity of subjects to patient populations, and relevance to the clinical question/topic.	Chapter 4: Search and Critical Appraisal of the Literature Chapter 8: Systematic Reviews and Clinical Practice Guidelines
Set Forth Evidence-Based Practice Recommendations			
Summarize recommendations about assessments, actions, interventions/treatments derived from the evidence synthesis with an evidence grade assigned to each.	Recommendations for practice are set forth based on the synthesis of the evidence. The strength of evidence for each practice recommendation needs to be clearly documented.	Use a standard grading schema.	Chapter 2: Models and Evidence Chapter 4: Search and Critical Appraisal of the Literature. Chapter 12: Planning for Success
Decision to Change Practice			
Based on critical appraisal and synthesis of evidence, decisions are made about practice changes.	Critical appraisal and synthesis may result in validating that current practices are aligned with the evidence or result in minor or major practice changes.	Consider the following: Consistent results from several well-designed studies Findings are consistent across systematic reviews, EBP guidelines, and critiqued research Benefits of applying the EBPs outweigh potential risks	Chapter 12: Planning for Success
Convert EBP Recommendations Into Local Standards, Policies, or Procedures			
	A written EBP standard (e.g., policy, procedure, guideline) for the organization or setting is necessary so that individuals in the setting know (1) that the practices are based on evidence and (2) the type of evidence (e.g., RCT, expert opinion) used in development of the practice.	Have EBP standard reviewed by key stakeholders for feedback. Focus groups are a useful way to provide discussion about the EBP and to identify key areas that may be potentially troublesome during the implementation phase.	Chapter 2: Models and Evidence Chapter 12: Planning for Success

TABLE 1.4   Overview of EBP Steps and Chapter Linkages—cont'd

EBP Step	Description	Factors to consider	Book chapter(s)
Implement the Practice Change			
Multiple implementation strategies are needed.	Use the Translating Research into Practice model to guide selection of implementation strategies. Trying the EBPs on a small scale first is recommended to determine whether process and outcome improvements occur as expected (Piloting).	Select implementation strategies that address each of the following areas: nature of the EBP topic (e.g., complexity); methods for Communicating the EBPs; and users of the EBPs Social context/setting for implementation.	Chapter 12: Planning for Success Chapter 13: Launching Implementation Chapter 14: Implementation Strategies for Stakeholders Chapter 15: Patient Centered Evidence-Based Practices
Evaluation			
Collection and analysis of data aligned with use of new EBPs; used to determine impact of the EBPs	Evaluation criteria are derived from the evidence sources and should include process and outcome indicators.	Use QI data when available. Focus on collecting essential data. Evaluation includes planned feedback to staff making the practice change.	Chapter 10: Understanding Statistics for Evidence-Based Practice Chapter 11: Evidence-Based Approaches for Improving Healthcare Quality Chapter 16: Evaluation of Evidence-Based Practice
Dissemination			
Plan for ways to share the results of the EBP implementation with internal and external audiences.	Make presentations to key stakeholder groups. Write executive summaries. Give presentations at regional and national conferences.	Consider use of active dissemination strategies. Know your dissemination options. Use social media and blogs.	Chapter 17: Dissemination

AHRQ, Agency for Healthcare Quality and Research; *CDC,* Centers for Disease Control and Prevention; *EBP,* evidence-based practice; *PICO,* problem/patients/populations, intervention, comparison, outcome; *QI,* quality improvement; *RCT,* randomized controlled trial.

BOX 1.1   Questions to Consider in Identification of Key Stakeholders

- How are decisions made in the practice areas where the evidence-based practice (EBP) will be implemented?
- What types of system changes will be needed?
- Who is involved in decision making?
- Who is likely to lead and champion implementation of the EBP?
- Who can influence the decision to proceed with implementation?
- What type of cooperation is needed from the stakeholders for the project to be successful?

improvements, to participate in organizational initiatives to improve care through implementation of the latest evidence, and to critically question current practices with an eye toward improving care through evidence application.

As the next generation of nursing leaders, you must acquire the knowledge and skills essential to carry out the work of EBP (AACN, 2006). Master's-prepared nurses are expected to do the following:

- lead interprofessional EBP teams;
- critically appraise and synthesize the evidence for use in practice;
- articulate to a variety of audiences the evidence base for practice decisions, including the credibility of sources of information and the relevance to the practice problem confronted;
- set forth EBPs for the local setting, based on evidence synthesis;
- use effective implementation strategies;
- apply the principles and tools of QI;
- direct EBP evaluation; and
- disseminate the impact of EBPs to internal and external audiences.

Nurses with doctorates of nursing practice are expected to be experts in EBP, possessing the preceding knowledge and skills of master's-prepared nurses. In addition, a doctorally prepared nurse is expected to do the following:

- be knowledgeable about the latest evidence for your patient populations;
- develop, implement, and evaluate the effect of EBP programs at the organization and system levels;
- design, direct, and evaluate QI methodologies to promote safe, timely, effective, efficient, equitable, and patient-centered care;
- explicate the return on investment of EBP;
- negotiate system changes that foster practice climates for EBP; and
- role model knowledge and skills of EBP.

Evidence is now available for a variety of topics to inform leadership and administrative decision making (e.g., staff turnover, staff performance, optimizing staffing patterns). Therefore the leaders of your health care system have an accountability to promote an organizational culture that makes evidence-informed leadership decisions and creates EBP environments to promote high-quality, safe patient care. This includes the following:

- creating and enacting an organizational mission, vision, and strategic plan that incorporates EBP;
- developing and implementing performance expectations for all staff that include EBP work;
- integrating the work of EBP into the governance structure of the health system;
- role modeling the value of EBPs through administrative behaviors; and
- establishing explicit expectations that nurse leaders create microsystems that value and support clinical inquiry.

It is our hope that you will accept this call to action. Whether as educators, administrators, leaders, or advanced practice nurses, we must possess the knowledge and skills to ensure health care is accessible, of the highest quality, and based on the latest evidence. The chapters in this text are designed to give you the knowledge and skills necessary about EBP for you to succeed in making a difference.

SYNTHESIS

The nursing profession has a robust history of using research evidence to improve patient care. As a nursing leader, you will be challenged to engage your colleagues in using an evidence-based approach as the foundation of their practice. Building effective teams is key to undertaking EBP and QI projects. The IPEC Competencies featured in Appendix G will be valuable for you to use as you collaborate to achieve successful EBP project outcomes. Understanding the roles and responsibilities of colleagues from different professions, including consumers, will increase the degree to which you respect and value their contributions. You will lead or be a member of intraprofessional and interprofessional teams where you will need to cultivate EBP champions who are committed to developing clinical questions, searching the literature for the best available evidence, critically appraising the evidence and using it to inform clinical decision making about implementing and evaluating tests of change. Meeting this challenge is essential for achieving the Triple Aim of improving population health, reducing the per capita cost of health care, and enhancing the experience of care. Quality improvement initiatives strive to address the components of the Triple Aim. QI models like Donabedian's Structure-Process-Outcome framework are often used with EBP initiatives. Evidence-based practice is a type of quality improvement. The Iowa Model of Evidence-based Practice is an EBP model that can be used to guide clinicians in completing EBP initiatives. Clinical, educational, and administrative leaders are called to action to lead organization and systems level change using EBP and QI to advance the quality of cost effective and satisfying health care based on the best available evidence.

KEY POINTS

- The application of evidence to improve quality of care and patient outcomes is central to health care improvement.
- Nursing has a rich history of using research in practice, pioneered by Florence Nightingale.
- The national agenda for EBP is clearly in the forefront of health care.

- EBP and conduct of research have distinct purposes, questions, approaches, and evaluative measures.
- A model commonly used to guide QI is Donabedian's Structure-Process-Outcome Framework, which addresses improving quality of care in these three fundamental components of health care.

- EBP is a type of QI that focuses on implementing evidence-based processes of care to improve patient outcomes and population health. Not all QI, however, is evidence-based.
- An emerging body of knowledge in translation science provides an empirical base for guiding the selection of implementation strategies to promote adoption of EBPs in real-world settings.
- EBP and translation science are not interchangeable terms.
- The Iowa Model of Evidence-Based Practice is an EBP model that has been widely disseminated and used in academic and clinical settings. It serves as a guide for clinicians in completing the steps of EBP.

- Consideration should be given to including on the EBP team a layperson who has experience with the selected topic. Involving consumers may increase their understanding of why certain EBPs are used in what circumstances and why they are important.
- Each of us is called to act within our practice organizations to lead EBP improvements, participate in organizational initiatives to improve care through implementation of the latest evidence, and critically question current practices with an eye toward improving care through evidence application.
- Performance expectations regarding EBP are explicated for master's and doctorate of nursing practice–prepared nurses.

REFERENCES

Agency for Healthcare Research and Quality. (2015). *2014 national healthcare quality and disparities report (AHRQ Publication No. 15–0007)*. Rockville, MD: U.S. Department of Health and Human Services. Retrieved from: http://www.ahrq.gov/research/findings/nhqrdr/nhqdr14/index.html.

Agency for Healthcare Research and Quality. (2016, November 8). *About the comparative health systems performance (CHSP) initiative*. Retrieved from: https://www.ahrq.gov/chsp/about-chsp/index.html.

Agency for Healthcare Research and Quality. (2016, November 8). *AHRQ research: examples of AHRQ's research and evidence that makes health care safer and improves quality*. Retrieved from: https://www.ahrq.gov/research/ahrq-research.html.

American Association of Colleges of Nursing. (2006). *The Essentials of Doctoral Education for Advanced Nursing Practice*. Washington, DC: American Association of Colleges of Nursing.

Armstrong, R., Waters, E., Dobbins, M., Anderson, L., Moore, L., Petticrew, M., et al. (2013). Knowledge transition strategies to improve the use of evidence in public health decision making in local government: intervention design and implementation plan. *Implementation Science*, 8(1), 121–131.

Berwick, D., (2008). The science of quality improvement. *JAMA*, 299(10), 1182–1184.

Best, M., & Neuhauser, D. (2005). W. Edwards Deming: father of quality management, patient and composer. *Quality and Safety in Health Care*, 14(4), 310–312.

Brooks, J., Titler, M. G., Ardery, G., & Herr, K. (2009). The effect of evidence-based acute pain management practices on inpatient costs. *Health Services Research*, 44(1), 245–263.

Brownson, R. C., Chriqui, J. F., & Stamatakis, K. A. (2009). Understanding the evidence-based public health policy. *American Journal of Public Health*, 99(9), 1576–1583.

Canadian Institutes of Health Research (CIHR). Knowledge Translation. Retrieved from: https://www.cihr-irsc.ca/e/

Centers for Disease Control and Prevention. (2016, May 2). *Centers for disease control and prevention*. Retrieved from: http://www.cdc.gov/.

Centers for Medicare & Medicaid Services. (2016). *CMS quality strategy 2016*. Baltimore, MD. Retrieved from: https://www.cms.gov/Medicare/Quality-Initiatives-Patient-Assessment-Instruments/QualityInitiativesGenInfo/Downloads/CMS-Quality-Strategy.pdf.

Conway, L. J., Pogorzelska, M., Larson, E., & Stone, P. W. (2012). Adoption of policies to prevent catheter-associated urinary tract infections in United States intensive care units. *American Journal of Infection Control*, 40(8), 705–710.

Cronenwett, L. R. (1995). Effective methods for disseminating research findings to nurses in practice. *Nursing Clinics of North America*, 30(3), 429–438.

Dickinson, S., & Shever, L. L. (2012). Evidence-based nursing innovations. *Critical Care Nursing Quarterly*, 35(1), 1.

Dobbins, M., Hanna, S. E., Ciliska, D., Manske, S., Cameron, R., Mercer, S. L., et al. (2009). A randomized controlled trial evaluating the impact of knowledge translation and exchange strategies. *Implementation Science*, 4(1), 61–77.

Dockham, B., Schafenacker, A., Yoon, H., Ronis, D. L., Kershaw, T., Titler, M. G., et al. (2016). Implementation of a psychoeducational program for cancer survivors and family caregivers at a cancer support community affiliate: a pilot effectiveness study. *Cancer Nursing*, 39(3), 169–180.

Donabedian, A. (1966). Evaluating the quality of medical care. *The Milbank Memorial Fund Quarterly, 44*(3), 166–206.

Eccles, M. P., & Mittman, B. S. (2006). Welcome to implementation science. *Implementation Science, 1*(1), 1–3.

Estabrooks, C. A., Derksen, L., Winther, C., Lavis, J. N., Scott, S. D., Wallin, L., et al. (2008). The intellectual structure and substance of the knowledge utilization field: a longitudinal author co-citation analysis, 1945–2004. *Implementation Science, 3*(1), 49–70.

Funk, S. G., Tornquist, E. M., & Champagne, M. T. (1989). A model for improving the dissemination of nursing research. *Western Journal of Nursing Research, 11*(3), 361–367.

Graham, I. D., Logan, J., Harrison, M. B., Straus, S. E., Tetroe, J., Caswell, W., et al. (2006). Lost in knowledge translation: time for a map? *Journal of Continuing Education in the Health Professions, 26*(1), 13–24.

Haughom, J. (2016). Five Deming principles that help healthcare process improvement. *Health Catalyst.* Retrieved from: https://www.healthcatalyst.com/wp-content/uploads/2014/11/Five-Deming-Principles-That-Help-Healthcare-Process-Improvement.pdf.

Henly, S., McCarthy, D., Wyman, J., Heitkemper, M., Redeker, N., Titler, M. G., et al. (2015). Emerging areas of science: recommendations for nursing science education from the council for the advancement of nursing science idea festival. *Nursing Outlook, 63*(4), 398–407.

Horsley, J. (1983). *Using research to improve nursing practice: a guide.* Philadelphia, PA: WB Saunders Company.

Institute of Medicine. (2009). *Initial national priorities for comparative effectiveness research.* Washington, DC: The National Academies Press.

Institute of Medicine. (2011). *Clinical practice guidelines we can trust.* Washington, DC: The National Academies Press.

Institute of Medicine. (2012a). *For the public's health; Investing in a healthier future.* Washington, DC: The National Academies Press.

Institute of Medicine. (2012b). *Living well with chronic illness: a call for public health action.* Washington, DC: The National Academies Press.

Institute of Medicine. (2013). *The CTSA program at NIH: opportunities for advancing clinical and translational research.* Washington, DC: The National Academies Press.

Institute of Medicine. (2015). *The current state of obesity solutions in the United States: workshop in brief.* Washington, DC: The National Academies Press.

Kelley, P. W. (2010). Research to practice in the military healthcare system. *Nursing Research, 59*(1), S1.

King, D., Barnard, K. E., & Hoehn, R. (1981). Disseminating the results of nursing research. *Nursing Outlook, 29*(3), 164–169.

Kirchhoff, K. T. (2004). State of the science of translational research: from demonstration projects to intervention testing. *Worldviews on Evidence-Based Nursing, 1*(s1), S6–S12.

Krueger, J. C. (1978). Utilization of nursing research: the planning process. *Journal of Nursing Administration, 8*(1), 6–9.

Krueger, J. C., Nelson, A. H., & Wolanin, M. O. (1978). *Nursing research: development, collaboration, and utilization.* Germantown, MD: Aspen.

Kueny, A., Shever, L., Lehan Mackin, M., & Titler, M. G. (2015). Facilitating the implementation of evidence-based practice through contextual support for nursing leadership. *Journal of Healthcare Leadership, 7,* 29–39.

Lindeman, C. A., & Krueger, J. C. (1977). Increasing the quality, quantity, and use of nursing research. *Nursing Outlook, 25*(7), 450–454.

Madsen, D., Sebolt, T., Cullen, L., Folkedahl, B., Mueller, T., Richardson, C., et al. (2005). Listening to bowel sounds: an evidence-based practice project. *American Journal of Nursing, 105*(12), 40–49.

Mark, D. B., Titler, M. G., & Latimer, R. W. (Eds.). (2014). *Integrating evidence into practice for impact Nursing Clinics of North America, 49*(3), 269–452.

Moore, J. E., Kane-Low, L., Titler, M. G., Dalton, V., & Sampselle, C. (2014). Moving towards patient centered care: women's decisions, perceptions, and experiences of the induction of labor process. *Birth, 41*(2), 138–146.

Moore, J. E., Titler, M. G., Kane-Low, L., Dalton, V. K., & Sampelle, C. M. (2015). Transforming patient-centered care: development of the evidence-informed decision-making through engagement model. *Women's Health Issues, 25*(3), 276–282.

National Institute of Research. (2017). *Dissemination and implementation research in health.* http:/ grants.nih.gov/grants/ guide/pa-files, 9/18/2017.

National Institute of Nursing Research. (2016). *The NINR strategic plan: advancing science, improving lives.* NIH publication #16-NR-7783. Bethesda, MD: National Institute of Nursing Research National Institutes of Health.

Nelson, E. C., Batalden, P. R., & Godfrey, M. M. (2007). *Quality by decision: a clinical microsystem approach.* San Francisco, CA: Jossey-Bass.

Newhouse, R., Bobay, K., Dykes, P. C., Stevens, K. R., & Titler, M. G. (2013). Methodology issues in implementation science. *Medical Care, 51*(4), S32–S40.

Nightingale, F. (1858). *Notes on matters affecting the health, efficiency, and hospital administration of the British Army.* London: Harrison & Sons.

Nightingale, F. (1859). *A contribution to the sanitary history of the British Army during the late war with Russia.* London: John W. Parker & Sons.

Nightingale, F. (1863a). *Notes on hospitals*. London, UK: Longman, Green, Roberts, & Green.

Nightingale, F. (1863b). *Observation on the evidence contained in the statistical reports submitted by her to the Royal Commission on the sanitary state of the army in India*. London, UK: Edward Stanford.

Northouse, L. L., Katapodi, M. C., Song, L., Zhang, L., & Mood, D. W. (2010). Interventions with caregivers of cancer patients: meta-analysis of randomized trials. *CA Cancer Journal Clinicians*, 60(5), 317–339.

Northouse, L. L., Kershaw, T., Mood, D. W., & Schafenacker, A. (2005). Effects of a family intervention on the quality of life of women with recurrent breast cancer and their family caregivers. *Psycho-Oncology*, 14, 478–491.

Northouse, L. L., Mood, D. W., Schafenacker, A., Kalemkerian, G., Zalupski, M., LoRusso, P., et al. (2013). Randomized clinical trial of a brief and extensive dyadic intervention for advanced cancer patients and their family caregivers. *Psycho-Oncology*, 22(3), 555–563.

Northouse, L. L., Mood, D. W., Schafenacker, A., Montie, J. E., Sandler, H. M., Forman, J. D., et al. (2007). Randomized clinical trial of a family intervention for prostate cancer patients and their spouses. *Cancer*, 110(12), 2809–2818.

Purtle, J., Peters, R., & Brownson, R. C. (2016). A review of policy dissemination and implementation research funded by the National Institutes of Health, 2007–2014. *Implementation Science*, 11(1), 1–8.

Rutledge, D. N., & Donaldson, N. E. (1995). Building organizational capacity to engage in research utilization. *Journal of Nursing Administration*, 25(10), 12–16.

Shever, L. L., & Dickinson, S. (2013). Mobility: a successful investment for critically ill patients. Foreword. *Critical Care Nursing Quarterly*, 36(1), 1–2.

Shever, L. L., Titler, M. G., Mackin, M. L., & Kueny, A. (2010). Fall prevention practices in adult medical-surgical nursing units described by nurse managers. *Western Journal of Nursing Research*, 33(3), 385–397.

Shuman, C. J., Liu, J., Montie, M., Galinato, J. G., Todd, M. A., Hegstad, M., et al. (2016). Patient perception and experiences with falls during hospitalization and after discharge. *Applied Nursing Research*, 31, 79–85.

Siu, A. L., Bibbins-Domingo, K., & Grossman, D. (2015). Evidence-based clinical prevention in the era of the Patient Protection and Affordable Care Act: the role of the US Preventive Services Task Force. *Journal of the American Medical Association*, 314(19), 2021–2022.

Squires, D., & Anderson, C. (2015). U.S. health care from a global perspective: spending, use of services, prices, and health in 13 countries. *Issue Brief (Commonwealth Fund)*, 15, 1–15.

Straus, E., Richardson, R. B., Glasziou, P., Richardson, W. S., & Haynes, R. B. (2011). Evidence-based medicine: how to practice and teach (4th ed.). New York, NY: Elsevier.

Sving, E., Gunningberg, L., Hogman, M., & Mamhidir, A.-G. (2012). Registered nurses' attention to and perceptions of pressure ulcer prevention in hospital settings. *Journal of Clinical Nursing*, 21(9–10), 1293–1303.

Tinkle, M., Kimball, R., Haozous, E. A., Shuster, G., & Meize-Grochowski, R. (2013). Dissemination and implementation research funded by the U.S. National Institutes of Health, 2005–2012. *Nursing Research and Practice*, 2013, 1–15.

Titler, M. G. (2010). Translation science and context. *Research and Theory for Nursing Practice*, 24(1), 35–55.

Titler, M. G. (2011). Nursing science and evidence-based practice. *Western Journal of Nursing Research*, 33(3), 291–295.

Titler, M. G. (2014). Overview of evidence-based practice and translation science. *Nursing Clinics of North America*, 49(3), 269–274.

Titler, M. G., Conlon, P., Reynolds, M. A., Ripley, R., Tsodikov, A., Wilson, D. S., et al. (2016). The effect of a translating research into practice intervention to promote use of evidence-based fall prevention interventions in hospitalized adults: a prospective pre-post implementation study in the U.S. *Applied Nursing Research*, 31, 52–59.

Titler, M. G., Herr, K., Brooks, J., Xie, X.-J., Ardery, G., Schilling, M., et al. (2009). Translating research into practice intervention improves management of acute pain in older hip fracture patients. *Health Services Research*, 44(1), 264–287.

Titler, M. G., & Moore, J. (2010). Evidence-based practice: a civilian perspective [Editorial]. *Nursing Research*, 59(1), S2–S6.

Ward, B. W., Schiller, J. S., & Goodman, R. A. (2014). Multiple chronic conditions among us adults: a 2012 update. *Preventing Chronic Disease*, 11, 130389.

Whittington, J. W., Nolan, K., Lewis, N., & Torres, T. (2015). Pursuing the triple aim: the first 7 years. *Milbank Quarterly*, 93(2), 263–300.

Wilson, D. S., Montie, M., Conlon, P., Reynolds, M. A., Ripley, R., & Titler, M. G. (2016). Nurses' perceptions of implementing fall prevention interventions to mitigate patient-specific fall risk factors. *Western Journal of Nursing Research*, 38(8), 1012–1034.

2

Models and Evidence

Geri LoBiondo-Wood, Marita Titler, Judith Haber

LEARNING OUTCOMES

After reading this chapter, you should be able to do the following:

- Differentiate among research, evidence-based practice (EBP), quality improvement, and translation science.
- Apply the steps of EBP using the Iowa Model.
- Analyze the characteristics of the EBP process with consideration of the risk/benefit and cost/benefit ratio.
- Compare selected EBP models.

KEY TERMS

Cost/benefit ratio	Meaning	Risk/benefit ratio
Diagnosis	Problem-focused triggers	Stakeholder
Evidence-based practice	Prognosis	Therapy
Harm	Quality improvement	Translation science
Knowledge-focused triggers	Research	

Evidence-based models are frameworks that provide a guide for clinical leaders and their teams as they decide to launch, implement, and complete an evidence-based project to improve quality of care. Think about evidence-based practice (EBP) models as you would think about building a house. As with a house, components of an EBP model provide the foundation, floor, walls, and roof or, in this case, all the component parts of the EBP process. Similarly, there are models for building quality improvement (QI) projects. A house is built in a specific sequence; so too, EBP and QI projects are designed, implemented, and evaluated following a specific sequence guided by the steps of a particular model. Evidence from research studies, published and unpublished, is used to inform clinical decision making about application of findings to practice.

Deciding when and how to use research findings disseminated in journals and at conferences to inform and support practice requires critical appraisal skills that provide a foundation for your clinical decision making.

Critical appraisal skills are an important set of skills to acquire or refine because not all research findings are ready for application to practice. As a clinical leader, you will be responsible for making decisions, or guiding your team to make decisions, about the strength, quality and consistency, and readiness of research evidence related to your project for applicability to practice. The purpose of this chapter is to present the Iowa Model, the EBP model that will be featured throughout this text, as well as a critical appraisal of principles that will help you evaluate research evidence to determine whether it validates current practice or positively or negatively supports minor or major changes in clinical practice.

COMPARING RESEARCH, EVIDENCE-BASED PRACTICE, AND QUALITY IMPROVEMENT

Evidence-based practice, quality improvement, and research are unique processes (see Chapter 1). Each of these processes has unique components that, although independent, complement each other. The unique yet complementary components of each requires an understanding of how these processes mesh with clinical expertise, patient values, and context. Clinical teams that raise clinical questions engage in the following processes:

- search and review the literature for research studies to answer their clinical question,
- critically appraise the evidence,
- synthesize the evidence, and
- make decisions about applicability of findings to practice.

These steps culminate in nursing practice that is evidence based. For example, to help you understand the importance of EBP, think about the systematic review and meta-analysis from van Driel et al. (2016), which assessed interventions to improve adherence to lipid-lowering medication (Appendix A). On the basis of their review and synthesis of the research literature, they identified that a combination of strategies, including provision of information, use of reminders, adherence reinforcement, and emphasis on the person's perspective, might lead to more effective adherence to the medications. However, they also identified the need for more long-term follow-up studies to identify interventions that promote long-term adherence. Whereas research supports or generates knowledge, EBP uses currently available research knowledge to improve health care delivery. The key similarity among these three processes is that each begins with a question. The difference among the three is that a research study actively tests a research question with a design and specific methodology (i.e., sample, instruments, procedures, and data analysis) appropriate to the research question or hypothesis and contributes to new, generalizable knowledge. EBP uses research findings as the basis of practice, and QI may or may not use research findings to improve quality of care (see Chapters 11–16). The EBP process uses a clinical question (see Chapter 3) to search the published literature for completed studies to bring about improvements in care. To successfully use EBP processes, you need to be able to critically appraise the literature. That is, you must be a knowledgeable consumer of research who can evaluate the strengths and weaknesses of research evidence and use existing standards to determine the merit and readiness of research for use in clinical practice (AACN, 2006; QSEN, 2017). In contrast, translation science, as discussed in Chapter 1, focuses on testing the implementation of interventions to improve uptake and use of evidence to improve patient outcomes and population health, as well as to clarify what implementation strategies work for whom, in what settings, and why (Titler, 2014).

Models of Evidence-Based Practice

Multiple models of EBP and translation science are available (Table 2.1). Common elements of EBP models are the following:

- Critical appraisal of evidence
- Synthesis of evidence
- Implementation
- Evaluation of patient care impact
- Consideration of the context/setting in which the evidence is implemented

Implementing evidence in practice must be guided by a conceptual model to organize the strategies being used and to clarify extraneous variables (e.g., behaviors, facilitators) that may influence adoption of EBPs (e.g., organizational size, characteristics of users). The model threaded throughout this text is the Iowa Model (Titler, 2001).

THE IOWA MODEL OF EVIDENCE-BASED PRACTICE

The Iowa Model of Evidence-Based Practice, as an example of an EBP model, is illustrated in Fig. 1.2. This model, based on a problem-solving approach, has been widely disseminated and adopted in academic and clinical settings since its inception (Titler et al., 2001). The steps of the model are as follows:

- Selection of a Topic
- Team Formation
- Evidence Retrieval
- Grading the Evidence
- Critical Appraisal and Synthesis of Evidence
- Proposing Evidence-Based Practice Recommendations
- Development of the Evidence-Based Practice
- Implementation and Dissemination of the Practice Change(s)
- Evaluation of the Change

Selection of a Topic

Use of the Iowa Model is activated when health care staff members question a current practice, categorized as a problem-focused trigger or a knowledge-focused

TABLE 2.1   Example of EBP Models

Model Name	Major Constructs/Concepts
Promoting Action on Research Implementation in Health Services (PARIHS) (Kitson, Harvey, & McCormack, 1998)	Three core elements for success: Knowledge (clarity about the nature of the evidence), Context (quality of the context), and Facilitation (type of facilitation needed to ensure successful change). Each element has multiple components to consider.
Advancing Research Through Close Clinical Collaboration (ARCC Model; Fineholt, Overholt, Melnyk, & Schultz, 2005)	Developed to promote EBP, establish a network of clinicians who support EBP, disseminate best evidence through research and conference. The model follows the steps of EBP: Ask a question, obtain best evidence, appraise the evidence, decide to implement change or not, and evaluate outcomes.
Ottawa Model of Research Use (Graham & Logan, 2004)	Three phases: (1) Assess barriers and supports while considering the evidence-based innovation, adopters' characteristics, and environment's structure and social context. (2) Monitor intervention and degree of use, considering implementation such as diffusion, dissemination and transfer of strategies, and innovation adoption. (3) Evaluate and monitor patient, practitioner, and system outcomes.
Knowledge to Action (KTA) Model (Graham, Tetroe, & KT Theories and Research Group, 2007)	KTA has seven cycles that lead to knowledge translation: Problem identification, adaptation of the knowledge use to the local context, assessment of barriers to knowledge use, selection, tailoring and implementing interventions to promote knowledge use, monitoring knowledge use, evaluating outcomes of use, and sustaining knowledge use.
Johns Hopkins Nursing EBP Model (Newhouse, Dearholt, Poe, Pugh, & White, 2005)	Uses the PET Process for EBP: P = Practice question, E = Evidence, and T = Translation. The three phases have related steps to accomplish the process.
Dobbins's Framework for Dissemination and Utilization of Research (Dobbins, Ciliska, Cockerill, Barnsley, & DiCenso, 2002)	The model has five stages of innovation: knowledge, persuasion, decision, implementation, and confirmation. Within each stage are factors to consider for transferring research to practice.

EBP, Evidence-based practice.

trigger. *Problem-focused triggers* are those identified by staff through quality improvement, risk surveillance, benchmarking, and financial data or recurrent clinical problems. *Knowledge-focused triggers* arise when health providers hear scientific presentations, read research articles or published EBP guidelines, and question practice. An example of a knowledge-focused trigger is how long before surgery a patient should be maintained NPO (nothing by mouth). An example of a problem-focused trigger is whether knee-high or thigh-high TED hose should be used postoperatively to prevent deep vein thrombosis (DVT). The problem-focused trigger in this case would be QI data from two quarters revealing an increase in postoperative DVT rates. Currently knee-high TEDs are the standard of care. The QI committee questions whether it would be better to switch to thigh-high TED hose in some or all cases to provide a more effective standard of care based

on a trigger/problem a question that is formulated (see Chapter 3). There are five types of clinical questions derived from the problem:

- Therapy—A therapy question focuses on determining the effect of an intervention(s) on patient outcomes.
- Harm—A harm question focuses on the potential harm of a symptom or group of symptoms, disorder, treatment, or intervention.
- Diagnosis—A diagnosis question focuses on the establishment of the power of a test to differentiate between those with the disease or problem and those who do not experience the problem.
- Prognosis—A prognosis question focuses on a patient's likely course for a disease state or factors that may alter a prognosis.
- Meaning—A meaning question focuses on the situation or processes related to how people experience, cope, or adapt to conditions, illnesses, or circumstances.

On the basis of the clinical question, studies are located and the findings from retrieved studies are combined with findings from existing scientific knowledge to develop and implement practice guidelines. If there is insufficient research to guide practice and conducting a study is not feasible, other types of evidence (e.g., case reports, scientific principles, theory) are used and/or combined with available research evidence to guide practice (see Chapter 4).

Forming a Team

A team needs to be formed from a unit or service area that is responsible for development, implementation, and evaluation of an EBP. The team members select a topic that guides them and should include interested stakeholders. A *stakeholder* is a key individual or group of individuals who will be directly or indirectly affected by the implementation of the EBP. For example, a team working on an evidence-based diabetes self-management initiative should be interprofessional and include pharmacists, nurses, and physicians. In contrast, a team working on the EBP aimed at decreasing postoperative anxiety for cardiac patients might include a psychologist, physician, psychiatric nurse practitioner, staff nurses, and assistive nursing personnel. Although not traditionally included in the team, engagement of patients, family members, and consumers as team members is becoming more common as patient-centered, whole-person care becomes the norm (Moore, Kane-Low, Titler, Dalton, & Sampselle, 2014; Moore, Titler, Kane-Low, Dalton, & Sampselle, 2015; Shuman et al., 2016). For example, a team focusing on end-of-life care in the pediatric intensive care unit may invite a parent who lost a child to participate on the team.

In addition to the team, additional stakeholders who can facilitate an EBP project or create barriers that preclude successful implementation should be identified. Some of these stakeholders may be members of the team. Others may not be team members but are key individuals within the organization or unit who can adversely or positively influence the adoption of the practice. Questions to consider in identification of key stakeholders include the following:

- How are decisions made in the area where the EBP will be implemented?
- What types of unit or system changes will be needed?
- Who is involved in decision making?
- Who is likely to lead and champion implementation of the practice?
- Who can influence the decision to proceed with implementation of the practice, either positively or negatively?
- What type of cooperation is needed from stakeholders for the practice change to be successful?

Failure to involve or keep supportive stakeholders informed may place success of the project at risk because they are unable to anticipate and/or defend the rationale for changing practice, particularly with resistors (e.g., nonsupportive stakeholders), who have a great deal of influence among their peer group.

An important early task for the EBP team is to use the PICO format to formulate the EBP or clinical question (Table 2.2; see also Chapter 3). Using the information in Example 1 in Table 2.2, the resultant EBP question would be, "What EBPs can be implemented to improve management of chronic pain and decrease pain intensity of adults with cancer patients admitted for chronic pain?" This helps set boundaries around the project and assists in evidence retrieval.

> **IPE TIP**
>
> Interprofessional collaboration is an essential feature of effective EBP and QI Teams. The value of input by stakeholders representing different internal and external constituencies are important to consider as you form each project team. Consumers, as external stakeholders, also provide valuable input that informs the team's understanding of satisfying patient experiences.

Evidence Retrieval

Once a clinical question (PICO) is developed, relevant research and related literature need to be retrieved (see Chapter 4). In addition to literature found in journals, it is also important to review evidence-based information found on websites such as from the Agency for Health Research and Policy (AHRQ; http://www.AHRQ.gov). AHRQ sponsors Evidenced-Based Practice Centers and a National Guideline Clearinghouse, where abstracts of EBP guidelines are available. Once the literature is located, it is helpful to classify the articles using an Evidence Hierarchy as illustrated in Fig. 2.1, as well as clinical (nonresearch background information), theory, policy articles, and EBP guidelines. Before critically appraising research, it is useful to first read background articles to incorporate a broad view of the topic and

TABLE 2.2   **Using PICO to Formulate the Evidence-Based Practice Question**

	Patient/Population/ Problem (P)	Intervention/ Treatment (I)	Comparison Intervention (C)	Outcome(s) (O)
Tips for building the question	How would we describe a group of patients like ours?	Which main interventions are we considering?	What is the main alternative to compare with the intervention?	What can we hope to accomplish?
Example 1	Pain management for adult cancer patients admitted to a hospital with chronic pain	Pain assessment pain tool Patient-controlled analgesia	Standard of care Nurse-administered analgesic	Regular (e.g., every 4 hours) pain assessment Less pain intensity Decreased length of stay
Example 2	Pain assessment in hospitalized children	Pain assessment tool designed for pain assessment in hospitalized children	Assess pain Yes/No question	Regular pain assessment with treatment of pain Fewer children experience pain

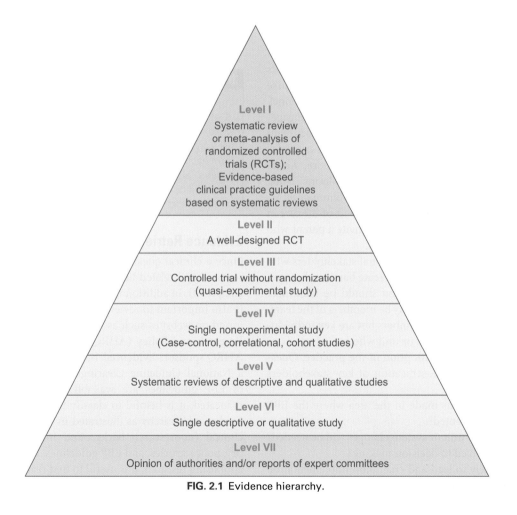

FIG. 2.1 Evidence hierarchy.

TABLE 2.3   GRADE Working Group Criteria

Quality of the Evidence (Balshem et al., 2011; Guyatt et al., 2011, 2013)

High: Very confident that the true effect lies close to that of the estimate of the effect. Scientific evidence provided by well-designed, well-conducted, controlled trials (randomized and nonrandomized) with statistically significant results that consistently support the recommendation.

Moderate: Moderately confident in the effect estimate: The true effect is likely to be close to the estimate of the effect, but there is a possibility that it is substantially different.

Low: Confidence in the effect estimate is limited: The true effect may be substantially different from the estimate of the effect.

Very Low: Very little confidence in the effect estimate: The true effect is likely to be substantially different from the estimate of effect.

Note: The type of evidence is first ranked as follows:
Randomized trial = high.
Observational study = low.
Any other evidence = very low.

Quality may be downgraded due to design flaws/threats to internal validity (risk of bias), important inconsistency of results, uncertainty about the directness of the evidence, imprecise or sparse data, and high probability of publication bias can lower the evidence grade.

Factors that may increase quality of evidence of observational studies:

(1) large magnitude of effect (direct evidence, $RR = 2–5$ or $RR = 0.5–0.2$ with no plausible confounders); very large with $RR > 5$ or $RR < 0.2$ and no serious problems with risk of bias or precision (sufficiently narrow confidence intervals); more likely to rate up if effect is rapid and out of keeping with prior trajectory; usually supported by indirect evidence;

(2) dose–response gradient;

(3) all plausible residual confounders or biases would reduce a demonstrated effect or suggest a spurious effect when results show no effect.

Strength of Recommendations (Andrews et al., 2013)

Strong: confident that desirable effects of adherence to a recommendation outweigh undesirable effects.

Weak: desirable effects of adherence to a recommendation probably outweigh the undesirable effects, but developers are less confident.

Note: strength of recommendation is determined by the balance between desirable and undesirable consequences of alternative management strategies, quality of evidence, variability in values and preferences (trade-offs), and resource use.

RR, Relative risk.
From the GRADE Working Group (http://www.gradeworkinggroup.org).

related concepts. It is helpful to read/critique articles in the following order:

1. Clinical and theory articles to understand the state of the practice and theoretical perspectives and concepts that may be encountered in critiquing studies
2. Meta-analyses, systematic and integrative reviews to understand the state of the science
3. Evidence-based practice guidelines and evidence reports
4. Research articles

Grading the Evidence

There is no consensus among professional organizations or in health care disciplines regarding the best system to use for grading the type and quality of research evidence or the grading schemas to denote the strength of a body of evidence (Balshem et al., 2011; NAM, formerly IOM, 2011). Identifying the level of evidence according to the design of the study is a key first step. The Evidence Hierarchy in Fig. 2.1 is useful for identifying the level of evidence provided by specific research designs. To truly understand the strength of the evidence, however, all components of studies reviewed need to be assessed for quality. A specific schema, the GRADE system, provides a structure and criteria for grading the quality and strength of evidence and formulating recommendations based on the evidence. Table 2.3 illustrates the GRADE system's schemas for assessing the quality of studies.

TABLE 2.4   Domains and Elements for Grading the Strength of Evidence

Quality	The aggregate of quality ratings for individual studies, predicated on the extent to which bias was minimized.
Quantity	Magnitude of effect, numbers of studies, and sample size or power.
Consistency	For any given topic, the extent to which similar findings are reported using similar and different study designs, including relevance, benefits, and harm.

Information posted on the GRADE website (http://www.gradeworkinggroup.org) is also important to help you understand the challenges of and approaches to assessing the quality of evidence and strength of recommendations. Important domains and elements to include in grading the strength of the evidence are defined in Table 2.4.

In grading evidence, two areas are essential to address: (1) the quality of the evidence (e.g., the individual studies, systematic reviews, meta-analyses); that is, the strengths and weaknesses of the individual studies; and (2) the overall strength of the synthesized body of evidence. Important domains and elements of any system used to rate the quality of individual studies are featured in Tables 2.3 and 2.4. Before the body of evidence can be evaluated, the team needs to evaluate the scientific merit of the studies and other evidence sources found in the literature search (see Chapter 4). Fig. 2.1 provides an Evidence Hierarchy used for grading the strength of specific research designs and the evidence they provide. Several highly respected EBP centers, such as the Centre for Evidence-Based Medicine (CEBM), provide internationally recognized critical appraisal tools that assist with evaluating the scientific merits of different types of research designs. Table 2.5 provides links to commonly used critical appraisal tools. Application of these critical appraisal tools to various design types and levels of evidence are described in Chapters 5–9.

Critical Appraisal and Synthesis of Evidence

Critical appraisal is the process of critiquing individual studies to identify their strengths and weaknesses. The next step in the critical appraisal process is to synthesize the overall strengths and weaknesses of the group of studies as a body of literature. The steps of critical appraisal require a working knowledge of the types of research designs and their components. When critiquing studies

and evidence-based guidelines (Chapters 5–9), the critical appraisal process should be a shared responsibility. It is helpful, however, to have one individual provide leadership for the EBP or QI project and design strategies for completing critical appraisals of pertinent studies. A group approach to critical appraisal is recommended because it:

- distributes the workload,
- helps those responsible for implementing the changes to understand the scientific base for the practice change,
- arms nurses with citations and research-based language to use in advocating for changes with peers and other disciplines, and
- provides novices with an environment to learn critical appraisal and application of research findings.

EBP TIP

Encourage staff participation in the appraisal process by enlisting members to work in teams to complete the steps of the critical appraisal processes.

Once individual studies are critiqued, the literature needs to be synthesized; that is, the overall strengths and weaknesses of the studies as a group need to be considered. A decision is made regarding use of each study in the synthesis of the evidence for application in practice. Factors that should be considered for inclusion of studies in the synthesis of findings are the:

- overall scientific merit,
- type of subjects enrolled (e.g., age, gender, pathology) and the similarity to the patient population to which the findings will be applied, and
- relevance of the study to the question topic.

For example, if the practice area is prevention of DVT in postoperative cancer patients, a descriptive study using a heterogeneous population of medical patients is not appropriate for inclusion in the synthesis of findings. Relevant studies would focus on DVT prevention in cancer patients who have undergone surgery. When synthesizing study findings, it is important to develop a synthesis summary table that includes the overall strengths and weaknesses of the studies (see Chapter 4). The synthesis summary table should include the critical information from each study, as well as other evidence sources such as practice guidelines reviewed. Essential information to include in a summary table is as follows (Table 2.6):

- Research questions/hypotheses
- Independent and dependent variables studied

TABLE 2.5   Evidence-Based Resources

Resource	Purpose
Centre for Evidence-Based Medicine (CEBM)	Provides education and the dissemination of evidence-based resources for promoting evidence-based practices in health care decision making through research and education.
Grading of Recommendations Assessment, Development, and Evaluation (GRADE)	Provides consensus resources on rating quality of evidence and strength of practice recommendations, system of rating quality of evidence and grading strength of recommendations in systematic reviews, health technology assessments, and clinical practice guidelines addressing alternative management options.
Critical Appraisal Skills Programme (CASP)	CASP provides critical appraisal skills training, workshops, and tools used to evaluate research for trustworthiness and relevance. CASP offers eight critical appraisal tools designed to be used for assessing research.

TABLE 2.6   Summary Table for Research Critiques

Citation	Research Questions/ Hypothesis	Design	Independent Variables and Measures	Dependent Variables and Measures	Sample Size Population n	Results	Strengths	Weaknesses/ Limitations/ Bias

Use of a summary table helps identify information across studies regarding findings and the types of patients to which study findings can be applied.

- Description of the study sample and setting
- Type of research design
- Methods used to measure each variable and outcome
- Study findings
- Strengths and weaknesses of each study
  Methods to make the critical appraisal process fun and interesting include the following:
- Use a journal club to discuss critiques completed by each member of the group.
- Pair a novice and expert to complete critiques.
- Elicit assistance from both undergraduate and graduate students who may be interested in the topic and want experience doing critiques, and are interested in the topic and process.

EBP TIP

A summary table is key because it serves to identify commonalities and differences across studies regarding study findings and the types of patients to which findings can be applied. A well-done table also provides a synthesis of the overall strengths and weakness of the studies as a group.

Proposing Evidence-Based Practice Recommendations

On the basis of the critique of practice guidelines and research synthesis (that is, the quality and consistency of the evidence found), the team works together to review the information and make recommendations for practice. The type and strength of evidence used to support the practice needs to be clearly delineated in the evidence table. Fig. 2.1 and Tables 2.3 and 2.4 are useful tools to assist with this activity.

After the studies are critiqued and synthesized, the next step is to decide whether the findings are appropriate for use in practice. Criteria to consider include the following:

- Relevance of evidence for the respective practice area
- Consistency of findings across studies and/or guidelines
- A significant number of studies and/or EBP guidelines with sample characteristics similar to those to which the findings will be used
- Consistency among evidence from research and other nonresearch evidence
- Feasibility for use in practice
- The risk/benefit ratio (risk of harm vs. the potential benefit for the patient)

Synthesis of study findings and other evidence may result in supporting current practice, making minor practice modifications, undertaking major practice changes, or developing a new area of practice.

Development of the Evidence-Based Practice

The next step is to document the evidence base of the practice using the agreed-upon grading schema. When critique results and synthesis of evidence support practice or justify a practice change, a written EBP standard (e.g., policy, standard of practice protocol, guideline) is warranted. This is necessary so care providers (1) know that the practices are based on evidence and (2) understand the type of evidence (e.g., randomized controlled trial, expert opinion) used in development of the practice.

It is imperative that once the EBP standard is written, key stakeholders have an opportunity to review it and provide feedback to the team responsible for developing it. Focus groups are a useful way to provide discussion about the EBP and to identify key areas that may be potentially troublesome during the implementation phase.

EBP TIP

A consistent approach to developing EBP standards and referencing the research and related literature is key.

Implementation and Dissemination of the Practice Change

If a practice change is warranted, the next steps are to pilot the practice change to ensure that the change is consistent with the patients, environment, and staff. Piloting the change allows staff the opportunity to provide feedback on the practice and modify it if necessary. Changes extend beyond writing a policy or procedure that is evidence based; it requires interaction among direct care providers to champion and foster evidence adoption, leadership support, and system changes.

Characteristics of an EBP that affect adoption include the relative advantage of the EBP; the compatibility with values, norms, work, and perceived needs of users; the complexity of the EBP topic; and the potential risk/benefit ratio and cost/benefit ratio that the change may affect. The *risk/benefit ratio* is the extent to which a potential change in practice may benefit individuals versus the potential impact of an intervention's harm or potential negative outcome(s) of a practice change. For example, EBP topics that are perceived by users as relatively simple (e.g., influenza vaccines for older adults) are more easily adopted in less time than those that are more complex (e.g., acute pain management for hospitalized older adults). The *cost/benefit ratio* is the analysis of health care resource costs relative to possible medical/health care benefit. The cost/benefit analysis is important in health care settings when identifying priorities where choices must be made based on costs—both monetary and potential side effects. For example, when decisions must be made regarding which medication should be prescribed for a disease or condition, care providers must evaluate not only the drugs' ability to affect the disease but which among the choice of drugs is both effective to treat the condition and more cost-effective. Chapters 12–15 detail implementation strategies that promote and sustain implementation.

Evidence-based change involves a series of action steps in a complex, nonlinear process. Implementing the change requires shifting the perceptions of users and stakeholders; understanding that the amount of time it takes time to integrate the change depends on the nature of the practice change. Merely increasing staff knowledge about an evidence-based practice and passive dissemination strategies is not likely to work, particularly in complex health care settings.

Evaluation of the Practice Change

Evaluation of a practice change provides an opportunity to collect and analyze data regarding use of the new EBP and then to modify the practice as necessary. It is important that the evidence-based change is evaluated, both at the pilot testing phase and when the practice is replicated in additional settings or sites of care. The importance of the evaluation cannot be overemphasized; it provides information for performance gap assessment, audit, and feedback and provides information necessary to determine whether the EBP should be retained, modified, or eliminated (see Chapter 16).

Evaluation should include both process and outcome measures (Titler et al., 2016). The process component focuses on how the practice change is being implemented. It is important to know whether staff members are using and implementing the practice as noted in the EBP guideline. Evaluation of the process also should note (1) barriers that staff encounter in carrying out the practice (e.g., lack of information, skills, or necessary equipment), (2) differences in opinions among health care providers, and (3) difficulty in carrying out the steps of the practice as originally designed (e.g., nasointestinal tubes). Outcome data are an equally important part of evaluation. The purpose of outcome evaluation using baseline and outcome measures is to assist in assessing whether the patient, staff, and/or fiscal outcomes expected are achieved.

SYNTHESIS

The steps of EBP require not only knowledge of the process but also consideration of the context in which a change is recommended. Health care organizations are currently experiencing multiple changes from all types of payers and care systems. Change in any system or level of care is never an easy process regardless of whether there is buy-in from the staff and administration. As the health care system undergoes systematic changes to primary care and integrated health care delivery systems, there is a need for health care professionals at all levels to work toward improving the quality, efficiency and effectiveness of patient care (Berwick, Nolan, & Whittington, 2008). Finding solutions requires not only the ability to search the literature but also having a keen awareness of the larger system changes, such as health care reform, that will filter down to all levels of health care delivery. Organizations such as AHRQ provide databased information of clinical support decision making.

Frameworks and care models such as the Chronic Care Model and Patient-Centered Medical Home (PCMH) also need to be understood and integrated into health care systems to improve patient care (AHRQ, 2017). To improve practice in all types of care environments, it is necessary for health care teams to mindfully incorporate strategies that consider the Triple Aim—that is, improving population health; reducing per capita costs; and improving the patient's experience of care, whether the patient is an individual, family, or community (Stiefel & Nolan, 2012). Resources in an organization need to be dedicated to implementing models that provide a framework to use in the pursuit of excellence, such as the Iowa Model; systems can be challenged to provide evidence that documents improvement through QI initiatives. Small but successful tests of change can then be scaled up for population-level implementation in hospitals or community-based organizations.

▌KEY POINTS

- Evidence-based practice and quality improvement models provide a guide for clinical leaders and their teams for designing EBP and QI projects to improve the quality of care.
- Evidence-based practice, quality improvement, and research have unique, independent, but complementary feature.
- An evidence hierarchy provides a schema for rating the strength of specific types of research designs.

- Evidence-based practice begins with formulating a clinical question derived from problem-focused or knowledge-focused triggers, using the PICO format.
- Five types of clinical questions focus on therapy, harm, diagnosis, prognosis and meaning.
- A clinical question guides the search for the best available evidence.
- Critical appraisal using standardized critical appraisal tools identifies the strengths and weaknesses of each individual research study.

- Synthesis refers to assessing the overall strengths and weaknesses of a group of studies.
- Evaluating the outcomes of an EBP Project occurs prior to making recommendations about applicability to practice.
- Recommendations for applying evidence to practice depend on the strength and quality of the evidence to support current practice, making minor changes

in practice, undertaking major practice changes, or developing a new area of practice.
- Evidence provides the foundation for developing or revising practice standards, protocols, and polices.
- Piloting an EBP practice change is an important step that allows staff to provide feedback and modify as appropriate.

REFERENCES

AACN. (2006). *The essentials of doctoral education for advanced nursing practice.*

Agency for Healthcare Research & Quality (AHRQ). (2017).

Andrews, J., Guyatt, G., Oxman, A. D., et al. (2013). GRADE guidelines:14. Going from evidence to recommendations; the significance and presentation of recommendations. *Journal of Clinical Epidemiology, 66,* 719–725.

Balshem, H., Helfand, M., Schuneman, H. J., et al. (2011). GRADE guidelines:3. Rating the quality of evidence. *Journal of Clinical Epidemiology, 64*(4), 401–406.

Berwick, D. M., Nolan, T. W., & Whittington, J. (2008). The triple aim: Care, health and cost. *Health Affairs, 27*(3), 759–769.

Dobbins, M., Ciliska, D., Cockerill, R., Barnsley, J., & DiCenso, A. (2002). A framework for the dissemination and utilization of research for health-care policy and practice. *The Online Journal of Knowledge Synthesis for Nursing, 9,* document no.7.

Fineholt-Overholt, E., Melynk, B. M., & Schultz, A. (2005). Transforming health care from the inside out: advancing evidence-based practice in the 21st century. *Journal of Professional Nursing, 21*(6), 335–344.

Grade Working Group. www.gradeworkinggroup.org.

Moore, J. E., Kane-Low, Titler, M. J., et al. (2014). Moving towards patient centered care: Women's decisions, perceptions, and experiences of the induction of labor process. *Birth, 41*(2), 138–146.

Moore, J. E., Titler, J. E., Kane-Low, L., Dalton, & Sampselle, C. (2015). Transforming patient-centered care: development of the evidence informed decision making through engagement model. *Women's Health Issues, 25*(3), 276–282.

Newhouse, R. P., Dearholt, S. L., Poe, S. S., Pugh, L. C., & white, K. M. (2005). Evidence-based practice: A practical approach to implementation. *Journal of Nursing Administration, 35*(1), 35–40.

Quality & Safety Education for Nurses. (2017). http://www.qsen.org/.

Schaffer, M. A., Sandau, K. E., & Diedrick, L. (2013). Evidence-based practice models for organizational change: overview and practical application. *Journal of Advanced Nursing, 69*(5), 1197–1209.

Shuman, C. J., Liu, J., Montie, M., et al. (2016). Patient perception and experiences with falls during hospitalization and after discharge. *Applied Nursing Research, 31,* 79–85.

Stiefel, M. K., & Nolan, K. (2012). *A guide to measuring the triple aim: Population health, experience of care, and per capita cost. IHI Innovation Series white paper.* Cambridge: MA: Institute for Healthcare Improvement. www.IHI.org.

Titler, M. G. (2014). Overview of evidence-based practice and translation science. *Nursing Clinics of North America, 49*(3), 269–274.

Titler, M. G., Conlon, P., Reynolds, M. A., et al. (2016). The effect of translating research into practice interventions to promote use of evidence-based fall preventions in hospitalized adults: a prospective pre-post implementation study in the US. *Applied Nursing Research, 31,* 52–59.

Van Driel, M. L., Morledge, M. D., Ulep, R., Shaffer, J. P., Davies, P., & Deichmann, R. (2016). Interventions to improve adherence to lipid-lowering medication (Review). *Cochrane Database of Systematic Reviews.*

3

Developing Compelling Clinical Questions

Judith Haber

LEARNING OUTCOMES

After reading this chapter, you should be able to do the following:

- Discuss the purpose of developing a clinical question.
- Compare the differences between a clinical question and a research question or hypothesis in relation to evidence-based practice.
- Differentiate between knowledge- and problem-focused triggers as sources of clinical questions.
- Apply the PICO framework to the formulation of clinical questions.
- Evaluate how the clinical question guides the search for evidence.

KEY TERMS

Clinical question	Knowledge-focused triggers	Problem-focused triggers
Hypothesis	PICO	Research question

INTRODUCTION

Whether you are a nurse practitioner, clinical specialist, clinical nurse leader, nurse educator, nurse manager, or a member of the quality improvement team at your health care organization, you are a clinical leader. Evidence-based practice (EBP) is a key component of the expertise you offer to your patients and staff. It provides the foundation for developing clinical questions that launch your search for health information that provides the best available evidence to inform health care and clinical decisions. High-quality, cost-effective care that provides a satisfying experience for patient, provider, and staff challenges health professionals to provide patient care that is informed by the latest and best evidence (Berwick et al., 2008). Increasingly, the external health care environment—including, but not limited to, patients, employers, certifying organizations, regulatory boards, insurers, and professional organizations—expects that evidence-based information guides clinical practice.

Clinical practice is kept up to date by searching for, retrieving, and critically appraising research studies, systematic reviews, and EBP guidelines that apply to practice issues encountered in clinical settings. Clinicians strive to navigate the abundance of clinical information available to health professionals; finding the right information, at the right time, using the right search strategy (see Chapter 4) is a challenge! Your search for information—that is, the best available evidence—is converted into focused clinical questions that are the foundation of EBP and quality improvement. The evidence, coupled with clinical judgment, as well as patient preferences and

---

BOX 3.1   PICO Question Components

- Patient/Population/Problem
  - Diagnosis
  - Age
  - Gender
  - Ethnicity/race
  - Marital status
- Intervention or Clinical Issue of Interest
  - Risk behavior (e.g., unprotected sex)
  - Therapy/intervention
  - Exposure to disease
  - Prognosis
- Comparison Intervention or Clinical Issue of Interest
  - No risk behavior (e.g., protected sex)
  - Alternative therapy/intervention, placebo, no intervention at all
  - No disease
  - Alternative prognosis
- Outcome
  - Risk of disease or condition
  - Expected/predicted outcome expected from therapy/intervention (e.g., decreased catheter-associated urinary infections)
  - Accuracy of diagnosis (e.g., sensitivity and specificity)
  - Rate of occurrence of adverse outcome (e.g., mortality)

BOX 3.2   PICO Question Formats

Therapy/Intervention

In _____ (population), what is the effect of _____ (intervention), compared with _____ (comparison intervention), on _____ (outcome)?

Diagnosis/Assessment

For _____ population, does _____ (tool or procedure) yield more accurate or more appropriate diagnostic/assessment information than _____ (comparison tool/procedure) about _____ (outcome)?

Prognosis

For _____ (population), does _____ (disease/condition), relative to _____ (comparison disease or condition) increase the risk for or influence _____ (outcome)?

Causation/Harm/Etiology

Does _____ (exposure or characteristic) increase the risk for _____ (outcome) compared with _____ (comparison exposure or condition) in _____ (population)?

Meaning or Process

What is it like for _____ (population) to experience _____ (condition, illness, circumstances?)
  Or:
What is the process through which _____ _____ (population) cope with, adapt to, or live with _____ (circumstance)?

---

contextual factors, combine to inform the most effective clinical decision making about practice (see Chapter 1). The purpose of this chapter is to highlight the importance of clinical questions, that is, how to develop and use them in searching for the best available evidence to find answers that inform clinical practice.

WHAT IS A CLINICAL QUESTION?

Clinical questions form the basis for searching the literature to identify supporting evidence from research to inform development or revision of clinical standards, protocols, and policies that guide professional nursing and interprofessional best practice. Clinical questions have four basic components:

- **P**opulation and problem
- **I**ntervention
- **C**omparison
- **O**utcome

These components, known as **PICO**, provide an effective format for developing focused and searchable clinical questions. PICO is a tool to help you formulate

the clinical question. Box 3.1 presents components of the PICO question. PICO question formats linked with types of clinical questions are illustrated in Box 3.2. PICO questions linked with types of designs are highlighted in Table 3.1. The significance of the clinical question becomes apparent as research evidence from the search is critically appraised. Research evidence, clinical judgment, and patient preferences are used to validate, develop, or revise best practices.

Identifying the **P**— patient population, problem, or setting—may seem obvious to you as a clinician or to

TABLE 3.1 Classifying Types of Clinical Questions and Kind of Study Providing Best Evidence

Clinical Question	Type of Question	Kind of Study Design Providing Best Evidence
How can the problem be prevented?	Prevention	Randomized Clinical Trial/Systematic Review
Will detecting the problem early, before symptoms, make a difference in my health?	Screening	Randomized Clinical Trial/Systematic Review Cohort Studies
How good is this test for detecting my problem?	Diagnosis	Cohort Studies
What is the likely outcome of this problem?	Prognosis	Cohort Studies
What proportion of the population is newly diagnosed with this problem each year?	Incidence	Cohort Studies
What proportion of the population is currently living with the problem?	Prevalence	Case Control/Cohort Studies
What causes the problem?	Etiology	Randomized Clinical Trials/Systematic Review
What should be done to treat this problem?	Therapy	Randomized Clinical Trials/Case-Control Studies
Will there be any negative effects from an intervention?	Harm	

your team. However, it is often stated too generally and may be misleading in terms of using the correct search terms when designing your evidence search. Using Box 3.1 will be helpful to you in focusing identification of the target population or setting. For example, limiting the population to a specific diagnostic subgroup (e.g., young men under 30 with testicular cancer) is appropriate when there is a rationale for doing so and the population is linked to the other components of the PICO question and search terms. When the setting is the focus of interest (e.g., group homes for psychiatric patients), the setting becomes the key focus of your search.

The **I**, the issue of interest, commonly the intervention, should reflect greater diversity than the traditional definition of an intervention. For example, it may include a treatment (e.g., new high-dose 1-week breast cancer radiation protocol), a diagnostic test (prostate-specific antigen test for prostate cancer), and exposure (e.g., human papilloma virus), risk factor (e.g., *BRCA* positive), or prognostic factor (e.g., cardiac stent[s] vs. coronary bypass surgery) survival rates. The **C**—the comparison intervention or issue of interest—needs to be relevant and linked to the **I**. Greater specificity for the **I** and the **C** will be associated with a more focused search strategy. When the **I** is a new intervention, you may have to do some background reading

before specifically identifying the **I** as well as the comparison. The comparison is usually the current standard of care, a placebo, or another intervention or combination of interventions. For example, the **I** may be examining the effect of using an antidepressant and cognitive behavioral therapy (CBT) compared with CBT alone for treatment of clinical depression. The **C**—the comparison intervention — may be the current standard of care or no intervention at all. For example, in this example, the current standard of care for the comparison intervention may be treatment with CBT alone. Because clinical depression is associated with the risk of suicide, it is unlikely that this would be a PICO question in which the comparison intervention would be no intervention at all.

Other clinicians may be focused on prognosis as an issue of interest. For example, a nurse practitioner who was developing an online health literacy FAQ for women newly diagnosed with breast cancer was interested in being able to provide an evidence-based answer about the differences in survival rates for women with breast cancer who had had a lumpectomy compared with traditional mastectomy.

The **O**—outcome—specifies the focus of the answer to the PICO question that will be revealed by the targeted search for and critical appraisal and synthesis of the evidence. Evidence from cohort research studies for the preceding example reveals that there was no significant difference in 5-year survival for women who had a lumpectomy compared with a mastectomy.

Sometimes a PICO question will specify more than one outcome. In a **P** population of men with type 2 diabetes who are 25% overweight, **I** what is the effect of prescribing Jardiance + metformin in **C** comparison to metformin alone on improvement of **O1** HgbA1c and **O2** weight loss?

EBP TIP

A well-developed PICO question guides a focused search for scientific evidence about assessing, diagnosing, treating, or providing patients with information about the prognosis for their specific health condition.

WHY ARE CLINICAL QUESTIONS IMPORTANT?

Busy clinicians, like you, can be overwhelmed by the volume of literature you have to access, sift through, and evaluate to identify the best practice supported by the strongest evidence that is applicable to your population and practice issue or problem. Moreover, no two patients are exactly alike, and colleagues may have differing opinions on the best approach to resolving a patient problem. When your team members ponder the clinical question they want to develop, it may be helpful to think about the purpose or objective of the evidence-based project they want to implement. The purpose of an evidence-based project includes what the clinical team aims to achieve with the initiative. When a purpose statement is used, it suggests the planned approach that will be used to guide the project. When the purpose of an evidence-based project is to ask a clinical question that compares the effectiveness of two interventions, the search for evidence will be linked to intervention or therapy studies that focus on testing the effectiveness of interventions queried in the PICO question. For example, if the purpose of an evidence-based project aims to answer whether, in a population of preoperative patients, the use of music compared with no music will have a significant effect on decreasing preoperative anxiety, the search for the best available evidence will focus on studies that are Level I systematic reviews, Level II randomized clinical trials (RCTs), or Level III quasi-experimental designs (see Chapter 4).

Clinical questions are important as they provide a structured format focused on finding an answer to a specific knowledge- or problem-focused trigger. Formulating the PICO question facilitates searching the literature efficiently to locate and retrieve the right information in a timely manner so that the best available information can be shared with your colleagues and patients (Chapters 4 and 17). Integrating a proactive evidence-seeking approach into your clinical practice style is essential to remaining at the cutting edge of clinical practice to provide high-quality, cost-effective care and satisfying patient and staff experiences (IHI, 2012).

IPE TIP

Teamwork is involved in developing a clinical PICO question. Team members may have differing perspectives about the focus of the clinical question. They need to respect and consider the value of each member's contribution to finalizing the PICO question and making sure it aligns with the aims of the EBP or QI project.

SOURCES OF CLINICAL QUESTIONS

Clinical questions originate from multiple sources, including the patient and family. The Iowa Model (see Chapter 1) EBP framework is widely disseminated and adopted in clinical settings; it guides clinicians to question current practices and whether patient care can be improved through the use of research findings. In this model, knowledge- and problem-focused "triggers" provide a template for clinicians to use when trying to think about and select an EBP project topic and develop a relevant clinical question (Titler et al., 2001).

Problem-focused triggers are those issues that are identified by clinical teams, quality improvement staff, or committees based on data that emerge from specific sectors of an organization or practice. Data sources for problem-focused triggers are as follows:
- Quality improvement data
- Risk management data
- Internal or external benchmarking data
- Financial data
- New or recurrent clinical problems
- Patients' concerns

An example of a problem-focused trigger would be a high 30-day hospital readmission rate for congestive heart failure patients discharged from inpatient units. These data would have a clinical as well as a financial impact on an organization and would likely be a priority EBP topic. The team charged with addressing this problem might generate a preliminary clinical question focused on a postdischarge transition care program using the PICO format. They would review and critically appraise the literature for relevant studies suggesting effective evidence-based transition care solutions involving e-health compared with the current standard of care (Titler et al., 2001).

Knowledge-focused triggers are ideas generated when, for example, clinical teams or quality improvement committees read research studies, listen to scientific papers presented at professional conferences, or encounter practice guidelines published by federal organizations such as the US Preventive Task Force or professional organizations such as the American Diabetes Association. Members of the team or committee may review and critically appraise the evidence reported in a research study or group of studies pertaining to use of motivational interviewing to promote lifestyle changes and glycemic control in patients with type 2 diabetes and determine how the evidence aligns with a clinical problem being encountered in the primary care diabetes program in their organization. Similarly, they may review a new Centers for Disease Control and Prevention (CDC) central line–associated bloodstream infection (CLABSI) guideline for prevention of CLABSIs that is relevant because of a recent spike in internal/external benchmarking data related to CLABSIs in the critical care units (CDC, 2011, CDC, 2016). Remember that focused clinical questions using the PICO format may emerge from these knowledge-focused triggers:

- New research or other literature
- National agencies or organizational standards and guidelines
- Philosophies of care
- Questions from institutional standards or policy committees

Problem- and knowledge-focused triggers are important because they are instrumental in defining the clinical issue in the form of an answerable clinical question. Asking the right questions and seeking evidence-based answers is correlated with evidence-informed decision making. Sometimes your clinical question may be a combination of knowledge- and problem-focused triggers. As clinicians, we strive to provide patient-centered care that addresses the whole person as partners in their care. This approach can lead to stronger patient engagement and activation (see Chapter 15). For example, patients feel validated when their providers are open to answering their clinical questions,

responding to their evidence challenges, and clarifying evidence whether it is obtained from scientific sources or the Internet. Consumers increasingly want to engage in an evidence-informed discussion with providers; it is an essential component of the Triple Aim: the satisfying patient experience (Berwick, 2008).

TYPES OF CLINICAL/PICO QUESTIONS

A well-developed PICO question has the following advantages:
- It helps to clarify the clinical problem and the information required to solve it.
- It helps to define the type of evidence needed from which type of study.
- It helps to provide terms to make searching for evidence more effective.

Classifying PICO questions according to the type of question being asked is one approach, as illustrated in Table 3.1. As Box 3.2 indicates, there are different clinical question formats depending on the type of clinical question being asked. For example, the clinical question, "What is the effectiveness of CBT compared with antidepressant therapy in decreasing depression in people with a cancer diagnosis?" suggests thinking about which therapy is most effective for treating this patient or patient population. Generally, the kind of studies that potentially provide the best evidence for answering this kind of therapy clinical question are RCTs (see Chapter 6) as illustrated in Table 3.1. Boxes 3.3 through 3.6 provide case studies using therapy, prognosis, diagnosis, and meaning clinical questions that illustrate how different types of clinical questions are used to address specific clinical issues. The examples and templates we have included are to develop your expertise in formulating clinical questions, the first stop on the EBP train! However, as you delve into the EBP literature, you will quickly realize that there are other types of clinical questions to ask and other ways to ask them; using the PICO format ensures that you will be able to search for and find the answer to your clinical questions effectively or have an evidence-based rationale for modifying your clinical question.

> ### EBP TIP
> Once you have developed a focused clinical question using the PICO format, you will search the literature for the best available evidence to answer your clinical question.

BOX 3.3   Case Study 1: Therapy Question

Larry H is a 55-year-old man who has a strong family history of type 2 diabetes (T2D). His maternal grandmother and grandfather were diagnosed with T2D in their 50s and his father at age 55. His father also had severe coronary artery disease (CAD), diagnosed after a myocardial infarction (MI). He had a fatal MI at age 72. Larry, although slim at 5′9″ and 160 pounds, loves sweets and can easily finish a package of cookies by himself in one sitting. He eats beef (red meat) almost every day and does not exercise. At his annual physicals for the past 5 years, he has had a fasting blood sugar of 120 to 130; each year his primary care provider cautions him to "watch his sugar intake."

At this year's physical, Larry has a new provider, a nurse practitioner (NP). As she completes his history and physical examination, including his current HgA1c of 6.8, she thinks about the clinical question that would guide the evidence-based information she would discuss with Larry about the potential to prevent, delay, or reverse the onset of T2D, given his risk factors and clinical data.

Keep in mind that a focused clinical question is important in conducting an effective search. The problem-focused triggers that come to mind are the robust family history of T2D and CAD, high sugar intake, beef at least five times per week, and no exercise. On the other hand, Larry does not fit the usual overweight T2D risk factor. On the basis of those problem-focused triggers, the NP

might develop the following clinical question: "In a population of high-risk middle-aged men (P), how do diet and exercise (I) compared with medication management with metformin (C), affect the HgbA1C over 6 months (O)? This clinical question would guide a search of the literature for research studies; probably therapy, cohort, or case-control studies; systematic reviews; or clinical practice guidelines that provide the best available evidence for developing an effective management plan.

Ideally, the NP would search for and find a systematic review (SR), a synthesis study that would include a sample of multiple randomized clinical trials that address this clinical question (see Chapter 8). As you recall from Chapter 2, systematic reviews provide Level I evidence. If critical appraisal of the systematic review indicates that it is a well-designed SR providing high-quality evidence, the NP would have confidence in having obtained an answer to the clinical question and applying the findings in practice. When an SR is not available, the research design that provides the strongest evidence for an individual study to answer this clinical question is a randomized clinical trial; it provides Level II evidence (see Chapter 6). The intervention and comparison groups are evaluated in relation to the outcome and the extent to which it was achieved. In this case, the outcome of interest is the effect of the lifestyle intervention of diet and exercise compared with medication on reduction of HgbA1c.

Feldman, A. L., Long, G. H., Johansson, I., Weinehall, L., Fharm, E., Wenger, P., . . . Rolandsson, O. (2017). Change in lifestyle behaviors and diabetes risk: evidence from a population-based cohort study with 10-year follow-up. *International Journal of Behavioral Nutrition and Physical Activity, 14*(1), 39; Tuomilehto, J., Lindstrom, J., Erikson, J. G., Valle, T. T., Hämäläinen, H., Ilanne-Parikka, P. . . . Finnish Diabetes Prevention Group. (2001). Prevention of type 2 diabetes mellitus by changes in lifestyle among subjects with impaired glucose tolerance. *New England Journal of Medicine, 344*, 1343–1350; Whittmore, R., Melkus, G., Wagner, J., Birthrup, V., Dziura, J., & Grey, M. (2009). Translating the diabetes prevention program to primary care: a pilot study. *Nursing Research, 58*(1), 2–12.

BOX 3.4   Case Study 2: Prognosis

Tamika is a 45-year-old woman who has been diagnosed with breast cancer; she had a lumpectomy and a lymph node dissection because she had a positive sentinel lymph node. She will also be treated with radiation and chemotherapy. Six weeks later, Tamika begins attending a breast cancer support group in her local community and listens to one of the women talking about swelling and pain in her arm that is called lymphedema. Tamika is very concerned because the woman had the same kind of surgery as hers. None of Tamika's care providers have mentioned lymphedema as a potential complication or side

effect of her treatment. At the next follow-up visit with her surgeon, she asks you, her nurse practitioner (NP), for information about lymphedema and asks whether there is any way to decrease her risk for developing it, preventing it, or improving it if it happens.

In this case, the clinical question focuses on prognosis, which helps clinicians, based on evidence, to predict a patient's or patient population's clinical trajectory over a specified timeframe. On the basis of research evidence, context, and patient preferences, clinicians are able to predict the likelihood that targeted outcomes will occur.

BOX 3.4   Case Study 2: Prognosis—cont'd

The difference between therapy and prognosis questions is that there is no random assignment to an intervention or comparison group because of ethical issues that preclude an randomized clinical trial design or because of other issues such as feasibility.

The problem-focused trigger that guides the NP's search for evidence to answer Tamika's question might focus on studies that report prevalence of lymphedema for women having lumpectomy and lymph node dissection followed by radiation and chemotherapy, as well as studies reporting evidence about programs for preventing and/or treating lymphedema and their benefit. The NP might develop the following prognosis clinical question that would guide her search: For women treated for breast cancer with lumpectomy and lymph node dissection, followed by radiation and chemotherapy (P), does choosing the Optimal Lymph Flow Program (Condition), relative to choosing self-administered breast arm exercises (Comparison Condition), reduce the risk for developing lymphedema (O)? The answer to

a prognosis question would need to include studies that followed groups of patients with a specific condition (e.g., breast cancer) who chose or were part of nonrandomly assigned treatments that were different for each of the groups (Optimal Lymph Flow Program vs. self-administered breast arm exercises) and where subjects in the groups are monitored over time to assess the likelihood of an outcome (lymphedema) occurring or not (no lymphedema). Cohort studies that provide Level III evidence are the most common type of study to answer a prognosis question. Case control studies that provide Level IV evidence are another design for answering prognosis clinical questions (see Chapter 7). You also may find a systematic review (see Chapter 8) of cohort studies examining the influence of lymphedema risk reduction and prevention programs in comparison to self-administered breast arm exercises that provides Level I evidence, but keeping in mind that this evidence summary is for cohort or even case-control studies that use less rigorous research designs.

Fu, M. R., Axelrod, D., Guth, A. A., Wang, Y., Scagliola, J., Hiotis, K., . . . El-Shammaa, N. (2016). Usability and feasibility of health IT interventions to enhance self-care for lymphedema symptom management in breast cancer survivors. *Internet Interventions*, *5*, 56–64; Fu, M. R., Axelrod, D., Guth, A. A., Rampertaap, K., El-Shammaa, N., Hiotis, K., . . . Wang, Y. (2016). mHealth self-care interventions: managing symptoms following breast cancer treatment. *mHealth, 2*, 28.

BOX 3.5   Case Study 3: Meaning

An interprofessional coronary care unit (CCU) team is having their monthly quality improvement (QI) meeting. The nurse manager and the physician hospitalist report that several family members have raised the question about whether their presence would be welcomed should their family member go into cardiac arrest and have to be resuscitated. The team's immediate response is to strongly oppose family presence despite letters from family members expressing how important it would be to them to be with their family member during this difficult situation, and, perhaps, during their loved one's last moments. One nurse practitioner (NP) states that because patient and family satisfaction are such important indicators of the patient experience, perhaps the team should take an evidence-based approach to inform their decision making about this policy. The team develops a clinical question that focuses on the qualitative meaning

of presence during resuscitation from the perspective of the resuscitation team members. In this example, the clinical question would have the following format: How do CCU resuscitation team members (P) with a critically ill family member (I) experience the presence of the patient's family during resuscitation (O)?

This clinical question differs from those in Case Studies 1 and 2. You must have noticed that the C is not included in this question. When posing a meaning question, there is no comparison because the clinical question focuses on the qualitative meaning of family presence during resuscitation to the CCU resuscitation team. The studies best suited to answer this clinical question are individual qualitative studies (Level VI evidence), such as phenomenological studies (see Chapter 9) or qualitative evidence summaries called *metasyntheses* that provide Level V evidence.

Hassankhani, H., Zamanzadeh, V., Rahmani, A., Haririan, H., & Porter, J. E. (2017). Family presence during resuscitation: a double-edged sword. *Journal of Nursing Scholarship, 49*(2), 127–134.

BOX 3.6 Case Study 4: Diagnosis

The gastroenterology team journal club at the Hospital ABC Cancer Center reviews a new study reporting that more adults aged 20 to 54 are dying from colorectal cancer (CRC), raising issues about earlier screening and better detection methods for younger patients. Epidemiological data reveals that CRC incidence has been increasing in the United States among adults younger than 55 years since the mid-1990s. They are also dying at slightly higher rates, even though the overall CRC death rate has been declining. The increase has been confined to white men and women. However, CRC rates among the African American population continue to exceed rates for white men and women.

This knowledge-focused trigger, gleaned from a new journal club research study, highlights the importance of asking a clinical question focused on diagnosis. On the basis of the knowledge-focused trigger, the team, including an NP, surgeon, medical and radiation oncologists, epidemiologist, and pharmacists, might develop the following clinical question: "In a population of white men and women aged 20 to 55 (P), is colonoscopy (I) compared with MRI (C) more accurate in diagnosing CRC (O)?" This clinical question would guide a search of the literature for research studies; probably therapy, cohort, or case-control studies; systematic reviews; or clinical practice guidelines that provide the best

available evidence for determining the diagnostic test with the greatest sensitivity and specificity. However, because these are new data, current diagnostic tests that are effective and age at which to begin screening to correctly identify CRC each time it is used may not exist. This highlights what may be an urgent need to find reliable diagnostic tools to accurately detect and screen for CRC in young people, especially those in high-risk groups such as those who have specific risk factors, including a family history of CRC, African American ethnicity, or chronic conditions such as inflammatory bowel disease, Crohn's disease, or colitis that raise the risk for CRC.

Ideally, the team would search for and find a systematic review (SR), a synthesis study that would include a sample of multiple randomized clinical trials (RCTs) that address this clinical question (see Chapter 8). As you recall from Chapter 2, SRs provide Level I evidence. If critical appraisal of the systematic review indicates that it is a well-designed SR providing high-quality evidence, the team would have confidence in having obtained an answer to the clinical question and applying the findings in practice. When an SR is not available, the research design that provides the strongest evidence for an individual study to answer this clinical question is an RCT; it provides Level II evidence (see Chapter 6).

Kekelidze, M., D'Errico, L., Pansini, M., Tyndall, A., & Hohmann, J. (2013). Colorectal cancer: current imaging methods and future perspectives for the diagnosis, staging, and therapeutic response evaluation. *World Journal of Gastroenterology, 19*(46), 8502–8514; Kijima, S., Sasaki, T., Nagata, K., Utano, K., Lefor, A. T., & Sugimota, H. (2014). Preoperative evaluation of colorectal cancer using CT, colonoscopy, MRI, and PET/CT. *World Journal of Gastroenterology, 20*(45), 16964–16975.

CLINICAL QUESTIONS DIFFER FROM RESEARCH QUESTIONS AND HYPOTHESES

Clinical questions differ from research questions and hypotheses in their approach. They may sound alike, but their purposes differ. Both research questions and hypotheses are key preliminary steps in conducting research studies and guide the design and implementation of a research study. Both are used by researchers to test the relationships between and among variables. Research questions are written as questions that address a gap or conflict in the literature. They test a measureable relationship between the independent and dependent variable that is examined in the study. The remainder of the study should flow

from the research question. The research question is answered by the findings of the study. A properly written research question will be clear and concise. It should contain the topic being studied (purpose), the variable(s), and the population. Hypotheses are used in research studies to predict the outcome(s) of the study. A hypothesis is predictive in nature and typically used when significant knowledge already exists on the subject, which allows the prediction to be made. Both research questions and hypotheses are commonly used in quantitative research. Guided by their *clinical questions*, clinicians search for and use evidence provided by the findings of research studies to answer clinical questions. Once found and retrieved, the evidence is critically appraised, and, based on the strength, quality, and consistency of the evidence, it is used to answer the clinical question by determining whether the evidence is applicable to clinical practice and to provide a basis for implementation of EBPs.

SYNTHESIS

Clinicians are increasingly concerned about ensuring that the care they provide is evidence-based. In your leadership role, you are being asked to provide evidence to support the quality and cost-effectiveness of the care provided for your patient population or program. Individual research studies, systematic reviews, and clinical guidelines are evidence-based products you will use to support your practice. Formulating clinical questions is fundamental to and the first step in the EBP process. Clinical questions convert situations and problems into answerable questions that you will use to guide your search for the best available evidence, coupled with clinical expertise and patient preferences that you will use to make a difference and act as a role model for colleagues. As you become confident as an EBP clinical leader, another aspect of your role will be to mentor other NPs, nurses, and colleagues from other professions to develop their clinical question and other EBP competencies.

QI CHECKPOINT

The quality improvement data at your hospital indicate that the prevalence of central line–associated bloodstream infections (CLABSIs) has increased in your hospital intensive care units (ICU) by 10% in the last two quarters. As a member of the ICU Quality Improvement Committee, collaborate with your committee colleagues from other professions to develop an interprofessional action plan. Deliberate to develop a clinical question to guide the quality improvement project.

▉ KEY POINTS

- Clinical questions form the basis of the search of the literature for supporting evidence from research to inform development or revision of clinical standards, protocols, policies, guidelines that guide clinical practice.
- Clinical questions are important as they provide a structured format focused on providing an answer to a problem-focused or knowledge -focused trigger.
- Clinical questions have four basic components that specify the population or problem (P), intervention (I), comparison (C), and the outcome (O), all of which are known as PICO, a tool to help formulate a clinical question.

- There are different types of clinical questions that focus on finding answers to issues related to therapy, prognosis, diagnosis, prevention, screening, harm, incidence, and prevalence.
- Specific types of clinical questions are associated with research study designs that provide the best available evidence.
- Clinical questions differ from research questions and hypotheses. Research questions and hypotheses guide the direction of research studies that generate evidence, whereas clinical questions use the evidence generated by research studies to inform clinical decision making.

REFERENCES

Berwick, D. M., Nolan, T. W., & Whittington, J. (2008). The triple aim: Care, health, and cost. *Health Affairs*, *27*(3), 759–769.

Centers for Disease Control. (2011). Guideline for prevention of intravascular catheter-associated bloodstream infections. https://www.cdc.gov/infection control/guidelines/bsi/index.html.

Centers for Disease Control. (2016). Checklist for prevention of central line associated blood stream infections. http://www./stor.org/stable/10.1086/676533.

Titler, M. G., Kleiber, C., Steelman, V. J., et al. (2001). The Iowa model of evidence-based practice to promote quality care. *Critical Care Nursing Clinics of North America*, *13*(4), 497–509. PMID.

4

Search and Critical Appraisal of the Literature

Susan Jacobs, Barbara Krainovich-Miller

LEARNING OUTCOMES

After reading this chapter, you should be able to do the following:

- Use the PICO format to ASK a clinical question identifying the Patient, Problem, or Population of interest AND the proposed Intervention as a first step toward conducting a literature search.
- Demonstrate competency in Boolean logic to construct a search query based on a PICO question.
- Recognize the range, scope, strengths, and limitations of digital repositories and tools to

GATHER, organize, evaluate, and synthesize evidence.
- ASSESS and APPRAISE the strength of evidence by evaluating the methodology described in a study and locating it on the evidence pyramid.
- Develop an evidence synthesis table.
- Recognize that acquiring evidence and critical appraisal is an iterative process of strategic exploration.
- Develop on ongoing engagement with search tools to discover, cite, distill, manage, and share results.

KEY TERMS

Altmetrics
Background question
Boolean connectors
Citation management tools
Controlled vocabulary
Evidence summary

Gray literature
Meta-analysis
Metaliteracy
Point-of-care tool
Primary source
PRISMA flow chart

Scoping search
Search bias
Secondary source
Snowballing
Synthesis
Systematic review

Discovering research evidence requires clinical leaders to search the literature both as background for the research they intend to conduct and in their role as research consumers. Knowledge of how and where to search, beyond Googling, often requires a new way of thinking that is transformative. Many users of the digital landscape have been informed by educational experiences along with misperceptions gained as customers responding to marketing approaches. As seekers of evidence to inform practice in the vast health sciences information ecosystem (Association of College & Research Libraries [ACRL], 2015), an understanding of searching and knowledge

practices, critical thinking, the underlying evidence hierarchy, and, overall, critical appraisal and avoidance of bias must accompany each step of the discovery process. The increasingly interconnected digital environment has extensive resources and search tools. The purpose of this chapter is to take a focused clinical question (see Chapter 3), translate it to searchable terms, select appropriate databases to leverage the evidence hierarchy (see Chapter 2), and begin to systematically synthesize and appraise the results (see Chapters 5–9). This process ensures that educators, administrators, clinicians, and their patients will benefit from the most recent and highest quality research evidence.

EVIDENCE IS HIERARCHICAL

Discovery of the published evidence requires a searcher to seek both primary sources, that is, original evidence, and secondary sources, which are derived from or are interpretations of primary sources.

Primary sources include:
- peer-reviewed research studies;
- systematic reviews that are meta-analyses;
- non–peer-reviewed articles and editorials;
- public health reports and news;
- clinical trials in progress;
- statistical data sets;
- websites, social media postings, and personal communications;
- expert opinions; and
- unpublished "gray" literature.
  Secondary sources include:
- textbooks;
- review articles that are narrative reviews, integrative reviews, and systematic reviews;
- preappraised studies and critiqued abstracts;
- evidence summaries and syntheses and point-of-care (POC) tools; and
- clinical practice guidelines.

All types of sources are important to consider and are highlighted in Table 4.1. Even the most experienced and knowledgeable scholar can face information overload and be in need of a road map or framework to begin discovery. Fundamental to the process of inquiry and engagement with the published literature is depicting the evidence of health care as hierarchical. A core idea for advanced practice nurses is to envision the evidence pyramid (see Fig. 2.1 in Chapter 2) and contextually situate a research study as a first step to evaluate the strength of the research evidence. Earlier chapters have introduced the evidence-based practice (EBP) steps; the current chapter focuses on the first steps: ASK, GATHER, and ASSESS/APPRAISE.

METALITERACY

Clinical leaders are challenged to gain competence with search tools to search for and retrieve research evidence, using multiple desktop or handheld applications, appraisal tools, and citation management tools (see Table 4.2). Managing digitized sources, leveraging search tool interfaces, and using the full functionality of multiple platforms requires metaliteracy, defined as an "ongoing adaptation to emerging technologies and an understanding of the critical thinking and reflection required to engage in these spaces" (ACRL, 2015). This challenging task has been compared with the "tacit knowledge" required to read, write, speak a language, or play an instrument (Meyer & Land, 2003). Competence in managing these multiple systems and platforms requires hands-on engagement, which requires practice entering search terms and viewing results. Critical thinking informs *each* step of the process in addition to being an important focus of Step 3, Assess/Appraise/Synthesize, covered in the second part of this chapter.

WHERE TO START

When entering any portal, your decision about *where to begin* the discovery of evidence for a clinical question is critical. It is important to avoid search bias, the skewed or insufficient retrieval of literature that results from a careless or incomplete search strategy or selection of the wrong database. Knowledge of the scope, unique characteristics, and functionality of any online database is crucial to your literature search. Evidence of a rigorous, comprehensive, documented literature review is often a requirement of the critical appraisal tool checklists that you will find listed in Table 4.2. Knowledge of the process of information creation (ACRL, 2015), peer review, research methodologies, and publication cycles are all essential as you decide where to locate and define what is meant by "evidence."

Why not Google?

As you embark on a search for evidence, you might raise the question, What about Google? Search engines such as Google, Google Scholar, or a licensed commercial web-scale tool may be useful as an instructive first step for strategic exploration to:
- immerse yourself in a new topic,
- locate a "known item" (an article by a certain author, in a given year, in a specific journal),
- gain a sense of the breadth or depth of a topic,
- identify evidence that is highly cited in the literature, and
- begin to appreciate the ambiguities introduced by a simple keyword search, identify synonyms, and become aware of "false hits."

TABLE 4.1 Background Sources of Evidence May Be Located in a "Review" Article, Practice Guideline, "Point-of-Care" (POC) Tool, Book, Report, Critiqued Abstract, or Other Evidence Summary

Background Source	Citation	Description
Topic summary located on a government website	Facts About ASDs. (n.d.). Retrieved from http://www.cdc.gov/ncbddd/autism/facts.html	From the Centers for Disease Control and Prevention website, a summary situates music therapy within potential treatments for autism spectrum disorder. Available free of charge.
Report	Kroger, A. T. (n.d.). General Recommendations on Immunization. Recommendations of the Advisory Committee on Immunization Practices (ACIP). Retrieved from https://www.cdc.gov/mmwr/preview/mmwrhtml/rr5515a1.htm.	From *MMWR (Morbidity and Mortality Weekly Report)*, a single report suggests music as a "distraction" method for alleviation of discomfort associated with vaccination. Available free of charge.
Evidence summary	Nguyen, D. H. (2017). Anxiety in adults undergoing surgical procedures: Music interventions [evidence summary]. *Joanna Briggs Institute EBP Database*. Retrieved from http://journals.lww.com/jbisrir/Pages.	From the *Joanna Briggs JBI Database of Systematic Reviews and Implementation Reports*, a three-page evidence summary concludes "that music be offered to surgical patients during the preoperative period to reduce patients' anxiety levels during and after surgery." Requires subscription.
Clinical practice guideline	National Guideline Clearinghouse. (2012). Depression in older adults. In: *Evidence-Based Geriatric Nursing Protocols for Best Practice*. Retrieved from https://guidelines.gov/summaries/summary/43922.	From the National Guideline Clearinghouse*, a guideline summary developed by the Hartford Institute for Geriatric Nursing situates "music therapy" as one form of "daily participation in relaxation therapies" for depression in older adults.
Abstract journal (with critically appraised commentary for a single published study)	Taylor-Piliae, R. (2002). Review: Music as a single session intervention reduces anxiety and respiratory rate in patients admitted to hospital. *Evidence-Based Nursing*, 5(3), 86–86.	*Evidence Based Nursing*, an "abstract" journal with studies critically appraised with expert commentaries. *Taylor-Piliae (2002) is a commentary on:* Evans, D. (2002). The effectiveness of music as an intervention for hospital patients: a systematic review. *Journal of Advanced Nursing*, 37(1), 8–18. Requires subscription, with selected free articles (http://ebn.bmj.com).
POC tool	Adler, A., & Pravikoff, D. (2016). Music Therapy and Anxiety. CINAHL Nursing Guide. EBSCO Publishing (Evidence-Based Care Sheet). Nursing Reference Center Plus.	Nursing Reference Center Plus, a POC tool, summarizes the evidence for music therapy and anxiety. The 18-item reference list cites 1 meta-analysis, 2 systematic reviews, 11 randomized controlled trials, 2 nonrandomized trials, and 1 review article. Requires subscription from: https://www.ebscohost.com/nursing/products/nursing-reference-center-plus.
Review article	Cole, L. C., & LoBiondo-Wood, G. (2014). Music as an adjuvant therapy in control of pain and symptoms in hospitalized adults: A systematic review. *Pain Management Nursing*, 15(1), 406–425.	A systematic review of music as an adjuvant therapy for pain control in hospitalized adults identified 17 randomized controlled trials that met the inclusion criteria and concluded that "the use of music is safe, inexpensive, and an independent nursing function that can be easily incorporated into the routine care of patients."

*As of this printing, the NGC will no longer be available due to ceased federal funding.

TABLE 4.2   Tools for Organizing, Citing, and Sharing Evidence

Tool/Resource	Examples[a]
Online database training tutorials	U.S. National Library of Medicine. (n.d.). PubMed Tutorial Training Material and Manuals https://www.nlm.nih.gov/bsd/disted/pubmedtutorial/cover.html CINAHL BASIC. http://support.ebsco.com/training/flash_videos/cinahl_basic/cinahl_basic.html?_ga = 2.153464443.218261045.1508804171–1270823217.1508266989 CINAHL ADVANCED. http://support.ebsco.com/training/flash_videos/cinahl_advanced/cinahl_advanced.html?_ga = 2.60624366.218261045.1508804171–1270823217.1508266989 Tutorials on APA Databases http://www.apa.org/pubs/databases/training/tutorials.aspx
Systematic review tools (collaborating, citation screening, filtering, critiquing, and sharing)	Covidence: https://www.covidence.org/ DistillerSR: https://www.evidencepartners.com/products/distillersr-systematic-review-software/ PRISMA: Diagram Generator http://prisma.thetacollaborative.ca/ SUMARI: https://www.jbisumari.org/
Citation management tools (build a personal repository of citations and a PDF library; output formatted in-text citations and reference lists)	Mendeley: http://www.mendeley.com (create free account) Refworks: http://refworks.com (institutional or individual subscription) Zotero: http://zotero.org (create free account) Endnote: http://endnote.com (individual purchase or via institutional download)
Alerting Services (via databases, publisher or journal websites)	My NCBI: http://ncbi.nlm.nih.gov Save PubMed searches, collections; create automatic e-mail alerts, and more (free of charge) KT + (Knowledge Translation +) McMaster University: https://plus.mcmaster.ca/kt/ E-mail alerts about new Quality-filtered KT Articles; includes alerting service from ACP Journal Club, Evidence Updates, Evidence-Based Nursing +, Evidence-Based Obesity +, Evidence-Based Rehab + Scopus: (via institutional subscription) https://www.elsevier.com/solutions/scopus Set up "My Alerts" to customize search alerts, Author citation alerts, and Document citation alerts. Web of Science Plus (via institutional subscription) Create a personal profile to set up citation alerts or search alerts in the Science Citation Index Expanded, Social Sciences Citation Index, and Arts & Humanities Citation Index. NYU Libraries. Research Guides: https://guides.nyu.edu/healthalerts Alerting Services, Health Sciences
Appraisal Tools	AGREE Enterprise: http://www.agreetrust.org/ Center for Evidence Based Medicine (CEBM): http://www.cebm.net/critical-appraisal/ Critical Appraisal tools PRISMA: http://prisma-statement.org/Default.aspx Transparent Reporting of Systematic Reviews and Meta-Analyses
Scholarly Metrics Tools	Altmetric: https://www.altmetric.com/about-our-data/our-sources/ Metrics and qualitative data aggregated from the web deliver a score assessing research impact; complements traditional, citation-based metrics PlumX Metrics: https://plumanalytics.com/learn/about-metrics/ Measures research output in the online environment; categorizes metrics into five separate categories: Usage, Captures, Mentions, Social Media, and Citations

[a]List is not intended to be exhaustive.

Yet a pitfall of a broad web-scale tool is that you, and other searchers, often retrieve an overwhelming and unmanageable number of hits. Search engines that index the "web" deliver results in one list, often masking what is freely available and what is behind the paywall of institutional access. Web-scale tools may mask the differences among scholarship and "user-generated" content (Knapp & Brower, 2014), ranked by an unknown algorithm that may skew toward advertised content. Results for a typical keyword search are often vast and unfiltered. For most topics related to scientific research and health care, results are too numerous, enticing you to randomly cherry-pick results from the top of a long list. Critical to understanding the digitized environment is that whereas a discovery platform (a "search box") is flat, the evidence for health care interventions is hierarchical, as shown in Fig. 2.1 in Chapter 2. Unfiltered search results from a general search engine may include a range of evidence, from raw data and opinion through randomized controlled trials or practice guidelines based on systematic reviews. Web-scale tools have little functionality for filtering results. Locating health care evidence requires more sophisticated and specialized search tools.

Imagine a scenario in which a clinical team seeks evidence for a knowledge-focused trigger question (see Chapter 1):

> *What is the best evidence to support the use of music therapy as an intervention to decrease anxiety in inpatients?*

The results from a Google search are shown in Table 4.3. The same search conducted in Google Scholar, a subset of Google prefiltered for resources, produces a smaller but still unwieldy number of hits. Notice the same search terms and number of hits in the specialized article databases PubMed/Medline and CINAHL. Both databases are bibliographic indexes of research for biomedicine, nursing, and allied health. The overall results and the advantages of using a specialized tool are obvious. Decision making that is biased on the basis of viewing the first few pages of results can unwittingly neglect valuable and relevant evidence, including the evidence not captured by the scope of the selected web search engine. As advanced practice nurses, graduate students, administrators, and educators, you must be open to a transformed view of the

landscape, a "conceptual gateway" or portal, other than a familiar tool like Google. "Getting lucky" with Google or Google Scholar and cherry-picking is a low value and risky practice!

BEYOND THE PUBLISHED EVIDENCE

Investigation of a clinical question may include going beyond the published research that is indexed commercially. Gray literature, defined as fugitive, ephemeral, invisible, or unpublished, is unevaluated and not peer-reviewed. It ranges from raw data, pamphlets, white papers, trial registries, conference proceedings, podcasts, and websites to research studies in progress or unpublished dissertations. Unpublished clinical trials are listed in an online repository called Clinicaltrials.gov, HSRProj (Health Services Research Projects in Progress, https://wwwcf.nlm.nih.gov/hsr_project/home_proj.cfm). Another example of a resource specific for nursing research is the Virginia Henderson Global Nursing e-Repository (Virginia Henderson Global Nursing e-Repository, 2017), a site available to researchers conducting research as well as consumers of research searching for trials in progress (see Table 4.4).

EBP TIP

Search on a topic of your choice in Google, Google Scholar, or another web-scale tool. How many hits do you retrieve from each source? Compare results with a search using the same terms in a specialized health care database such as PubMed/Medline or CINAHL.

ASK a Background Question

Your first step in searching the literature for a clinical question is to ASK one or more broad background questions, those questions that lead you to investigate information about a disease, a condition, or a treatment that is derived from a knowledge-focused trigger. For example, asking the initial question may entail investigating the current "state of the science"; tracing the development of a theory; seeking the history of a disease or an intervention across diverse populations or settings; conducting a reconnaissance of the breadth and depth of the literature on a general topic; seeking general guidelines, evidence summaries, syntheses, or reports;

TABLE 4.3   Comparing Results for a Search on a "Population" (Inpatients) AND "Intervention" (Music Therapy) in Web-Scale Search Engines and Article Databases (PubMed/Medline and CINAHL)

Search engine/Search string	Number of hits	Notes, features, filters
Google Music therapy AND inpatients (most used search engine on the World Wide Web)	>430,000	Phrase search ("verbatim"), limits available for publication date, images, shopping, videos, and news
Google Scholar Music therapy AND inpatients (a subset of Google that indexes scholarly literature)	>24,200	Limits available for publication date, relevance ranking Links customizable to local library Article metrics Scholar profile
PubMed/Medline: Music therapy AND inpatients (The US National Library of Medicine's PubMed interface to the MEDLINE database of citations and abstracts in the fields of medicine, nursing, dentistry, veterinary medicine, health care systems, and preclinical sciences. Available: https://www.ncbi.nlm.nih.gov/pubmed.)	83	Mapping disambiguation to standard thesaurus term: "music therapy" [MeSH Terms]. Limits available for Article type, Age groups, Publication date, clinical queries, topic-specific queries and more.
CINAHL Music therapy AND inpatients (Cumulative Index to Nursing and Allied Health Literature indexes nursing and allied health literature, including nursing journals and publications; covers a wide range of topics including nursing, biomedicine, health librarianship, alternative/complementary medicine, and consumer health. Available: https://health.ebsco.com/products/the-cinahl-database (Requires institutional subscription)	330	Mapping disambiguation to standard thesaurus terms: Music Therapy AND Inpatients Limits available for "Peer-reviewed," "Research," other Publication types, Age groups, Publication date, Clinical queries, and more.

TABLE 4.4   Core Databases Indexing the Literature

Database/Access	Description	Sample Citation
CINAHL (Cumulative Index to Nursing and Allied Health Literature) https://health.ebsco.com/products/the-cinahl-database (Requires institutional subscription)	An index of nursing and allied health literature, including nursing journals and publications from the National League for Nursing and the American Nurses Association; covers a wide range of topics including nursing, biomedicine, health sciences librarianship, alternative/complementary medicine, and consumer health and 17 allied health disciplines. Indexes more than 3,100 journals.	Thompson, M., Moe, K., & Lewis, C. P. (2014). The effects of music on diminishing anxiety among preoperative patients. *Journal of Radiology Nursing, 33*(4), 199–202. (A "research" article in CINAHL)
PubMed (MEDLINE) http://www.ncbi.nlm.nih.gov/pubmed (Available free of charge)	The premier source for bibliographic coverage of biomedical topics, including health administration. (Free public access to citations and abstracts; citations may include links to full text content in PubMed Central or open-access journals on publisher sites.)	Kushnir, J., Friedman, A., Ehrenfeld, M., & Kushnir, T. (2012). Coping with preoperative anxiety in cesarean section: Physiological, cognitive, and emotional effects of listening to favorite music. *Birth: Issues in Perinatal Care, 39*(2), 121–127.

(Continued)

TABLE 4.4 **Core Databases Indexing the Literature—cont'd**

Database/Access	Description	Sample Citation
PsycINFO http://www.apa.org/pubs/databases/psycinfo (Requires institutional subscription)	Bibliographic records, ranging from 1806 to the present, centered on psychology and related disciplines, including medicine, psychiatry, nursing, sociology, pharmacology, physiology, and linguistics.	Spintge, R. (2012). Clinical use of music in operating theatres. In R. MacDonald, G. Kreutz, & L. Mitchell (Eds.), *Music, health, and wellbeing* (pp. 276–286). New York, NY: Oxford University Press.
Embase http://www.elsevier.com/solutions/embase-biomedical-research (Requires institutional subscription)	Biomedical and pharmaceutical database indexing journals from more than 90 countries in drug research, pharmacology, pharmaceutics, toxicology, clinical and experimental human medicine, health policy and management, public health, occupational health, environmental health, drug dependence and abuse, psychiatry, forensic medicine, and biomedical engineering/instrumentation Selective coverage for nursing, dentistry, veterinary medicine, psychology, and alternative medicine.	Beccaloni, A. M. (2011). The medicine of music: A systematic approach for adoption into perianesthesia practice. *Journal of Perianesthesia Nursing.* (A narrative literature review)
Science Citation Index and Social Science Citation Index (Web of Science) http://ipscience.thomsonreuters.com/product/web-of-science (Requires institutional subscription)	Multidisciplinary research platform with linked content citation metrics from multiple sources.	Wang, S. M., Kulkarni, L., Dolev, J., & Kain, Z. N. (2002). Music and preoperative anxiety: A randomized, controlled study. *Anesthesia and Analgesia, 94*(6), 1489–1494.
Global Dissertations and Theses http://www.proquest.com/products-services/pqdtglobal.html (Requires institutional subscription)	Repository of graduate dissertations and theses from universities in 88 countries.	Hillmer, M. G. (2007). *Survey of nurses' attitudes and perceptions toward music therapy in the hospital setting.* Master's thesis, University of Kansas. Retrieved from https://search.proquest.com/central/docview/304857271/abstract/C2B097734CB45EEPQ/1
ProQuest Central http://www.proquest.com/libraries/academic/databases/ProQuest_Central.html (Requires institutional subscription)	Large multidisciplinary database that includes scholarly sources as well as newspapers and popular periodicals.	Cooke, M., Chaboyer, W., Schluter, P., & Hiratos, M. (2005). The effect of music on preoperative anxiety in day surgery. *Journal of Advanced Nursing, 52*(1), 47–55.
Scopus https://www.elsevier.com/solutions/scopus (Requires institutional subscription)	Multidisciplinary index of peer-reviewed journals and conference proceedings covering science, technology, medicine, social sciences, and arts and humanities.	Nilsson, U. (2008). The anxiety- and pain-reducing effects of music interventions: A systematic review. *AORN Journal, 87*(4), 780,782,785–794,797–807.

along with lower-level background data or statistics. A scoping search identifies the existing evidence or a gap in research, and informs the focus for developing a refined PICO question (Straus, Glasziou, Richardson, & Haynes, 2010).

A recommended practice is to identify the two or three main concepts, such as those highlighted below from the previous scenario:

What is the best evidence to support the use of music therapy as an intervention to decrease anxiety in inpatients?

To begin to scope for background information, consider the secondary sources that may have aggregated or synthesized the topic in the form of a quality evidence summary, a current textbook, or a recent "review" article (a type of publication). Background evidence for a nursing intervention related to music therapy in health care may also be found by using point-of-care tools (POC). Often available for handheld devices, POC tools are designed to aid decision support for clinicians by synthesizing evidence for common clinical problems, diseases, drugs, and therapies. Summarized high-quality evidence, preappraised synopses, care sheets, and patient-level handouts can be invaluable for advanced practice nurses "at the bedside" as well as for graduate student research. Examples of POC tools include the following: Nursing Reference Center Plus (EBSCO Industries, Inc., 2017), UpToDate (Wolters Kluwer Health, 2017), and Clinical Key (Elsevier, Inc., 2017). A POC resource such as McMaster University's Nursing +, available free with registration, offers "one-stop" access to preappraised evidence, and an article alerting service matched to area of specialization (McMaster University, Health Information Research Unit, 2017). An example of a specialized POC tool is Natural Medicines, a source that synthesizes evidence for complementary and alternative therapies (Therapeutic Research Center, 2017b). To support the question posed earlier, the resource includes a professional monograph on "Music Therapy" that synthesizes background, safety, effectiveness, administration, adverse effects, mechanism of action, and includes a reference list for more exploration, plus patient-level handouts in Spanish, French, and English (Therapeutic Research Center, 2017a).

Initial exploration of added examples of background sources such as those in Table 4.1 may generate related questions, such as the following:

- What is the most recent nursing and biomedical evidence summarizing the value of music therapy?
- Are there recent guidelines for using music therapy?
- What are staff or patients' attitudes about music therapy or the broader field of complementary and alternative therapies?
- What statistics summarize the most recent data on music interventions in health care?
- Are "review" articles or evidence summaries available?
- Is there an evidence summary in a POC tool?

A search for "music therapy" as an intervention may retrieve overviews on anxiety or pain outcomes, healing, length of stay, and other measurable criteria, or it may point you to individual research studies in journals with a narrower focus on evidence in:

- a specialized setting such as a neonatal intensive care unit (NICU) or long-term care facility;
- a specialized population such as children with autism spectrum disorder, adults with schizophrenia, adolescents with depression, or patients with opioid use disorders; or
- patients undergoing a specific procedure such as cesarean section or heart catheterization.

One strategy for locating background evidence is to locate a systematic review or evidence summary. A systematic review, sometimes called a review, is a type of research method in which researchers find all of the relevant studies, published and unpublished, on a topic or question and present a state-of-the-science conclusion in the form of an evidence summary. A meta-analysis, a type of systematic review, is a research method that takes the results of multiple studies in a specific area, quantitatively analyzes the findings as an aggregate, and presents a quantitative conclusion about the strength of the evidence provided by the group of studies and may make recommendation about the applicability of the findings. The terms "systematic review" and "meta-analysis" are often used interchangeably. You should keep in mind that although a meta-analysis is a systematic review, not all systematic reviews are meta-analyses (see Chapter 8 for an in-depth discussion of systematic reviews). In contrast, an evidence summary is a short summary of available evidence that may provide presynthesized data as well as recommendations for research and clinical practice. Fig. 4.1 is an example of a systematic review article, which also happens to be a meta-analysis. A review article, like any study, still requires that it be appraised for quality, but locating one may provide a useful summary and starting point for your search; the article's reference list can often supply a comprehensive review of previous evidence as of the date published.

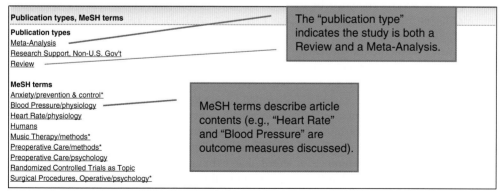

Cochrane Database Syst Rev. 2013 Jun 6;(6):CD006908. doi: 10.1002/14651858.CD006908.pub2.

Music interventions for preoperative anxiety.

Bradt J[1], Dileo C, Shim M.

⊕ Author information

Abstract

BACKGROUND: Patients awaiting surgical procedures often experience significant anxiety. Such anxiety may result in negative physiological manifestations, slower wound healing, increased risk of infection, and may complicate the induction of anaesthesia and impede postoperative recovery. To reduce patient anxiety, sedatives and anti-anxiety drugs are regularly administered before surgery. However, these often have negative side effects and may prolong patient recovery. Therefore, increasing attention is being paid to a variety of non-pharmacological interventions for reduction of preoperative anxiety such as music therapy and music medicine interventions. Interventions are categorized as 'music medicine' when passive listening to pre-recorded music is offered by medical personnel. In contrast, music therapy requires the implementation of a music intervention by a trained music therapist, the presence of a therapeutic process, and the use of personally tailored music experiences. A systematic review was needed to gauge the efficacy of both music therapy and music medicine interventions for reduction of preoperative anxiety.

OBJECTIVES: To examine the effects of music interventions with standard care versus standard care alone on preoperative anxiety in surgical patients.

SEARCH METHODS: We searched the Cochrane Central Register of Controlled Trials (CENTRAL) (The Cochrane Library 2012, Issue 7), MEDLINE (1950 to August 2012), CINAHL (1980 to August 2012), AMED (1985 to April 2011; we no longer had access to AMED after this date), EMBASE (1980 to August 2012), PsycINFO (1967 to August 2012), LILACS (1982 to August 2012), Science Citation Index (1980 to August 2012), the specialist music therapy research database (March 1 2008; database is no longer functional), CAIRSS for Music (to August 2012), Proquest Digital Dissertations (1980 to August 2012), ClinicalTrials.gov (2000 to August 2012), Current Controlled Trials (1998 to August 2012), and the National Research Register (2000 to September 2007). We handsearched music therapy journals and reference lists, and contacted relevant experts to identify unpublished manuscripts. There was no language restriction.

SELECTION CRITERIA: We included all randomized and quasi-randomized trials that compared music interventions and standard care with standard care alone for reducing preoperative anxiety in surgical patients.

DATA COLLECTION AND ANALYSIS: Two review authors independently extracted the data and assessed the risk of bias. We contacted authors to obtain missing data where needed. Where possible, results were presented in meta analyses using mean differences and standardized mean differences. Post-test scores were used. In cases of significant baseline differences, we used change scores.

MAIN RESULTS: We included 26 trials (2051 participants). All studies used listening to pre-recorded music. The results suggested that music listening may have a beneficial effect on preoperative anxiety. Specifically, music listening resulted, on average, in an anxiety reduction that was 5.72 units greater (95% CI -7.27 to -4.17, P < 0.00001) than that in the standard care group as measured by the Stait-Trait Anxiety Inventory (STAI-S), and -0.60 standardized units (95% CI -0.90 to -0.31, P < 0.0001) on other anxiety scales. The results also suggested a small effect on heart rate and diastolic blood pressure, but no support was found for reductions in systolic blood pressure, respiratory rate, and skin temperature. Most trials were assessed to be at high risk of lack of blinding. Blinding of outcome assessors is often impossible in music therapy and music medicine studies that use subjective outcomes, unless in studies in which the music intervention is compared to another treatment intervention. Because of the high risk of bias, these results need to be interpreted with caution.None of the studies included wound healing, infection rate, time to discharge, or patient satisfaction as outcome variables. One large study found that music listening was more effective than the sedative midazolam in reducing preoperative anxiety and equally effective in reducing physiological responses. No adverse effects were identified.

AUTHORS' CONCLUSIONS: This systematic review indicates that music listening may have a beneficial effect on preoperative anxiety. These findings are consistent with the findings of three other Cochrane systematic reviews on the use of music interventions for anxiety reduction in medical patients. Therefore, we conclude that music interventions may provide a viable alternative to sedatives and anti-anxiety drugs for reducing preoperative anxiety.

Fig. 4.1 A PubMed/MEDLINE citation from the Cochrane Database of Systematic Reviews. (From https://www.ncbi.nlm.nih.gov/pubmed/23740695.)

Once a scoping search has established the summarized current evidence or state of the science for an intervention, identified a gap in the literature, or pointed to an area for further research, a *narrower* question may be identified. Discovery of research evidence is an "iterative" process of inquiry as described in Fig. 4.2. A knowledge-focused trigger can lead to developing a more sharply focused PICO question.

ASK A "PICO" QUESTION

After a strategic scoping search of background sources and an initial assessment, and critical appraisal of the results, a narrower focus may generate a clinical question that guides searching for primary studies for the most current research findings. The previous section emphasized the value of evidence summaries, review articles, and POC tools among the many sources of pre-aggregated research evidence; the most current research studies are generally found in peer-reviewed journals, which are indexed in specialized health sciences article databases. PubMed/Medline, CINAHL, EMBASE, PsycINFO, and others, described in Table 4.4, comprehensively index published studies from journals. Citations are described ("tagged") with metadata drawn from a controlled vocabulary, which is an online thesaurus of terms that disambiguate and facilitate more precise retrieval using search terms. These core databases are the essential sources of research studies that you should consider as primary tools for evidence discovery. Unlike Google or other large web-scale repositories, each database has a defined scope of subject and publication year coverage and a standard indexing scheme. Databases allow you as a searcher to seek terms tagged as subjects

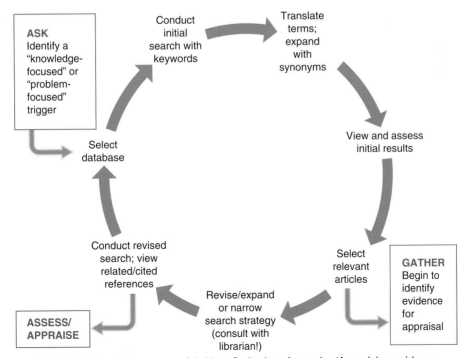

Fig. 4.2 The iterative process of Asking, Gathering, Assessing/Appraising evidence.

or key words in abstracts, for preliminary assessment of content and level of evidence. Standard categorical limits for article type, research design, specialized populations, age groups, and more are available to filter search results, described later in the chapter. When you need to locate evidence for related specialized health care topics, such as health economics or public policy, health care ethics, advanced technologies, news reports, or any of a range of interdisciplinary subjects that involve nursing and health care, a health sciences librarian can suggest additional database sources.

The unique features of each database, how to search, access, save results, apply limits, and access the full text of articles are generally covered in online tutorials and "help" screens within context. Recommended search tutorials and learning tools are listed in Table 4.2.

Database search interfaces vary, but all rely on the use of Boolean connectors, AND and OR, depicted schematically in Fig. 4.3.

A Simple Search, Translating a PICO Question

A focused clinical question most commonly seeks an answer about the efficacy of a specific nursing intervention. Framing an answerable question (ASK) is best done by structuring a clinical question using the PICO template to define a PROBLEM (or participant of interest, or a population) and a proposed INTERVENTION (Straus et al., 2010) (see Chapter 3).

On the basis of the earlier background question, discovering the evidence for the efficacy of music therapy for anxiety in a variety of settings or situations, a refined clinical question focuses on the problem of anxiety in a

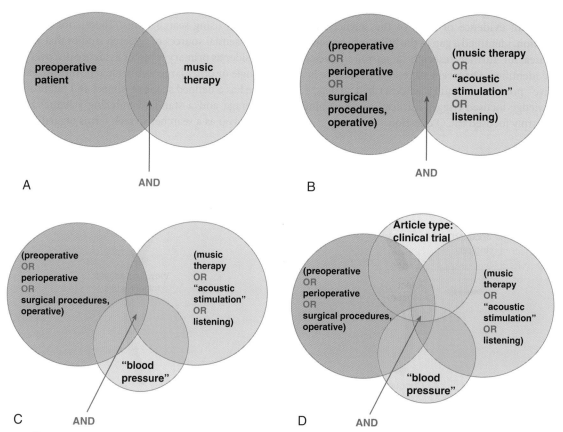

Fig. 4.3 (A) An *initial* search strategy translates the PICO elements (Problem, Patient or Population of interest, AND an Intervention) into a keyword search. (B) An *expanded* search strategy identifies synonyms for both the "P" and the "I." Synonyms are connected with "OR" and nested in parentheses to expand a search query to include *any* of the alternate terms. (C) A revised search strategy can *narrow* the results to studies that contain a selected comparative or outcome measure, such as "blood pressure." (D) A filtered search further narrows results to studies that meet a higher standard of evidence, in this example, the publication type: "clinical trials."

population of *preoperative* patients, and music therapy as an intervention:

What is the evidence for using music therapy as an intervention to decrease patients' preoperative anxiety?

P = preoperative patient prone to anxiety

I = music therapy

C = another relaxation technique such as meditation, pharmacological therapy, no therapy

O = lower anxiety level

Using the PICO framework to construct a search strategy, you are encouraged to start an article search with the **P** (**Patient, Problem, or Population**) AND the **I** (***Intervention*) *only*.** (Search terms for the *Comparison* and *Outcome* and other inclusion/exclusion criteria may be added later, as you browse abstracts and review full text of articles.)

Using the connectors AND and OR (also known as the "building blocks method") (Goodman, Gary, & Wood, 2014), an initial search strategy is shown in the Venn diagram in Fig. 4.3, depicting the set of results that include *both* search terms. Inclusion of terms for comparative and outcome measures may be too limiting for the initial broad search and risks omission of studies; adding comparative and outcome terms may not be necessary if placebo or no treatment is the comparison.

EBP TIP

Search the specialized health sciences databases using Boolean logic:

- Use **AND** to connect the **P** (Problem, Patient, Participant of interest, or Population) AND the **I** (Intervention) as a first step to conducting an article search.
- Use **OR** to expand each term with synonyms.
- Remember: AND narrows a search; OR expands synonyms and retrieves more.
- Use standard database filters for Age Group, Publication Type, Date of Publication, and more.

An Advanced Search: Expanding the Quest for Evidence

As initial search results are evaluated, identify the most germane studies and harvest synonyms for one or both search terms. Synonyms may be seen in the title, abstract, or metadata of relevant results and used to expand one or both of the initial search terms with the Boolean OR connector. For example, synonyms for the term "music" might be *acoustic stimulation* OR *listening*, as shown schematically in Fig. 4.3. Abstracts may mention terms such

as "playlist," "iTunes," or "smartphones" and thus generate ideas for further expanding your search terms (Cumino et al., 2017; Keilani et al., 2017; Sucala et al., 2017). As initial results are reviewed, notice the standard descriptive subject terms. For example, in PubMed, notice the "MeSH" terms; in PsycInfo notice the "Descriptors;" in CINAHL notice the "Subject headings." The descriptive metadata seen in a relevant citation or located in online database thesauri, define and disambiguate terms, as well as situate terms hierarchically. The metadata provide the links ("breadcrumbs") to similar articles. A hierarchy of PubMed "MeSH" metadata indicates a broader category that includes music therapy. The term "Sensory Art Therapies" (https://www.ncbi.nlm.nih.gov/mesh/68026421) situates "music therapy" as one among other subordinate terms such as "art therapy," drama therapy," "play therapy," "color therapy," and more. Hence, a search on Sensory Art Therapies retrieves all the citations tagged with any of the narrower terms. This feature is known as "automatic explosion" and is an important feature of many article databases (U.S. National Library of Medicine, 2017). When an initial article search retrieves too few results, perhaps indicating a topic that is too narrow, searching a broader term, as described, is often a helpful strategy. A pitfall of increasing or broadening search results in this manner will inevitably also retrieve "false hits," off topic or irrelevant results, hence some manual filtering is necessary. You are advised to seek results with "high sensitivity," which may result in "low precision" but is a critical practice for a comprehensive literature search (Higgins & Green, 2011). Searching is iterative; rather than a linear process of retrieval, one study leads to an idea that sparks a quest for a related question or line of inquiry. Using the example of music therapy for a population of preoperative patients, you may explore *other* uses of music therapy, perhaps for a population such as patients with depression, infants in the NICU, or for caregivers. Your literature search also may take a direction toward identifying evidence on *outcomes other than decreasing anxiety*, such as the benefits of a music intervention for cognition, sleep quality, or hypertension or for pain management

Expanding the search from the most relevant studies, conduct snowballing (following reference lists backward and following articles that cite an article following publication) to explore links to related records or similar articles (Goodman et al., 2014). Notice the "cited reference" search feature in selected databases, which allows the searcher to follow a focal article forward in time to view citing articles;

the "times cited" is one article metric, among others, that can evaluate the impact of a study. **Altmetrics**, the non-traditional impact of a study, tracked by many publishers at the article level, may measure downloads, captures (bookmarks, favorites, watchers, and other indications a reader wants to return to an item), "mentions" in news outlets, blogs, tweets, and other social media ("Altmetric for Researchers," 2015; Haustein, Peters, Sugimoto, Thelwall, & Larivière, 2014). All are additional indicators of scholarly impact and another way to link to related research from a publication. An Altmetric rainbow "donut" appearing on a publisher's article page provides both a graphic and numeric score of the combined "attention" the research study has received ("The donut and Altmetric Attention Score," 2015). Librarians can suggest additional resources for assessing metrics at both the article level and the journal level (M. Smith, 2017). See Table 4.2.

> ### EBP TIP
>
> The scope of each article database (described in Table 4.4) covers a broad range of journals. For advanced practice topics, searching *both* CINAHL and PubMed/Medline provides coverage across most of the premier journals addressing nursing and biomedical topics and the psychosocial aspects of health care. An important adjunct is the PsycINFO database providing additional coverage of journals in the behavioral sciences. EMBASE provides more international journal coverage. The Web of Science (WOS) provides a broad scope across both science and the social sciences; WOS and Scopus are examples of two multidisciplinary databases with functionality to follow cited references forward in time.

When searching the literature, the process of "strategic exploration" helps identify synonymous concepts to broaden search results. Table 4.4 describes the core article databases that index the nursing literature.

Narrowing Search Results: Filtering

Viewing evidence in the context of the evidence pyramid in Chapter 2, you are reminded to notice the categorical limits or filters available in electronic databases. Once a comprehensive search strategy has been conducted, a manual review of citations, viewing study titles and abstracts, can inform your next steps. You might decide to narrow retrieved citations by using AND to add a selected PICO "comparative" or "outcome" term. In Fig. 4.3 notice the search terms narrowed with "blood

pressure." A physiological measure, such as systolic blood pressure, noted in one study, is an example of an outcome measure that you could use to further narrow the search for research on the effectiveness of music therapy for preoperative anxiety (Kushnir et al., 2012). Notice the MeSH terms in the systematic review shown in Fig. 4.1. "Blood pressure," "heart rate," and "anxiety" are all outcome measures that were determined to be measured in the review; these are suggestions for narrowing the literature search with a C (comparative) or O (outcome) term.

> ### EBP TIP
>
> The following strategies can help revise (troubleshoot) database searches:
>   **Too few results?**
> * Expand one or more of your search terms connecting synonyms with "OR."
> * Consult the online database thesaurus to ensure you are using standard terms; consider alternate terms; consider alternate spellings; use standard terms along with keywords or natural language.
> * View the database thesaurus hierarchy of terms; consider a broader term to improve recall (e.g., "sensory art therapies" is a broader MeSH term that includes "music therapy").
> * Use truncation to expand a term by searching for the root; for example, music* retrieves music, musical, musician, etc.
> * Try another database; the psychosocial aspects of health care are indexed more comprehensively in CINAHL and PsycINFO, to name just two resources.
> * Follow the "breadcrumbs"; from a relevant citation, notice links to "Similar Articles"; follow citations in a reference list; locate cited references.
>   **Too many results?**
> * Use the database "focus" feature to narrow results to citations where one or more terms have been designated the major subject of the article.
> * Make use of categorical filters for Article Type, Methodology, Age Group, Year of Publication, Population groups (e.g., "Human"; filtering for article type can be a first step toward raising the level of evidence that correspond with higher levels in the evidence pyramid).
> * Explore the "clinical queries" feature available in PubMed/Medline, PsycINFO, and CINAHL.
> * Narrow with subheadings; investigate the subheading structure of database thesauri, (e.g., a standard subheading such as "music therapy—therapeutic use").
> * Revisit background sources, syntheses, or POC tools.
> * Add a comparative or outcome term to the strategy (see Fig. 4.3C).

Filtering by research methodology is a powerful technique for you to use to raise the level of evidence and increase precision of results. Fig. 4.3 depicts the Patient/Problem and Intervention, further refined, filtered, in this example to include only studies tagged for Publication type: "clinical trials." The health sciences databases include filters that correspond to many publication types that align with higher levels of evidence, such as randomized controlled trials, meta-analysis, practice guideline, and more. (Filtering for publication type as described earlier is not the same as the "quality filtering" that takes place with critiquing the methodology of a study.)

More sophisticated and specialized research methodology filters have been developed for EBP and available in PubMed, CINAHL, and PsycINFO. Known as "clinical queries," they are preformulated limits ("hedges") that assist searchers of evidence related to questions of prognosis, diagnosis, etiology, and clinical prediction guidelines; as a searcher, you are given the option to select a "broad, sensitive" approach or a "narrow, specific" approach to retrieval (National Center for Biotechnology Information, U.S. National Library of Medicine, 2017). You also may find that the clinical queries are helpful in identifying evidence for nonintervention PICO questions discussed in Chapters 9, 12, and 13. Another set of preformulated search queries is the topic-specific PubMed queries that assist with searches in selected disease categories, health services research, history of medicine, complementary medicine, consumer health topics, and more (PubMed® Special Queries, 2016). Like any automated tool, you should use them in conjunction with other search strategies and search methods because no one size fits all, and knowledge of how the filter works is essential.

IPE TIP

ASK a librarian! The process of searching the literature is always enhanced and improved by consulting with a search expert. Consult with the health sciences librarian at your institution to discuss the PICO question and available resources, and to develop a suggested initial search. Given the complexity of searching the literature, the expertise and guidance of a health sciences librarian can be invaluable, allowing the searcher to focus on interpretation of the evidence and critical decision making (Higgins & Green, 2011; Homan, 2010; Smith & Noble, 2016).

Organizing, Evaluating, and Sharing the Evidence

As a body of evidence is gathered and evaluated in context, the search may take on a new direction, pointing to the interrelatedness of elements of evidence (Meyer & Land, 2003). With practice and guidance, a searcher acquires experience and expertise with the features and idiosyncrasies of each article database contents, as well as the platform interface and refinements. Many databases allow customizing a personal account to save both search strategies and citations (e.g., a PubMed "My NCBI" account) enabling saving search strategies, automated email alerts, setting individual preferences, and a helpful feature to track "recent activity." Journal table of contents and topic "alerting services" are available (see Table 4.2).

As you develop your clinical question, you will want to take advantage of citation management tools such as Endnote, Zotero, Mendeley, and Refworks, among others (see Table 4.2). These are platforms for downloading citations from library catalogs, article databases, websites, and more to build a personal data/article repository. The other invaluable feature of these tools is to assist you in writing, citing, and formatting written papers, with a functionality to insert citations, format a reference list for a selected publication style, and complement note-taking to avoid plagiarism. Advanced screening tools for collaborative project management, screening results of a literature review based on inclusion and exclusion criteria, with features for data extraction, are available via subscription (Covidence, 2017; Systematic Review and Literature Review Software by Evidence Partners, 2017). A PRISMA flow chart, a graphical depiction of the process of identifying, screening, determining eligibility, and applying exclusion criteria during the process of creating an integrative or systematic review, can be very useful as a graphical depiction of your search. Creating this diagram provides a snapshot of the sources searched, the numbers of citations screened and critiqued after duplicates were removed, and filters and inclusion criteria, and it is often a requirement for publishing the results of a systematic review or an integrative review (PRISMA Diagram Generator, n.d.) (see Table 4.2).

ASSESS/APPRAISE/SYNTHESIZE

The PICO question threaded throughout the first part of this chapter demonstrated how developing an answerable PICO question provided the foundation for efficiently searching, filtering, and retrieving an initial body of evidence. Once your literature search has been conducted and refined, you will determine whether the retrieved studies that meet your search criteria provide the highest available level of evidence to answer your PICO question (see Chapter 3). Next you will critically appraise each of the individual studies to determine whether the studies, as a group, provide sufficient, quantity, consistency, and quality of evidence to change practice or if further research needed. Critical appraisal involves evaluating the strengths and weaknesses of each research study or guideline (AGREE Enterprise, 2014). An overview of critical appraisal is addressed in Chapter 2; critical appraisal criteria as sources of bias for specific quantitative and qualitative designs are found in Chapters 5 to 9. Fig. 2.1 is an example of an Evidence Table that you and your team or journal club can use to enter the salient features of each study (e.g., Design, Sample, Method, Findings, Limitations), including their strengths and weaknesses. There may be other features that you as a clinician find useful to include in an evidence table.

When the individual studies have been critically appraised, a synthesis of the overall strengths and weaknesses of the studies as a group should be developed. The purpose of synthesizing a body of critically appraised evidence is to establish the state of the science for answering your PICO question and provide an evidence-based foundation on which to base practice and standards of care.

Recommendations to validate current practice or to adopt a sustained change in practice requires a careful evaluation and synthesis of the evidence, one that challenges you as clinicians, educators, and administrators to inform your decision making with the best available evidence (Krainovich-Miller, Haber, Yost, & Jacobs, 2009; AHRQ, 2013, Nov.18). Table 4.5 illustrates the features that can be included in a synthesis evidence table. A frequently asked question is, "How many studies do I need to include in my synthesis?" Ideally, synthesis of a group of studies provides a sufficient quantity of high-quality, consistent evidence to make one of the following recommendations: 1) validate current practice, 2) make a minor change in practice, or 3) make major change in practice. The synthesis also may reveal evidence that is inadequate or too weak to support a recommendation for a practice change. There is a debate (Suri, 2013) about the practice of including only high-quality studies, such as systematic reviews (see Chapter 8) and randomized clinical trials (see Chapter 6) to answer a PICO question and include in an evidence synthesis. On one hand, you

and your team always search for studies that provide the highest level and strongest evidence. On the other hand, the state of the science may be that there is a paucity of high-quality studies. Observational studies, those that use a cohort or case control design, may be those that offer the strongest evidence (see Chapter 7). As such, inconsistent findings and/or studies with multiple threats to internal and external validity may represent the "best available evidence." In that case, an evidence synthesis is particularly important because you will use it to inform your decision making about clinical issues as well as allocation of financial and human resources.

> ### EBP TIP
>
> Remember that the PICO question drives what is included and considered in the synthesis of individual studies.

Points to consider when developing your synthesis table that include, but are not limited to, the following:

- Decide which study components to include in the synthesis table.
- Include verbatim information from each study.
- Avoid synthesis bias by not paraphrasing or interpreting what was stated by the researcher.
- Organize the synthesis table by using a specific strategy, including but not limited to listing studies in chronological order, according to their Level of Evidence, or by design type.
- Include all of the critically appraised studies in the evidence table.
- Compare and contrast similar components across studies to determine the overall strength or weakness of that component (e.g., compare sampling strategies or type of design).

The synthesis table, as presented in Table 4.5, enables you and your team to view, at a glance, the critical appraisal data from each study as well as the comparison information that keeps you focused on comparing and contrasting the overall strengths and weaknesses of the studies as a group. When your project team completes the synthesis and considers the studies as a whole, you will draft an evidence synthesis summary that includes your recommendation about applicability for adoption in practice.

The evidence synthesis summary should consider issues such as the following:

- Design
- Clinical significance versus statistical significance
- Fidelity

TABLE 4.5   Evidence Synthesis Summary Table

Study Citation	Study Design and Level of Evidence	Risk of Bias	Study Sample	Data Collection[a]	Intervention	Outcomes	Strength, Quality of Findings
Thompson et al., 2014	Quasi-experimental Level III	No blinding No random assignment Evidence of fidelity	N = 137 men and women	Pre/post test using VAS	Music or no music before invasive or noninvasive surgery; no premedication	Significant decrease in preop anxiety	Low No harm
Bradt et al., 2013	Systematic Review/meta-analysis Level I	High risk for bias—no blinding; Some studies had no random assignment Some had no evidence of fidelity	26 RCTs and Quasi-experimental studies met the inclusion criteria	State Scale of STAI or VAS	Music or no music before surgery; no premedication	Significant decrease in preop anxiety across studies	Low r/t high risk for bias across studies
Ni et al., 2012	RCT Level II	No blinding No evidence of fidelity	N = 183 adult males and females randomly assigned to intervention or control group using computer generated program	State Scale of STAI	Music or no music before ambulatory day surgery; no premedication	Significant decrease in preoperative anxiety	Low No harm
Lee et al., 2011	RCT Level II	No blinding; No evidence of fidelity	N = 111 Males and females randomly assigned to an intervention or control group using a table of random numbers	VAS	Music or no music before surgery; no premedication	Significant decrease in preop anxiety	Low No harm

[a]Including outcome measures.
RCT, Randomized controlled trial; *STAI,* State-Trait Anxiety Inventory; *VAS,* visual analog scale.

- Effect size
- Impact on patient outcomes
- Implementation cost
- Ethical issues, if any, related to proposed practice change

For example, in the PICO question regarding use of a music intervention to decrease adult patients' preoperative anxiety, the evidence synthesis, as illustrated in Table 4.5, highlights that the evidence provided by the studies were of low to moderate quality, had a number of moderate threats to internal validity indicating evidence of bias, and had limitations in external validity, limiting generalizability. The studies provided no evidence of blinding, had inconsistent evidence of power analysis and intervention fidelity, and used different music modalities. However, all of the studies consistently reported a significant decrease in preoperative anxiety. The evidence synthesis concluded that no negative effects were noted, and as such, listening to music may help reduce anxiety in patients waiting for surgery. The recommendation was that preoperative patients can be offered this inexpensive music intervention and should be able to choose the type of music to listen to while waiting to go to surgery.

> ### EBP TIP
>
> When developing an evidence synthesis aimed at answering a clinical question, you need to carefully consider the consistencies as well as the inconsistencies across studies. You will become skilled at identifying what gaps have been filled, what gaps still exist, and what researchers need to focus on to improve the evidence base to answer a specific clinical question.

Once the evidence synthesis is completed, it can be used to inform clinical decision making to improve health outcomes. The evidence synthesis in Table 4.5 reveals that the studies were not high quality. However, the evidence reveals that the preoperative music intervention significantly reduced preoperative anxiety across studies; it is inexpensive, and does no harm. As such, your team might decide to implement a pilot QI program to test implementation of a similar intervention in your clinical setting.

SYNTHESIS

Overall, a focused search of the literature includes an iterative process of evidence-based practice that supports the process of ASK, GATHER, ASSESS/EVALUATE/SYNTHESIZE. Your search of the literature needs to follow a road map for translating background queries and focused clinical questions into a search for evidence, using the suggested core databases and gray literature resources to search for the best available evidence. Critically appraising individual studies and synthesizing the overall strengths and weaknesses of the studies as a group requires practice and repeated, continual engagement to gain competency navigating among multiple tools, platforms, and knowledge practices. Recognizing the complexity of searching the literature and avoiding bias is a challenge for lifelong learning, a valuable skill that informs clinical decision making to support high-quality, cost-effective, and satisfying evidence-based care.

▮ KEY POINTS

- Research evidence is discovered by searching the published and unpublished literature
- When searching the literature, you need to seek primary and secondary sources
- Evidence is hierarchical; evidence hierarchies provide a first step to evaluate the strength of research evidence
- Background sources of evidence include reports, evidence summaries, clinical practice guidelines, abstracts, point of care tools, and review articles
- Tools for organizing, citing, and sharing evidence are important for promoting collaboration on EBP and QI Projects

- Formulating broad background questions using secondary sources and point of care tools advance identifying a clinical question
- Core databases like CINAHL, PubMed, PsychINFO, and Embase are essential in searching for primary and secondary sources that provide evidence for developing and answering a clinical PICO question
- Searching electronic databases is an iterative process that begins with selecting a database and conducting an initial search with key terms and expanded using synonyms

- Selecting and critically appraising relevant articles and documents is essential for determining gaps and revising, expanding or narrowing the search strategy
- Citation management tools are platforms for downloading citations to build a personal data/article repository that assists you in writing, citing, and formatting written papers.
- PRISMA flowcharts, provide a graphical format for identifying screening, eligibility, and applying

exclusion criteria when conducting a systematic review or completing a review.
- Synthesis of evidence pertaining to answering the PICO question, identifies the overall strengths and weaknesses of the body of literature obtained from the search and following critical appraisal of each study.
- Synthesis of the evidence provides the basis for making recommendations about applicability of findings for practice.

REFERENCES

AGREE Enterprise. (2014). *AGREE II Training Tools*. Retrieved from: http://www.agreetrust.org/resource-centere///agree-ii-training-tools.

AHRQ. (2013, November 18). *Grading the Strength of a Body of Evidence When Assessing Health Care Interventions for the Effective Health Care program of the Agency for Healthcare Research and Quality: An Update/ Effective health Care*. Retrieved from: https://effectivehealthcare.ahrq.gov/topics/methods-guidance-grading-evidence/methods/.

Altmetric for Researchers. (June 1, 2015). Retrieved from: https://www.altmetric.com/audience/researchers/.

Association of College & Research Libraries (ACRL). (February 2, 2015). *Framework for Information Literacy for Higher Education*. Retrieved from: http://www.ala.org/acrl/standards/ilframework.

Bradt, J., Dileo, C., & Shim, M. (2013). Music interventions for preoperative anxiety. *Cochrane Database of Systematic Reviews* (6), CD006908.

Covidence. (2017). *Covidence*. Retrieved from: https://www.covidence.org/.

Cumino, D. O., Vieira, J. E., Lima, L. C., Stievano, L. P., Silva, R. A. P., & Mathias, L. A. S. T. (2017). Smartphone-based behavioural intervention alleviates children's anxiety during anaesthesia induction: A randomised controlled trial. *European Journal of Anaesthesiology, 34*(3), 169–175.

EBSCO Industries, Inc. (2017). *Nursing Reference Center Plus | Evidence-Based Nursing Resources | EBSCO*. Retrieved from: https://www.ebscohost.com/nursing/products/nursing-reference-center.

Elsevier, Inc. (2017). *ClinicalKey*. Retrieved from: https://www.clinicalkey.com/#!/.

Goodman, J. S., Gary, M. S., & Wood, R. E. (2014). Bibliographic search training for evidence-based management education: a review of relevant literatures. *Academy of Management Learning & Education, 13*(3), 322–353.

Haustein, S., Peters, I., Sugimoto, C. R., Thelwall, M., & Larivière, V. (2014). Tweeting biomedicine: An analysis of tweets and citations in the biomedical literature. *Journal of the Association for Information Science and Technology, 65*(4), 656–669.

Higgins, J. P., & Green, S. (2011). Cochrane handbook for systematic reviews of interventions. Retrieved from: http://handbook.cochrane.org/.

Homan, J. M. (2010). Eyes on the prize: reflections on the impact of the evolving digital ecology on the librarian as expert intermediary and knowledge coach, 1969–2009. *Journal of the Medical Library Association: JMLA, 98*(1), 49–56.

Keilani, C., Simondet, N., Maalouf, R., Yigitoglu, A., Bougrine, A., Simon, D., et al. (2017). Effects of music intervention on anxiety and pain reduction in ambulatory maxillofacial and otorhinolaryngology surgery: a descriptive survey of 27 cases. *Oral and Maxillofacial Surgery, 21*(2), 227–232.

Knapp, M., & Brower, S. (2014). The ACRL framework for information literacy in higher education: implications for health sciences librarianship. *Medical Reference Services Quarterly, 33*(4), 460–468.

Krainovich-Miller, B., Haber, J., Yost, J., & Jacobs, S. K. (2009). Evidence-based practice challenge: teaching critical appraisal of systematic reviews and clinical practice guidelines to graduate students. *Journal of Nursing Education, 48*(4), 186–195.

Lee, K., Chao, Y., Yiin, J., Chiang, P., & Chao, Y. (2011). Effectiveness of different music-playing devices for reducing preoperative anxiety: a clinical control study. *International Journal Of Nursing Studies, 48*(10).

McMaster University, Health Information Research Unit. (2017). *NURSING+ | Search*. Retrieved from: https://plus.mcmaster.ca/np/Search.

Meyer, J., & Land, R. (2003). *Threshold concepts and troublesome knowledge: linkages to ways of thinking and practising within the disciplines*. Edinburgh: University of Edinburgh. Retrieved from: https://www.dkit.ie/zh-hans/system/files/Threshold_Concepts__and_Troublesome_Knowledge_by_Professor_Ray_Land_0.pdf.

National Center for Biotechnology Information, U.S. National Library of Medicine. (2017). *PubMed Help Clinical Queries Filters*. Retrieved from: https://www.ncbi.nlm.nih.gov/books/NBK3827/#pubmedhelp.Clinical_Queries_Filters.

Ni, C., Tsai, W., Lee, L., Kao, C., & Chen, Y. (2012). Minimising preoperative anxiety with music for day surgery patients–a randomised clinical trial. *Journal Of Clinical Nursing, 21*(5/6), 620–625.

PRISMA Diagram Generator. (n.d.). Retrieved from: http://prisma.thetacollaborative.ca/.

PubMed® Special Queries. (2016). *[Procedures]*. Retrieved from: https://www.nlm.nih.gov/bsd/special_queries.html.

Smith, J., & Noble, H. (2016). Reviewing the literature. *Evidence-Based Nursing, 19*(1), 2–3.

Smith, M. (2017). Research guides: scholarly metrics: home. Retrieved from: http://guides.nyu.edu/c.php?g=277165&p=1847189.

Straus, S. E., Glasziou, P., Richardson, W. S., & Haynes, R. B. (2010). *Evidence-Based Medicine: How to Practice and Teach It, 4e* (4th ed.). Edinburgh: Churchill Livingstone.

Sucala, M., Cuijpers, P., Muench, F., Cardoș, R., Soflau, R., Dobrean, A., et al. (2017). Anxiety: There is an app for that. A systematic review of anxiety apps. *Depression and Anxiety, 34*(6), 518–525.

Suri, H. (2013). *Towards methodologically inclusive research syntheses: expanding possibilities*. Milton Park, Abingdon, Oxon: Routledge.

Systematic Review and Literature Review Software by Evidence Partners. (2017). *DistillerSR*. Retrieved from: https://www.evidencepartners.com/.

The donut and Altmetric Attention Score. (July 9, 2015). Retrieved from: https://www.altmetric.com/about-our-data/the-donut-and-score/.

Therapeutic Research Center. (2017a). *Music Therapy [Monograph]*. Retrieved from: Natural Medicines database.

Therapeutic Research Center. (2017b). *Natural Medicines*. Retrieved from: https://naturalmedicines.therapeuticresearch.com/databases/health-wellness/professional.aspx?productid=1304.

Thompson, M., Moe, K., & Lewis, C. P. (2014). The Effects of Music on Diminishing Anxiety Among Preoperative Patients. *Journal of Radiology Nursing, 33*(4), 199–202.

U.S. National Library of Medicine. (May 2017). *Glossary [Training Material and Manuals]*. Retrieved from: https://www.nlm.nih.gov/bsd/disted/pubmedtutorial/glossary.html.

Virginia Henderson Global Nursing e-Repository. (2017). Retrieved from: http://www.nursinglibrary.org/vhl/.

Wolters Kluwer Health. (2017). *UpToDate*. Retrieved from: https://www.uptodate.com/contents/search.

5

Principles of Assessing Research Quality

Geri LoBiondo-Wood

LEARNING OUTCOMES

After reading this chapter, you should be able to do the following:

- Analyze how a study's design type affects evaluation and interpretation of the findings.
- Compare and contrast elements that affect the evaluation and fidelity of a study's findings.
- Identify threats to internal validity.
- Analyze how threats to internal validity can affect interpretation of a study's findings.
- Identify external validity threats.
- Analyze conditions that affect external validity and interpretation of a study's findings.
- Identify links between study design and evidence-based practice.

KEY TERMS

Bias	Generalizability	Maturation
Constancy	History	Measurement effects
Control	Homogeneity	Mortality
Control group	Independent variable	Randomization
Dependent variable	Instrumentation	Reactivity
Experimental group	Internal validity	Selection bias
External validity	Intervening variable	Testing
Extraneous variable	Intervention fidelity	

After the development of a PICO question and search of the literature, the next phase of a practice change involves critically appraising the identified studies. How a researcher structures, implements, or designs a study affects the study's results, appraisal, and, ultimately, application of the results to practice. Understanding the implications and usefulness of a study for evidence-based practice (EBP), requires understanding key research design issues. This chapter provides an overview of key issues related to assessing the strength and quality of quantitative research designs. Chapters 6 through 8 present specific design types and important critical appraisal principles for assessing scientific quality and practice applicability of quantitative designs

related to threats to control and internal and external validity. Evaluation of research findings requires an evaluation of individual studies as well as a synthesis evaluation of a collective group of studies investigating the same topic (see Chapter 4).

ISSUES RELATING TO MAXIMIZING APPLICABILITY OF FINDINGS TO PRACTICE

Let's suppose that you have developed an intervention-focused PICO question, during your search of the literature, you locate and retrieve several randomized controlled trials (RCTs). You may think, "Eureka!

My search is complete; now I can answer my clinical question." Actually, this is not the case. You will need to evaluate each study to assess its overall scientific quality, including the design, sample type and size, measurement instruments, data collection, and data analysis methods. You will also need to evaluate the studies as a collective group by synthesizing the overall strengths, quality, and consistency of the evidence provided by the studies retrieved (see Chapter 4). When thinking about your synthesis, keep in mind that you may have a collection of studies that include different design types and methods to answer the same PICO question. The overall goal is to critically appraise each component of the individual studies found in your search, synthesize the findings across studies, and then determine applicability of the findings to practice. This chapter presents quantitative design elements that affect the application of findings to practice.

Elements of quantitative research designs include the following:

- Assessing how the research team conceptualized and tested the hypothesis or research question
- Assessing how the research team maintained control in the study
- Assessing threats to internal and external validity

The design, coupled with the methods and analysis, provides control for the study. Control is defined as the measures that the researcher uses to hold the conditions of the study consistent, thereby minimizing possible bias (any influencing factor that may change a study's results) in selection of subjects, randomization or assignment to experimental groups and control groups, and error in the measurement of the dependent variable(s) (outcome variable). Control measures help to control threats to the study's internal and external validity and applicability of findings to practice. Internal validity is the degree to which one can infer that the intervention, rather than another condition or variable, resulted in the outcome or observed effects. External validity is the degree to which findings can be generalized to other populations or environments. As you review studies for application to practice, you will need to make judgments about the quality of the studies. Be aware that it may not be possible to avoid validity threats, both internal and external. You will need to assess how the threats were minimized, how seriously they affect the credibility of the findings, and how the researchers, in the discussion of the findings of the article, account for any internal or external validity

issues that may have occurred. Control is weighted and assessed according to the level of the designs (see the discussion on evidence hierarchy in Chapter 2).

An example that demonstrates how the design can address a research question and maintain control is illustrated in the study by Lowe et al. (2017; Appendix B), the aim of which was to evaluate the impact of erythropoiesis-stimulating agents on behavioral measures in premature children. Subjects who met the study's inclusion criteria were randomly assigned to one of the three groups, using a computer-generated permuted block method and stratified by center. The interventions were clearly defined. The authors also discuss how intervention fidelity—faithfulness or constancy of the intervention as planned—was maintained during the delivery of the intervention and data collection. By establishing subject eligibility (inclusion criteria), methods for selection of subjects for study inclusion (e.g., random selection), and clearly describing and designing the experimental intervention, the researchers demonstrated that they had a well-developed plan and were able to consistently maintain the study protocol. A variety of considerations, including the chosen type of design, affect a study's successful completion and utility for EBP. These considerations include the following:

- Objectively conceptualized research question or hypothesis addressing gaps in the science
- Homogenous sample
- Data collection constancy
- Intervention fidelity
- Internal validity
- External validity

Statistical principles are associated with the mechanisms of control, but it is more important that you have a clear conceptual understanding of these mechanisms. As you will recall from Chapter 2, a study's design type is linked to a level of evidence. As you appraise the design, you must also take into account other aspects of a study's design and implementation. These aspects are reviewed in this chapter. How the elements of control are applied depends on the type of design (see Chapters 6–9).

AN OBJECTIVELY CONCEPTUALIZED RESEARCH QUESTION

Objectivity in a study begins with a review of the scientific literature. Researchers assess the depth and breadth of available knowledge about a question that, in turn, affects the design chosen. For example, the research question "What is the optimal length of a teaching program to promote adherence to oral cancer medication?" may suggest an experimental design (RCT; Chapter 6), whereas the question "What are the symptoms and coping strategies of children with cancer?" suggests an observational design (Chapter 7).

> **EBP TIP**
>
> When reading a study, the literature review that incorporates all aspects of the question allows you to judge the objectivity of the research question and whether the design matches the question.

HOMOGENOUS SAMPLE

The characteristics of a study's subjects such as age, sex, and health history are common extraneous variables or variables that may confound a study's outcome. Extraneous variables may also be referred to as *confounding variables*. For example, in the study by Lowe et al. (2017; Appendix B), the researchers ensured homogeneity of the sample by including subjects in both groups (premature infants vs. full-term children) who currently were between the ages of 3.5 and 4 years of age. This step limits the generalizability or application of the outcomes only to similar populations when applying the outcomes (see Chapter 6). As you read studies, you will often find that researchers limit their statements about generalizability of the findings to like samples.

As a control for these and similar problems, the researcher's subjects should demonstrate homogeneity or similarity with respect to minimizing extraneous variables relevant to the particular study (see Chapter 6). Extraneous variables are not fixed but must be reviewed and decided on according to the study's purpose. By using a sample of homogeneous subjects, based on inclusion and exclusion criteria, a researcher has a straightforward approach to maximizing control.

DATA COLLECTION CONSTANCY

A critical component of control is constancy in data collection. The concept of constancy refers to the methods used to maintain sameness in data collection. That is, data should be collected in the same way from each subject under the same conditions. This means that environmental conditions, timing of data collection, data collection instruments, and data collection procedures used to collect data are the same for each subject. The degree to which researchers maintain constancy in data collection is known as fidelity. In observational studies or nonexperimental studies, constancy of data collection is achieved through the use of a homogenous sample and consistent data collection procedures. If a study includes an intervention, data collection constancy and implementation (or delivery of an intervention as planned) help to ensure intervention fidelity.

INTERVENTION FIDELITY

Researchers choose a design that is consistent with the research question or hypothesis and maximizes the degree of control, fidelity, or uniformity of the study methods. Control is maximized by a well-planned study that considers each step of the research process and the potential threats to internal and external validity. Intervention studies are used to test whether a treatment or intervention affects patient outcomes. Observational studies do not test an intervention or manipulate the **independent variable** and thus do not have a control group. The use of a control group in intervention studies is related to the aim of the study (see Chapter 6).

In studies that test an intervention, manipulation of the independent variable is used as a means of control. This refers to the administration of a program, treatment, or intervention to only one group within the study and not to the other subjects in the study. The first group is known as the experimental group or intervention group, and the other group is known as the control group. In a control group, the variables under study are held at a constant or comparison level.

Researchers choose a design that is consistent with the research question and maximizes the degree of control, **fidelity,** or uniformity of the study methods. Control is maximized by a well-planned study that considers each step of the research process and the potential threats to internal and external validity. Control is accomplished by ruling out other variables, termed intervening variables, that compete with the independent variables as an explanation for a study's outcome. An intervening variable is a variable that may occur during a study that contributes to the change of the dependent variable or outcome. For example, in a study that aims to test an intervention to improve cancer patients' adherence to a medication trial, an intervening variable may be an antianxiety medication given to some patients during the medication trial. An **extraneous,** mediating, or intervening variable is one that interferes with interpretation of the dependent variable. An example would be the effect of the stage of cancer and depression during different phases of cancer treatment.

In a study that tests interventions (interventions studies; see Chapter 6), intervention fidelity (also referred to as treatment fidelity) is a key concept. Fidelity means trustworthiness or faithfulness. Intervention fidelity means that the researcher standardized the intervention and demonstrates how the intervention was administered to each subject in the same manner under the same conditions. A study designed to address issues related to a study's fidelity maximizes results, decreases bias, and controls preexisting conditions that may affect outcomes. The elements of control and fidelity differ based on the design type and the variables tested. Thus, when various research designs are critically appraised, the issue of control is always raised but with varying levels of flexibility. The issues discussed here will become clearer as you review the various design types discussed in Chapters 6 and 7.

Means of controlling for intervention fidelity includes the following:
- Use of a homogeneous sample
- Use of consistent data collection procedures
- Training and supervision of interventionists
- Manipulation of the independent variable and intervention fidelity
- Randomization

EBP TIP

As you review studies, assess whether the study included an intervention and whether there is a clear description of the intervention and how it was controlled. If the details are not clear, the intervention may have been administered differently among the subjects, affecting the interpretation and strength of the results.

CRITICAL APPRAISAL CRITERIA

When reviewing studies, assess whether the researchers clearly identified controls that enhance generalizability from the sample to the specific population.

The elements of *intervention fidelity* (Breitstein, Robbins, & Cowell, 2012, French et al., 2015; Gearing et al., 2011; Nelson, Corday, & Hulleman, 2012; Preyde & Burnham, 2011) are as follows:
- Design: Allows an adequate testing of the hypothesis(es) in relation to the underlying theory and clinical processes
- Training: Training and supervision of the data collectors and/or interventionists to ensure that the intervention is delivered as planned and in a consistent manner
- Delivery: Assessing whether the intervention is delivered as intended, including that the "dose" (as measured by the number, frequency, and length of contact) is well-described for all subjects, the dose is the same in each group, and there is a plan for possible problems
- Receipt: Verifying the treatment was delivered and understood by the subject
- Enactment: Assessing whether the intervention the subject performs is completed as intended

This type of control strengthens the investigators' ability to draw conclusions, discuss limitations, and cite the need for further research. When interventions are implemented, researchers should describe the training and supervision of interventionists completed to ensure fidelity. All study designs should demonstrate constancy (fidelity) to the methods of data collection. Studies that test an intervention require particular attention to intervention fidelity.

EBP TIP

The lack of manipulation of the independent variable does not mean a weaker study. The type of question, amount of theoretical development, and research that has preceded the study affect the researcher's design choice. If the question is amenable to a design that manipulates the independent variable, it increases the power of a researcher to draw conclusions; that is, if all of the considerations of control are equally addressed.

INTERNAL VALIDITY

Internal validity assesses whether the change in the dependent variable or study outcome was related to the *independent variable*. When conducting a study, researchers consider the potential impact of internal validity threats on findings as one or more sources of bias. Clinicians must evaluate whether the study's findings are valid before implementation in practice. To establish internal validity, the researcher rules out other factors or threats as rival explanations of the relationship between the variables—essentially, sources of bias. There are a number of threats to internal validity. You should note that the threats to internal validity are mainly assessed in intervention studies but also can compromise outcomes of all quantitative studies. The overall strength and quality of a study's findings should be considered to some degree in all studies. How these threats may affect specific designs is addressed in Chapters 6 through 8. Threats to internal validity include history, maturation, testing, instrumentation, mortality, and subject selection bias. Table 5.1 provides definitions and examples of internal validity threats. Generally, researchers will discuss the threats to validity that they encountered in the discussion or limitations section of a research article.

> **EBP TIP**
>
> More than one threat can be found in a study, depending on the study design. Finding a threat to internal validity in a study does not invalidate a study's results but should be acknowledged in the study's "Results" or "Discussion" or "Limitations" section.

> **EBP TIP**
>
> Avoiding threats to internal validity can be difficult. This reality does not render studies that have threats useless, however. Take them into consideration and weigh the total evidence of a study for not only its statistical meaningfulness but also its clinical meaningfulness.

EXTERNAL VALIDITY

External validity is an assessment of the generalizability of a study's findings to additional populations and environmental conditions. External validity questions under what conditions and with what types of subjects the same results can be expected to occur.

The factors that may affect external validity are related to selection of subjects, study conditions, and type of observations. These factors are termed *selection effects*, *reactive effects*, and *testing effects*. You will notice the similarity in the names of the factors of selection and testing to those pertaining to threats to internal validity. When assessing a study's internal validity threats, you assess for their potential as they relate to the testing of *independent* and *dependent* variables within a study. External validity threats are assessed in terms of the *generalizability* or use of the study findings in other populations and settings. The threats to internal and external validity can interact with each other. It is important to remember that the interaction of these threats varies with the design and methods of the study. Problems of internal validity are generally easier to control. Generalizability issues are more difficult because it means that the researcher is assuming that other populations are similar to the one being tested. As more controls are designed into a study, internal validity improves, but generalizability is likely to decline.

> **EBP TIP**
>
> Generalizability depends on who actually participates in a study. Not everyone who is approached actually participates, and not everyone who agrees to participate completes a study. As you review studies, think about how well the subjects reflect the population of interest.

Selection Effects

Selection refers to the generalizability of the results to other populations. An example of selection effects occurs when the researcher cannot attain the ideal sample population. At times, the numbers of available subjects may be low or not accessible. Therefore the type of sampling method used and how subjects are assigned to research conditions affect the generalizability to other groups: the external validity.

Examples of selection effects are reported when researchers note the following:

"Limitations of this study include the small number of children in each of our groups, which limits

TABLE 5.1	**Internal Validity Threats—Definitions and Examples**	
Threat	**Definition**	**Example**
History	In addition to the independent variable, another specific event that may have an effect on the dependent variable may occur either inside (during the study) or outside the experimental setting.	A study tested a partial weight-bearing activity intervention for athletes recovering from lower leg injuries at two sites. During the study's final month, a new, partial weight-bearing treadmill, the Super G, was introduced to some of the patients at one site only, leaving the researchers to question the outcomes from the center that instituted the added intervention. Data from the one hospital (cohort) were not included in the analysis.
Maturation	Can occur in studies that test an intervention or variables over time and refers to the developmental, biological, physiological, or psychological processes within an individual as a function of time and are external to a study's event, differences between the two testing periods rather than the experimental treatment.	Hjertstedt, Barnes, and Sjostedt (2013) evaluated the effects of a community-based geriatric dentistry rotation on oral health literacy and found that the interactions during multiple home visits with dental students can positively affect oral health literacy. They noted that the changes in oral care may have been due to subjects' knowledge of time and day of the dental students' repeat home visits and solicitation of information on brushing practices since the last visit. Another example: Suppose one wishes to evaluate the effect of an intervention in a group of elder subjects in a dementia center over a period of time. The investigator would record the subjects' abilities before and after the intervention. Between the pretest and posttest, the subjects' health and dementia status can change. The growth or change may be unrelated to the study and may explain differences between the two testing periods.
Testing	Taking the same test repeatedly could influence subjects' responses the next time the test is completed. The effect of taking a pretest on the subject's posttest score is known as testing. The pretest may sensitize an individual and improve the posttest score. Individuals generally score higher when taking a test on a second occasion, regardless of the treatment. The differences between posttest and pretest scores may not be a result of the independent variable but rather of the experience gained through the testing.	Thomas et al. (2017) discussed how parent self-report of skill attainment in seeking services for their children may have influenced responses on actual skill attainment level.
Instrumentation	Changes in the measurement of the variables or observational techniques may account for changes in the measurement obtained.	In a study of obesity and disability in young adults, Lee et al. (2017) acknowledged that "our measures of disability are not directly comparable to more traditional measures of disability used in studies of older adults." Another example: Researchers may wish to study several types of cardiac monitoring to compare the accuracy of the different monitor types. To prevent instrumentation threat, a researcher must check the calibration of the monitors according to the manufacturer's specifications before and after data collection.

TABLE 5.1	Internal Validity Threats—Definitions and Examples—cont'd	
Threat	Definition	Example
Mortality	The loss of study subjects from the first data collection point (pretest) to the second data collection point (posttest). If the subjects who remain in the study are not similar to those who dropped out, results could be affected. Subject loss may be from the sample as a whole, or, in a study that has both an experimental and a control group, there may be differential loss of subjects. Differential loss of subjects means that more of the subjects in one group dropped out than in the other group.	In a community intervention study designed to achieve healthy eating standards, evaluation of 2-year changes in outcomes in types of food and beverages served revealed that over the study period, 30% of the participants dropped out of the study.
Selection bias	If the precautions are not used to gain a representative sample, selection bias could result from how the subjects were chosen. To avoid selection bias, subjects can be randomly assigned to groups. In a nonexperimental study, even with clearly defined inclusion and exclusion criteria, selection bias is difficult to avoid completely.	Lowe et al. (2017; Appendix B) controlled for selection bias within the sample by including subjects in both groups (premature infants vs. full-term children) who were between the ages of 3.5 and 4 years at the time of the study.

generalizability of the findings. Also there was a difference in neurological development al impairments between groups that may have impacted behavior."

(Lowe et al., 2017; Appendix B).

These remarks caution you about potentially generalizing beyond the type of sample in a study, but also point out the usefulness of the findings for practice and future research aimed at building the research in this area.

Reactive Effects

Reactivity is defined as the subjects' responses to being studied. Subjects may respond to the investigator not because of the study procedures but merely as an independent response to being studied. This is also known as the Hawthorne effect, which is named after Western Electric Corporation's Hawthorne plant, where a study of working conditions was conducted. The researchers developed several working conditions (i.e., turning up the lights, piping in music loudly or softly, and changing work hours). They found that no matter what was done, the workers' productivity increased. They concluded that production increased as a result of the workers' realization that they were being studied rather than because of the experimental conditions.

In a study by Hjertstedt et al. (2013), the investigators tested a pre–post oral health intervention with a group of elder adults in the community. The investigators noted that the subjects knew ahead of time about the data collectors' upcoming visits and may have made an extra effort to brush their teeth immediately before the visit, thereby introducing a Hawthorne effect.

Measurement Effects

Administration of a pretest in a study affects the generalizability of the findings to other populations and is known as measurement effects. Pretesting can affect the posttest responses in a study (internal validity) and affects the generalizability outside the study (external validity). For example, suppose a researcher wants to conduct a study with the aim of changing attitudes toward breast cancer screening behaviors. To accomplish this, an education program is incorporated on the risk factors for breast cancer. To test whether the education program changes attitudes toward screening behaviors, tests are given before and after the teaching intervention. The pretest on attitudes allows the subjects to examine their attitudes regarding cancer screening. The subjects' responses on follow-up testing may differ from those of individuals who were given the education program and did not see the pretest. Therefore, when a study is conducted and a pretest is given, it may "prime" the subjects and affect the ability to generalize to other situations.

> ### EBP TIP
>
> When reviewing a study, be aware of the internal and external validity threats. These threats do not make a study useless—but actually more useful—to you. Recognition of the threats allows researchers to build on data and allows you to think through what part(s) of the study can be applied to practice. Specific threats to validity depend on the design type.
>
> There are other threats to external validity that depend on the type of design and methods of sampling used by the researcher, but these are beyond the scope of this text. Campbell and Stanley (1966) offer detailed coverage of the issues related to internal and external validity.

SYNTHESIS

Quantitative Research

Evaluating a study's design requires you to have knowledge of the overall implications that the choice of a design may have for the study as a whole. When investigators ask a research question, they (1) design a study, (2) decide how the data will be collected, (3) decide which instruments will be used, (4) identify the sample's inclusion and exclusion criteria, (5) determine how large the sample needs to be to diminish threats to the study's validity, and (6) choose the appropriate method of analyses. These choices are based on the nature of the research question or hypothesis. Minimizing threats to internal and external validity of a study enhances the strength of evidence. In this chapter, the meaning, purpose, and important factors of design choice, as well as the vocabulary that accompanies these factors, have been introduced.

Several criteria for evaluating the design related to maximizing control, minimizing threats to internal and external validity, and, as a result, sources of bias can be drawn from this chapter. When evaluating the potential threats of internal and external validity of quantitative designs, it is important to refer back to the research question or hypothesis and aims of the study.

■ KEY POINTS

- How a researcher structures, implements, or designs a study affects the study's results, appraisal, and, ultimately, application of the results to practice.
- Evaluation occurs by synthesizing the overall strengths, quality, and consistency of the evidence provided by the studies retrieved.
- Control measures help manage threats to the study's internal and external validity and applicability of findings to practice.

- Internal validity is the degree to which one can infer that the intervention, rather than another condition or variable, resulted in the outcome or observed effects.
- External validity is the degree to which findings can be generalized to other populations or environments.
- Studies reviewed for an evidenced-based practice project need to be evaluated for quality individually as well as a collective group.

REFERENCES

Breitstein, S., Robbins, L., & Cowell, M. (2012). Attention to fidelity; Why is it important? *Journal of School Nursing*, 28(60), 108–407.

Campbell, D., & Stanley, J. (1966). *Experimental and quasi-experimental designs for research*. Chicago, IL: Rand-McNally.

French, C. T., Diekemper, R. L., Irwin, R. S., et al. (2015). Assessment of intervention fidelity and recommendations for researchers conducting studies on the diagnosis and treatment of chronic couch in the adult: CHEST Guideline and Expert Panel Report. *Chest*, 148(1):32–54.

Gearing, R. E., El-Bassel, N., Ghesquiere, A., et al. (2011). Major ingredients of fidelity: a review and scientific guide to improving quality of intervention research implementation. *Clinical Psychology Review, 31,* 79–88.

Hjertsedt, J., Barners, S. L., & Jostedt, S. (2013). Investigating the impact of a community-based geriatric dentistry rotation on oral health literacy and oral hygiene of older adults. *Gerontologist, 31,* 296–307.

Lee, H., Pantazis, A., Cheng, P., Dennisuk, L., Clarke, P. J., & Lee, J. M. (2017). The association between obesity and disability incidence in young adolescents. *Journal of Adolescent Health, 59,* 472–478.

Lowe, J. R., Rieger, R., Moss, N. C., Yeo, R., Winter, S., Patel, S., et al. (2017). Impact of erythropoiesis-stimulating agents on behavioral measures in children born premature. *Journal of Pediatrics,* 1–6.

Nelson, M. C., Corday, D. S., Hulleman, C. S., Darrow, C. L., & Somner, E. C. (2012). A procedure for assessing intervention fidelity in experiments testing educational and behavioral interventions. *The Journal of Behavioral Health Services & Research, 39*(4), 374–395.

Preyde, M., & Burnham, P. V. (2011). Intervention fidelity in psychosocial oncology. *Journal of Evidence-Based Social Work, 8,* 379–396.

Thomas, K. C., Stein, G. L., Williams, C. S., Perez-Jolles, M., Sleath, B. L., Martinez, M., et al. (2017). Fostering activation among Latino parents of children with mental health needs: An RCT. In: *Psychiatry Services in Advance,* 68(10):1068–1075.

6

Intervention Studies

Susan Sullivan-Bolyai, Carol Bova

LEARNING OUTCOMES

After reading this chapter, you should be able to:

- Describe the purpose of intervention studies
- Compare and contrast intervention study designs
- Identify potential threats to internal and external validity related to intervention studies
- Critically appraise the strengths and weaknesses of intervention studies

- Synthesize evidence from intervention studies based on answering a PICO question
- Debate the contributions of intervention studies to evidence-based practice
- Apply findings from intervention studies to decision making for clinical practice

KEY TERMS

After-only design
Blinding
Control
Concealment
CONSORT Diagram
Crossover design
Double blind
Double blind
Efficacy

Effectiveness
Exclusion criteria
Experimental arm
Intent-to-treat method
Intervention dose
Intervention fidelity
Intervention studies
Manipulation
Pilot study

Power analysis
Pragmatic trials
Quasi-experimental design
Randomized clinical trial
Randomization (random assignment)
Single blind
Solomon four-group design
Triple blind

INTRODUCTION

Clinicians use research evidence to inform their decisions about how to best care for and communicate with their patients, families, and colleagues to achieve the highest quality, most cost-effective, and most satisfying experience of care. It is a challenge to determine which studies are most important for you and your colleagues to use as busy practitioners for clinical decision making. Because researchers often propose various and sometimes contradictory conclusions while studying the same or similar issues, you often feel challenged to determine which study findings are most applicable to inform patient care.

Intervention studies, often called randomized controlled (clinical) trials and abbreviated as RCT, reflect the strongest design type for an individual study, located at Level II on the Evidence Hierarchy (See Chapter 2). Because RCTs maximize control by having intervention and control groups as well as randomization, they are the most appropriate type of design to answer questions about the effectiveness and efficacy of interventions focused on testing cause-and-effect relationships. Other types of intervention studies include quasi-experimental designs, located at Level III on the Evidence Hierarchy. Quasi-experimental designs differ from RCTs in that they either lack a comparison group or randomization and, as such, have a higher risk of bias. The Decision-Making Algorithm for Intervention Studies highlights some of the factors that influence a researcher choosing an RCT or a quasi-experimental design (see Chapter 5).

As you follow the steps of the Iowa Model (Titler et al., 2001; see Chapter 1) for your evidence-based project that uses data from Intervention Studies, you may include several different types of intervention studies. You must evaluate each type of study using the parameters of their respective design elements as described in this chapter. Clinical leaders must not assume that the evidence provided by intervention studies is always strong enough to be translated into practice by automatically applying the findings to a patient care problem. Clinicians must evaluate—that is, critically appraise—the strength, quality, and consistency of evidence provided by intervention studies before making a decision about applying it to practice. The purpose of this chapter is to provide an overview of intervention studies, related types of clinical questions, and an overview of research designs associated with intervention studies and the questions and issues to raise while critically appraising experimental and quasi-experimental designs.

Experimental and Quasi-Experimental Design

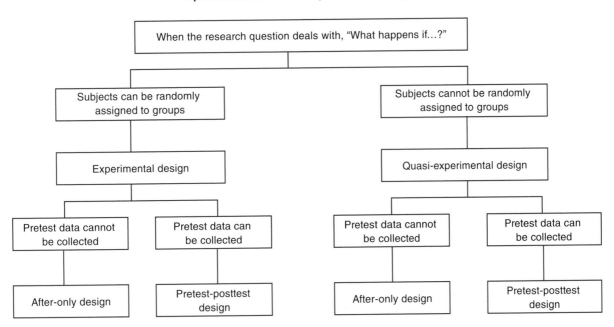

PURPOSE OF INTERVENTION STUDIES

A research design is a road map that outlines the components of the study used to test a research question or hypothesis. The purpose of intervention studies is to answer research questions or hypotheses related to the efficacy and effectiveness of an intervention. Efficacy, or how well the intervention performs under ideal and controlled conditions like a research study, has to be established first before an effectiveness trial is undertaken. Efficacy is established by implementing an RCT. Effectiveness refers to an intervention's performance under "real-world" conditions, sometimes called a pragmatic trial. Intervention studies exist on a continuum with a progression from efficacy trials to effectiveness trials. An efficacious intervention must be readily available. Providers must identify the target population for which the intervention is appropriate and then recommend the intervention, and patients must accept and adhere to the intervention. For example, several studies highlight how highly efficacious screening for colorectal cancer is underused and, as such, contributes to poor effectiveness in clinical practice that moderates the effect of the intervention (Singal, Higgins, Waljee, 2014; Klabunde, Brown, Ballard-Barbush et al., 2010).

As a clinical leader focused on evidence-based practice and quality improvement, you search the literature for intervention studies that potentially provide answers to the clinical questions being raised by you as an individual clinician or by your clinical team (See Chapter 4). Your clinical question, using the PICO format, might ask about the effectiveness of one intervention in comparison to another for a targeted patient population with a specific diagnosis or condition. For example, if you are a family nurse practitioner, you may be interested in finding out whether the Gardasil vaccine decreases the incidence of human papillomavirus (HPV) in females between the ages of 11 and 26. You will search for, retrieve, and critically appraise the strengths and weaknesses of studies to identify those that provide the strongest evidence to support your clinical decision making about how effective Gardasil vaccine is as a standard of care for this patient population. You may use this evidence in your patient and family teaching about the importance of this vaccine in the prevention of HPV.

TYPES OF INTERVENTION STUDIES

Randomized controlled trials. RCTs, commonly called intervention or therapy studies, use an experimental design and are the gold standard for testing an intervention. As individual studies, RCTs are located at Level II on the Evidence Hierarchy; a well-designed and implemented RCT should have a low risk of bias. RCTs compare the efficacy and/or effectiveness of different interventions and vary in format. For example, an RCT can involve one treatment group being exposed to an intervention under investigation and a comparison/control treatment group receiving another intervention, such as the current standard of care, to determine which yields the better outcome. The control group also can involve an intervention group that is receiving no intervention, such as a placebo. An RCT is characterized by three essential features:

- control
- randomization
- manipulation

These three properties help to reduce threats to internal and external validity (see Table 6.1 and Chapter 5).

Control refers to a measure that researchers use to maintain consistent conditions in the study to decrease

threats to internal and external validity and minimize bias (See Table 6.2). Bias includes any factors that may influence or change a study's results.

Randomization, or random assignment, is the distribution of subjects, by chance, to either the experimental or the control group. Sometimes the intervention and control group(s) are called the "arms" of the study. RCTs have at least two arms; one is the intervention and one is the control or comparison group. There can be more than two arms. For example, in an RCT investigating the effect of psychoeducation and telephone counseling in comparison to the current standard of care on the physical, emotional, and social adjustment of women with breast cancer and their partners, there were multiple intervention groups and a control group (Budin, Hoskins, Haber et al., 2009). The rationale for the random assignment is to equalize the extraneous variables that occur in the real world of clinical practice so that the two groups are equivalent in terms of demographic variables such as age, gender, socioeconomic status, race, ethnicity, health status, diagnosis, or other factors at baseline that potentially could affect the study outcomes. Manipulation is the process of "doing something." It means using a different dose of "something," in one group (the intervention group) and not the other group (the control group). Researchers compare the effect of different types of treatment by manipulating the independent variable at least for subjects randomly assigned to the intervention arm of the study. Examples may include participation in a palliative care support group, participation in an exercise intervention, or taking a new drug or treatment.

Although RCTs are the standard design for testing interventions, they have a series of limitations that must be understood. RCTs are designed to provide robust internal validity, which often reduces external validity (see Chapter 5). Sidani and Braden (2011) suggest that some of the limitations of an RCT design may include the following:

- No representative samples due to self-selected samples of research participants
- Highly selective settings that do not mimic the real world
- Results that reflect group findings and not how individuals will respond to the intervention
- RCTs sometimes purposefully exclude complexities in practice and community settings that might be effective when applied more broadly in "real life" clinical settings

TABLE 6.1	**Watch List for Threats to Validity (Internal, External, and Statistical Conclusion)**	
Type of Validity	**Threat**	**What to Watch for**
Internal	History: An event that occurs as the study is being conducted that could influence the outcome (the event could be global, national, local, or personal to individual research participants)	When was the study conducted? Were there any important events that could influence the study outcomes? Were new treatments made available during the study period? Did the researcher address this issue at all (try to collect data about it, control for it, or consider it in the analyses)?
Internal	Maturation: Changes that occur within individuals during the course of the study (i.e., changes in functioning, knowledge, cognition, developmental milestones, fragility, progression of disease state)	Did the study design take into account issues of maturation (especially in studies done with children and elders)? Was the sample randomly assigned? Were there any differences in the characteristics of the groups that indicate maturation might be an issue (e.g., more adolescents in one group than in the other)?
Internal	Testing: Changes in response to measures that are caused by repeating the administration of the same measures multiple times	Are baseline and follow-up measures spaced far enough apart to prevent memory of prior responses? Are measures too brief so that easy recall is likely? Are number of data collection points supported by clear rationale? Note: Use of the Solomon four-group design reduces this threat.
Internal	Instrumentation: Changes to the instrument over time during the study (e.g., also can refer to changes in equipment such as changing scales to measure weight without calibration or changing to a new interviewer with minimal experience)	Is equipment being used in the study, and if so, is it calibrated each time it is used? Is there adequate training of all study personnel, including interviewers and observers? How often did the interviewers/observers change during the course of a study? Is there evidence that random checks were performed to make sure equipment and/or interviewers/observers were applying measures consistently?
Internal	Statistical regression to the mean: A tendency for those with extremely high and low scores on the baseline test to gradually move their scores toward the mean value	Did the researchers describe the distribution of scores at baseline and indicate any extremely high or low scores? Did the researchers discuss doing any statistical analyses to evaluate the effects for the total sample, as well as those with very high or low scores at baseline? Note: Randomization is used to reduce this threat and equalize groups.
Internal	Selection effect: When the research participants differ in some important ways from those who did not participate in the study, or between study groups, and this difference may potentially influence the study outcomes	Did the researchers describe a reliable means of randomizing research participants to groups? Did the researchers describe whether the intervention and control groups were the same or different on baseline characteristics? Did the researchers attempt to control for any differences in baseline characteristics by group in the main study analyses?

Continued

TABLE 6.1   Watch List for Threats to Validity (Internal, External, and Statistical Conclusion)—cont'd

Type of Validity	Threat	What to Watch for
Internal	Mortality, also known as attrition: When research participants drop out of the study	Did the researchers describe how many research participants in each group dropped out of the study? Was the dropout rate different between the two groups? Was the power calculation done to estimate the potential attrition rate? Was there a plan in place to reduce attrition? Did the researchers compare the characteristics of those who dropped out with those who completed the study? If there was a difference, did the researcher attempt to control for this in the final analyses? Did the researchers conduct an intent-to-treat analysis?
Internal	Contamination: When some or all of the components of the intervention are shared with or experienced by the control group	Did the researchers discuss how they controlled for any possible contamination between groups? Were separate individuals delivering the intervention and control conditions? Did research participants from both groups have the opportunity to interact with each other?
External	Interaction of selection and treatment effects: When research participants are different from the target population in important ways, and this difference has the potential to influence how they respond to the intervention being studied (i.e., more positively or more negatively)	Are the inclusion/exclusion criteria clearly outlined? Is the recruitment site located in a setting that may attract only a certain subgroup of study participants? How many research participants are approached, and how many decline to participate in the study? Did the researchers detail the study participant characteristics so you can judge how the results might be applied to the target population?
External	Interaction of setting and treatment effects: When the study setting is unique in some way or may attract only a certain type of subject	Is the setting unique in any important way that might influence how research participants evaluate the intervention? If there are multiple sites, did the researchers describe these settings and analyze the data by setting to evaluate any effect of the setting on study outcomes?
External	Interaction of history and treatment effect: When the period in history in which the study is conducted may be unique in some way that would reduce the likelihood that an attempt to replicate the findings would be successful	Did the researchers report the dates when data were collected? Is there anything historical about this time period related to the research study that might reduce the generalizability of the findings? Was there an extraneous variable occurring during the study period (e.g., television, radio, or social media ads)
Statistical conclusion	Low or no statistical power	Was a power analysis done and reported? Was an adequate sample recruited and retained?
Statistical conclusion	Assumptions underlying statistical tests are not met	Did the researchers use the correct statistical procedures for answering the research questions? Did the researchers provide enough data to know whether normal distributions were present when parametric analyses were performed? Did the researchers need to transform data, and did data meet statistical assumptions? Did the researchers use nonparametric analyses when data were not normally distributed?

TABLE 6.1 Watch List for Threats to Validity (Internal, External, and Statistical Conclusion)—cont'd

Type of Validity	Threat	What to Watch for
Statistical conclusion	Fishing expedition: When researchers do multiple comparisons without accounting for the probability of committing a Type I error; exploring the data and doing analyses that are not originally planned	Did the researcher stick to the original analysis plan? Is the analysis plan consistent with the conceptual/theoretical framework? If multiple tests were performed, was the *p*-value adjusted to account for the multiple comparisons (i.e., Bonferroni correction)?
Statistical conclusion	Unknown or poor reliability of scales used in the study: Random error associated with the reliability of a scale—the lower the reliability, the larger the amount of random error present; thus, it is essential to know the reliability of each scale for each study	Did the researchers report the reliability of all scales used in the study in their sample? Were any of the alphas for the scales less than 0.7?

TABLE 6.2 Design Choice and Evaluating Quality

Design	Properties	Quality Criteria
True Experimental Design		
Randomized controlled trial Pre-posttesting	Randomization	Evidence that baseline data collection occurred followed by randomization (random assignment)
	Control	Both groups receive a constant (for example, the same basic standard of care) to limit bias
	Manipulation	The experimental group receives the "something"—key ingredient that is hypothesized to make a change in the outcome variable
		Examine the recruitment and retention rates
Posttest only	Randomization, manipulation, less control but used in studies where baseline might be impossible (e.g., postoperative pain management)	Same as earlier but no baseline to compare for change over time, thus threatening that groups could be different
Solomon four-group design	Randomization, control, manipulation with four groups of two each for experimental and two for control (only one experimental and one control receiving pretest) to better control testing threat to internal validity	Same as pre- and posttest Sample size accommodates four groups, but mortality (dropout) may be larger
Crossover design	Can also be called a "wait-list control" design, where subjects are randomly selected to receive the intervention first versus second (or at a later point in time)	Both groups receive the experimental treatment at different time points

Continued

TABLE 6.2 **Design Choice and Evaluating Quality—cont'd**		
Design	**Properties**	**Quality Criteria**
Factorial MOST	First, uses a screening phase where individual intervention components (such as education, social support) are selected to be included and tested; second, based on factorial analysis, some components will be chosen and further tested in a refining phase (optimized), while others will be rejected based on the data results. Finally, what might be considered a phase 4 trial (in a real-world setting, looking at effectiveness long-term, after intervention has suggested efficacy) or confirming phase; optimized intervention components from previous phase are tested	Clear description of each phase with results that inform the next phase Evidence of rigorous development of intervention "pieces"
Factorial SMART	An innovative design that builds interventions based on different phase outcomes by identifying the best pieces of the intervention (time-based) using a priori analysis outcome decision rules	Clear description of each phase with results that inform the next phase Evidence of rigorous development of intervention "pieces" and moving on to include or eliminate based on empirical evidence
Quasi-Experimental		
Nonrandomized control design	Missing either randomization or control inherent in an experimental design	Evidence that the characteristics of the intervention group and control groups are measured and then compared (even if not randomly assigned) and attempt is made to control for the main differences in the analyses

MOST, Multiphase optimization strategy; *SMART,* sequential multiple assignment randomized trial.

EBP TIP

Randomized clinical trials (RCTs) provide Level II evidence and have a lower risk of bias.

EBP TIP

Quasi-experimental designs provide Level III evidence and have a higher risk of bias because randomization is absent.

Other types of experimental designs that are considered intervention or therapy studies are the Solomon four-group, posttest only, and crossover designs. The Solomon four-group design has four groups (two experimental and two control). Two groups are identical to those used in the classic experimental design described earlier, plus two additional groups, including an experimental after-group and a control after-group. Subjects are randomly assigned to one of four groups before baseline data are collected. This design results in two groups that receive only a posttest rather than a pre- and posttest. This design, although complex to implement and at higher risk for attrition, provides an opportunity to minimize testing bias that may have occurred because of exposure to the pretest (also called pretest sensitization). Moreover, with two additional intervention groups, a larger sample is needed that would increase the time and cost to implement the study. Ishola and Chipps (2015) used the Solomon four-group design to test a mobile phone intervention to improve pregnant women's mental health outcomes in Nigeria. They hypothesized that those who received the mobile phone intervention would have greater psychological flexibility, defined as the ability to be present and act when necessary. The subjects were randomly assigned to one of four groups:

1. Pretest-mobile phone, intervention-immediate posttest
2. Pretest-no mobile phone, intervention-immediate posttest
3. No pretest-mobile phone, intervention-posttest only
4. No pretest-no mobile phone, intervention-posttest only

The study found that although psychological flexibility improved in the mobile phone intervention groups, this effect was influenced by a significant interaction between the pretests and the intervention. This means that pretest sensitization was present and a source of bias. The findings of this study present an application question similar to the findings of a group of intervention studies in Chapter 4 investigating the effect of music on preoperative anxiety. Should clinicians consider applying evidence to a practice change where the evidence contains bias? In Chapter 4, the studies were not high quality. However, the evidence revealed that the preoperative music intervention significantly reduced preoperative anxiety across studies; it was inexpensive, and did no harm. Like that team, you might decide to implement a pilot QI program to test implementation of a similar intervention in your clinical setting.

The **after-only design** is a less frequently used and weaker design composed of two randomly assigned groups, but unlike the classic experimental design, neither group is pretested. The independent variable is manipulated for the **experimental arm** but not for the control group. Randomly assigning subjects to the intervention and control arms is assumed to be sufficient to ensure lack of bias so that the effect of the intervention can be determined in comparison to the control group. However, control over extraneous variables is limited. As such, caution should be exercised when interpreting the results of a posttest-only intervention study because the outcomes could be related to some factor other than the intervention. This design is useful when pretesting of outcomes is not possible (e.g., when testing the effectiveness of a postoperative pain management intervention). A **crossover design** is considered a repeated measures design in which subjects serve as their own controls. Subjects are randomized to one of two groups; one group initially receives the intervention, and the other group serves as the control. At a predetermined point, the subjects in each group cross over so that subjects receiving the intervention switch to the control group and those in the control group now receive the intervention. The two trial periods in which the subjects receive different treatments whose effects are being compared must be separated by a washout phase that is sufficiently long to rule out any carryover effect. All subjects eventually receive the intervention. This design requires a smaller sample size and is efficient in terms of time and cost. Of course, the weakness and challenge in interpreting the findings is that the influence of the first condition and treatment assigned could influence the response when subjects cross over to the other group if there is not a sufficient washout period (i.e., a span of time when no intervention is occurring).

MOST and SMART designs. More recently, two factorial designs (multiphase optimization strategy [MOST] and sequential multiple assignment randomized trial [SMART]) have been proposed as alternative approaches to RCTs (Collins et al., 2014). Too often, intervention studies result in nonsignificant findings. This happens for many reasons, including poor design, inadequate power, and recruitment and retention issues. However, nonsignificant findings may occur due to our inability to deconstruct a complex multiple-component intervention to determine the effective component. Two intervention frameworks recently have been introduced that show promise in determining which components within an intervention are most effective and efficient for improving clinical outcomes (Wilbur, Kolanowski, & Collins, 2016). These frameworks are based on engineering principles to effect change. Collins et al. (2014) have developed these models to extract which key ingredients in a bundled intervention make a difference over time. MOST uses a factorial design to pull apart the components and test them in varying combinations. For instance, using peer mentors, parent education vignettes, and human patient simulator teaching experiences as one entire intervention does not get at the individual value of each component. However, with this 2^3 factorial design with eight experimental conditions (not to be confused with an eight-arm RCT), one can offer different combinations to test and analyze which of the eight experimental conditions works best in a select sample.

The other adaptive intervention that allows tailored components based on patient responses is SMART (Collins et al., 2014; Lei, Nahum-Shani, Lynch, Oslin, & Murphy, 2012; Wilbur et al., 2016). This design takes into account individual patient responses, adherence to treatment, and personal preferences to be used in tailoring the intervention. For example, patients with cancer require sequences of treatments based on their response to previous treatment to promote optimal outcomes. Guidelines for these individualized sequences of treatment are known as dynamic treatment regimens where the initial treatment and subsequent modifications depend on the response to the previous treatments, disease progression, and other patient characteristics and behaviors. Both innovative designs may help us identify what is most helpful in meeting our patients' and families' health care needs.

Pragmatic trial designs. Pragmatic trials evaluate the effectiveness of an intervention previously tested for efficacy in traditional experimental designs (Patsopoulos, 2011). With a pragmatic trial, the focus is on whether the intervention is doable and effective in a real-world clinical setting compared with other accepted clinical practice treatments. An example would be comparing yoga exercise outcomes to surgical outcomes in patients with chronic back pain. These trials are considered pragmatic because they are practical and realistic. They typically have limited inclusion/exclusion criteria (if any), exert minimal control over extraneous variables, have all practitioners apply the comparison treatment, and include data from all study participants in the final analysis.

Quasi-experimental design. Quasi-experimental intervention studies similarly test for change through manipulation of the independent variable. However, they lack one of the three key properties of an experimental design—typically, randomization or presence of a control group. There are times when randomizing participants to groups may not be feasible, or a control condition cannot be created. In these instances, there are several different quasi-experimental designs that are useful. For example, Pickham, Shin, Chan, Funk, and Drew (2012) conducted a quasi-experimental nonequivalent control group study to evaluate nurses' knowledge and ability to perform QT/QTc interval monitoring in a single hospital. Subjects were not randomly assigned, but nurses did complete a baseline pretest evaluation to serve as a form of control of prior knowledge. The nurses participated in a one-hour QT education class (intervention), and the same posttest evaluation was conducted after the education session was completed. The results demonstrated significant improvement in posttest scores after the intervention. However, because the research participants were not randomly assigned to the intervention or a control condition, there is no way to truly know whether the scores on the evaluation would have improved without the intervention (e.g., just from the experience of taking the test). The basic problem with quasi-experimental designs is weakened confidence in making causal assertions that the results occurred because of the intervention. Instead, the results may be caused by other extraneous variables. Threats to internal validity, such as selection effect, testing, and mortality, are common with this type of design. For example, in an after-only nonequivalent control group design, it

may be difficult to support the assertion that two non-randomly assigned groups are comparable at the outset of a study because there was no way to assess its validity. However, it is practical, cost-efficient, and more easily executed in real-life clinical settings.

Pilot studies. A pilot study is defined as a small sample study conducted as a prelude to a larger scale study, often called the "parent study." The pilot study uses the same design as is planned for the larger-scale study. A major purpose of conducting a pilot study is to implement it using similar methods and procedures that yield preliminary data to determine the feasibility of a larger scale study and establish if sufficient scientific evidence exists to justify subsequent and more extensive research and gives more experience to the research team (Whitehead, Sully, and Campbell, 2014).

> ### EBP TIP
>
> It is unclear what level of evidence is produced by pilot or feasibility studies. It depends largely on the purpose of the pilot study and how it was conducted. Therefore, be cautious when reviewing the published results of pilot and feasibility studies because the evidence they produce is only preliminary and applicable to a future full-scale trial.

TYPES OF DATA IN INTERVENTION STUDIES

Types of data found in intervention studies are collected directly from individuals about the effect of the intervention being tested on a clinical, educational, organizational, or financial outcome. Data also may be collected from organizational units. Whatever the type of data, it is essential that it be collected using a systematic and consistent plan to maximize fidelity.

When you think about the type of data analysis that is appropriate for intervention studies, consider that the focus of the analysis would be on testing differences in outcomes between the intervention and the control group and testing the treatment effect of the intervention. Researchers conducting RCTs are interested in determining whether the randomly assigned intervention and control groups are different after the introduction of the experimental treatment and how large the treatment effect is. For example, a two-group, randomized clinical trial protocol by Vorderstrasse, Melkus, Pan, Lewinski, and Johnson (2015) proposed testing the effect of a virtual environment (LIVE) in comparison to a traditional web-based site on diet and physical activity and metabolic outcomes in a sample of 300 adults with type 2 diabetes who had no serious complications or comorbidities. In the protocol, a moderate effect size was selected to detect the treatment effect based on their pilot data and the literature in behavioral diabetes interventions. They proposed that testing for clinical significance would involve at least a moderate effect and assumed a 20% attrition rate. As such, they needed 240 participants to test for the main effect with an 80% probability of rejecting the null hypothesis with effect sizes of .44 or greater. Remember that intervention studies should report the total number of subjects assigned to each group and the total number of subjects included in the data analysis and reporting of outcomes.

Statistical tests like t-tests, analysis of variance, and the intent-to-treat method are among the tests and methods for continuous data used to assess the differences between the experimental and control arms of an RCT. Statistics like odds ratios, numbers needed to treat, numbers needed to harm are used for analyzing dichotomous data; effect size, confidence intervals, and level of significance are other commonly reported intervention statistics that you will see reported as in the example earlier in the chapter. Chapter 10 will provide more in-depth content about data analysis for intervention studies.

CRITICALLY APPRAISING INTERVENTION RESEARCH

Intervention studies are considered to provide the strongest research evidence to make causal assertions that inform clinical decision making about applicability of research findings to clinical practice. However, there is no guarantee that the study design or the evidence provided by the findings of an RCT is strong enough to be translated into practice. Clinical leaders and their teams need to beware of automatically applying findings from intervention studies in practice. Rather, each study needs to be critically appraised to determine its strengths and weaknesses. If there is more than one study, a synthesis of the overall strengths and weaknesses of the studies needs to be completed as a group (see Chapter 4) before determining applicability of the findings. Standardized critical appraisal tools for RCTs such as those from the Center for Evidence-Based Medicine (CEBM) or the Critical Appraisal Skills Programme (CASP) provide

---

BOX 6.1 Critical Appraisal Criteria for Intervention Studies

Critical Appraisal of Internal and External Validity

- How was control maximized, and how were sources of bias minimized?
- How was randomization to intervention and control groups implemented?
- Were clinicians, recruiters, and subjects blinded to study group assignment?
- Was there a CONSORT (Consolidated Standards of Reporting Trials) diagram that accounted for recruitment, enrollment, and attrition?
- Were the intervention and control groups equivalent on demographic and clinical variables at baseline?
- How was intervention fidelity appropriately carried out to ensure consistency in data collection and implementation of the intervention and control group protocols?
- Was there evidence of training, monitoring, and supervision of interventionists?
- Were the subjects analyzed in the group to which they were randomly assigned?
- Was there evidence of reliability and validity for the instruments used to measure the outcomes?
- Were there sources of bias related to testing or maturation?

Critical Appraisal of the Statistical Conclusions

- Was the data analysis appropriate for the research question or hypothesis (e.g., t-test, ANOVA, ANCOVA)?
- Were all of the clinical outcomes measured?
- How large is the treatment effect (e.g., numbers needed to treat, numbers needed to harm, effect size, significance level)?
- How precise is the intervention or treatment effect (e.g., OR and confidence intervals)?
- What is the risk/benefit and cost/benefit of the intervention?
- How representative is the sample?
- To what extent are the study findings generalizable?
- How feasible is the intervention in my clinical setting?
- How does implementation of the intervention align with the values and preferences of my patient population?

---

a choice of evidence-based tools for you to select. The critical appraisal criteria in Box 6.1 also provide an evidence-based, user-friendly guide for you and your team to use. Table 6.1 provides a watch list for threats to internal and external validity and statistical conclusions.

Threats to internal and external validity are the benchmark criteria to use in critiquing whether a study's outcomes were truly the cause of the effect of the intervention on the dependent variable outcome(s) (see Chapter 5). Keeping a sharp, discerning eye out for potential threats to both internal and external validity helps you determine whether the results of the studies you are considering to incorporate into your evidence-based practice are legitimate and do no harm. You are in effect saying, "Are the conclusions in this publication rigorous and efficacious or effective? Are there other reasons why changes may have occurred due to extraneous or confounding variables?" Table 6.1 is a *watch list* for you to use when critiquing intervention studies. When thinking about threats to internal validity, you want to have confidence that the intervention study you read actually suggested a strong relationship between the independent variable and clinical outcomes.

Random assignment of subjects to either the intervention arm or the control arm of an RCT is the strategy researchers use to maximize the likelihood that the intervention being tested produces an outcome that is not caused by chance but by the intervention, and this strategy reduces selection bias. The randomization method should be identified. For example, in the Lowe et al. (2017), study in Appendix B, randomization of the participants born preterm to erythropoiesis stimulating agent (ESA) or placebo groups was performed during their initial hospitalizations using a computer-generated, permuted block method, stratified by center. Randomization also maximizes the probability that the intervention and control groups will be equivalent at baseline; statistical assessment of the equivalence of the two groups at baseline on key variables (e.g., age, gender, race/ethnicity, socioeconomic status, diagnosis, health status) is important for you to note and is usually presented in a format like Table 11 in the Lowe et al. study. However, in this study, despite the use of appropriate randomization procedures, there were differences in the children in neurodevelopmental impairments between the groups. More children in the ESA group had a full scale IQ < 70 or mild cerebral palsy ($P < .01$). Lack of equivalence at baseline is a point to consider when evaluating the results of this study.

Recruitment bias also must be critically appraised. A best practice is to have designated recruiters who are not researchers and are independent of the study. Otherwise, it is possible that recruiters may treat those being recruited to the intervention group differently than those

going into the control group. Therefore random assignment for each consenting subject should be concealed until the recruitment process is complete. **Concealment** is a method of protecting the randomization process to make sure the group assignment is not readily known by anyone before the subject is assigned to a group. Sealed envelopes can be used to conceal random assignment information. Ideally, the random assignment is best handled by a central research office that is separate from the researchers. **Blinding**, sometimes called masking, is the process of concealing from the researchers, recruiters, interventionists, and subjects and/or data collectors what treatment the subjects are receiving in the study. **Single blind** occurs when the subject does not know which intervention he or she is receiving. **Double blind** means that neither the subject nor the researcher knows to which arm the subject is assigned (i.e., the intervention or the control arm of the study). In the Lowe et al. (2017) study in Appendix B, caregivers of the child subjects and investigators (except the research pharmacists and coordinators administering the medication) were masked to the treatment assignment of the children. **Triple blind** occurs when the researcher, interventionist, and subjects do not know which arm is receiving the experimental treatment versus the placebo. The degree to which blinding is part of the study design is a function of the outcome being studied. For example, a Lyme disease vaccine trial featured triple blinding; the investigator, research nurse, and subjects were blinded, and the vaccine and placebo vials looked exactly the same by creating a "sham" look-alike (Sigal, Zahradnik, Lavin et al., 1998).

Several aspects related to the intervention study sample pose potential sources of bias related to internal and external validity. You may recall from Chapter 5 that threats to external validity compromise your confidence in the generalizability of the study findings, even for use in your clinical setting.

The sample size in any intervention study must be evaluated carefully. Intervention studies typically use standard power calculation procedures to make sure they enroll and retain an adequate number of research participants to address the study hypothesis. A power calculation should be evident in the article; it is used to determine the number of participants needed to detect a small, medium, or large treatment effect; that is, whether there is a difference between the intervention and control condition at a predetermined level of significance (e.g., $P < .05$ or $P < .01$). **Power analysis** is calculated to estimate the sample size needed to detect the treatment effect and calculated to reduce the probability of making a Type II error; that is, the likelihood of accepting that the intervention did not work when it really did. Studies that have high attrition rates because they are conducted longitudinally or with severely ill patient populations are more likely to have unavoidably high attrition and end up with a sample too small to accurately detect a significant treatment effect. In that case, do not be surprised if you note that in anticipation of attrition, the researchers overenrolled the number of subjects originally calculated in the power analysis. Generally, an attrition rate of 15% to 20% is acceptable, but power analysis provides the statistical projection based on the desired effect size. Sometimes replacement recruitment continues with researchers trying to match new subjects on demographic variables with those subjects who have dropped out. For example, in the RCT protocol by Vorderstrasse et al. (2015), sample size calculations were based on power to reject the null hypothesis for the primary aim, which stated that "the trajectories of dietary behavior and physical activity are equivalent for the LIVE and control groups across the 52 weeks after randomization using a variance covariance matrix of fixed effects for a variety of sample and effect sizes." They assumed a 20% attrition rate.

Subjects should be analyzed in the groups to which they were randomly assigned. In the data analysis component of the RCT protocol by Vorderstrasse and colleagues (2015), subjects were retained in their originally assigned groups; this aligned with their planned use of the intent-to-treat method. Another strategy is to use a method that assumes the worst outcome for those who withdrew, repeats the analysis, and compares the outcomes. If the outcomes reveal the same treatment effect, the validity of the study findings can be regarded as uncompromised (see Chapter 10). The Lowe et al. study in Appendix B had a small number of children in each of the groups, which is a source of bias related to external validity that limits the generalizability of the findings.

On another note, you want to critically appraise whether subjects were analyzed in the group to which they were randomly assigned. Despite the best efforts of the interventionists, subjects may not complete one or more data collection points. For example, in an RCT by Budin et al. (2008), investigating the effect of a psychoeducation and telephone counseling intervention in comparison to standard care in promoting emotional, social, and physical adjustment for women with breast cancer and their partners, there were five data collection points over one year from diagnosis through ongoing recovery. Twenty percent of subjects did not complete one or more data collection points. Some dropped out of the study after completing one or more data collection points; others just missed or did not complete or return their questionnaire packets within the appropriate time frame. The intent-to-treat method was used to analyze data according to the group to which the subject was randomly assigned. Intent-to-treat preserves the comparability of the intervention and control groups, and minimizes Type I errors (see Chapter 10).

When critically appraising that section of an RCT or quasi-experimental design, you will expect that inclusion and exclusion criteria have been clearly identified so that a homogenous sample, likely a convenience or purposive sample, can be recruited. You want to note if there is a **CONSORT diagram** (http://www.consort-statement.org/), like Figure 1 in the 2017 study by Lowe et al. in Appendix B that evaluates whether the number of participants originally enrolled in the trial have completed the study. Issues can occur during a trial that can affect the power to detect a true difference between the intervention and the control conditions, including attrition of participants in the trial, poor reliability of measures, and poor intervention fidelity.

Intervention studies require precise measurement of independent variables (predictors) and dependent variables (outcomes). You will assess measurement instruments used for evidence of reliability and validity. The most common type of reliability is internal consistency reliability. With this type of reliability, a report of an alpha of .70 is considered minimally acceptable (DeVellis, 2017). Content validity is the most common type of validity you will see presented in research articles. Construct validity is more often referred to in citations from original psychometric studies. Use of valid and reliable measures increases the likelihood that if a true difference exists between the intervention and the control condition, it is accurately captured. Measures that are reliable and valid are required to reduce threats to internal and external validity. When evaluating intervention studies, it is important to pay close attention to how the researchers report the measures they used to determine the outcomes.

Intervention fidelity, also called treatment fidelity, refers to processes used to make sure that the research intervention and all related activities were delivered exactly as planned to ensure that any treatment effect found or not found is a result of the intervention and not of alterations in execution of the study. For example, fidelity includes development of an intervention manual, training, monitoring, and supervision of research staff, measuring the consistency with which it is delivered, ensuring that there is consistent adherence to data collection protocols, and confirming that the intervention was delivered and received using a standardized protocol. Activities to maximize fidelity need to be documented by a research team. For example, if there are multiple interventionists delivering the same intervention at different data collection sites, what is the evidence that training continued until there was a high level of interrater agreement across interventionists and that periodic booster sessions were conducted to monitor and prevent drift? Drift is a gradual change in how consistently the intervention and control groups' conditions are implemented during an RCT (Bova et al., 2017). The aim is to maintain a high level of adherence to the intervention protocol, which enhances the validity of study findings (Lebert et al., 2017). **Intervention dose**, another important component of intervention fidelity, is the amount of the "something" that is given to the study participants to create a change in the dependent variable(s) (Reed et al., 2007). This information should be readily available in the intervention articles you are reviewing. It may be referred to as number of sessions, time spent with the interventionist, materials or interactions that occurred, or a combination of several change agents.

The execution of intervention fidelity procedures can

> ### EBP TIP
>
> When thinking about critically appraising intervention fidelity, assess whether:
> - an intervention manual was developed and used,
> - all research personnel were trained on the careful execution of the intervention,
> - the consistency with which the researchers executed the intervention was monitored, and
> - adherence to the protocol (e.g., dose, timing) through supervision and booster sessions was measured.

be used as a quality control process to monitor intervention drift; that is, moving away from the strict standards of how an intervention is executed over time (Bova et al., 2017). Intervention studies need to report how they implemented processes to control for intervention fidelity throughout the trial.

Statistical versus clinical significance is another important critical appraisal concept. When you are critically appraising the findings of an intervention study, it is important for you, individually or as a team, to consider the clinical significance of the statistically significant differences that are reported; the two are not necessarily equivalent. In the Lowe et al. RCT (Appendix B), there was a statistically significant improvement in cognition for children in the ESA group compared with the control group. The treatment effect was most beneficial to the socioeconomic composite (SEC) group; that is, those children from low socioeconomic backgrounds. Despite the beneficial effect of the ESAs, the ESA-treated born preterm did not completely catch up with children born full-term on any of the cognitive outcome measures. Even though there were statistically significant differences between the groups, the clinical significance is minimized because the small sample limits generalizability. In addition, the groups were not equivalent at baseline on neurodevelopmental impairments, and the data comprised behavioral ratings rather than direct observation of the children and mother-child interactions. Although the evidence provided by the findings is consistent with the literature and has implications for the treatment of children born preterm with ESAs as one component of their medical regimen, confirmation in a larger study is recommended before translating the evidence into practice. One such trial is in progress, evaluating the neuroprotective effects of high-dose Epo, and will provide additional evidence about the effect of ESAs on the neurodevelopment of infants born preterm. When findings are consistent across different settings, clinical leaders can be more confident that the findings are clinically and statistically significant and ready for application in practice.

> ### IPE TIP
>
> As a clinical leader, you and your team need to assess whether the outcomes measured are clinically relevant for your clinical population, clinical setting, and available resources. You and your team need to use your clinical expertise and judgment—combined with the best available evidence, patient values, and preferences—to inform your decision about whether the outcomes of a study or group of studies are clinically important and applicable to improving patient care.

Ethical considerations are an important component when planning, conducting, and evaluating intervention trials. Stating that the study was evaluated by an institutional review board is one common requirement, but it is not sufficient to know whether the trial was conducted in an ethical way. The process of randomly assigning human beings to one treatment or another is fraught with ethical concerns. As you read an intervention study, it is important that you think through the ethical challenges posed by the specific study and decide whether the researchers did a good job of managing the ethical issues.

> **EBP TIP**
>
> Some helpful questions to ask yourself as you review these studies include the following:
> - What process was used to obtain informed consent?
> - Is there evidence that the researchers had equipoise about the different treatment arms?
> - Was the use of a placebo, sham intervention, or attention-control condition justified?
> - Was there any way to link data back to individual participants? (This could be an issue when qualitative results on a small sample are reported.)
> - Were the researchers transparent in reporting any difficulties, challenges, or limitations related to study execution or the study findings?

SYNTHESIS

Intervention studies provide the strongest level of evidence for designs of individual research studies. You are fortunate when your search of the literature reveals intervention studies that can be used to answer your PICO question. As a clinical leader, you and your team need to use your critical appraisal skills to determine the overall strengths and weaknesses of the study or studies and whether the findings of an intervention study or a group of studies can be applied to your patient population and clinical setting. A cost–benefit analysis may need to be completed and added to your team's overall appraisal before a final decision is made about implementing a change in practice (see Chapter 10). Because the goal of evidence-based practice is to achieve positive clinical outcomes and improve quality of life (Sidani, Miranda, Epstein, & Fox, 2009), it is important for you as a clinical leader to participate in translating evidence about new interventions into practice.

▌ KEY POINTS

- Intervention studies, also called RCTs, provide the strongest Level II evidence for an individual study.
- Quasi-experimental designs are intervention studies that provide Level III evidence but lack randomization or a control group.
- Intervention studies are characterized by three features: control, randomization, and manipulation.
- Newer study designs are emerging that may help researchers identify the most important components of nursing interventions and show how well these new interventions work in the real world of clinical care.

- Critical appraisal of intervention studies is a multi-step process that focuses on assessing how effectively the researchers minimized bias by controlling threats to internal and external validity.
- Results of intervention studies need to be critically appraised based on whether the data analysis is appropriate for answering the research question and significance of the evidence.
- Synthesizing the overall strengths and weaknesses of a group of intervention studies will inform clinical decision making about applicability of the findings to practice.

REFERENCES

Bova, C., Jaffarian, C., Crawford, S., Quintos, J. B., Lee, M., & Sullivan-Bolyai, S. (2017). Intervention fidelity: Monitoring drift, providing feedback and assessing the control condition. *Nursing Research, 66*, 54–59.

Budin, W. C., Hoskins, C. N., Haber, J., et al. (2008). Breast cancer: Education, counseling and adjustment among patients and partners: A randomized clinical trial. *Nursing Research, 57*(3), 199–213.

Collins, L. M., Trail, J. B., Kugler, K. C., Baker, T. B., Piper, M. E., & Mermelstein, R. J. (2014). Evaluating individual intervention components: Making decisions based on the results of a factorial screening experiment. *Translational Behavioral Medicine, 4*(3), 238–251.

DeVellis, R. F. (2017). *Scale development: Theory and applications* (4th ed.). Los Angeles: Sage.

Klabunde, C. N., Cronin, K. A., Breen, N., Waldron, W. R., Ambs, A. H., & Nadel, M. R. (2011). Trends in colorectal cancer test use among vulnerable populations in the United States. *Cancer Epidemiol Biomarkers Prev, 20*, 1611–1621.

Lebet, R., Hayakawa, J., Chamblee, T. B., Tala, J. A., Singh, N., Wypij, et al. (2017). Maintaining interrater agreement of core assessment. *Nursing Research, 66*(4), 323–329.

Lei, H., Nahum-Shani, I., Lynch, K., Oslin, D., & Murphy, S. A. (2012). A "SMART" design for building individualized treatment sequences. *Annual Review of Clinical Psychology*, 8, 21–48.

Lowe, J. R., Rieger, R. E., Moss, N. C., Yeo, R. A., Winter, S., Patel, S., et al. (2017). Impact of erythropoiesis-stimulating agents on behavioral measures in children born preterm. *Journal of Pediatrics*, 184, 75–80.

Patsopoulos, N. A. (2011). A pragmatic view on pragmatic trials. *Dialogues in Clinical Neuroscience*, 13(2), 217–224.

Pickham, D., Shin, J. A., Chan, G. K., Funk, M., & Drew, B. J. (2012). Quasi-experimental study to improve nurses' QT-interval monitoring: Results of QTIP study. *American Journal of Critical Care*, 21(3), 195–200.

Reed, D., Titler, M. G., Dochterman, J. M., Shever, L. L., Kanak, M., & Picone, D. M. (2007). Measuring the dose of nursing intervention. *International Journal of Nursing Terminologies and Classifications*, 18(4), 121–130.

Sidani, S., & Braden, C. J. (2011). *Design, evaluation, and translation of nursing interventions*. West Sussex, UK: Wiley-Blackwell.

Sidani, S., Miranda, J., Epstein, D., & Fox, M. (2009). Influence of treatment preferences on validity: A review. *Canadian Journal of Nursing Research*, 41(4), 52–67.

Sigal, L. H., Zahradnik, J. M., Lavin, P., et al. (1998). A vaccine consisting of recombinant *Borrelia burgdorferi* outer-surface protein A to prevent Lyme disease. *New England Journal of Medicine*, 339, 216–222.

Singal, A. G., Higgins, P. D. R., & Waljee, A. K. (2014). A primer on effectiveness and efficacy trials. *Clinical and Translational Gastroenterology*, 5(1), e452.

Titler, M. G., Kleiber, C., Steelman, V. J., Rakel, B. A., Budreau, G., Everett, L. Q., et al. (2001). The Iowa model of evidence-based practice to promote quality care. *Critical Care Nursing Clinics of North America*, 13(4), 497–509.

Titler, M. G., Conlon, P., Reynolds, M. A., Ripley, R., Tsodikov, A., Wilson, D. S., et al. (2016). The effect of a translating research into practice intervention to promote use of evidence-based fall prevention interventions in hospitalized adults: A prospective pre–post implementation study in the U.S. *Applied Nursing Research*, 31, 52–59.

Vorderstrasse, A. A., Melkus, G. D., Pan, W., Lewinski, A. A., & Johnston, C. M. (2015). Diabetes learning in virtual environments. *Nursing Research*, 64(6), 485–493.

Whitehead, A. L., Suly, B. G. O., & Campbell, M. J. (2014). Pilot and feasibility studies: Is there a difference from each other and from a randomized controlled trial? *Contemporary Clinical Trials*, 38, 130–133.

Wilbur, J., Kolanowski, A. M., & Collins, L. M. (2016). Utilizing MOST frameworks and SMART designs for intervention research. *Nursing Outlook*, 64(4), 287–289.

7

Observational Studies

Geri LoBiondo-Wood

LEARNING OUTCOMES

After reading this chapter, you should be able to do the following:

- Apply critical appraisal criteria to observational studies.
- Differentiate between the types of observational studies.
- Synthesize evidence from observational studies based on a PICO question.
- Summarize information from observational studies to formulate clinical decisions based on evidence.
- Apply findings from observational studies to formulate evidence-based clinical decisions.

KEY TERMS

Case series
Case control study
Cohort study
Cross-sectional study

Exposure
Longitudinal study
Observational study
Outcome

Repeated measures study
Retrospective study

INTRODUCTION

A critical focus for supporting your practice based on evidence is the ability to assess and implement interventions in a specific population that will lead to improvement of health care outcomes. A key benchmark for evidence-based practice (EBP) is intervention studies, but often, health care practice issues do not lend themselves to intervention studies. For example, assume that you are providing care for an adolescent population with cancer-related fatigue from undergoing chemotherapy. You may be interested in the amount of fatigue, variations in fatigue, and timing of patient fatigue in response to chemotherapy. You and your team would not be interested in therapy studies addressing interventions to relieve fatigue until you understand the patterns of fatigue over the course of treatment. Reviewing the evidence from intervention studies would not answer your clinical question. Instead, you and your team would need to examine the factors that contribute to the variability

in adolescent cancer-related fatigue by reviewing observational studies. Observational studies are used when researchers intend to explore events, people, or situations as they naturally occur, or test relationships and differences among variables. Observational studies construct a picture of variables at one point or over a period of time, and the variables are not manipulated or randomized as in a randomized clinical trial (RCT). The purpose of this chapter is to provide an overview of observational designs with questions and issues to raise when critically appraising observational studies for evidence-based practice decision making.

OBSERVATIONAL STUDIES

The major types of observational studies are: Cohort, Case Control, Cross-Sectional, and Survey. When you are reading studies classified as observational, it is key to remember that the researchers did not directly control or manipulate the variables, but measured them as they naturally occurred. Observational studies are considered nonexperimental designs because the researcher does not actively manipulate the variables nor does the researcher randomly assign subjects to groups. Data for observational studies may be gathered on one or several occasions. The data can be gathered prospectively; that is, moving forward in time, looking back in time, or working in a cross-sectional manner. As you review observational studies, the concepts of control and potential sources of bias (see Chapter 5) must be considered.

Observational studies are classified by the features of the study's design and data collection timing, and provide Level IV evidence (see Chapter 2). The information yielded by these types of studies is critical to developing a practice that is based on evidence and may also represent the best evidence available to answer either research or clinical questions.

The variables or conditions in observational studies are referred to as exposure and outcomes. An exposure, past, present, or future, can be either a harmful or beneficial condition that can affect the outcome of illness or health. An outcome is the consequence of the exposure.

Observational research is used when researchers wish to assess exposure to a condition and when manipulation is neither theoretically nor ethically possible, nor the aim of the study. Cigarette smoking and its relationship to lung cancer is a classic example of an observational study. For ethical reasons, individuals cannot be randomized to smoking or nonsmoking groups. Only the outcomes of long-term cigarette use versus nonuse in existing groups can be measured. As you evaluate observational studies, be aware of the sources of bias and internal and external validity issues that may affect study outcomes. Observational studies also are used to provide preliminary data for RCTs.

The conduct of observational studies in health care is appealing. Vast existing data sources, such as electronic chart data or health-related data banks, can be used to study clinical issues. As described in Chapters 3 and 5, there are different types of PICO questions. Answering a PICO question requires a search of the best evidence. Randomized controlled trials and quasi-experimental designs (see Chapter 6) are the gold standard for answering PICO questions about the efficacy or effectiveness of an intervention, but not all PICO questions are focused on the efficacy or effectiveness of an intervention.

TABLE 7.1	**Types of PICO Questions for Observational Studies**
Design	**PICO Question Type**
Cohort	Prognosis, Etiology, Diagnosis, Harm, Intervention
Case Series	Harm, Etiology, Prognosis, Diagnosis
Case Control	Intervention, Prognosis, Case Control

Questions related to diagnosis, prognosis, harm, and etiology may best be answered by reviewing Observational Studies (see Chapter 3). The types of PICO questions related to observational designs are listed in Table 7.1. As you follow the steps of the Iowa Model (Titler et al., 2001) (see Chapter 1) for your evidence-based project, you will most likely include several types of observational studies that must be evaluated within the parameters of their respective design elements as described in this chapter. Before discussing the observational design types that you will review and critically appraise for your evidence-based practice project, it is important to understand the principles underpinning observational study designs. When reviewing observational studies, you will find that the classifications of the designs are, at times, used interchangeably to categorize the components of a study. Fig. 7.1 provides a Decision-Making Algorithm for Observational Studies.

PURPOSE OF OBSERVATIONAL STUDIES

Several key overall concepts are operative in observational studies. One key concept is that the independent variable is not manipulated. It is observed and measured quantitatively, but not manipulated. Observational studies can use data from large data sets or collect data directly from subjects. Data may be collected once or on several occasions.

Observational studies are valuable when relationships, differences, and comparisons need to be assessed. Observational studies also are used to assess comparative effectiveness of interventions. Observational studies are useful when researchers wish to make comparisons among various treatments and randomization of subjects is not possible, practical, or ethical. Large observational studies provide an avenue for researchers to obtain data from a diverse array of patients, providers, and treatment

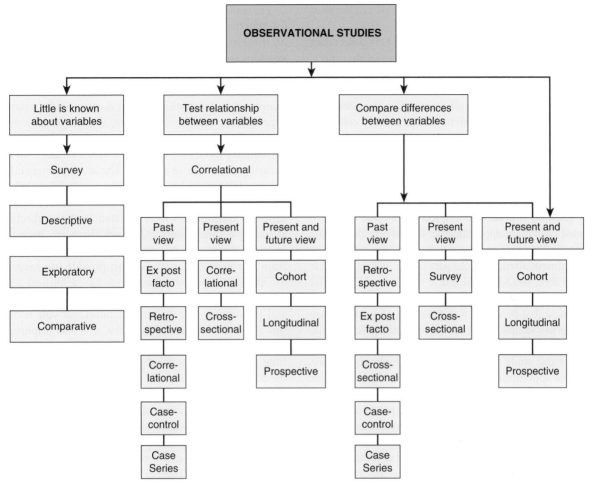

Fig. 7.1 Decision-Making Algorithm for Observational Studies.

facilities (Jagi et al., 2014). Observational studies can test treatments retrospectively, cross-sectionally, or prospectively when studying cohorts in relation to an outcome of interest when a clinical trial and randomization are not possible. Because observational studies lack some of the elements of control, issues related to internal validity such as sampling, instrumentation, and testing must be closely assessed (see Chapter 5). As stated earlier, cohort studies are useful when your clinical question is focused on diagnosis, harm, causation, or prognosis.

EBP TIP

When conducting an EBP project, more than one design may be found and used to answer your PICO question.

TYPES OF OBSERVATIONAL STUDIES

Cohort Studies

Cohort studies also are known as longitudinal, prospective, **repeated measure,** or retrospective studies. Cohort studies are those in which investigators compare or assess the differences or associations between and among subjects who have been exposed or not exposed to an outcome. Cohort studies can be prospective or retrospective. In a prospective cohort study, researchers assess a group of subjects experiencing an exposure; that is, either an intervention or a condition. The sample or study subjects are followed from a present point in time to an outcome at a future point in time (Sessler & Imrey, 2017; Song & Chen, 2010). Data are collected at multiple time points and subjects are not randomized into the study.

In a retrospective cohort study, researchers collect data from a sample of subjects who have previously experienced a disease or condition and identify variables that are thought to be predictive of the disease or outcome identified. Retrospective studies offer researchers the advantage of having data from different groups already collected. The disadvantage of retrospective studies is that the data may be incomplete, inaccurate, or measured in a manner that is not ideal for answering a research or clinical question (Hulley et al., 2013). For example, assume that you are working in an outpatient setting and the focus of your clinical question is understanding the factors that influence missed outpatient appointments. Identifying the factors from the literature can potentially help improve patient appointment attendance. As part of the literature search in this area, you found an article that assessed potential demographic, disease, and practice factors extracted from chart data that predicted nonattendance in primary care settings in a sample of 550,083 subjects (Ellis, McQueenie, McConnachie, Wilson, & Williamson, 2017). The purpose of this study was to assess individuals who missed multiple appointments to identify potential risk markers for vulnerability and poor health outcomes. By including this article and other similar studies, you potentially could identify patient and practice factors that contribute to the likelihood of patients missing practice appointments.

Data for cohort studies are collected at multiple time points. Subjects are not randomized in cohort studies. Subjects are chosen based on inclusion criteria. Examples of inclusion criteria may be disease, age, or treatment. Cohort studies may include subjects who have a condition or disease or may be healthy at the beginning of the study. Because cohort studies include multiple data collection points, attrition—or subject loss—may be a problem. Consequently, it is important to assess if there was loss of subjects to follow up in the overall sample, or if more than one group was in the study, was there differential loss of subjects in one of the groups? In addition to attrition, the measures of the variables may have changed over time. Each of the threats to internal validity outlined in Chapter 5 is important to assess in each study reviewed. You may find that a study did not have mortality issues, but selection issues were a problem. The subjects in cohort studies are not randomized. The lack of randomization also requires an assessment of the threats to external validity (see Chapter 5).

For example, assume you are considering an EBP intervention project for individuals who have sustained an involuntary job loss, and you want to review interventions that have been tested. When conducting your literature review, you find the cohort study by Haynes et al. (2017). In this study, the researchers prospectively examined social rhythms, sleep, dietary intake, energy expenditure, waist circumference, and weight gain over 18 months in a group of individuals who had sustained involuntary job loss. Participants were evaluated on six occasions over the 18 months. The study overenrolled subjects to account for attrition and missing data. When reviewing studies such as this, it is key to assess subject dropout, testing, and issues related to data collection at multiple time points. Although there are issues to consider if using such a study in an EBP project, data from this and similar studies can provide information for the development of evidence-based clinical programs aimed at implementing supportive interventions and prevention of negative outcomes. As you review this and other studies in this area, it is also important to assess how the variables were measured at multiple time points. Was there subject attrition or loss during the course of the study and if so, at what point(s) in the study? Synthesizing the findings—that is, the overall strengths and weaknesses of this and other similar studies—can help you decide what interventions to include in your support program.

A cohort study can provide both prospective and retrospective data. The Nurses' Health Study (NHS I) is a prospective, longitudinal study of nurses' health and health habits. This large study of 121,700 registered nurses began in 1976 and has expanded to two additional iterations, NHS II and NHS III (Bao et al., 2016). In these studies, nurses were sent questionnaires at specific time intervals and queried about their health status and health risk factors related to cancer, cardiovascular disease, and other disease processes. Initially, the study only included female nurses, but it was later expanded to male nurses. The data from this study enable researchers to prospectively gather information on several health issues, such as cardiovascular disease risk factors, cigarette smoking, and diet. Retrospectively, researchers have used this data to study the impact of cigarette smoking and diet on health over time. Data from these studies have assisted and will continue to assist care providers in developing new evidence-based avenues of health assessments and interventions in diabetes and cancer care and further aid development of evidence-based health care strategies for both women and men.

Another example of a retrospective cohort study was conducted by Kok et al. (2017). The study assessed the impact of obesity in cirrhotic patients with septic shock. In this study, the research team was able to assess the relationship of obesity using body mass index (BMI), septic shock, and mortality in a sample of 362 cirrhotic patients. The data obtained were from 1995 to 2015, taken from 28 medical centers across the United States and Canada. As you review the study, you find that it did not include data regarding presence or absence of ascites, potential variability in the sample in terms of treatment, or lack of a more accurate method of assessing obesity other than BMI (Kok et al., 2017). The authors acknowledged that the data do not imply causation but only that an association about the impact of obesity in cirrhotic patients with septic shock could be inferred. The researchers also acknowledged the lack of a more accurate method of assessing obesity other than BMI (Kok et al., 2017).

The studies reviewed point to several of the components of cohort studies, which often cannot be avoided. Because the exposure is not controlled in cohort studies and the samples are not randomized, it is difficult to conclude that the outcomes are truly due to the intervention. When samples are not randomized, it is important to note that researchers can use various statistical procedures to assess for differences in the samples. Other previously identified issues to be aware of that may influence the results of cohort studies are:

- Missing data
- Subjects' similarity
- Sample size
- Reliability of the data collection measures
- Time points of data collection

As you critically appraise cohort studies, remember that they provide useful information for practice. However, it is always important to assess how the variables were measured and identify each of the internal and external validity issues that can affect a study's outcome.

Case Control Studies

Case control studies are those designed to assess the association between an exposure (independent variable) and an outcome (dependent variable). Subjects with the outcome of interest are compared with subjects without the outcome. Examples of exposure can be variables such as drug usage, symptoms, and diagnosis. Examples of outcomes may be a disease or a psychological or physiological condition. Case control studies also may be labeled as *ex post facto, retrospective,* or *comparative.* Case control studies can help identify risk factors related to disease or health conditions. Data from subjects in these studies are typically retrospective; that is, data are abstracted from charts or other databases. Subjects who have the intervention or condition are the controls, and those who do not have the intervention are the cases. Subjects in case control studies are *not* randomized to a group. Although the data are retrospective, these designs can assist you in identifying risk factors related to health and illness outcomes.

Assume you are working in a neonatal intensive care unit, and your team is interested in the best means for identifying risk factors for early-onset Group B streptococcal sepsis in neonates to reduce the health consequences of sepsis. The PICO question leads you to a case control study that was conducted by Santhanam et al. (2017). The objective of this study was to identify the perinatal risk factors for early onset (EOS) of Group B streptococcus (GBS) sepsis in neonates after implementation of a risk-based maternal intrapartum antibiotic prophylaxis (IAP) strategy. Subjects or cases were all babies admitted to the neonatal unit between 2004 and 2013 who were found to have invasive GBS within 72 hours of birth. Babies born before and after the case were considered the controls. The data related to multiple perinatal risk factors for GBS infection were abstracted from records and not from neonates currently being treated in the ICU. The authors concluded that data from this study support the utility of IAP in newborns. The study found that the number of vaginal examinations was a significant risk factor, as were caesarean section and urinary tract infection. When considering the data for application to practice from case control studies such as this, it is essential to assess how similar the sample was in each group, especially since the data were gathered over a long period (2004–2013); how and when the data were collected from the patients' records; and what the IAP policies and interventions were at the time of data collection, since practice changes over time.

Another example is a retrospective case control study conducted by Dabrowski et al. (2017). The aim of this multicenter study was to identify gender differences in risk factors for the development of cancer between men and women with type 2 diabetes. The study included 118 women and 98 men who developed cancer and the same number of subjects who had type 2 diabetes but did not develop cancer. If considering these findings for practice, it would be important to note that the data for the 216 subjects were gathered from charts at different centers over an extended period (January 1998 to September 2016). Additionally, when the subjects were broken down in groups for analysis, there were small numbers of subjects in each cancer diagnosis group related to gender. Also, smoking habits were categorized into never smokers, past smokers and current smokers and reported in percentages. These categories do not provide an indication of the multiple aspects of cigarette smoking, such as number of cigarettes or packs per week and type of cigarette smoked. Also, all comorbidities were classified into three categories: hypertension, hyperlipidemia, and cardiovascular disease. The data from these and other retrospective studies are not useless, but must be understood within the context of current practice and knowledge.

As is the case in both studies identified in this section, data were collected over long periods of time and, over time, policies change, as do interventions and practice. When assessing case control studies, as these studies highlight, it is critical to assess not just the design type but the methodology used in the studies.

EBP TIP

When evaluating observational studies, it is important to assess whether the sample is representative of the population, especially if more than one group is being studied.

Case Series

Case series designs are studies that collect data from a consecutive sample of patients treated in a similar manner without a control group or comparison group. As you read case studies, it is important to understand that these studies include one group only and have no control group, and the sample is one of convenience. Assume you and your clinical team are interested in interventions that would support compensatory memory after a traumatic brain injury (TBI) in your patients. In your search of the literature, you find a case series study conducted by Bos, Babbage, & Leathem (2017)

that aimed to investigate the efficacy of a memory notebook and a smartphone as compensatory memory aids after traumatic brain injury. Individuals with traumatic brain injury commonly experience difficulties with prospective memory. The researchers postulated that an electronic memory notebook could potentially assist prospective memory. The study's methods included one group of seven subjects. Each subject's memory was assessed to establish a no-intervention baseline, followed by training and the intervention with either a smartphone alone or a memory notebook followed by a smartphone. Participants who used a smartphone demonstrated improvement in their ability to complete memory tasks within the assigned time frame. The study results also supported that smartphone use provided additional benefits over a memory notebook. In this study, the participants were not randomized to the study and the sample was one of convenience; the group comprised those willing to participate and the sample size was very small. Although the study identified the potential of smartphone use in the neurorehabilitation sample, it would be important to assess if other studies were completed in this area before a practice change could be instituted. Other studies in this area may have used different designs and larger samples, but similar methods.

When you are conducting an EBP project and you locate case series studies related to your clinical question, it is important to review and consider each of the threats to internal and external validity. Case series also may be labeled as *longitudinal* because the data may be collected from the same group over a period of time. Case series also may be referred to as *case reports*.

Survey Studies

Studies classified as surveys provide information in areas where little is known, often ask broad questions, and generally have large sample sizes. Survey studies can be classified as descriptive, exploratory, or comparative. These terms can be used alone, interchangeably, or together to describe a study. Surveys can be implemented by mail or phone or in person. Surveys focus on studying attitudes, preferences, and behaviors, and assist in establishing patterns and gaining information in an area where little is known. Surveys collect detailed descriptions of variables and use the data to justify and assess conditions and practices or make plans for improving health care practices. You will find that the terms *exploratory, descriptive, comparative,* and *survey* are used alone, interchangeably, or together to describe this type of study design. A survey is used to search for information about the characteristics of particular subjects, groups, institutions, or situations or about the frequency of a variable's occurrence, particularly when little is known about it. Variables in surveys can be classified as opinions, attitudes, or facts. Surveys are useful because they can provide data for the development of intervention studies. Surveys also can be described as comparative when used to determine differences between variables. Survey data can be collected with a questionnaire or an interview and can have large or small samples of subjects drawn from defined populations. Surveys can be either broad or narrow and can be composed of people or institutions. Surveys relate one variable to another or assess differences between variables, but do not determine causation.

The advantages of surveys are that a great deal of information can be obtained from a large population in a fairly economical manner, and that survey research information can be surprisingly accurate. If a sample is representative of the population, even a relatively small number of subjects can provide an accurate picture of the population.

Survey studies do have disadvantages. The information obtained in a survey tends to be superficial. The breadth, rather than the depth, of the information is emphasized. A practice change would not be based on survey data alone.

An example of a survey is a study conducted by Shen et al. (2017). The purpose of the study was to explore the patterns and modes of information and communication sharing among family members on topics related to family well-being. The survey queried 2017 respondents to gain information on family communication patterns. This study found that the most common method of family information sharing was face-to-face, followed by instant messaging and phone, followed by social media sites and video calls. Although this survey included a large number of subjects, the majority were women (92%) and well educated. Data collected were mainly responses to yes/no questions, and the results were reported in categories (i.e., age was categorized as 18–24, 25–44, 45–64, and > 65 years). Although the data reported were categorized, the study's results do provide information for clinicians on information delivery methods that may be useful for specific patient populations. Survey studies such as the Shen study can provide useful background information

for a clinical project, but would require more specific data from other observational studies to answer a clinical question.

> **EBP TIP**
>
> Evidence gained from a survey may be coupled with clinical expertise and applied to a similar population to develop an educational program, to enhance knowledge and skills in a clinical area (e.g., a survey designed to measure the nursing staff's knowledge and attitudes about evidence-based practice where the data are used to develop an evidence-based practice staff development course).

> **EBP TIP**
>
> When you are establishing evidence for practice, each step of a study must be assessed. The design type is one element of assessment. Be aware that possible sources of bias can be introduced at any point in the study.

TYPES OF DATA AND DATA ANALYSES IN OBSERVATIONAL STUDIES

Data found in observational studies can be collected directly from individuals at one or more data points, or data may come from sources such as patient charts, registries, claims, or databases such as Surveillance, Epidemiology, and End Results (SEER), which provides information on cancer incidence, prevalence, and survival statistics in the United States. Observational studies also use data from sources such as Medicare and Medicaid and other large clinical databases. Data also are obtained from self-report questionnaires. These may be continuous data, such as pulse rates or blood pressure readings. Data may also be from questionnaires that require a subject to respond to questions on a Likert scale from "strongly agree" to "strongly disagree." Survey data also can be categorical or dichotomous, such as a "yes" or "no" response.

Data for observational studies such as age, gender, medications, and disease characteristics also are abstracted from patient records. Information found in cohort studies includes actively collected questionnaire data that measure psychosocial variables from a sample or samples of individual subjects who meet a study's inclusion criteria. As you review the data found in cohort studies, consider the data sources, time of data collection, how the data collection was standardized, and whether the measures were reliable and valid.

The sample and sample size in the studies reviewed within this chapter also must be evaluated. Chapter 6 discusses sample size in relationship to testing an intervention. Not all observational studies will have a sample size calculation. For example, surveys do not, but you will find a sample size calculation in a cohort study.

EBP TIP

When you are reviewing cohort studies, remember that the lack of randomization and manipulation of the variables can affect the results and your interpretation of the results.

Data analyses found in observational studies include both descriptive and inferential data (see Chapter 10). The descriptive data will describe the subjects and the study's variable characteristics, while the inferential statistics aid the researcher in drawing conclusions about the data that can be applied to the sample. When you are conducting an EBP project, the data analysis will differ from study to study, based on the variables' level of measurement, the instruments used, and the sample size (see Chapter 10). Because the data analyses vary from study to study, it is important to evaluate not just the statistic used but the issues previously identified, such as sample, instruments, and time period of data collection.

When you are evaluating studies for an EBP, consider the clinical significance as well as the statistical significance (see Chapter 10). The results of the data analysis in each study set the stage for the interpretation, discussion, and limitations sections that follow the results. The "Results" section should reflect analysis of each research question and/or hypothesis tested. The information from each hypothesis or research question should be presented sequentially. The tests used to analyze the data should be identified. If the exact test that was used is not explicitly stated, the values obtained should be noted. The researcher does this by providing the numerical values of the statistics and stating the specific test value and probability level achieved.

CRITICALLY APPRAISING OBSERVATIONAL STUDIES

When moving through the steps of the Iowa Model of Evidence-Based Practice (Titler et al., 2001) and

conducting an EBP project, it is key to assemble the relevant research and related literature to move to effective evidence-based practice changes. It is important to critique each study individually and collectively for strengths and weaknesses. You will find that working with a team to assemble and evaluate the literature will help you move through the steps of the Iowa Model (Titler et al., 2001) more efficiently. When you locate multiple studies related to your clinical question, it may be useful to pair a novice and expert to complete the critiques.

The variables or conditions in observational studies are not controlled using random assignment or manipulation as they are in RCTs. As such, these designs place the interpretation of findings at a higher risk for bias related to the threats of internal and external validity. It is important that you ask several key questions about each study that you review related to your clinical question (Table 7.2). Because observational studies lack the control associated with RCTs, it is important to assess for bias in each step of the study. The assessment of bias requires a review of each of the threats to internal validity (See Chapter 5). First, since the samples in these studies are generally convenience samples and subjects are not randomized into groups, it is important to assess the specific inclusion and exclusion criteria, and assess whether the subjects are similar or dissimilar in relation to the study objectives and demographics at baseline and in all the key elements of treatment or disease condition. Assessment of the measurement of variables is also key. Points to assess are:

- Were the data collected in real time?
- Did data collection depend on subjects' recall (which can lead to recall bias)?
- Were the instruments reliable and valid?
- Were the instruments administered in the same manner to all subjects?
- Were the conditions of data collection similar for all subjects to maximize fidelity?
- If a study collected data on several occasions, was there subject loss?
- How many subjects were approached to participate, and how many agreed?

Subjects may be lost to follow-up if the data collection takes more time than a subject is willing to give. Subject dropout and incomplete questionnaire data may be issues, especially if there are multiple data collection periods. Understanding the questionnaires also can be an issue for subjects. How many questionnaires

TABLE 7.2 Critical Appraisal and Sources of Bias—Observational Studies

Study Component	Potential Source of Bias
Design	Was the design consistent with the research problem or hypothesis studied?
Sample	Observational studies do not include randomization of subjects to groups. Review the inclusion criteria and assess how the subjects' characteristics were alike or dissimilar at baseline on key variables related to the study questions and relevant demographics.
	Was the sample representative of individuals experiencing the same condition or health issue?
	Were the overall characteristics of the subjects alike?
	If more than one group, were their characteristics alike?
	Was the sample size adequate?
	Was the sample representative of the disease or condition being studied?
	Was a sample size calculation using power analysis reported?
	If a cohort study, was there subject attrition?
	If there was a comparison group, were the groups similar to each other regarding data collection points?
	How did the researchers control for bias in the sample?
Instruments	Were the instruments reliable, valid, and consistent with the variables measured?
Data Collection	What were the sources of data?
	Were the data collected consistent with the research question or hypothesis?
	If data were collected over time, was the follow-up adequate and were the time periods valid? Were the data sources the same for all subjects?
	Were the data collection procedures consistent to maximize fidelity?
	If more than one group of subjects, were the groups similar and the data collected at the same time?
	If the data were collected longitudinally as in a cohort, longitudinal, repeated measures study, was the follow-up adequate for the outcome to occur, and were the data collected at the same time for all groups?
Data Analysis	Was there missing data (especially important in cohort studies)?
	Was the analysis consistent with the question?
	Was the follow-up period adequate for the outcomes to occur?
	Was the analysis adjusted for confounding variables?
Findings	Were internal and external validity threats identified and discussed?
	Were the limitations of the study addressed?

were they asked to complete, and what was the length of each? Lengthy questionnaires can contribute to missing data and increase bias in study results. It is difficult to control confounding variables in observational studies. If confounding variables affected the study's outcome, it would be important for researchers to address this in the findings and conclusions sections of the article.

Because there are different types of observational studies with different strategies for sampling, data collection, and analysis, it is important to assess each study. Standardized critical appraisal tools such as those offered by the Center for Evidenced-Based Medicine (CEBM) and Critical Appraisal Skills Programme (CASP) offer tools geared to assessing specific types of designs. For example, the CASP website offers checklists for diagnostic, case control, and cohort studies.

The checklist questions will help guide you through the process of evaluating the different types of designs you will encounter as you answer your PICO question. As you review studies in this category, also consider the key concepts of critical appraisal identified within this chapter and in Box 7.1 and Table 7.2.

IPE TIP

Collaboration is an essential feature of EBP projects. Critical appraisal of studies is most effectively accomplished by having at least two team members critically appraise each study using a CASP or CEBM critical appraisal tool to establish interrater agreement by having them compare their respective critiques and arrive at a consensus about the strength and quality of the evidence.

EBP TIP

Generalizability of studies from one sample to another depends on who participated in a study. When you are reviewing studies, the sample from each study must also be assessed. As you review studies, think about how well the subjects represent the population of interest.

BOX 7.1   Critical Appraisal for Observational Studies

- Was the risk for the dependent variable or outcome the same for the exposed and control groups?
- Were the inclusion and exclusion criteria clearly identified?
- If there was a comparison group, how alike were the subjects in each group in terms of subject characteristics and time of data collection?
- If there was a comparison group, were the subjects in both groups similar in terms of predictive factors related to the study's outcomes?
- When were the data collected for the groups? Practice and interventions change rapidly, so data from studies that are several years old may not be relevant to current therapies.
- Were the data from the groups collected simultaneously?
- Where were the studies conducted, and were the settings similar to your setting?
- Were there any intervening variables?
- What were the threats to internal and external validity (see Chapter 5)?
- Were the data sources from charts or directly from subjects?
- If data were collected from subjects, was subject recall the basis of data collection?
- Are the results relevant to my patients?
- How strong is the relationship between independent variable/exposure and the dependent variable/outcome?

SYNTHESIS

Observational studies do not control interventions as do RCTs. As such, it is important to interpret the results of observational studies with caution. What strengthens the findings of observational studies is ensuring that all components of a study are clearly identified and consistent. Included in the assessment of individual observational studies is consideration not only of the design

but also of the appropriateness of the measures, including the reliability and validity of the measures, sample size, sample characteristics, and analyses. Synthesis of the overall strengths and weaknesses of the findings of a group of observational studies advances your clinical team's ability to make recommendations about the applicability of findings to your clinical population and setting. This will be enhanced by a final assessment that includes the evaluation of similar studies conducted in the same or similar populations, using similar methods that concur with each other.

■ KEY POINTS

- Observational studies lack randomization.
- Observational studies can be prospective, retrospective, cross-sectional, or longitudinal.
- Observational studies also include case control and survey studies.
- If an intervention is included, subjects are not randomized to the intervention nor are the methods controlled as in an RCT.
- Bias or threats to internal and external validity need to be considered in each study reviewed.

REFERENCES

Bao, Y., Bertola, M. L., Lenart, E. B., Stampfer, M. J., Willett, W. C., Speizer, F. E., et al. Origins, methods, and evolution of the Three Nurses' Health Studies. *American Journal of Public Health*, *106*(9), 1573–1581.

Bos, H. R., Babbage, D. R., & Leathem, J. M. (2017). Efficacy of memory aids after traumatic brain injury: A single case series. *Neurorehabilitation*, *41*(2), 463–481.

Dabroski, M., Szymanska-Garbacz, E., Miszczyszyn, Z., Derezinski, T., & Czupryniak, L. (2017). Differences in risk factors of malignancy between men and women with type 2 diabetes: A retrospective case control study. *Oncotarget*, *8*(40), 66940–66950.

Ellis, D. A., McQueenie, R., McConnachie, A., Wilson, P., & Williamson, A. E. (2017). Demographic and practice factors predicting repeated non-attendance in primary care: A national retrospective cohort analysis. *The Lancet*, *2*, e551–e559.

Jagsi, R., Bekelman, J. E., Chen, A., Chen, R. C., Hoffman, K., Shih, Y. C. T., et al. (2014). Considerations for observational research using large data sets in radiation oncology. *International Journal of Radiation Oncology, Biology, Physics*, *90*(1), 11–24.

Haynes, P. L., Silva, G. E., Howe, G. W., Thomson, C. A., Butler, E., Quan, S. F., et al. (2017). Longitudinal assessment of daily activity patterns on weight change after involuntary job loss: The ADAPT protocol. *BMC Public Health, 17*, 793.

Hulley, S. B., Cummings, S. R., Browner, W. S., Grady, D. G., & Newman, T. B. (2013). *Designing Clinical Research* (4th ed.). Wolters Kluwer Lippincott Williams & Wilkins.

Kok, B., Karvellas, C. J., Abraides, J. G., Jalan, R., Sundaram, V., Gurka, D., et al. (2017). *The impact of obesity in cirrhotic patients with septic shock: A retrospective study*. Liver international Epub ahead of print12/17.

Sessler, D. I., & Imrey, B. (2015). Clinical research methodology 2: Observational clinical research. *Anesthesia & Analgesia, 121*(4), 1043–1051.

Shen, C., Wang, M. P., Chu, J., Wan, A., Viswanath, K., Chan, S. S. D., et al. (2017). Sharing family life information through video calls and other information and communication technologies and the association with family well-being: Population-based survey. *JMIR Mental health, 4*(4), e57.

Santhanam, S., Arun, S., Rebekah, G., Ponmudi, N., Chandran, J., & Jana, A. K. 2107. Perinatal risk factors for neonatal early-onset group-B streptococcal sepsis after initiation of risk-based maternal intrapartum antibiotic prophylaxis—A case control Study. *Journal of Tropical Pediatrics, 0.* 1–5.

Titler, M. G., Kleiber, C., Steelman, V., Rakel, B. A., Budrea, G., Everett, L. Q., et al. (2001). The Iowa Model of evidence-based practice to promote quality care clinical care. *Nursing Clinics of North America, 13*(4), 497–509.

8

Systematic Reviews and Clinical Practice Guidelines

Judith Haber, Barbara Krainovich-Miller

LEARNING OUTCOMES

After reading this chapter, you should be able to do the following:

- Differentiate among specific types of systematic reviews.
- Assess the quality of evidence from systematic reviews using standardized critical appraisal tools and criteria.
- Determine clinical relevance of a systematic review's conclusion and recommendation.

- Determine applicability of systematic review recommendations for clinical practice.
- Judge the quality of clinical practice guidelines using standardized critical appraisal tools and criteria.
- Differentiate among clinical practice guidelines developed by professional healthcare organizations and single health care institutions.

KEY TERMS

AGREE II tool
Clinical practice guidelines
Effect size
Fail safe number
Forest plot
Funnel plot
GRADE

Gray literature
Integrative review
Meta-analysis
Narrative review
Publication bias
Rapid review
Realist review

Review
Scoping review
Sensitivity analysis
Systematic review
Test for heterogeneity

Public and private agencies, payors, accreditation bodies, and certification organizations (e.g., Centers for Medicare and Medicaid Services (CMS), Joint Commission, and Magnet Commission) require that organizations demonstrate how they meet the Triple Aim of providing high-quality, cost-effective, and satisfying care experiences. Clinical leaders and their organizations are challenged to document how an evidence-based approach is used to meet those standards. Given the growth in the breadth and depth of clinical research, it is a challenge for you as a clinical leader, and your team, to critically appraise studies that offer the strongest evidence and remain current about clinical practice guidelines, based on the best available evidence, that inform adoption or revision of practices in your clinical setting.

Systematic Reviews and Clinical Practice Guidelines offer clinicians a strategy for translating the best available evidence into clinical practice. Both focus on assessing multiple studies that answer a clinical question (see Chapters 3 and 4). A review is an evidence summary that synthesizes information from quantitative and qualitative research studies, as well as theoretical and conceptual published and unpublished papers (Grant & Booth, 2009). You will note that there is no emphasis on a formal quality assessment of the included literature. Often, a review article aims to map out and categorize existing literature on a specific topic and identify gaps in the literature from which to support further reviews, systematic reviews, evidence-based practice, and quality improvement projects or scholarship initiatives.

TABLE 8.1	Systematic Review and Meta-Analysis
Systematic review	Assessment of a group of quantitative studies with similar designs based on a focused clinical PICO question uses systematic and explicit methods and criteria to search for, identify, critically appraise, and analyze relevant data from the selected studies to summarize and communicate the findings and implications for applicability of evidence in a focused area (Liberati et al., 2009; Moher, Shamser et al., 2015).
Meta-analysis	Statistical approach to analyzing the data from a group of studies included in a systematic review allows statistical integration and combination of data across studies to quantify the effect using a larger sample size, thereby generating a more accurate estimate of the magnitude of the effect that informs an answer to a PICO question (Reith & Malone, 2001).

TABLE 8.2	Types of Reviews
Integrative review	Critical appraisal of the literature in an area of interest that does not include a statistical analysis due to the limitations of the study designs or the heterogeneity of the designs and samples. A systematic approach using explicit criteria is often used (Whittemore & Knafl, 2005).
Narrative review	Review of the literature that includes studies that support an author's perspective and provide a broad background discussion in a focused area of interest. A systematic approach to searching for and appraising papers is often not used (O'Hara, Campbell, & Schmidt, 2015).
Scoping review	A preliminary search and assessment of the potential size and scope of available research literature, including ongoing research. It aims to determine the value of undertaking a full systematic review (Grant & Booth, 2009).
Rapid review	A research methodology that uses shorter time frames than other evidence-based summaries. It provides a timely and valid view of evidence but sacrifices rigor. As such, RRs are both review and assessment, and respond to urgent clinical and public health-related questions (Khangura, Konnyu, Cushman, Grimshaw, & Moher, 2012).
Realist review	Provides explanatory analysis aimed at discerning what works for whom, in what circumstances, and how. Sources can include theoretical, policy, and research literature that combine theoretical understanding with empirical evidence and focus on the context in which an intervention is applied, the mechanisms by which it works, and the outcomes it produces. It is intended to provide the policy and practice community with a rich, yet practical, understanding of complex social interventions when they are planning and implementing programs at a local, regional, or national level (Pawson, Greenhaigh, Harvey, & Walshe, 2005).

Different types of reviews include, but are not limited to, meta-analysis, integrative, and scoping reviews. A systematic review is a collection of research studies based on a clearly focused question that uses a defined search strategy to locate, assess, critically appraise, and synthesize relevant evidence to determine clinical practice recommendations. Other types of evidence reviews, such as rapid, realist, and narrative, also can be found in the literature. The different types of systematic reviews and review types are highlighted in Tables 8.1 and 8.2. Definitions and examples of these reviews and how they differ are described in Table 8.3.

Clinical practice guidelines are systematically developed statements or recommendations that link research and practice and provide an evidence-based best practice guide for clinicians. Systematic reviews of randomized controlled trials (RCTs) are considered to provide Level I evidence on the Evidence Hierarchy, found at the top of the evidence pyramid (see Chapter 2). Clinical Practice Guidelines are based on evidence ranging from Level I meta-analyses to those at Level VIII based on expert opinion.

In Chapters 6 and 7, you were introduced to quantitative designs focused on intervention and observational studies and shown how to critically appraise those studies for quality and applicability to practice. The purpose of this chapter is to expose you to systematic reviews and clinical practice guidelines that assess and/or provide

TABLE 8.3   Examples of Reviews

Type	Example
Integrative review	The purpose of Nurse Practitioner-Led Transitional Care Interventions: An Integrative Review (Mora, Dorrejo, Carreon, & Butt, 2017) was to answer the research question: In community-dwelling adults above age 65, can an NP-led intervention versus standard care decrease hospital readmissions? The authors conducted a literature search and used the integrative review methodology of Whittemore and Knafl (2005) and PRISMA (Moher, Tetzlaff, Altman, & PRISMA Group, 2009). Synthesis of three RCTs, one meta-analysis, and four nonrandomized studies suggests that the interventions, although not exclusively led by NPs, decreased hospital readmission rates. However, the level of evidence is insufficiently high for generalizability and warrants further study.
Narrative review	The objective of the narrative review, Interventions to Promote the Use of Advance Directives: An Overview of Systematic Reviews (Velazquez, Lorda, Portero et al., 2009), was to provide a general overview of research literature in the specific area of patient advance directive completion. The method was to identify, appraise, and synthesize the results of systematic reviews of the literature employing various types of interventions to increase advance directive completion rates. A systematic search of the published and gray literature was conducted; studies were evaluated by two judges for inclusion based on specific criteria. Assessment of quality was not specified, and a statistical analysis of the data was not indicated for this narrative review.
Scoping review	A scoping review is a type of narrative review. Exercise as a Treatment for Fibromyalgia: A Scoping Review (Fink & Lewis, 2017) explored how exercise can reduce pain and promote physical function in adults who have painful conditions due to FMS. The aim was to summarize and disseminate evidence-based findings using a rigorous and transparent method and to identify gaps in the literature. A search strategy with inclusion/exclusion criteria was identified, studies were analyzed for inclusion by two independent judges, and a PRISMA flow diagram summarized the results of the literature search. A method for evaluating the quality of evidence was specified. The evidence was assessed in narrative form without a quality assessment although the studies included in the review were RCTs and meta-analyses. Recommendations for practice based on the "consistent message" across studies were as follows: Exercise alleviates pain and improves physical function in FMS patients, it should be done daily, and it should be individually tailored to meet the needs and tolerance of the patient.
Rapid review	Bryant and Gray (2006) conducted a rapid review demonstrating the positive impact of information support on patient care in primary care. A rapid literature review aimed to identify and summarize key papers that librarians might consult in making the case for investment in information support highlighted the gaps in research evidence. They reported that there was a small body of evidence to demonstrate the positive impact of library and information services on the direct care of patients. They concluded that there is relatively limited research evidence of the impact of information and library services in primary care in comparison with hospital settings.
Realist review	Mukumbang, Van Belle, Marchal, and van Wyk (2017) conducted a realist review of the literature on group-based HIV/AIDS treatment and care models in Sub-Saharan Africa. It is acknowledged that differentiated care models have the potential to manage large volumes of patients on ART. Various group-based models of ART service delivery aimed to decongest local health facilities and increase patient adherence to care guidelines. However, there is little understanding of how these care models work to achieve intended outcomes. The aim of this study was to review the theories explaining how and why group-based ART models work using a realist evaluation framework. They concluded that although they could distill the components of the group-based programs, they could not identify a salient program theory based on the Intervention-Context-Actor-Mechanism-Outcome analysis.

ART, Antiretroviral therapy; *FMS,* fibromyalgia; *PRISMA,* Preferred Reporting Items for Systematic Reviews and Meta-Analyses; *RCTs,* randomized controlled trials.

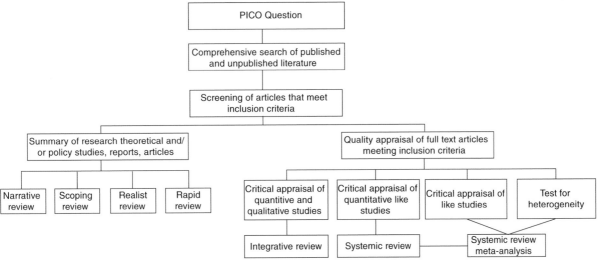

Fig. 8.1 The decision-making algorithm.

evidence from multiple studies focused on answering a specific clinical question. They provide a bridge between research and practice and offer a vital link for developing and implementing quality improvement initiatives.

TYPES OF REVIEWS

Based on a clearly focused clinical question, a systematic review represents a summation and assessment of a group of research studies found in the literature. A systematic review uses systematic and explicit criteria and methods to search for, identify, select, critically appraise, and analyze relevant data from the selected studies to summarize findings in a focused area and make recommendations about applicability of the evidence to practice (Liberati et al., 2009; Moher, Shamseer et al., 2015; Cochrane Handbook for Systematic Reviews, 2016).

Reviews also are guided by a focused question that may target a clinical, policy, or education topic or issue. The Decision-Making Algorithm in Fig. 8.1 provides a guide to assist you in deciding which type of systematic review is appropriate to answer a specific PICO question. A meta-synthesis is a review comprised of qualitative studies that is addressed in Chapter 9.

A plethora of review article types has emerged in clinical and nonclinical disciplines that aim to demonstrate that the authors have searched the literature extensively using a clearly defined search strategy. Review articles cover a wide range of subject matter, including case study, qualitative, and quantitative research findings. Theoretical works and policy reports also can be used as the focus of a review to inform organizational or policy decision making. Tables 8.2 and 8.3 provide definitions and examples of different types of reviews.

Systematic reviews are guided by a PICO question. They use search strategies to identify quantitative studies that address the same clinical question. The goal is to locate relevant studies that provide the strongest evidence with which to answer your clinical question and assess the strengths and weaknesses of the evidence in each study. In your search to find the best available evidence, you and your team will strive to locate RCTs. However, the reality of evidence-based practice is that cohort and case-control studies may provide the strongest level of evidence and design type to answer your clinical question.

Systematic reviews often are completed by clinical teams comprising clinicians, health science librarians, epidemiologists, and statisticians. Each study is critically appraised for validity and reliability—that is, quality, quantity, and consistency of the evidence, using standardized evaluation criteria and tools. The review uses rigorous inclusion and exclusion criteria, an explicit and reproducible search methodology to identify all studies that meet the eligibility criteria, and assessment of the methods and findings from the included studies (Moher et al., 2009) (see Chapter 4). When completing the critical appraisal of a systematic review using one of the standardized critical appraisal tools identified in the IT Resource Box, the following issues are addressed for each study:

- A focused clinical question
- Search strategy
- Sampling issues (e.g., inclusion, exclusion criteria, and sampling strategy)
- Methods and instrumentation
- Sources of bias related to internal and external validity
- Data analysis
- Findings
- Applicability of findings to practice

More than one person on the team will evaluate the studies independently to be included or excluded from the review, sometimes called data extraction. A comprehensive search strategy will include both published and unpublished studies (often called gray literature; see Chapter 4). Similarly, you will note that at least two members of the team serve as independent judges to rate the quality of the studies using a standardized tool such as Consolidated Evidence for Reporting Trials (CONSORT) for the RCT studies and Strengthening the Reporting of Observational Studies in Epidemiology (STROBE) for cohort studies. Once the studies in a systematic review (SR) are assessed for quality and synthesized according to a quality score or focus, practice recommendations are made and presented. The components of the SR are the same as a meta-analysis except there is no statistical analysis of the studies (Fig. 8.2 and Table 8.4).

> **EBP TIP**
>
> A systematic review is an example of a secondary source because it uses previously conducted research studies. The individual studies that make up a systematic review, covered in Chapters 6, 7, and 9, are examples of primary sources.

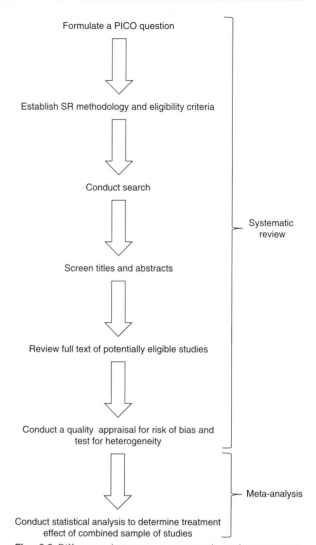

Fig. 8.2 Difference between a systematic review or meta-analysis.

Formulate a PICO question

Establish SR methodology and eligibility criteria

Conduct search

Screen titles and abstracts

Review full text of potentially eligible studies

Conduct a quality appraisal for risk of bias and test for heterogeneity

Conduct statistical analysis to determine treatment effect of combined sample of studies

Systematic review

Meta-analysis

An example of an SR was conducted by Bryant, Alonzo, and Schmillen (2017). The purpose of the SR was to review self-care interventions for adults with heart failure and describe direct provider involvement versus no direct provider involvement on patient self-care behaviors. The review appropriately was based on a PICO question, had predetermined inclusion/exclusion criteria, had a detailed search strategy, and used the Preferred Reporting Items for Systematic Reviews and Meta-Analyses (PRISMA) and the PRISMA Checklist to ensure appropriate reporting of results to minimize bias. A strength of the SR was that assessment of studies

TABLE 8.4	**Systematic Review Components With or Without Meta-Analysis**
Introduction	• Review of background, rationale for conducting the SR, and a clear clinical (PICO) question
Methods	• Search strategy described, inclusion and exclusion criteria identified, databases used for obtaining published and unpublished studies (gray literature), how studies and data were selected and extracted, at least two independent judges specified
	• Description of methods to assess quality and risk of bias, obtaining a quality appraisal score for each individual study and an overall quality score
	• Description of summary methods used to assess the findings descriptively and/or quantitatively
Results	• Number of studies screened and characteristics (e.g., design types)
	• Risk of bias in each study
	• Narrative or quantitative reporting of results for all outcomes being investigated for strength, quality, quantity, and consistency of evidence
	• Table of Evidence (TOE)
Discussion	• Synthesis of findings including the strength, quality, and consistency of the evidence for each outcome, limitations of the studies, conclusions and recommendations for application of findings for practice
	• Synthesis Table of Evidence (TOE)
Funding	• Sources of funding for the systematic review

SR, Systematic review.

for inclusion in the SR was completed independently by the two researchers. Based on grounding in the PICO question and the inclusion/exclusion criteria, 29 studies were selected. Quality appraisal of the studies was completed using the CONSORT for the RCT studies and STROBE for observational studies. The review included 29 studies, of which 23 were RCTs. The remainder were quasi-experimental, cohort, mixed methods, or single-group designs. Studies included heart failure interventions, measurement of a self-care behavioral change as the outcome, and identification of provider involvement in the research. The majority of the studies' quality was moderate to low, which can affect validity. Weaknesses of the studies reviewed included the heterogenous nature of the study designs, interventions and their delivery (lack of consistent provider involvement), confounding strategies between studies, and limited generalizability that precluded statistical analysis of the studies as would be done with a meta-analysis. The authors appropriately concluded that there was a lack of data and quality of research studies to answer the PICO question and demonstrated a significant gap in the literature. Additional rigorous explanatory research that focuses on the patient and provider interactions, including self-care communication strategies is needed.

The individual studies in a systematic review are assessed and presented in a Table of Evidence (TOE) (see Chapter 2); the studies as a group are synthesized in a Synthesis Table of Evidence that highlights the overall strengths and weaknesses of the studies (see Chapter 4). Conclusions are based on your evaluation of the synthesized evidence:

• Does the SR answer my clinical (PICO) question?
• Was the SR unbiased in its methodological quality?
• Are the SR results clinically important?
• Are the results useful and applicable to practice?

If you and your team have decided that the evidence is valid and important, you need to think about how it applies to your clinical question. For example, does your patient or population have characteristics similar to or different from those in the study? Is it feasible to apply the evidence in your practice setting in terms of resources or patient preferences? Recommendations can be made using standardized systems such as the Grading of Recommendations Assessment, Development, and Evaluation (GRADE) system (see Chapter 4). **GRADE** recommendations range from a strong recommendation based on high-quality evidence to a weak recommendation based on very low-quality evidence. You can download the GRADE Handbook (2013) that walks you through making recommendations about applicability to practice based on the extant evidence provided by the systematic review you and your team have critically appraised.

Six recommended standards for SR teams are (Eden et al., 2017):

• Establish the review team with appropriate expertise of users and stakeholders.
• Ensure user and stakeholder input.

- Manage bias and conflict of interest of the reviewers and stakeholders.
- Formulate the topic for the review.
- Provide for peer review of the review protocol.
- Make the review publicly available.

IT RESOURCES

Examples of systematic review standardized critical appraisal tools to make sense of evidence include but are not limited to:

- Center for Evidence-based Medicine (CEBM)—Systematic Review Critical Appraisal Worksheet (cebm.net)
- Critical Appraisal Tools Programme (CASP)—Systematic Review Checklist (casp-uk.net)
- Joanna Briggs Critical Appraisal Tools—Checklist for Systematic Reviews and Research Syntheses (joannabriggs.org)
- Strengthening the Reporting of Observational Studies in Epidemiology (STROBE) Checklists (www.strobe-statement.org)
- Newcastle-Ottawa Assessment Scale–used for critical appraisal of nonrandomized studies included in systematic reviews and meta-analyses (www.ncbi.nln.nih.gov>appb-fm4)

These are free to download and can be used by evidence-based practice teams or individual clinicians.

Regardless of the type of systematic review you are reading, it is important that the authors clearly explain the methods used and that those methods can be replicated (Moher, Stewart et al., 2015). Although systematic reviews are highly useful, they must be reviewed and critiqued carefully for scientific rigor and applicability of the evidence to support continuing a practice or making a minor or major change in practice.

Meta-analysis is a quantitative epidemiological technique and is considered a subset of systematic review (Haidich, 2010). Meta-analysis is used to statistically assess a group of systematically collected and completed studies to derive conclusions about that body of research. The unique component of a meta-analysis is that, in addition to meeting the criteria for a systematic review, it includes a statistical analysis. Systematic methods including a quantitative component are used to minimize bias, thereby providing more reliable findings from which conclusions can be drawn and clinical decisions made. Outcomes of a meta-analysis may include a more precise quantitative estimate of the effect of treatment or risk factor for disease, or other outcomes, than any individual study contributing to the summarized results of all studies included in the pooled analysis. A meta-analysis is a complex and time-consuming undertaking. It is completed by an interprofessional team including, but not limited to, clinicians, statisticians, epidemiologists, public health experts, health science librarians, and informatics experts. You will find that although the components of a meta-analysis sound complicated, your role as a clinician, educator, or administrator does not require an in-depth understanding of statistics. Your job is to read, understand, and most importantly, interpret the findings of a meta-analysis; determine whether the results are of sufficient quality and consistency to consider applying them to practice; and think about their relevance for your patient, student or staff resources, and setting.

The protocol for a meta-analysis, like all systematic reviews, begins with and includes a research or clinical (PICO) question and search strategy. For example, in the meta-analysis in Appendix A by van Driel and colleagues (2016), the objective of the review was to assess the effects of interventions aimed at improving adherence to lipid-lowering drugs, focusing on measures of adherence and clinical outcomes. The clinical question asked, "Which interventions help improve people's ability to take lipid-lowering drugs more regularly?"

Components necessary to incorporate into a meta-analysis are:

1. Method for locating studies to be included in the analysis
2. Methods for evaluating the quality of the studies
3. Statistical testing of the combined sample for assessment of the effect

The clinical question will guide establishment of your search strategy. Identifying the inclusion/exclusion criteria is the first step. You will find that meta-analyses strive to include studies of similar design that provide the strongest evidence and, as such, predominantly include randomized clinical trials that provide Level II evidence. For example, in the van Driel (2016) meta-analysis, the search strategy inclusion and exclusion criteria included only randomized clinical trials of parallel-group or crossover designs (see Chapter 6). Identifying electronic databases and search terms used by databases such as PUBMED, EMBASE, PsychINFO, CINAHL, and the Cochrane Register of Controlled Trials (CENTRAL) is extremely important in searching the published literature.

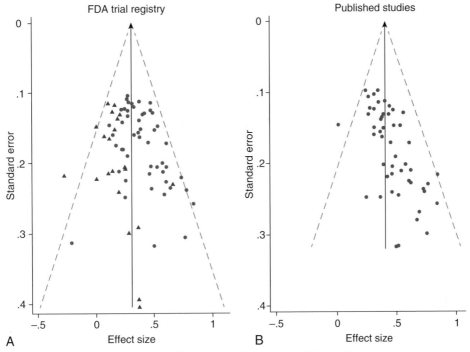

Fig. 8.3 A and B funnel plots illustrating publication bias.

You will observe that the search results are like an inverted pyramid; the search starts off by locating many more studies than are used in the meta-analysis. Limits that decrease the number of studies include design type, language restrictions, and funding source. Based on the inclusion/exclusion criteria, studies are screened for inclusion by at least two independent judges.

The inclusion of unpublished studies, often called gray literature, in the search strategy is more common in meta-analyses than in other types of SRs. Inclusion of unpublished studies is thought to decrease publication bias associated with including only published studies (Mavridis & Salanti, 2014). Evidence synthesis of published studies might only produce publication bias, which is misleading results, since the set of published data may not be a representative sample of the overall evidence. For example, it has been found that commercially funded research is more likely to be published if the research findings are positive, whereas publicly funded research is more likely to be published irrespective of the results (Higgins, 2013). To overcome publication bias, mandatory registration of trials has been advocated regardless of publication status. Unpublished clinical trials can be found in the Clinical Trials

Register (ClinicalTrials.gov; www.anzctre.org.au/) (see Chapter 4).

Publication bias can be assessed using a funnel plot. This is a graph based on odds ratios (ORs) (see Chapter 10) that detects small study treatment effects. Lack of observed studies in certain regions of the plotted data that correspond to nonsignificant results may indicate that studies with nonpositive findings have not been published. If you examine Fig. 8.3A and B, you will see an example of symmetrical and asymmetrical funnel plots. Fig. 8.3A illustrates a symmetrical funnel plot of a Federal Drug Administration (FDA) registry of 73 published and unpublished studies comparing 12 antidepressants to placebo (Turner, 2008). Fig. 8.3B illustrates an asymmetrical funnel plot of 50 studies published in scientific journals, skewed to the right side of the vertical axis, suggesting publication bias. Unpublished data, which can include studies, conference proceedings, abstracts, and personal communications, usually have not been through a peer review process.

Another test, the Fail-Safe Number, also is used to correct for publication bias. Meta-analysis teams need to be concerned about studies that have been conducted but not published because of negative or neutral results.

Risk of bias graph: review authors' judgments about each risk of bias item presented as percentages across all included studies

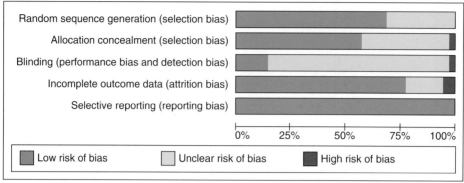

Fig. 8.4 Risk of bias graph.

One way to assess for publication bias is to report the fail-safe N that uses an odds ratio (OR) (see Chapter 10) to calculate the number of studies reporting no treatment effect that would need to be included in the analysis to reduce the pooled odds ratio to a nonsignificant value. When the fail-safe N is small, the results of the meta-analysis are uncertain and easily could change if a small number of unpublished studies with negative treatment effects were identified and included in the meta-analysis statistical testing. On the other hand, if the fail-safe N is large, many studies would be needed to overturn the treatment effect results and you would feel much more confident about the reported findings.

It is also very important to examine whether and how the researchers assessed the quality of the studies selected for inclusion in the meta-analysis. Measuring the quality of the studies is essential since bias exists in all study designs, even though researchers attempt to minimize it. Even research from established teams published in high-impact journals can have methodological flaws, biases, and limited generalizability and applicability. Using a quality appraisal tool to evaluate sources of bias allows uniformity in the critical appraisal process of the findings and conclusions (Smith & Noble, 2014). You want to document that quality appraisal of studies was completed by at least two independent judges using a standardized quality assessment tool. For example, van Driel and colleagues performed a risk of bias assessment using the Cochrane "Risk of Bias" Tool (Higgins, 2011). Risk of bias categories included:

- **selection bias** by assessing the method of random assignment and process of allocation concealment

- **performance and detection bias** or blinding of participants, providers, and outcomes assessors
- **attrition bias** or assessing how incomplete data were managed
- **reporting bias** or assessing whether all intended outcomes were reported

Each study was rated "high risk," "low risk," or "unclear risk" for each of those bias risk domains. In Appendix A, Figure 2 provides a methodological quality summary for the studies included in the van Driel meta-analysis. Fig. 8.4 illustrates a Risk of Bias graph based on the bulleted risk categories mentioned previously. Others like Reith and Malone (2001) modified the Chalmers (1981) quality assessment tool for clinical trials and each study received an individual quality score where points were assigned to each category based on evidence of randomization, blinding, fidelity, statistical reporting, identification of withdrawals, and study funding or sponsorship. A higher score indicated a higher quality study.

EBP TIP

When studies other than randomized controlled trials are included in a systematic review, quality appraisal tools specific to the design types should be used. For example, Strengthening the Reporting of Observational Studies in Epidemiology (STROBE) is used for quality appraisal of observational designs with high quality (7–8 criteria met), moderate quality (4–6 criteria met), and low quality (1–3 criteria met). The New Castle-Ottawa Quality Assessment Scale can be used in SRs for the quality appraisal of cohort and case-control studies.

Quantitative synthesis by testing the effect of the intervention is what differentiates a meta-analysis from other types of systematic reviews. Examining the heterogeneity of studies is a key component of a meta-analysis. The test of heterogeneity, sometimes referred to as the test of homogeneity, is calculated often using the Chi Square to determine that the hypothesis that each study is measuring is similar across studies and for the same population. If the null hypothesis is supported, and the studies do not differ significantly from each other at the $p < .05$ level of significance, the studies would be considered similar and appropriate for a combined statistical analysis. If the null hypothesis was rejected, then the studies would be considered too diverse or heterogenous to be pooled legitimately and analyzed statistically as a pooled sample in a meta-analysis, and might conclude as a nonquantitative systematic review (see Chapter 10). When results from the test of heterogeneity reject the null hypothesis, revealing that at least some of the studies are significantly different from the others in terms of design, results, or influence in the analysis, sensitivity analysis can be used to examine the effect of those studies that are "outliers."

Evaluating the treatment effect is an important component of a meta-analysis. The focus of combining studies in a meta-analysis is determining the treatment effect or effect size for each study. The effect size is a measure of the degree to which the null hypothesis is false; that is, the treatment makes a significant difference. Various statistics are used to calculate effect sizes, including t-tests, F-values, and correlation coefficients. One commonly used effect size measure that you will see reported in the literature and that you need to be able to interpret is Cohen's D, which derives the effect size for continuous data (e.g., HgbA1c levels) by subtracting the mean of the treatment group from the mean of the control group in each study and dividing by the pooled standard deviation. Cohen (1988) classifies effect sizes of 0.2 as small, 0.5 as moderate, and 0.8 as large. In the case of binary or dichotomous variables (e.g., quit smoking vs. did not quit smoking), the odds ratio (OR) and 95% confidence intervals (CI) are used to express the magnitude (size) of the treatment effect (see Chapter 10).

Once individual study effect sizes have been calculated, the effect sizes are pooled to obtain a pooled treatment effect or effect size that is reported in different ways, depending on the types of variables (continuous or dichotomous) involved and related statistical tests used. One of the most common graphics you will see is the forest plot, which features a visual reporting of the individual study ORs and the CIs as well as the pooled OR and CI for the combined studies, as illustrated in Fig. 8.5. An advantage of a meta-analysis is that combining the results of a group of studies results in a larger sample size, so you have more power to detect the magnitude of the effect of the intervention. The question you and your team need to answer is, "How large and precise is the treatment effect?"

The meta-analysis by van Driel (Appendix A) provides dichotomous data for the PICO question, "Which interventions improve people's ability to take lipid-lowering medications more regularly?" Results were reported as OR with 95% CIs. For continuous data, mean difference and standard deviations of pre- and post-measures were reported. For analysis, the types of interventions were categorized. For example, Fig. 8.5 reports ORs and CIs for seven individual RCTs, and pooled data for the seven studies comparing the effect of intensified treatment versus usual care in improving adherence to lipid-lowering medication. If you inspect Fig. 8.5, you will see on the left side the subgroup of studies all testing the same hypothesis and the sample size in the intensified versus the usual care groups. In the middle of Fig. 8.5, you will see the vertical axis line of no effect (1) that reports the individual effect and OR (little squares), and the individual study CI (horizontal line with each little square). The larger the square, the larger the contribution of that study to the measure of effect. On the right of the vertical axis is the weight contributed by each study and the CI for each study. Studies with smaller samples generally contribute less to the estimates of overall effect (Haidich, 2010). The summary combined treatment effect (OR) is located at the bottom of the vertical axis as a diamond, with its vertical points representing the pooled effect and the horizontal points representing the CI for the overall effect. Analysis of the data reveals that five of the seven studies report ORs favoring the effect of intensified treatment; the combined OR at the bottom of the vertical axis reveals that intensified patient care has an overall significant effect on improving medication adherence at 6 months compared to usual care at a 95% confidence level. Chapter 10 addresses data analysis for systematic reviews in greater depth.

Comparison 1: Intensified patient care vs. usual care; Outcome 1: Medication adherence at ≤ 6 months

Review: Interventions to improve adherence to lipid-lowering medication

Comparison: 1 Intensified patient care vs. usual care

Outcome: 1 Medication adherence at ≤ 6 months

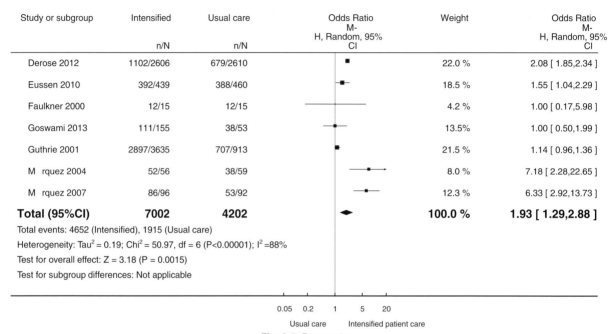

Study or subgroup	Intensified n/N	Usual care n/N	Odds Ratio M- H, Random, 95% CI	Weight	Odds Ratio M- H, Random, 95% CI
Derose 2012	1102/2606	679/2610		22.0 %	2.08 [1.85,2.34]
Eussen 2010	392/439	388/460		18.5 %	1.55 [1.04,2.29]
Faulkner 2000	12/15	12/15		4.2 %	1.00 [0.17,5.98]
Goswami 2013	111/155	38/53		13.5%	1.00 [0.50,1.99]
Guthrie 2001	2897/3635	707/913		21.5 %	1.14 [0.96,1.36]
M rquez 2004	52/56	38/59		8.0 %	7.18 [2.28,22.65]
M rquez 2007	86/96	53/92		12.3 %	6.33 [2.92,13.73]
Total (95%CI)	**7002**	**4202**		**100.0 %**	**1.93 [1.29,2.88]**

Total events: 4652 (Intensified), 1915 (Usual care)

Heterogeneity: Tau^2 = 0.19; Chi^2 = 50.97, df = 6 (P<0.00001); I^2 =88%

Test for overall effect: Z = 3.18 (P = 0.0015)

Test for subgroup differences: Not applicable

0.05   0.2   1   5   20

Usual care   Intensified patient care

Fig. 8.5 Forest plot.

EBP TIP

As a DNP student beginning your DNP project, you should include in your search strategy search terms and filters to locate meta-analyses that provide the highest level of evidence to answer your PICO question.

Integrative Reviews

An integrative review is a critical appraisal of the literature in an area that does not include a statistical analysis due to the limitations of the study designs or the heterogeneity of the designs and samples. A systematic approach still is used to locate and evaluate the studies (see Chapter 4). Integrative reviews are the broadest category of reviews and can include theoretical literature, research literature, or both. An integrative review can include quantitative or qualitative research, or

both. When a review includes studies using qualitative and quantitative designs, it is called a mixed-methods review.

An example of an integrative review was conducted by Blakeman and Stapleton (2017), who explored the extant literature for key features of prodromal and acute myocardial infarction (MI) fatigue experienced by women. Based on Whittemore and Knafl's (2005) approach and the Theory of Unpleasant Symptoms, they conducted a comprehensive search, screening, and analysis of the evidence. The search revealed diverse types of evidence that included nonexperimental and qualitative studies (all of which were considered to provide Level II evidence) and doctoral dissertations. They used the Johns Hopkins Nursing Evidence-Based Practice Model (Dearholt & Dang, 2012) for their quality appraisal of the 21 studies that met the inclusion criteria. Results were summarized by fatigue characteristics such as frequency, quality, distress and intensity, and timing. They concluded that fatigue is the most common prodromal MI symptom experienced by women and is also a common acute symptom. The authors appropriately point out the limitations posed by inconsistent nomenclature or tools to differentiate reporting of fatigue when assessing women, and they highlight the need for additional research to fully explore fatigue and understand the multidimensional nature of MI-related fatigue. The high rate of morbidity and mortality that is exacted by MI makes the evidence reported by this team especially relevant to clinical practice and the assessment of women who often present with atypical prodromal symptoms of myocardial infarction.

If you and your team have decided that the evidence is valid and important, you need to think about how it applies to your clinical question. For example, does your patient or population have characteristics similar to or different from those in the study? Is it feasible to apply the evidence in your practice setting in terms of resources or patient preferences? Recommendations can be made using standardized systems such as GRADE (see Chapter 4). GRADE recommendations range from a strong recommendation based on high-quality evidence to a weak recommendation based on very low-quality evidence. You can download the GRADE Handbook (2013) that walks you through making recommendations about applicability to practice, based on the extant evidence provided by the systematic review you and your team have critically appraised.

Critically Appraising Systematic Reviews

When you are critically appraising an integrative review, systematic review, or meta-analysis, remember the differences between the types of methods. Using a specific search strategy, reviews provide a broad overview of the literature related to a focused PICO or clinical question. A weakness is that it often does not include quality appraisal of individual conceptual or policy literature or of quantitative and/or qualitative studies included in the review. Systematic reviews without a meta-analysis, as illustrated in Fig. 8.2, also begin with a focused PICO or clinical question, should use an exhaustive search strategy that targets the published and gray literature, and should use independent judges to screen studies for inclusion and quality appraisal. The unique feature of a systematic review that is a meta-analysis is the statistical analysis to determine a single combined pooled estimate of effect, with a related CI for each relevant outcome.

Judging the credibility of integrative reviews, systematic reviews, and meta-analyses is essential. We will focus on critical appraisal of systematic reviews and meta-analyses in the following discussion. Use the Critical Appraisal Box as a guide for what we will discuss in this section of the chapter. The strengths and weaknesses of data for each critical appraisal component can be extracted and summarized in a TOE similar to the example in Chapter 2.

Critical appraisal begins by assessing whether the study poses a clearly stated question. For example, can you tell from reading the question what type of question is being asked, and what is the exposure, such as a therapy or diagnostic test, and are the outcome(s) of interest clearly stated?

The search strategy is the next SR critical appraisal component. A high-quality search is comprehensive and exhaustive. It identifies clearly stated inclusion and exclusion criteria, search terms, key words, MESH terms used by specific databases, and filters to narrow the search and align with inclusion and exclusion criteria. A high-quality search includes published and unpublished literature using major bibliographic databases such as PubMed, Cochrane, CINAHL, and EMBASE, as well as dates searched. The search also should include evidence that the researcher attempted to minimize publication bias by reviewing reference lists from relevant studies, contacting experts particularly to inquire about unpublished studies, review of conference proceedings, and search of the Clinical Trials Register (see Chapter 4). As discussed earlier in the chapter, funnel plots (see Fig. 8.3A and B) may be used to illustrate that publication bias has been evaluated. Make sure that at least two independent judges have screened the identified studies and arrived at a consensus about those to be included in the SR.

It is important for you and your team to determine whether a quality appraisal to evaluate the quality of the included studies was completed by at least two independent judges using a standardized quality appraisal tool appropriate to the type of clinical question and design. It is common for each study to have a quality rating, either numerical or high/medium/low, and for there to be an overall quality rating for the combined group of studies. When you are critically appraising a systematic review or meta-analysis, you will want to document the individual and collective quality appraisal data on your TOE. For example, in the SR by Bryant and colleagues (2017) assessing the impact of provider involvement on heart failure self-care, the quality assessment based on CONSORT and STROBE identified 10 studies as providing high-level quality of evidence, 10 moderate-level, and 9 low-level.

Do not assume that because a systematic review is comprised of RCTs or includes a meta-analysis, you will have confidence in the strength and quality of the evidence provided by the results. When you and your team critically appraise the SR, common reasons for low confidence include:

- An unfocused clinical/PICO question that guided implementation of the SR
- Lack of description of a detailed search strategy that included published and unpublished literature
- Studies with high risk of bias
- Small sample size for individual and pooled studies
- Studies that differ in hypotheses or research questions tested
- Study subjects who may differ in important ways from those in whom we are interested
- Inconsistent results across studies

You will find that the studies included in an SR will vary in design and results. This may result in a descriptive evaluation of the studies in a systematic review. In the Bryant et al. (2017) SR, combining studies for analysis was problematic because of the heterogenous nature of the designs, type of educational delivery, and confounding strategies between studies. When studies are similar enough in design and hypothesis being tested or research question being answered, they potentially can be combined for quantitative analysis in a meta-analysis.

When you and your team are critically appraising an SR that includes a meta-analysis, it is important to assess whether the appropriate criteria were met to justify proceeding with the statistical testing of effect associated with meta-analysis. The main question is whether the results were similar from study to study. The results of the studies should be similar or homogenous. As discussed earlier in the chapter, the test for heterogeneity estimates whether the differences are significant; the chi square test should report a $p > .05$ difference supporting that the results of the studies are similar. If the test for heterogeneity reveals that there is a significant difference, a sensitivity test can be used

to systematically eliminate studies that account for the differences until the test for heterogeneity reveals the required homogeneity of the studies to be included in the effect analysis.

In the van Driel (2016) meta-analysis in Appendix A, heterogeneity was evaluated by first assessing the comparability of included studies in terms of population, setting, and outcomes using the Chi Square statistic. They also performed sensitivity analysis for the pooled results by removing studies that contributed to heterogeneity. The effect size is calculated using odds ratios and confidence intervals for dichotomous data and t-tests, F-values, and correlation coefficients for continuous data. Forest plots, like the one in Fig. 8.5, provide for visual interpretation of the overall and/or subgroup results. Subgroup analyses are particularly common when no overall effect is found. Subgroups may be analyzed by type of design, intervention, setting, or quality.

When the results are reported, you want to think about whether the evidence provided by the findings aligns with the authors' conclusions. Consider whether the conclusions are justified by the strength, quality, and consistency of the evidence. Remember that the essence of evidence-based practice is integrating the best available evidence with patient preferences (values, choices, resources, and concerns) and clinical judgment. There are high- and low-quality systematic reviews just as there are for individual studies. Clinical leaders must evaluate whether the conclusions and recommendations are justified and appropriate for informing clinical practice decisions based on the strength and quality of the evidence presented in the SR. For example, the authors of the van Driel meta-analysis in Appendix A appropriately concluded that the evidence in their review demonstrates that intensification of patient-care interventions improves short- and long-term medication adherence as well as total cholesterol and LDL-cholesterol levels. They also concluded that the studies generally were of low risk to bias; using the GRADE system, the evidence for outcomes was rated high quality for long-term adherence (>6 months) and reduction in total cholesterol and moderate quality for short-term medication adherence and LDL cholesterol (up to 6 months). For the outcome total cholesterol levels (<6 months), the evidence was downgraded to low quality. As such, the recommendation supported implementation of team-based intensification of patient care interventions for improving outcomes related to this clinical issue.

Final critical appraisal considerations are pragmatic and focus on applicability:

- Is the study population similar to that of my patients?
- What are the risks and benefits of implementing the findings in my setting for my patient population?
- Is it feasible to implement the findings in my setting?

- Does my organization have the resources to implement the findings reported in this SR? What is the cost/benefit?
- What are the values and preferences of my patients and their families?

CRITICAL APPRAISAL CRITERIA

1. Does the review explicitly address a focused clinical/PICO question?
2. Does the PICO question match the studies included in the review?
3. Are the inclusion and exclusion criteria clear and comprehensive?
4. Was the search for relevant studies exhaustive, including both published and gray literature?
5. Were there at least two independent judges assessing whether the studies met the criteria for inclusion in the review?
6. What is the level of evidence provided by the studies included in the review?

7. Was a quality appraisal conducted according to specific criteria to assess for risk of bias?
8. If the studies were critically appraised individually, were the strengths and weaknesses clearly reported?
9. Were the appropriate analyses completed to determine whether a meta-analysis could be conducted?
10. If a meta-analysis was conducted, how large was the effect, and did the review address confidence in effect estimates?
11. Was a synthesis reported for the overall strengths and weaknesses of the included studies?
12. Are the conclusions and recommendations relevant and supported by the review?

CLINICAL PRACTICE GUIDELINES

Clinical Practice Guidelines (CPGs) are systematically developed statements and recommendations intended to optimize care and link research and practice by providing a guide for practitioners. "CPGs are informed by a systematic review of evidence and include an assessment of the benefits and harms of alternative care options." (IOM, 2011, p. 25–26). CPGs are being developed globally and used to reduce health care service variability and improve resource utilization and clinical outcomes. CPGs are developed by organizations such as the U.S. Preventive Services Taskforce (USPTF), clinical specialty organizations, and providers. Guidelines also are used by clinicians at the point of care or system-level administrators conducting cost/benefit analyses to improve clinical outcomes, reduce cost of care, and create satisfying patient and provider experiences. In the Iowa Model (see Chapter 2), CPGs often function as knowledge-focused triggers that, coupled with internal quality improvement (QI) data from problem-focused triggers, propel clinical teams and QI committees to consider critically appraising a new CPG (see Chapter 2). For example, based on QI data for a sample of adult patients at high risk for diabetes, the QI team of a large primary care system was considering a policy change

regarding allocation of fiscal resources for a routine diabetes screening and lifestyle modification program for adults at high risk for diabetes as part of cardiovascular risk assessment. Their search for a recent CPG found that in 2015, the USPSTF updated its 2008 recommendation statement that found insufficient evidence to assess the benefits and harms of diabetes screening for asymptomatic adults who did not have hypertension (Siu, 2015). Siu (2015) reports that since the 2008 recommendation, six new lifestyle intervention studies that incorporate long-term follow-up consistently have shown the benefit of lifestyle modifications to prevent or delay diabetes progression and improve clinical outcomes. As such, the newer evidence led the USPSTF to conclude that there is a moderate net benefit to measuring blood glucose in adults who are at increased risk for diabetes, and it recommends screening (B recommendation) as part of cardiovascular risk assessment in adults aged 40 to 70 years who are overweight or obese. It also is recommended (B recommendation) that clinicians offer or refer patients with abnormal blood glucose levels to intensive behavioral counseling to promote a healthy diet and physical activity (Siu, 2015). Based on the USPSTF Grade B recommendation, the clinical team was confident about the benefit and decision to recommend allocation of resources to offer screening and lifestyle modification. A cost/benefit analysis would be the next step in the decision-making process.

It is important to understand the issues surrounding emergence of CPGs and the factors contributing to their use or lack of use by nurse practitioners, physicians, and other health care professionals. The rapid growth in guideline development has resulted in a wide variation in the rigor of CPGs and reporting of how the guideline was formulated and how the recommendations are graded. Keep in mind that CPGs can range from scientifically rigorous based on Level I meta-analysis evidence to Level VII expert opinion. Pragmatically, CPGs sometimes are developed and written in complicated formats that clinicians and organizations find challenging to implement, which limits effectiveness in influencing clinical practice and improving patient outcomes. Because CPGs vary in quality, it is essential that health care teams and organizations appraise the quality of a CPG to determine whether it should be implemented in a primary care practice, home care setting, or acute care institution. The IOM (2011) has identified 8 standards for developing trustworthy CPGs:

1. Establishing transparency
2. Management of conflict of interest
3. Guideline development group composition
4. Clinical practice guideline (systematic review intersection)
5. Establishing evidence foundations for and rating strength of recommendations
6. Articulation of recommendations
7. External review
8. Updating

EBP TIP

Many CPGs are very long and address multiple clinical issues. You and your team may find that only specific sections of a CPG apply to your specific clinical issue, type of practice, and setting.

Completing a CPG appraisal will enhance your team's position in making a convincing argument to your health care colleagues and/or administrators about why or why not to adopt a CPG as a policy or practice standard. For example, the evidence-based CPG in Linear Growth Measurement of Children (Foote, Brady, Burke et al., 2009) used the USPSTF recommendation rating system for each recommendation made with related supporting rationale and evidence documentation. Ratings for recommendations ranged from A for components of the height measuring instruments to E for use of a tape measure to gauge the height of infants and children. The E recommendation rating states, "There is good evidence to support exclusion of the practice" (p. 2). The accompanying rationale and evidence documentation states, "Using a tape measure by any method to obtain a length measurement results in poor intraexaminer and interexaminer reliability" (p. 2).

The National Comprehensive Cancer Network (NCCN), a consortium of 21 cancer centers worldwide, is an organization that develops guidelines. The NCCN CPGs are accessible at www.nccn.org. For example, the NCCN sponsored guideline for Supportive Care has multiple CPGs within that broad category, including cancer-related fatigue, antiemesis, and survivorship.

Guidelines should be informed by the best available evidence and provide clinicians with an algorithm for clinical management or decision making for specific diseases (e.g., diabetes), conditions (e.g., obesity, hypertension), or treatments (pain management). Evidence-based practice guidelines are those developed using the scientific process. This includes convening an interprofessional team of experts in the field who are charged with developing guidelines and making recommendations using a scientific protocol similar to the steps of a systematic review (see Table 8.4). Ideally, evidence-based CPGs should comprise Level I systematic reviews (SRs) that are meta-analyses providing high-quality supporting evidence. When systematic reviews are not extant, teams developing an evidence-based CPG search the literature for the best available evidence provided by individual studies using Level II, III, and IV RCTs and quasi-experimental, cohort, and case-control designs.

For a variety of reasons, not all areas of clinical practice have a sufficient research base. You will observe that expert-based practice guidelines that provide Level VII evidence are developed by consensus panels and expert opinion groups. When this approach is used, nationally known experts in a field are convened to develop a CPG based on their opinions along with research evidence

BOX 8.1 Criteria for Developing a CPG

- Developed by a knowledgeable, multidisciplinary panel of experts and representatives from key affected groups
- Considers important patient subgroups and patient preferences, as appropriate
- Includes a structured abstract about the guideline and its development
- Includes systematically developed statements that include recommendations and strategies that assist clinicians and patients in making decisions about appropriate care for specific clinical conditions
- Produced under the sponsorship of government agencies at the local, state, or federal level
- Produced under the sponsorship of professional organizations (e.g., medical, nursing, pharmacy), public or private foundations, or health plans
- Guided by a systematic literature search and review of the existing scientific evidence published in peer review journals
- Includes critical appraisal of scientific evidence using standardized critical appraisal tools
- Includes graded recommendations based on the strength and consistency of evidence
- Developed, reviewed, or revised within the past 5 years

available to date. If only limited research is available for inclusion, a rationale should be presented for the practice recommendations made.

Like research studies, CPGs must be critically appraised by clinical teams like yours before adoption and implementation. Despite the limitations of CPGs as they evolve as scientific tools, there has been significant progress in improving evidence-based guideline development, implementation, and evaluation as important components of clinical decision making.

Clinical Practice Guidelines frequently are located on organizations' websites and are either open-access or available only to members. More accessible CPGs have been available through the Agency for Healthcare Research and Quality, which has supported the National Guideline Clearinghouse (NGC) (www.ahrq.gov>cpi>guideline.gov). As of this printing, the NGC will no longer be available due to ceased federal funding. Use of the above link will redirect you to a new guideline repository, when established. Box 8.1 provides a summary of the key features and criteria for development of a CPG. The next two IT Resource Boxes provide a

selected list of digital databases and organization websites where you can locate CPGs. These lists provide only a small sample of the abundantly available CPG dissemination and development resources.

IT RESOURCES

Selected Databases for Locating Clinical Practice Guidelines

- PubMed: Access through your health care setting's library or at http://www.ncbi.nlm.nih.gov/pubmed
- Guideline summaries: Access at https://www.guideline.gov/search?f_DocType = 0&fLockTerm = Guideline%20Summaries
- TRIP database: Turning Research into Practice can be accessed at https://www.tripdatabase.com/
- SCOPUS: Access via free onsite registration at https://www.scopus.com/home.url/
- United States Preventive Taskforce (USPTF): http://www.the communityguide.org/index/html
- Primary Care Clinical Practice Guidelines: http://medicine.ucsf.edu/education/resed/ebm/practiced.guidelines.html
- Cochrane Library: https://www.cochranelibrary.com/
- International Guideline Network: https://www.g-i-n.net/
- International Guidelines Library: http://www.g-i-n.net/library/international-guidelines-library/international-guidelines-library

IT RESOURCES

Selected Specialty Clinical Practice Guidelines Databases

- American College of Physicians: http://www.acponline.org/clinical_information/guidelines
- American Academy of Pediatrics: http://aappolicy.aapublications.org/
- American Psychiatric Nurses Association: https://www.apna.org.pages
- Oncology Nursing Society: http://www.ons.org
- University of Iowa Gerontological Nursing Interventions Research Center: http://www.nursing.uiowa.edu/excellence/nursing.interventions/
- American College of Cardiology: http://www.acc.org/quality and science/clinical/statements.htm
- Veterans Administration: https://www.va.gov/health/
- Ministry of Health Services, British Columbia, Canada: http://www.gov.bc.ca/health/

IMPLEMENTING CLINICAL PRACTICE GUIDELINES IN CLINICAL PRACTICE

Locating and reviewing a guideline in a clinical area can be overwhelming. Even after a guideline has been located, it can be a challenge to wade through the lengthy document and determine the critical clinical information. Usually the background information including the sponsoring organization, funding source, guideline development panel, and dates covered by the literature review is evident. Evidence-based CPGs also include the system used for quality appraisal and recommendations (e.g., USPSTF rating system).

Even more challenging is locating the relevant sections of the guideline and assessing whether there is transparency about the rigor of the evidence review and critical appraisal, whether the evidence supporting the recommendations is explicit, and identifying the benefits and harms associated with the intervention or management protocol. CPGs based on low-quality evidence such as expert opinion have the potential to be of no benefit or even harmful to patients, so they need to be appraised carefully before implementation (Alonso-Coello et al., 2010).

The 2017 Guidelines for the Prevention, Detection, Evaluation, and Management of High Blood Pressure in Adults (Whelton, Carey et al., 2017), is an update of the classic Seventh Report of the Joint National Committee on Prevention, Detection, Evaluation and Treatment of High Blood Pressure (JNC7), published in 2003. Developed jointly by the American College of Cardiology and the American Heart Association, it provides a good example of an interprofessional CPG representing experts from a broad array of backgrounds that demonstrates strong transparency about the rigor of its method, critical appraisal of the evidence, and recommendations. This CPG is comprehensive and incorporates new information regarding blood pressure (BP)-related risk of cardiovascular disease (CVD), ambulatory BP monitoring, home BP monitoring, BP thresholds to initiate antihypertensive drug treatment, BP goals of treatment, and strategies to improve hypertension treatment. The format for grading the quality of evidence and strength of recommendations appropriately appears at the beginning of the guideline. Presented in "modular knowledge chunk format," the CPG sections are accompanied by

the strength of the evidence and recommendation. For example, the recommendation that reads "Out-of-office BP measurements are recommended to confirm the diagnosis of hypertension and for titration of BP-lowering medications in conjunction with telehealth counseling or clinical interventions" is supported by Level A evidence (e.g., >1 RCT, meta-analysis of RCTs) and a Level 1 recommendation (strong). In comparison, a recommendation about BP treatment threshold and use of CVD risk states, "Use of BP-lowering medications is recommended for primary prevention of CVD in adults with no history of CVD and with an estimated 10-year risk of ASCVD <10% and a systolic (SBP) blood pressure of 140 mmHg or higher or a diastolic (DBP) blood pressure of 90 mmHg or higher." This was based on a Level A strong recommendation, but only C-LD level of evidence (e.g., nonrandomized observational or registry studies, meta-analyses of such studies), which was the best available evidence.

Despite the proliferation of RCTs conducted over the past four decades, there remains a paucity of high-quality RCTs and meta-analyses that provide strong and consistent evidence to inform CPG development and recommendations. The recommendations are based on the strength of the evidence for each of the questions identified at the beginning of the CPG. As you read CPGs, even those from prestigious groups like the USPTF, you may be surprised that few recommendations are based on Level A evidence. Remember that evidence-based CPG recommendations are based on the best available evidence per the quality appraisal model used for a specific CPG (Box 8.2). Some CPG panels choose to make recommendations based on expert opinion when the evidence is poor or lacking. When expert opinion is used, it should be identified as such and aggregated using a systematic protocol.

CPGs also do not necessarily provide a "cookie-cutter" approach with a "one size fits all" formula (Alonso-Coello et al., 2010; Kung et al., 2012; Mickan et al., 2011). Use of a CPG must be for the right person, at the right time, and in the right way (Haynes, 1993). Thinking about how useful the recommendations are to your patient population, you may use the section(s) of a CPG that apply to your patient population while considering patient preferences and available resources. Keep in mind that it is nearly impossible

---

> **BOX 8.2 Examples of Clinical Practice Guidelines Appraisal Tools**
>
> - AGREE II Tool (Brouwers et al., 2010): https://www.agreetrust.org/
> - AGREE GRAS (Brouwers et al., 2017); shortened version of AGREE II: https://www.agreetrust.org/resource-centre/agree-ii-grs-instrument/
> - Johns Hopkins Nursing Evidence-Based Practice Non-Research Evidence Appraisal Tool to assess non-evidence-based CPGs: https://www.hopkinsmedicine.org/evidence-based-practice/docs/appendix_f_nonresearch_evidence_appraisal_tool.pdf.
> - Johns Hopkins Nursing Evidence-Based Practice Research Evidence Appraisal Tool (2012) to assess evidenced-based CPGs: https://www.hopkinsmedicine.org/evidence-based-practice/_docs/appendix_e_research_evidence_appraisal_tool.pdf

for clinicians to keep up with the proliferation of individual research studies; that is why evidence-based CPGs are so important to clinicians who seek to provide high-quality, cost-effective, satisfying care to their patients.

Implementation of CPGs in clinical settings involves both an individual and system-level commitment. Despite the increasing availability of high-quality CPGs, their use remains low. Abrahamson, Fox, and Doebbeling (2012) identified the top three barriers that inhibit nurses from using CPGs:

- Lack of orientation and education
- Amount of time it takes to implement them
- Workload issues such as lack of staffing

Resources such as the Iowa Model (see Chapter 2) provide a framework for the development of a CPG implementation plan. Assessing your organization's readiness to implement a best practice guideline is a critical step and must involve all relevant levels of administrative and clinical leadership (Titler et al., 2001). Studies report effective CPG implementation and improvements in clinical outcomes when a multilevel plan is developed and implemented (Abrahamson, Fox, & Doebbeling, 2012; Campbell et al., 2015) (see Chapters 12 and 13). Essential ingredients for success in transferring evidence into practice include:

- Organizational support
- Unit-based champions

- A positive clinical milieu
- Resources to facilitate day-to-day implementation
- Interactive professional development sessions that focus on education and skill building
- Integration of the CPG into the electronic health record with required prompts, reminders, and point-of-care clinical decision tools
- Changing organizational policies to reflect the CPG as a required standard of care
- Incentives to disseminate a new CPG as a best practice internally and externally

In your role as a clinical leader, you can be an EBP mentor who supports interprofessional teamwork, collaboration, and unit-based champions. You can play a pivotal role as a liaison between the team charged with CPG implementation and administrative leadership. Evaluating the impact of the CPG on clinical and financial outcomes is an important factor in promoting organizational adoption and sustainability. The Iowa Model provides a framework for you and your team to monitor and evaluate the CPG structure, process, and outcome data (see Chapter 16). Quality improvement data and feedback provide evidence of whether the CPG is being used in practice and how it is affecting patient care. Disseminating the results of a CPG implementation project internally and externally is another area for staff development (see Chapter 17). For example, coaching your staff, especially the unit-based champions, to develop short but compelling CPG presentations to educate about and market to internal and external stakeholders is an excellent leadership skill to cultivate. Strategically planned presentations are excellent vehicles for obtaining organizational leaders' buy-in, which is vital to ensuring sustainability. Ongoing administrative support and staff engagement are critical elements in supporting long-lasting practice changes associated with improved clinical outcomes and evidence of organizational effectiveness.

> **IPE TIP**
>
> Use of the IPEC Competencies in Appendix G provides a useful framework for your team in developing the trust, respect, and effective communication skills a CPG team needs to undertake implementation of a CPG in a practice setting.

CRITICAL APPRAISAL OF CLINICAL PRACTICE GUIDELINES

Appraising Clinical Practice Guidelines

As evidence-based clinical practice guidelines proliferate, it becomes increasingly important to critically appraise them regarding the methods used for guideline formulation and their potential applicability.

CPGs vary in quality; there is probably no such thing as a perfect CPG for a patient's medical diagnosis (Kung et al., 2012; Mickan et al., 2011). The findings of a systematic review by Alonso-Coello and colleagues (2010) concluded that although the quality of CPGs was improving, quality scores as measured by the Appraisal of Guidelines Research and Evaluation (AGREE) (2001) Instrument have remained moderate to low over the last two decades. Locating an appropriate guideline to use is a function of the ability to critically appraise the scientific rigor of a guideline. Critical areas that should be assessed when critically appraising CPGs include the following:

- Date of publication or release and authors
- Endorsement of the guideline
- Clear purpose of the guideline, what it covers, and patient population and subgroups for which it was designed
- Types of evidence (research, theoretical) used in guideline development
- Inclusion criteria for types of research studies used in formulating the guideline
- Description of the method or model for grading the evidence
- Search terms and retrieval methods used to acquire evidence in the guideline
- Practice statements supported by citations
- Practice recommendations supported by graded recommendations
- Comprehensive reference list
- Review of the guideline by external experts
- Evidence of whether the guideline has been used or tested in practice. If yes, in what types of settings, and with which patient groups and subgroups?

In a well-known study, the Institute of Medicine (IOM, 2011) also identified eight attributes of guideline development:

1. Validity
2. Reliability and reproducibility
3. Clinical applicability
4. Clinical flexibility
5. Clarity
6. Documentation
7. Development by a multidisciplinary team
8. Plans for periodic review and update

Evidence-based practice guidelines that are formulated using rigorous methods provide a useful starting point for understanding the evidence base of practice. Although information in well-developed national guidelines is a starting point, it is usually necessary to localize the guideline using institution-specific, evidence-based policies, procedures, or standards before applying a guideline in a specific setting.

The Siering et al. (2013) systematic review of 40 appraisal tools for evaluating CPGs concluded that although these tools vary in quality and length, the most comprehensively validated one is the Appraisal of Guidelines Research and Evaluation II (AGREE II) instrument (https://www.agreetrust.org/). Siering and colleagues also noted that the research or clinical question dictates which appraisal tool should be used. The **AGREE II** instrument is one of the most widely used appraisal tools to evaluate the applicability of a guideline to practice (Brouwers et al., 2010). AGREE II was developed to help assess guideline quality, provide a methodological strategy for guideline development, and inform practitioners about information that should be reported in guidelines and how it should be reported. As you can see from the list in Box 8.2, AGREE II is available online and is very user-friendly. It focuses on six domains with a total of 23 questions rated on a seven-point scale and two final assessment items that require appraisers to make overall judgments about the guideline based on how they rated the 23 questions. Along with the instrument itself, the AGREE Enterprise website offers excellent guidance on tool usage and development that you will find very helpful, especially when you begin your CPG critical appraisal journey. Table 8.5 highlights the structure and content of the six domains of the AGREE II tool.

A recent update indicates that the AGREE II tool has been reformatted and renamed the AGREE Global Rating Scale (AGREE GRS) to facilitate clinician use. You can download it as a PDF at https://www. agreetrust.org/resource-centre/agree-ii-grs-instrument/. The AGREE GRS tool is shorter, has been tested since 2012, and has acceptable validity, but its sensitivity to detecting differences is low. Therefore, the AGREE Trust still recommends the use of the valid and reliable AGREE II tool.

EBP TIP

The quality of a clinical practice guideline (CPG) is only as good as the quality of the evidence used to support it. It is essential to critically appraise a CPG using the Appraisal of Guidelines Research and Evaluation II (AGREE II) tool before implementation to determine its quality and fit for your patient population.

Another important point to consider is the grading of the recommendations. Guidelines are inconsistent in how they rate the quality of evidence and strength of recommendations. As a result, CPG users like you are challenged to understand the information that grading systems are trying to communicate (Guyatt et al., 2008). Although there is a variety of rating frameworks, the Grading of Recommendations Assessment, Development, and Evaluation (GRADE) system is increasingly becoming the gold standard for rating CPG recommendations (www.gradeworkinggroup.org). For a detailed discussion of the GRADE rating system, consult the online GRADE Handbook (http://gdt.guidelinedevelopment.org/app/handbook/handbook.html). The U.S. Preventive Services Task Force (USPSTF) is another esteemed recommendation rating system (www.uspreventiveservicestaskforce.org/), as is the one developed by the Agency for Health Research and Quality (AHRQ) (www.ahrq.gov). Clinicians make health care decisions by weighing the potential benefit and/or harm of alternative treatment options based on the best available evidence. CPG recommendations and quality ratings provide an estimate of the confidence clinicians can have in expected advantages or disadvantages of the intervention effect. Clinical leaders need to carefully assess the quality of evidence that provides the rationale for recommendations. A classic example is that for a decade, guidelines recommended that clinicians encourage postmenopausal women to use hormone replacement therapy (HRT) to decrease cardiovascular risk. Had a rigorous system for rating the quality of recommendations been used, it would have revealed that the evidence came from observational studies with inconsistent evidence of low quality. Ultimately, randomized clinical trials showed that HRT does not reduce cardiovascular risk and may even increase it in some cases (Rossouw et al., 2002). In contrast to the earlier recommendation, the 2017 Final Recommendation Statement by the USPSTF cites a "D" recommendation against the use of combined estrogen and progestin for the primary prevention of chronic cardiovascular conditions in postmenopausal women. A "D" recommendation indicates a high degree of certainty that the service has no net benefit and that the harm outweighs the benefit. Critical appraisal of CPGs is implemented using a standardized critical appraisal tool like the AGREE II instrument and applying the criteria to the attributes of the guideline. The answers to the questions and the accompanying score reveal data about the strength and quality of the evidence provided by the CPG.

CRITICAL APPRAISAL CRITERIA

Clinical Practice Guidelines

1. Is the date of publication, release, or update cycle current?
2. Are the authors of the clinical practice guideline (CPG) clearly identified and appropriate to the guideline?
3. Were the authors representative of key interprofessional stakeholders in this specialty?
4. Who sponsored and/or funded development of the CPG?
5. Are the CPG problem, purpose, and population clearly addressed?
6. Was there a clearly identified CPG development methodology?
7. Was a clearly identified method used to grade the evidence and make recommendations?
8. Was there an explicit search strategy?
9. Did the CPG team conduct a comprehensive review and critical appraisal of the literature?
10. Were all the relevant outcomes specified?
11. Was each recommendation stated explicitly and accompanied by strength of evidence and a graded recommendation?
12. Are the recommendations clinically relevant?
13. Was the CPG subjected to peer review and testing?
14. Will the recommendations be helpful in caring for my patient population?
15. Does my health care organization or practice have the resources to implement the recommendations of this CPG?
16. Does implementation support current practice or require a minor or major change in practice?
17. Can the outcomes be measured in my clinical setting?

TABLE 8.5   Structure and Content of AGREE II's Six Domains

Structure of Domain	Content of Items
Domain 1: Scope & Purpose	Is the overall aim of the CPG clear, including specific health-related questions and its specific population (items 1–3)?
Domain 2: Stakeholder Involvement	Were the appropriate health professionals involved in its development, and does it represent the intended users (items 4–6)?
Domain 3: Rigor of Development	Was an appropriate and clear method used to search and synthesize evidence, including recommendations and methods for updating them (items 7–14)?
Domain 4: Clarity of Presentation	Is the language of the CPG clear, organized, and appropriately formatted, including recommendations (items 15–17)?
Domain 5: Applicability	Are facilitators and barriers to implementing the CPG and necessary resources identified (items 18–21)?
Domain 6: Editorial Independence	Are the recommendations unbiased in relation to the funding source or member's organizational affiliation (items 22–23)?

Critical appraisal is not just about evaluating the quality of the evidence and strength of the recommendations. As you can see in critical appraisal criteria 14 to 17, you and your team must assess whether the CPG will be helpful in providing care for your patient population (e.g., age, gender, comorbidities). Beyond considering whether the guideline applies to your patient population, is it feasible to implement it in your practice setting? For example, a CPG on fall prevention in the hospital setting is not the same as fall prevention in a home or long-term care setting. A guideline for adult asthma management is not the same as asthma management in children. As a clinical leader, you also must be aware of the financial resources needed to implement a practice change; you need to determine whether they are available in your practice setting. Finally, you want to make sure that the outcomes of implementing a CPG are measurable in your clinical setting so it can be integrated into your quality improvement program.

SYNTHESIS

Systematic reviews and clinical practice guidelines are powerful sources of evidence and recommendations with which to guide clinical, educational, or administrative practices. Evidence-based practice requires that you determine whether you and your team would consider proposing a change in practice based on the strength and quality of evidence provided by a systematic review and coupled with your clinical expertise and patient preferences. Systematic reviews, especially meta-analyses comprising multiple randomized controlled trials, offer stronger evidence in estimating the magnitude of the effect of an intervention. The strength of evidence is a key component of building a practice based on evidence. Clinical practice guidelines vary widely in the rigor with which they are developed and the strength of evidence to support recommendations. However, well-developed guidelines and their recommendations do inform practice and provide an important approach to making evidence-informed changes that enable clinicians to provide high-quality, cost-effective and satisfying care to their populations.

KEY POINTS

- A systematic review is guided by a focused clinical/PICO question and uses electronic searches to identify quantitative studies that use similar designs to answer a clinical question.
- A review is a type of systematic analysis guided by a focused clinical question. It includes an extensive search of the literature and can include a theoretical review of the literature or a review of both qualitative and quantitative research literature.
- Meta-analysis is a quantitative epidemiological study design, a subset of systematic reviews that quantitatively summarizes the findings of a group of studies using the same design to obtain an estimate of the impact of an intervention.

- Standardized tools for critically appraising a systematic review and meta-analysis are available from the Center for Evidence-Based Medicine (CEBM), the Critical Appraisal Skills Programme (CASP), and the Cochrane Collaboration.
- CPGs are systematically developed statements or recommendations that link research and practice.
- There are two types of CPGs, evidence-based and expert-based.
- Evidence-based guidelines search the research literature, assess the strength and quality of the evidence provided by the studies that meet the inclusion criteria, and make graded recommendations to guide practice.

- Expert-based guidelines are developed when the research literature is sparse. A panel of experts in an area of interest develops the CPG based on their expert opinions and critical appraisal of existing research.
- The AGREE II Tool is the gold standard instrument for critical appraisal of clinical practice guidelines.
- Clinicians need to determine whether the findings of systematic reviews and clinical practice guidelines are relevant for their patient populations, applicable in their clinical settings, and financially feasible to implement.
- Systematic review and clinical practice guideline teams should be interprofessional and represent diverse stakeholders including patients.

REFERENCES

Abrahamson, K. A., Fox, R. L., & Doebbeling, B. N. (2012). Facilitators and barriers to clinical practice guideline use among nurses. *American Journal of Nursing, 112*(7), 26–35.

AGREE Collaboration. (2001). *Appraisal of Guidelines for Research and Evaluation(AGREE) Instrument.* http://www/agreecollaboration.org.

Alonso-Coello, P., Irfan, A., Soia, I., Gich, I., Delgado-Noguera, M., Rigau, D., Tort, S., Bonfill, X., Burgers, J., & Schünemann, H. (2010). The quality of clinical practice guidelines over the last two decades: A systematic review of guideline appraisal. *Quality and Safety in Health Care (QualSaf Health Care, 19*(e58), 1–7.

Blakeman, J. R., & Stapleton, S. J. (2018). An integrative review of fatigue experienced by women before and during myocardial infarction. *Journal of Clinical Nursing, 00*, 1–11.

Brouwers., et al. (2010). AGREE IITool. https://www.agreetrust.org/.

Brouwers, et al. (2017). AGREE GRAS. https://www.agreetrust.org/resource-centre/agree-ii-grs-instrument/.

Bryant, R., Alonzo, A., & Schmillen, H. (2017). Systematic review of provider involvement in heart failure self-care. *Journal of the American Association of Nurse Practitioners, 29*(11), 682–694.

Campbell, J. M., Umapathysivam, K., Xue, Y., & Lockwood, C. (2015). *Evidence-based practice point-of-care resources: A quantitative evaluation of quality, rigor, and content.*

Center for Evidence-based Medicine Critical Appraisal Tools. (2016). www.cebm.net/critical-appraisal.

Cochrane Handbook for Systematic Reviews. (2016). http://www.cochrane-handbook.org.

Cohen, J. (1988). *Statistical power analysis for the behavioral sciences.* (2nd ed.). New York, NY: Academic Press.

Chalmers, T. C., Smith, H., Blackburn, B., et al. (1981). A method for assessing the quality of a randomized control trial. *Controlled Clinical Trials, 2*, 31–49.

Cluzeau, F. A., Littlejohns, P., Grimshaw, J. M., Feder, G., & Moran, S. E. (1999). Development and application of a generic methodology to assess the quality of clinical guidelines. *International Journal of Quality Health Care, 11*, 21–28.

Critical Appraisal Skills Programme. (2017). CASP systematic Review Checklist. http://www.casp-uk.net/.

Dearholt, S., & Dang, D. (2012). *Johns Hopkins nursingevidence-based practice model and guidelines* (2nd ed.). Indianapolis: INL Sigma Theta Tau International.

Fink, L., & Lewis, D. (2017). Exercise as a treatment for fibromyalgia: A scoping review. *The Journal for Nurse Practitioners, 13*(8), 546–551.

Foote, J. M., Brady, L. H., Burke, A. L., et al. (2009). Evidence-based Clinical Practice Guideline on Linear Growth Measurement of ChildrenDes Moines, IA. Blank children's Hospital: Unity Point Health.

Grant, M. J., & Booth, A. (2009). A typology of reviews: An analysis of 14 review types and associated methodologies. *Health Information and Libraries Journal, 26*, 91–108.

Guyatt, G. H., Oxman, A. D., Vist, G. E., et al. (2008). GRADE: An emerging consensus on rating quality of evidence and strength of recommendations. *British Medical Journal, 336*, 924–926.

Haynes, R. B. (1993). Where's the meat in clinical journals. *ACP Journal Club, 119*, A22–A23.

Haidich, A. B. (2010). Meta-analysis in medical research. *Hippokratia, 14*(Suppl. 1), 29–37.

Higgins, J. P. T., & Green, S. (2011). Cochrane Handbook for Systematic Reviews of interventions version 5.1.0. http://www.cochrane-handbook.org.

Institute of Medicine. (2011). Consensus report: Clinical practice guidelines we can trust. http://data.care-statement. org/wp-content/uploads/2016/12/IOMGuidelines-2013-1.pdf. Accessed January 13, 2018.

Khangura, S., Konnyu, K., Cushman, R., Grimshaw, J., & Moher, D. (2012). Evidence summaries: The evolution of a rapid review approach. *Systematic Reviews*, *1*(10), 1–10.

Kung, J., Miller, R. R., & Mackowiak, P. A. (2012). Failure of clinical practice guidelines to meet institute of medicine standards. *Archives of Internal Medicine*, *172*(21), 1628–1633.

Liberati, A., Altman, D. G., Tetzlaff, J., et al. (2009). The PRISMA statement for reporting items for systematic reviews and meta-analyses of studies that evaluate health care interventions: Explanation and elaboration. *Annals of Internal Medicine*, *15*(4), w65–w94.

Mavridis, D., & Salanti, G. (2014). Exploring and accounting for publication bias in mental health: a brief overview of methods. *Evidence-based Mental Health*, *17*, 11–15.

Mickan, S., Burls, A., & Glasziou, P. (2011). Patterns of 'leakage' in the utilisation of clinical guidelines: A systematic review. *Postgraduate Medical Journal*, *87*, 670–679.

Moher, D., Liberati, A., Terzlaff, J., & Altman, D. D. (2009). Preferred reporting items for systematic reviews and meta-analyses: The PRISMA statement. *PLOS Medicine*, *62*(10), 10006–10010. https://doi.org/101016/j.jclinepi. 2009.06.005.

Moher, D., Shamseer, L., Clarke, M., et al. (2015). Preferred reporting items for systematic review and meta-analysis protocols (PRISMA-P) 2015 Statement. *Systematic Reviews*, *4*(1), 1.

Mora, K., Dorrejo, X. M., Carreon, K. M., & Butt, S. (2017). Nurse practitioner-led transitional care interventions: An integrative review. *Journal of the American Association of Nurse Practitioners*, *29*(12), 773–790.

Mukumbang, F. C., Van Belle, S., Marchal, B., & vanWyk, B. (2017). An exploration of group-based HIV/AIDS treatment and care models in Sub-Saharan Africa using a realist evaluation. *Implementation Science*, *12*(1), 107–115.

O'Hara, C. B., Campbell, I. C., & Schmidt, U. (2015). A reward-centered model of anorexia nervosa: A focussed narrative review of the neurological and psychophysiological literature. *Neuroscience and Biobehavioral Reviews*, *52*, 131–152.

Pawson, R., Greenhaigh, T., Harvey, G., & Walshe, K. (2005). Realist review—a new method of systematic review designed for complex policy interventions. *Journal of Health Service Research Policy*, *10*(Suppl. 1), 21–34.

Reith, C. H., & Malone, D. C. (2001). Understanding the fundamental concepts for interpreting or conducting meta-analyses. *Formulary*, *36*, 594–609.

Rossouw, J. E., Anderson, G. L., Prentice, R. L., LaCroix, A. Z., Kooperberg, C., Stefanick, M. L., et al. (2002). Risks and benefits of estrogen plus progetin for secondary prevention of coronary heart disease in postmenopausal women: Principal results from the Women's Health Initiative randomized controlled trial. *Journal of the American Medical Association*, *288*, 321–333.

Siering, U., Eikermann, M., Hausner, E., Hoffmann-Eber, & Neugebauer, E. A. (2013). Appraisal tools for clinical practice guidelines: A systematic review. *PLOS ONE*, *8*(12), e82915. http://journals.plos.org/plosone/article?id = 10. 1371/journal.pone.0082915.

Siu, A. (2015). Screening for abnormal glucose and Type 2 diabetes mellitus: U.S. preventive services task force recommendations statement. *Annals of Internal Medicine*, *163*(11), 861–871.

Smith, J., & Noble, H. (2014). Bias in research. *Evidence-based Nursing*, *17*(4), 100–101.

Velazquez, M., Lorda, P., Portero, R., et al. (2009). Interventions to promote the use of advance directives: An overview of systematic reviews. *Patient education and counseling*, *80*(210), 10–20.

vanDriel, M. L., Ulep, R., Shaffer, J. P., Davies, P., & Deichmann, R. (2016). Interventions to improve adherence to lipid-lowering medications. *Cochrane Database of Systematic Reviews* Issue 12. https://doi.org/1002/14651858. CD004371.pub4.

Whelton, P. K., Carey, R. M., Aronow, W. S., et al. (2017). 2017 ACC/AHA/AAPA/ABC/ACPM/AGS/APhA/ASH/ASPC/NMA/PCNA Guideline for the3 Prevention, Detection, Evaluation, and Management of High Blood Pressure in Adults. *Journal of the American College of Cardiology*. https://doi.org/10.1016/j.jacc.2017.11.006.

Whittemore, R., & Knafl, K. (2005). The integrative review: Updated methodology. *Journal of Advanced Nursing*, *52*(5), 546–553.

9

Qualitative Studies

Dona M. Rinaldi

LEARNING OUTCOMES

After reading this chapter, you should be able to do the following:

- Describe the importance of qualitative research in evidence-based practice.
- Synthesize the value and rigor of qualitative research.
- Incorporate the role of critical appraisal of qualitative studies as it relates to evidence-based practice.
- Apply qualitative measures of rigor when critiquing qualitative research findings.

- Apply critical appraisal criteria to evaluate a qualitative study.
- Synthesize evidence provided by a group of qualitative studies.
- Evaluate metasynthesis of qualitative findings and how this approach can strengthen internal and external validity.
- Integrate qualitative evidence and clinical judgment in the planning and implementation of safe patient care.

KEY WORDS

Auditability
Case study
Confirmability
Credibility
Data saturation
Dependability

Emic
Ethnography
Etic
Grounded theory
Metasynthesis
Phenomenology

Purposive sampling
Qualitative research
Transferability
Trustworthiness

INTRODUCTION

Evidence-based practice (EBP) is acknowledged as important in professional nursing practice and has made significant contributions to patient care and outcomes over the past two decades. EBP integrates the best available research evidence, patient preferences, and clinical expertise to provide patient care that achieves the best outcomes for patients in any given clinical situation. Fundamental to reliable patient care is the development of your skill set to include critical thinking, process and outcome evaluation, and synthesis of all evidence available in an effort to make sound clinical decisions in your professional nursing practice (Baillie, 2015; Ferguson & Day, 2005; Cesario, Morin, & Santo Donato, 2002). Qualitative research is explanatory, descriptive, and inductive in nature and comprises methods that help us formulate an understanding of phenomena and their context answered by discovery-oriented research questions. As noted in Chapter 1, the current state of knowledge related to EBP provides you and your colleagues with well-defined criteria with which to appraise quantitative research. Criteria to evaluate qualitative findings have been evolving but may not be as transparent as quantitative critiquing guidelines. This is intrinsically related to the subjective nature of the findings and the ongoing dialogue concerning rigor in qualitative research. It is important for you to note that the evidence hierarchy presented in Chapter 1, Fig. 1.1 does include qualitative studies; however, they are ranked as providing weaker, Level VI evidence. As long as hierarchical evidence pyramids are used to rank the level of evidence provided by specific types of designs, the strength of evidence provided by qualitative studies will continue to be misrepresented because the linear approach used to evaluate quantitative studies such as randomized controlled trials does not align with the nonlinear nature of qualitative research. This supports the need for a different paradigm for critically appraising the strength and quality of the evidence provided by the findings of qualitative studies so the evidence provided by the findings are valued as important data that inform clinical practice about the patient experience.

The purpose of this chapter is to describe the significance of qualitative research as it relates to EBP. Qualitative research methods are defined, strategies to determine scientific rigor are addressed, and guidelines for critical appraisal and synthesis of qualitative research findings are described.

Qualitative research findings have a place in EBP and are an important component of quality improvement (QI). Findings from qualitative research can be linked to the Institute for Healthcare Improvement (2016) Triple Aim Initiative. These include improving the patient experience of care, including quality and satisfaction; improving the health of populations; and reducing the per capita cost of health care (Berwick, 2008). Describing the patient experience in a systematic fashion can lead to measurable improvement in health care services and the health status of targeted patient populations. The National Academy of Medicine, formerly called the Institute of Medicine (IOM), defines quality in health care as a direct correlation between the level of improved health services and the desired health outcomes of individuals and populations (IOM, 2001, 2015).

Qualitative research methodologies provide a relationship between what patients and health care teams aspire to in terms of improving health care services. One component of QI is the focus on the patient experience. An important measure of quality is the extent to which patients' needs and expectations are met. This directly connects to qualitative methodologies in which researchers are working to operationalize theoretical explanations of life experiences derived from actual patient experiences. One example might be found in transgender patient care, where the nursing literature is mostly silent, contributing to confusion, discomfort, and misunderstandings regarding how to provide the best evidence-based care for this population. In a study by Carabez, Eliason, and Martinson (2016), patients described feeling uncomfortable, judged, and exposed to harsh consequences of being transgender. The findings also revealed nurses' discomfort with and lack of knowledge about people who identify as transgender and their health care needs. Zunner and Grace (2012) noted that transgender patients frequently report encountering verbal abuse and condescending and humiliating treatment from health care providers. If we are to provide effective evidence-based care for this population, qualitative research will be critical to developing the thematic elements about the lived health care experiences of this patient population that will contribute evidence upon which to develop best practices that inform high-quality, cost-effective, and satisfying care tailored to this patient population. Qualitative methodologies could be used to develop comprehensive training about gender diversity, transgender identities, and the complications presented by binary constructs of male or female patients (Carabez, Eliason, & Martinson, 2016).

The Institute for Healthcare Improvement (2016) has described a Triple Aim Initiative that includes Experience of Care, Population Health, and Per Capita Cost. Qualitative research can contribute to the attainment of the Triple Aim by better describing health care needs and understanding of needs from the perspective of the lived experience. Describing the patient's lived experience can improve patient care, making it more satisfying and more coordinated, ultimately leading to a decrease in the burden of illness.

> **EBP TIP**
>
> Seek out educational opportunities and research conferences to improve your understanding of qualitative research and its relevance to your role as a clinical leader.

QUALITATIVE METHODOLOGIES AND WORLDVIEW

Researchers using qualitative methodologies approach their work with a worldview that is holistic; values subjectivity; and believes that each individual attributes meaning to their experience based on past, present, and possibly future experiences. For example, Ranjbar, Joolaee, Vehadhir, and Bernstein (2017) studied the development of moral competency in Iranian nursing students. Using a constructivist grounded theory method, they found that during the student's education experience three levels of moral development occurred that helped the formation of a professional identity. The levels included moral transition, moral reconstruction, and professional morality. This model provides insight into the development of professionalism in nursing, something that concerns every faculty member. Their study emphasizes how the worldview of students, in terms of professionalism, changes based on past, present, and possibly future experiences.

Qualitative research methods are selected to describe phenomena about which little is known. These methods capture meaning as it is lived and pays close attention to the experience as lived by the participants. An example of capturing meaning as it is lived can be understood in the work of Kuhnke, Bailey, Woodbury, and Burrows, (2014). Their qualitative research focused on understanding diabetic foot ulcers and amputation. People living with diabetes are at high risk for foot complications, lower extremity trauma, injury, ulceration, infection, and potential amputation. Findings of the study have the potential to improve patient care, prevent comorbidities, and improve quality of life with fewer complications.

In the preceding example, qualitative research explores and describes more fully the complexities of diabetes and their meaning to patients. The approach seeks to understand what is occurring for the patient and the family as it is lived. Equally important to the data gathered in qualitative research is how the findings enable clinicians to appreciate how different qualitative research approaches can explore the meaning of illness from the lived experience of the individual with acute or chronic illness (Kuhnke et al., 2014). Thousands of reports of well-conducted qualitative studies exist on topics germane to nursing practice. Findings from qualitative research provide valuable insights into understanding and improving patient care from both nurse and patient perspectives.

The intended goal of qualitative research is to describe phenomena relevant to nursing that is lacking in theoretical information or requires a better understanding of a particular phenomenon. You cannot study an issue using quantitative research methods if you don't have a theoretical basis to develop your study (van Manen, 2017b; Nelson, 2008). Qualitative research methods are often used when few studies are available on one particular topic or when the researcher wants to obtain an alternate view of an issue (Meadows-Oliver, 2016). The sample size in qualitative studies is small. The sampling method is often described as **purposive**; that is, the sample is homogeneous and reflects the population being studied. Subjects are often identified as participants or key informants. The common data collection method is interview with verbatim transcription of exactly what the participants have said. When no new data emerges, often referred to as *saturation*, data collection ends. **Data saturation** is determined by the researcher when no new information emerges from the informants. All data collection procedures result in large amounts of narrative data with the descriptive phrases, words, and quotes of the participants. Findings of the study have the potential to improve patient care, prevent comorbidities, or lead patients to recovery that is free of complications.

Raw data are a narrative compilation of exactly what both researcher and participant said during the interview that is then transcribed verbatim. Data analysis processes are systematic and rigorous to ensure that findings can be confirmed with qualitative analytic methods (Russell & Gregory, 2003).

Qualitative research is most valuable when expressing patients' stories and should be applied in areas where there is a need to build theory that may then lead to quantitative studies and instrument development (Stevens, 2005; Thorne, 2006). For example, Rice (2009) discussed the importance of qualitative research to EBP for psychiatric/mental health nurse practitioners, nurses, and colleagues. He noted that for psychiatric patients, "Recovery is not complete until patients make sense of their experiences and integrate an understanding of events within their lives" (Rice, 2009, p. 200). Rice (2009) further emphasized that the absence of interventions on the subjective aspects of mental illness is the result of failed attempts of dominant quantitative research methods to address the subjectivity of the human condition.

The intended purpose of qualitative research and the types of data analysis used in these projects are significantly different from those of quantitative studies. Qualitative approaches:
- must be appropriate for the phenomenon being studied,
- must be relevant to the PICO question,
- focus on the values and opinions most important to patients and families, and
- are patient-centered and can deepen patients' understanding (Newman, Thompson, & Roberts, 2006).

The qualitative paradigm is used to explore the meaning of experience that can be missed by quantitative studies. Qualitative studies build conceptual frameworks and theoretical understanding of the phenomenon being studied. By examining issues crucial to patients and families, it provides more complete information regarding the best evidence on which to build professional nursing practice and support satisfying experiences of care for individuals, families, and communities (Nelson, 2008). Caring for the transgender patient is an example of a topic that needs a theoretical foundation that can be built from qualitative methods. How can we possibly know what various populations need in terms of health care if we do not listen to the stories of their experiences as patients?

There are a variety of approaches to qualitative research (Fig. 9.1). The most commonly used, described in this chapter, are phenomenology, grounded theory, ethnography, and case study methods. Metasynthesis of qualitative research is also addressed. It is important for you to remember that when qualitative researchers

develop their expertise and select a methodology, they immerse themselves in the seminal work related to each method.

> ### EBP TIP
>
> Incorporate evidence from qualitative research into clinical practice to support patient satisfaction by developing your critical appraisal skills for evaluating qualitative research

PHENOMENOLOGY

Phenomenology is a qualitative research method derived from philosophy with the purpose of describing particular phenomena, or the appearance of things, as lived experience. The phenomenological term "lived experience" is critical for the understanding of phenomenological reflection, meaning, analysis, and insights. Data are collected via interviews guided by open-ended questions and prompts, then transcribed verbatim.

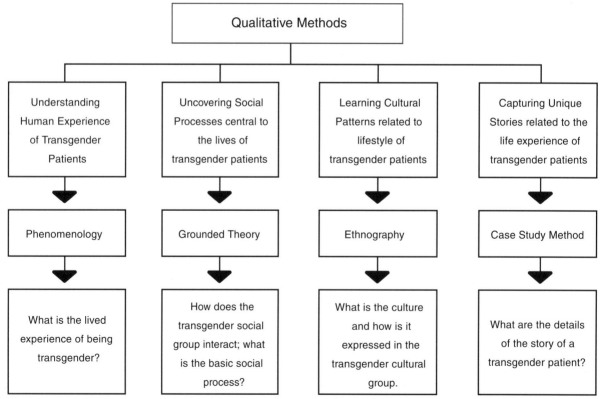

Fig. 9.1 Decision-Making Algorithm: Qualitative Research Methods to Study Transgender Patient Needs

Lived experiences are the data of phenomenological research; interviews with informants continue until data saturation occurs. The researcher then "dwells" with the data, reading and rereading the raw data until common thematic elements emerge. Developing a rich, thick description of the phenomenon under investigation is important for health care providers and help to identify health care needs. The primary goal of phenomenology is to peel back the layers of current beliefs to eventually get to the true raw description of the phenomenon (Van Manen, 2017). In the phenomenological study "Living My Family's Story: Identifying the Lived Experience in Healthy Women at Risk for Hereditary Breast Cancer," the authors' purpose was to explore how women at high risk for hereditary breast cancer incorporate living with knowledge of this risk into their lives (Underhill, Lalli, Kiviniemi, Murekeyisoni, & Dickerson 2012). The authors' findings make important contributions to the Institute for Healthcare Improvement (2016) Triple Aim since the thematic elements can inform clinical decision-making and interventions to improve the clinical experience of women who describe living with a "gray cloud over my head" and reduce per capita cost by supporting referrals to high-risk early intervention programs.

GROUNDED THEORY

Grounded theory research is used to generate theories about clinical practice and understanding about multiple aspects of health care. Grounded theory as a method is rooted in sociology; specifically, symbolic interactionism, which describes the relationship between people and society. The approach is inductive and has clearly developed systematic procedures designed to develop a theory or basic social process. The emergent theory is based on observations and perceptions of the social processes and evolves during data collection and analysis (Corbin & Strauss, 2015). The constant comparative method of data analysis, an iterative approach, is used to examine data from interviews, identify gaps in understanding from the data, and conduct additional interviews until data saturation occurs. For example, Hyatt and colleagues (2015) explored soldiers and their family reintegration experiences, as described by married dyads, after a combat-related traumatic brain injury. To better understand the basic social processes that shape behavior and develop interventions that

meet the family-centered needs of this population, the researchers asked a broad research question that permitted in-depth understanding and explanation of the behavior: "How do soldiers and their spouses identify the special challenges, sources of support, and overall rehabilitation process of post–mild traumatic brain injury family reintegration?" In contrast to phenomenology, the primary purpose of grounded theory research is to develop a theory that emerges from the data about the relevant social processes, which can then be applied to clinical practice.

ETHNOGRAPHY

Ethnography is associated with anthropology, the work of describing culture and the people of a particular culture. The purpose of ethnographic research is to discover and understand the social and psychological culture within a group of people. Within ethnography, culture is defined as the collective understanding and influences of shared behaviors and understandings and the deeper influences being placed on the group being studied.

Derived from the Greek term *ethnos*, meaning people, race, or cultural group, the ethnographic method focuses on the scientific description and interpretation of cultural or social groups and systems (Malik, McKenna, & Griggiths, 2016). The goal of the ethnographer is to understand the participants' views of their world, or the emic view. The **emic** view, the insiders' view, is contrasted with the **etic** view, the outsiders' view. The ethnographer's approach requires that the researcher enter the world of the study participants to observe what happens, listen to what is said, ask questions, and collect whatever data are available. Data can include artifacts of the culture such as clothing, jewelry, cooking implements, and ceremonial objects. Researchers use the method to study cultural variations in health and patient groups as subcultures within the larger culture of health care. For example, Grassley and colleagues (2015) studied nurses' support of breastfeeding on the night shift. Their approach is called institutional ethnography, which has as its goal to explore how social experiences and processes, in this case those of everyday work, are organized and mediate the context of nurses' everyday work. They were interested in identifying the interpersonal interactions and institutional structures that affect their ability to offer breastfeeding support and to promote exclusive breastfeeding on the nightshift.

CASE STUDY

Case study research is rooted in sociology and focuses on describing elements of an individual case, both the commonalities and the peculiarities. A single case may be an individual, a family, a community, or an organization (Stake, 2000). Case studies emphasize a holistic approach to the research that may lead to identification of patterns consistent across a set of cases that contribute to a more global understanding of a particular problem. The selection of cases can range from those that are most common to those that are most unusual. Stake (2000) advocates choosing cases that provide the best opportunity for learning. Case study data are gathered using interviews; field observations; and review of documents, diaries, and transcripts for evidence to describe and explain the complexity of a case (Stake, 2000). Although researchers pose questions to begin a case study data collection, the initial questions are never all-inclusive. Instead, the researcher uses an iterative process of "growing questions" in the field. As data are collected, other questions emerge and serve to guide the researcher's quest to untangle the complexities of the case. Schmidt and Haglund (2017) used a case study format to describe compassion fatigue using one nurse's experience as an example. From their work they developed a process called Personal Reflective Debrief for emergency department nurses. The method, when implemented, was found to promote resiliency in an environment where the reality of compassion fatigue is of imminent concern.

IPE TIP

Qualitative research teams are comprised of internal stakeholders, the research team members, and external stakeholders, the key informants who are partners in dialogue and discovery. Through observation and dialogue, the meaning of the lived experience, culture, social process, or historical period are revealed and represent a cohesive mutual representation of reality.

METASYNTHESIS

Metasynthesis, sometimes call a metasummary, is a rigorous synthesis of a critical mass of qualitative research evidence that relates to answering a specific research question. Metasynthesis reviews attempt to overcome possible biases at all stages by following a rigorous methodology. Metasyntheses involve further extraction and further abstraction of qualitative findings and include calculation of the manifest frequency effect sizes (Sandelowski & Barroso, 2003a). The methods include constant comparison, taxonomic analysis, the reciprocal interpretation of in vivo concepts, and the use of imported concepts to frame data (Sandelowski & Barroso, 2003b). Inferences about the findings are derived from taking all of the reports in a sample of studies as a whole to offer a cohesive description or explanation of the phenomenon while retaining the essence and unique contribution of each study (Sandelowski & Barroso, 2007). Researchers must make several decisions when preparing a metasynthesis, including:

- formulating a qualitative research question;
- identifying, selecting, and critically appraising relevant studies;
- abstracting, synthesizing, and lending further interpretation to the body of study findings; and
- drawing overall conclusions.

Equally important is the need to examine the validity of the results and decide how you and your team can apply the metasynthesis findings to patient care and quality improvement (Finfgeld-Connett, 2010; Flemming, 2007a, 2007b).

Metasynthesis of qualitative findings, similar to systematic reviews, may be the best way to integrate evidence across a wider range of scientific methodologies. In particular, this approach may help clinical leaders and their teams work within the qualitative evidence-based movement with greater assurance that scientifically sound reference points have not compromised the complexity, richness, and diversity inherent in clinical practice. Newer approaches to research synthesis and integration hold promise for increasing confidence about what might constitute a qualitatively derived evidentiary knowledge claim (Thorne, 2009). Qualitative synthesis has the ability to create a systematic logic within which findings from distinct studies in a field can be rigorously integrated into stronger and more generalizable knowledge claims (Butler, Hall, & Copnell, 2016; Thorne, 2009). Qualitative data from a metasynthesis provides stronger qualitative evidence that you and your team can use to validate and support the Triple Aim and patient experience and use in evidence-based QI initiatives aimed at improving the clinical experience of individuals, families, and communities.

EBP TIP

Volunteer to participate in the development of a metasynthesis related to a clinical question of interest to you or your clinical team.

KEY DIFFERENCES IN QUALITATIVE METHODOLOGIES

Sampling strategies in qualitative research have as their primary goal the collection of raw data, from individuals experiencing the phenomena being studied, with the goal of describing the phenomena from the perspective of the individuals actually living it (Duggleby & Williams, 2016). The specific sampling strategy, usually purposive, is driven by the phenomenon under investigation. Box 9.1 highlights common types of sampling strategies used in qualitative studies. For example, if a researcher was interested in the lived experience of having an implantable cardiac defibrillator, the researcher would need to sample individuals with defibrillators. Sampling is purposeful in that participants are selected because they can best inform the research question and have experience with the phenomenon under investigation. However, you will notice that sample size in qualitative studies is expected to be small; a predetermined sample size is not the norm.

> **EBP TIP**
>
> Often the standard of saturation is used to determine sample size. When you can say to yourself, "I am no longer hearing anything new," then the assumption is made that saturation has been reached. Choose participants carefully, ensuring that those selected can best inform the question.

Data gathered via qualitative research methods include thoughts, feelings, behaviors, and actual lived experiences as told by the individuals experiencing the phenomenon under investigation. By listening to patients' voices, scientific evidence can be enriched through narrative data that may not be heard or fully understood by filling out questionnaires or computing statistics (Flemming, 2007a). Whereas quantitative research methods strive to eliminate or control for contextual elements, qualitative research methods encompass these elements and construct studies that examine relevant issues related to individual life experiences (van Manen, 2017). Appraising the best evidence to inform practice should include qualitative findings as a source of critical evidence. However, thorough evaluation of qualitative findings is essential if they are to be incorporated into patient care and EBP (Hunt & Lahore, 2011; Kearney, 2001). Data collection ends when the

> **BOX 9.1 Common Types of Sampling Strategies Used in Qualitative Research**
>
> **Purposive sampling**—the intentional selection of participants or events consistent with the focus of the study
> **Snowball sampling**—recruitment of participants from social networks of informants already enrolled in the study
> **Convenience sampling**—recruitment of participants who meet the study inclusion criteria and volunteer to enroll in the study

researcher is no longer hearing anything new or different and is referred to as saturation, as noted earlier.

> **EBP TIP**
>
> Practice interviewing skills and have them evaluated by an expert before beginning data collection.

DATA ANALYSIS

Qualitative data are words rather than numbers. As such, they are analyzed by interpretation rather than mathematical manipulation. Meaning is extracted from the repetitive patterns of words emerging from the raw data that coalesce into thematic patterns that provide a rich description that explains the behavior or experience. This is where it becomes critically important that the researcher use a systematic process to describe thoroughly to the reader the process of how the researcher arrived at their conclusions (Davies, Dodd, Walsh, & Murray, 2010). By doing so, the researcher establishes the authenticity and trustworthiness of the data.

> **EBP TIP**
>
> Consider how you can apply qualitative findings to your clinical decision-making and QI.

SCIENTIFIC RIGOR IN QUALITATIVE RESEARCH

Criteria for determining the trustworthiness of qualitative research were introduced by Lincoln and Guba in the 1980s when they replaced terminology for achieving rigor, reliability, validity, and generalizability with dependability, credibility, and transferability. Strategies for achieving trustworthiness were also introduced. The literature reflects ongoing discussion of these

TABLE 9.1   Process-Related Differences in Qualitative Research

Qualitative Research Methods Naturalistic Paradigm	Quantitative Research Methods Positivist Paradigm
Grounded in qualitative methods, research conducted within this paradigm reflects a research process that lends focus to the complexities of phenomena as they exist in the world.	Grounded in quantitative methods, research conducted within this paradigm allows researchers to conduct studies that are more fundable and seek the facts of social phenomena.
Methods are generated from the disciplines of anthropology, psychology, history, and philosophy.	Methods are derived from logical positivism and empiricism.
The focus is on understanding and describing phenomena as they are experienced.	The focus is on controlling and predicting: Can we control the outcome?
Qualitative data collection methods include participant observation, interview, and retrospective description.	Quantitative data collection methods include experiments, quasi-experiments, physiological, and psychological and sociological measures
Knower and known are interactive and inseparable. The researcher is the instrument.	Knower and known are independent.
Approaches are subjective, holistic, and process-oriented.	Approaches are objective and outcome-oriented.
Data are thick and rich, providing for detailed analysis. Hundreds of pages of verbatim transcripts comprise the data.	The purpose is to predict relationships achieved by testing and validating hypotheses with a given statistical probability.
Data collection and analysis occur over an extended period of time. Interviews may need to be repeated two or three times to clarify information and ensure accuracy of analysis.	Data are analyzed through statistical inference.
Sample sizes in qualitative research are small due to rich, thick data gathered and the depth of analysis required. The researcher determines when to end collection of data. This is generally referred to as "saturation," or the point at which no new information is being noted during the data collection phase.	Quantitative designs use power analysis to ensure that enough subjects are recruited so that differences between groups can be detected.
The purpose is to develop theory.	The purpose is to test theory.

original criteria (Morse, 2016); however, this sentinel work remains in use today.

To conduct research that reflects precision and rigor, regardless of the paradigm, the researcher must first select the methodology most appropriate to study the research problem at hand (see Fig. 9.1). Qualitative approaches are used to describe the "why," whereas quantitative approaches address what has occurred, how many times something occurred, relationships among variables, or the effect of an intervention on an outcome (see Chapters 6–8). Qualitative approaches describe experiences about which little is known in the form of individuals' thoughts, feelings, and behaviors instead of numbers. Data are gathered in settings where what is being studied is actually occurring. Process is of primary concern rather than outcomes (Mayan, 2015). Table 9.1 lists methodological differences between qualitative and quantitative research studies.

EBP TIP

As a clinical leader, think about a bias you may have about a clinical situation or patient population. Talk through your bias with a neutral party or write your assumptions, bias experiences, and beliefs in a journal. Qualitative researchers suspend or bracket their biases to maximize their objectivity before launching a qualitative research study.

The criteria to critique the quality and rigor of quantitative and qualitative research are extremely different and grounded in each paradigm's specific end goals. In quantitative research, rigor is judged in terms of a study's validity, reliability, generalizability, and objectivity (see Chapter 5). Quantitative results are intended to be free from bias, to be replicable across contexts, and to generalize from the sample under study to the full target population. Qualitative research has its own, separate measures of quality: credibility, transferability, dependability, and confirmability as defined in Table 9.2 (Lincoln & Guba, 1985).

TABLE 9.2 Comparison Criteria: Critical Evaluation of Authenticity and Trustworthiness of Data

Quantitative Language	Qualitative Language	Definition	Example Techniques
Internal Validity: the degree to which it can be inferred that the experimental treatment, rather than an uncontrolled condition, resulted in the observed effects	Credibility, dependability/ **auditability**	When the exhaustive description is returned to the participants to review, they recognize it as their reality. The findings make sense to the participants.	Prolonged time in the field: evidence is supplied that indicates the researcher spent prolonged engagement in the field collecting data. Triangulation: two or more theories, groups of participants, methods instruments, or investigators were included. Peer debriefing: the researcher and the research are peer reviewed by another researcher who can challenge the method and offer guidance. The research can be audited in such a way that the reader can follow the line of thinking used by the researcher in the development of thematic elements and exhaustive description. Here, the researcher should offer raw data and demonstrate how that data were translated in the researcher. Audit trail of decision-making occurs throughout the research process.
External Validity/Generalizability: the degree to which the findings of a study can be generalized to other populations or environments.	Transferability	The purpose of qualitative research is theory development. The important question to be asked is whether or not the findings may be transferred to another similar setting.	Thick, rich descriptions of the setting and participants: findings are recognized by participants and possibly those not included in the study, but with similar experiences.
Objectivity	**Confirmability**	Provides confirmation of the researchers influence.	Bracketing. Journal writing, reflecting the researcher's thoughts and interpretations during data collection; also referred to as reflexivity.
Reliability	Authenticity and trustworthiness of the data/ credibility	Do the participants recognize the experience as their own? Has adequate time been allowed to fully understand the phenomenon?	Exhaustive description and synthesis of raw data with development of thematic elements is returned to the participants for them to validate accuracy of interpretation.
Generalizability	Transferability/ fittingness	Are the findings applicable outside the study situation?	Comprehensive descriptions of the setting and participants are produced.

Adapted from Lincoln and Guba (1985) and Baillie (2015).

Ensuring credibility refers to the conscious effort to establish confidence in an accurate interpretation of the meaning of the data (Carbonic, 1995). Do the results of the research reflect the experience of participants or the context in a believable way (Lincoln & Guba, 1985)? Does the explanation fit the description (Janesick, 1994)? Thorne (1997) identified the need to ensure that interpretations are trustworthy and reveal some truth external to the investigators' experience. Authenticity is closely linked to validity and involves the portrayal of research that reflects the meanings and experiences that are lived and perceived by the participants (Sandelowski, 1986).

Because qualitative research is based on entirely different epistemological and ontological assumptions compared with quantitative research, quantitative validity criteria are inappropriate for evaluation purposes (Hammersly, 1992). For example, the important distinction between internal and external validity in quantitative research holds less meaning and applicability within a framework where generalizability to populations is not a significant research goal (see Chapter 5). Leininger (1994) contended that quantitative validity criteria applied to qualitative research are awkward, confounding, and confusing (Hannes et al., 2010).

The expansion, proliferation, and evolution of qualitative research approaches have created a tension that has influenced validity criteria. Phenomenology, ethnography, grounded theory, and case study methods set the stage for the development of numerous other qualitative methods applicable to nursing science. The philosophical movements of feminism, postmodernism, and critical social theory also have contributed to creative approaches to science from an interpretive perspective. Much discussion has ensued regarding the alignment of philosophy, epistemology, and methodology. The divergence of the interpretive perspective from the positivistic perspective required in-depth analysis. Selecting research methods was viewed not simply as a technological choice; rather, methods were proposed to be based on philosophical, ideological, ethical, and political assumptions (Moccia, 1988).

> **EBP TIP**
>
> Work diligently and consistently to incorporate qualitative research into clinical practice.

Creativity must be preserved within qualitative research, but not at the expense of the quality of science. Creative work supports the discovery of the not yet known, going beyond previously established knowledge and challenging accepted thinking (Marshall, 1990). Table 9.3 provides a detailed summary of critiquing guidelines for qualitative research.

Promoting and evaluating scientific rigor in qualitative research is critical if these methodologies are to be used by clinicians in EBP. Criteria for assessing quality in qualitative research must differ from that of quantitative research. There is a range of techniques that can be used to promote, evaluate, and critique in qualitative research and, when consistently applied, provide practitioners with solid evidence to inform their practice. Remember that qualitative critiquing criteria are no less rigorous than those used to assess quantitative data; they are simply different and require different steps and measures to ensure quality data. You will note that the primary methods used to control internal validity in qualitative studies are those aimed at controlling bias relative to the researcher and the subjects. Qualitative researchers use bracketing as a method of recognizing and setting aside their knowledge or opinions about the study. Additional steps may include:

- prolonged engagements in the field,
- persistent observation,
- peer debriefing,
- member checks,
- audit trails,
- mixed methods, and
- establishing interrater reliability as data are analyzed and thematic elements emerge.

These steps are key for increasing both the dependability and credibility of the researcher's findings. The strongest qualitative evidence will emerge from studies that incorporate most of these common methods to enhance internal validity. See Table 9.3 for qualitative critique guidelines.

SYNTHESIS

From a philosophical viewpoint, the study of humans is deeply rooted in descriptive modes of science. With regard to safe patient care and accountability, remember that EBP has clear roots in quantitative and qualitative research. This has enlivened the debate about what constitutes evidence and reinvigorates the conversation about

TABLE 9.3 Critical Appraisal of Qualitative Research

Stylistic Considerations	1. Was the report well-written, grammatically correct, and well-organized? 2. Was there sufficient detail to enable critical appraisal? 3. Is there evidence that the researcher has the qualifications, knowledge, and expertise to conduct the research? 4. Does the abstract give a clear summary of the study. including the main findings and recommendations?
Statement of the Phenomenon of Interest	1. Was the title clear, accurate, and related to the research question? 2. What is the phenomenon of interest, and is it clearly stated for the reader? 3. What is the justification for using a qualitative method? 4. Is there a clearly defined qualitative research method?
Purpose	1. Is the purpose of the study appropriate for the research question? 2. Does the researcher describe the projected significance of the work to nursing?
Ethical Considerations	1. Is protection of human participants addressed? 2. Did the author address institutional review board approval? 3. Were the participants fully informed about the nature of the research? 4. Did the researcher address participant autonomy and confidentiality? 5. Were participants protected from harm?
Method	1. Is the method used to collect data compatible with the qualitative research question? 2. Is the qualitative method adequate to address the phenomenon of interest? 3. If a particular approach is used to guide the inquiry, has the researcher completed the study according to the processes described?
Sampling	1. What type of sampling is used? Is it appropriate given the particular method? 2. Are the informants who were chosen appropriate to inform the research? 3. Were the participants and setting adequately described and appropriate for Informing the research? 4. Was saturation achieved?
Data Collection	1. Is data collection focused on human experience? 2. Does the researcher describe data collection strategies (i.e., interview, observation, field notes)? 3. Were the data gathered of sufficient depth and richness? 4. Were the questions asked and observations made and recorded in an appropriate way? 5. Is saturation of the data described? 6. What are the procedures for collecting data?
Data Analysis	1. Are the data analysis strategies consistent with the qualitative method? 2. Has the researcher remained true to the data? 3. Does the reader follow the steps described for data analysis?

Authenticity and Trustworthiness of Data	1. Does the researcher address the credibility, auditability, and fittingness of the data?
	Credibility
	  • Do the participants recognize the experience as their own?
	Auditability
	  • Can the reader follow the researcher's thinking?
	  • Does the researcher document the research process?
	Fittingness
	  • Are the findings applicable outside the study situation?
	  • Are the results meaningful to individuals not involved in the research?
	  • Is the strategy used for analysis compatible with the purpose of the study?

Findings	1. Are the findings presented within a context? 2. Is the reader able to comprehend the essence of the experience from the report of the findings? 3. Are the researcher's conceptualizations true to the data? 4. Does the researcher place the report in the context of what is already known about the phenomenon? Was the existing literature on the topic related to the findings?

Continued

TABLE 9.3	**Critical Appraisal of Qualitative Research—cont'd**
Conclusions, Implications, and Recommendations	1. Do the conclusions, implications, and recommendations give the reader a context in which to use the findings?
	2. How do the conclusions reflect the study findings?
	3. What are the recommendations for future study? Do they reflect the findings?
	4. How has the researcher made the significance of the study explicit to nursing theory, research, or practice?
References	Were all the books, journals, and other materials referred to in the study accurately referenced?

the merits of qualitative research and its contribution to EBP (Meadows-Oliver, 2009). As a clinical leader, you want to think about the contribution to the Triple Aim (Institute for Healthcare Improvement, 2016) that is made by evidence from qualitative research studies; the three aims provide rich data about the patient experience and the context of care and also help to build theories about those lived experiences and social processes associated with being a patient. The purpose of qualitative research is about understanding phenomena and finding meaning through examining the pieces that make up the whole.

Evidence from the most commonly used qualitative nursing research methods—grounded theory, case study, ethnography, and phenomenology—provide valuable insights into why clinical practice may or may not work, help us consider patient preferences when designing best practice guidelines, and influence our QI strategies about how to provide a satisfying patient experience.

KEY POINTS

- Qualitative research findings are important components of EBP and QI.
- The purpose of qualitative research is to understand phenomena and find meaning by examining pieces that make up the whole.
- Qualitative research findings are linked to the component of the Triple Aim related to improving the patient's experience of care, including quality and satisfaction.
- Researchers using qualitative methods have a holistic worldview, value subjectivity, and believe that individuals attribute meaning to their experiences.
- Four types of qualitative methods include phenomenology, grounded theory, ethnography, and case study.
- The qualitative equivalent of a systematic review is a metasynthesis, sometimes called a metasummary.

- Qualitative research methods do not include a predetermined sample size; data collection continues until data saturation occurs.
- Qualitative data collection includes thoughts, feelings, observations, behaviors, and actual lived experiences as told by the informants experiencing the phenomenon under consideration.
- Qualitative data are words or artifacts, not numbers, that are analyzed by interpretation; narrative presentation of data is the norm.
- Scientific rigor is determined by critical appraisal criteria focused on dependability, credibility, transferability, and trustworthiness.

REFERENCES

Baillie, L. (2015). Promoting and evaluating scientific rigor in qualitative research. *Nursing Standard, 29*(46), 36–42.

Butler, A., Hall, H., & Copnell, B. (2016). A Guide to Writing a Qualitative Systematic Review Protocol to Enhance Evidence-Based Practice in Nursing and Health Care. *Worldviews on Evidence-Based Nursing, 13*(3), 241–249.

Carabez, R. M., Eliason, M. J., & Martinson, M. (2016). Nurses' Knowledge About Transgender Patient Care: A Qualitative Study. *Advances in Nursing Science (ANS), 39*(3), 257–271. *Advances in Nursing Science, 40*(2), 105–106.

Cesario, S., Morin, K., & Santa-Donato, A. (2002). Evaluating the level of evidence of qualitative research. *JOGNN: Journal of Obstetric, Gynecologic & Neonatal Nursing, 31*(6), 708–714.

Duggleby, w., & Williams, A. (2016). Methodological and Epistemological Considerations in Utilizing Qualitative Inquiry to Develop Interventions. *Qualitative Health Research*, 26(2), 147–153.

Davies, D., Dodd, J., Walsh, E., & Muncey, T. (2010). Qualitative research as evidence: criteria for rigour and relevance. *Journal of Research in Nursing*, 15(6), 497–508.

Finfgeld-Connett, D. (2010). Generalizability and transferability of meta-synthesis research findings. *Journal of Advanced Nursing*, 66(2), 246–254.

Flemming, K. (2007A). Research methodologies. Synthesis of qualitative research and evidence-based nursing. *British Journal of Nursing*, 16(10), 616–620.

Flemming, K. (2007B). The knowledge base for evidence-based nursing: a role for mixed methods research? *Advances in Nursing Science*, 30(1), 41–51.

Hannes, K., Lockwood, C., & Pearson, A. (2010). A Comparative Analysis of Three Online Appraisal Instruments' Ability to Assess Validity in Qualitative Research. *Qualitative Health Research*, 20(12), 1736–1743.

Hyatt, K. S., Davis, L. I., & Barroso, J. (2015). Finding the new normal: Accepting changes after combat-related mild traumatic brain injury. *Journal of Nursing Scholarship*, 47, 300–309.

Institute for Healthcare Improvement, The Triple Aim. http://www.ihi.org/Engage/Initiatives/TripleAim/Pages/default.aspx. Accessed November 24, 2017.

Kearney, M. (2001). Focus on research methods. Levels and applications of qualitative research evidence. *Research in Nursing & Health*, 24(2), 145–153.

Kuhnke, Bailey, Woodbury, & Burrows, (2014).

Lincoln, Y. S., & Guba, E. G. (1985). *Naturalistic inquiry*. Beverly Hills, CA:Sage.

van Manen, M. (2017). Phenomenology in Its Original Sense. *Qualitative Health Research*, 27(6), 810–825.

Meadows-Oliver, M. (2009). Does qualitative research have a place in evidence-based nursing practice? *Journal of Pediatric Healthcare*, 23(5), 352–354.

Nelson, A. (2008). Addressing the threat of evidence-based practice to qualitative inquiry through increasing attention to quality: a discussion paper. *International Journal of Nursing Studies*, 45(2), 316–322.

Newman, M., Thompson, C., & Roberts, A. (2006). Helping practitioners understand the contribution of qualitative research to evidence-based practice. *Evidence Based Nursing*, 9(1), 4–7.

Ranjbar, H., Joolaee, S., Vehadhir, A., & Bernstein, C. (2017). Becoming a nurse as a moral journey: A constructivist grounded theory. *Nursing Ethics*, 24(5), 583–597.

Rice, M. (2009). The importance of qualitative research to EBP. *Journal of the American Psychiatric Nurses Association*, 15(3), 200–201.

Sandelowski, M., & Barroso, J. (2003a). Creating metasummaries of qualitative findings. *Nursing Research*, 52, 226–233.

Sandelowski, M., & Barroso, J. (2003b). Toward a metasynthesis of qualitative findings on motherhood in HIV positive women. *Research in Nursing and Health*, 26, 153–170.

Sandelowski, M., & Barroso, J. (2007). *Handbook for synthesizing qualitative research*. Philadelphia, PA: Springer.

Schmidt, M., & Haglund, K. (2017). Debrief in Emergency departments to improve compassion fatigue and promote resiliency. *Journal of Trauma Nursing*, 24(5), 317–322.

Stake, R. E. (2000). Case studies. In N. K. Denzin, & Lincoln (Eds.), *Handbook of qualitative research* (2nd ed.). Thousand Oaks, CA: Sage.

Thorne, S. (2006). Reflections on 'Helping practitioners understand the contribution of qualitative research to evidence-based practice'. *Evidence Based Nursing*, 9(1), 7–8.

Thorne, S. (2009). The role of qualitative research within an evidence-based context: can metasynthesis be the answer? *International Journal of Nursing Studies*, 46(4), 569–575.

10

Understanding Statistics for Evidence-Based Practice

Carl Kirton, Leah Shever

LEARNING OBJECTIVES

After reading this chapter, you should be able to do the following:

- Discuss the significance of levels of measurement for data analysis.
- Explain the concept of probability as it applies to data analysis and interpretation of study findings.
- Differentiate between descriptive and inferential statistics.

- Distinguish between Type I and Type II error and their effects on a study's outcomes.
- Compare and contrast statistical tests used for specific types of research designs.
- Critically appraise statistics used for data analysis and report of findings in published research studies.
- Evaluate the strength and quality of the evidence provided by the findings of a research study and determine its applicability to practice

KEY TERMS

A priori
Absolute risk reduction
Clinical meaningfulness
Confidence interval
Continuous data
Descriptive statistics
Dichotomous data
Inferential statistics
Interval data
Likelihood ratio
Mean
Median

Mode
Negative predictive value
Nominal data
Nonparametric statistics
Numbers needed to treat
Null hypothesis
Null value
Odds ratio
Ordinal data
Parametric statistics
Positive predictive value
Prevalence

Probability value (*P*-value)
Power analysis
Range
Ratio data
Receiver Operating Characteristics (ROC) curve
Relative risk
Sensitivity
Specificity
Standard deviation
Type I error
Type II error

INTRODUCTION

Statistics are powerful tools that enable us to use data to make meaningful interpretations that can be applied to evidence-based clinical care. When used appropriately, they can describe, explain differences and relationships, and even predict outcomes of interest. Statistics also can be misinterpreted and misrepresented when not well understood. When considering the strength and quality of evidence to make a practice change, it is also important to understand the logic and information provided by the data in each of the studies you review. As you review studies, you will find different types of descriptive and inferential statistics that need to be considered. The consistency and appropriateness of the research design, methods, and statistical analyses are also important considerations when evaluating research literature. A research study of high quality will have a research design, methods, and statistical analyses that align with the research question(s) or hypotheses. This chapter is an introduction to basic concepts, statistical tests, and interpretation of findings for applicability to clinical practice.

BASIC CONCEPTS APPLIED TO AN EVIDENCE-BASED PROJECT: DATA

The collection of data to answer a PICO question (see Chapter 3) is fundamental and an essential part of the evidence-based (EB) or quality improvement (QI) project. Not all data are the same; it is essential that practitioners understand the type of data that is being reviewed or collected. Categorizing data helps to determine the type of analysis to be conducted during the analysis phase of the project. The theory of "levels of measurement" was proposed by Stanley Smith Stevens in 1946 (Stevens, 1946). He wrote that all measurement in science was conducted using four different types of scales that he called "nominal," "ordinal," "interval," and "ratio." The level of measurement of variables in an EB or QI project will influence the type of statistics that are possible to compute in the data analysis phase of the EB project.

Levels of Measurement

Nominal data, also referred to as categorical data, are not numerical and there is no established hierarchy between values. An example is the state you reside in. There is no numeric value associated with it, and there is no hierarchy between states like Michigan and Iowa. One does not hold a greater value than another. A specific type of nominal data is when there are only two options, such as yes/no, present/not present, or history of/no history of. When nominal data have only two possible options, they are referred to as dichotomous data.

The next level of data is ordinal, which is a set of data that has some type of hierarchy but the intervals between values may not be easily interpretable. An example is satisfaction level, where the choices are highly satisfied, neutral, and not satisfied. It is easy to see that there is a hierarchy, or rank, associated with these data

but how people interpret the difference between "highly satisfied" and "neutral" may differ because the interval is subject to interpretation.

Interval data are the level of data where the values are numeric, there is a hierarchy to the data, and the intervals between categories have consistent—set values that are easily understood across multiple individuals. The zero remains arbitrary and not absolute. An example would be temperature on a Fahrenheit scale where degrees have a common, set value so the difference between 20 and 30 degrees is the same value as the difference between 40 and 50 degrees.

The last type of data is ratio data, which has all of the same characteristics as interval data but includes absolute zero. This means that when a variable has a value of 0, there is a complete absence of that variable. An example is weight, where if a variable has a value of 0, that means it has no weight. However, when 0 represents a temperature, it is not absolute 0 because it is not possible to have an absence of temperature. See table below for data types, descriptions, and examples.

Examine Fig. 10.1, which is the Table II *Demographic Table* from the study by Lowe (Lowe et al., 2017) in Appendix B. Lowe lists nine factors (data or variables) to describe the study population. Gestational age, test age, income, maternal age, number of family moves, and number of children <6 years of age in the home are all ratio types of data because these data have different magnitudes at different levels and, as in the case of age, there is a true zero point. Maternal education, primary language, and ethnicity are measured at the nominal level of data because the response to the question fits a nonnumerical category and there is no established hierarchy between the categories.

Why is this discussion so important? Nominal and ordinal data are analyzed using what are called nonparametric or distribution-free statistical methods. On the other hand, interval and ratio scales are, if at all possible, to be analyzed using the typically more powerful parametric statistical methods. During the planning phase of your evidence-based project or QI project, the project team (sometimes with the support of a data analyst or statistician) selects an appropriate method of analysis for the study variables.

What about the critical appraisal process? How important to this process is understanding the statistics used? Most critical appraisal tools do not expect that the average reader is an expert in statistical design and

Table II. Demographic data

Factors		Placebo n = 14	ESA n = 35	Term n = 22	Placebo vs ESA	ESA vs term
Gestational age, wk	RATIO	27.64 (1.52)	27.37 (1.74)	39.05 (1.35)	.40	<.001
Test age, mo		48.79 (3.26)	48.64 (3.69)	45.04 (2.10)	.72	<.001
Income*		4.00 (1.92)	4.59 (2.10)	5.09 (1.68)	.24	.74
Maternal education†		4.50 (1.09)	4.85 (1.20)	5.43 (1.38)	.24	.34
Maternal age, y		24.57 (4.11)	27.92 (6.87)	29.91 (7.62)	.02	.74
Number of family moves		2.29 (1.94)	1.31 (1.28)	1.22 (1.41)	.01	.69
Number of children <6 y of age in home		2.07 (1.39)	1.59 (0.75)	1.65 (0.78)	.11	.19
Primary language					.10	.72
English	NOMINAL	100%	83%	86%		
Spanish		0%	17%	14%		
Ethnicity					.92	.05
Hispanic	NOMINAL	36%	37%	64%		
Non-Hispanic		64%	63%	36%		

Values shown are mean (SD) or percentiles.
*Income: <$10,000; $10,000–20,000; $20,000–30,000; $30,000–40,000; $40,000–50,000; $50,000–60,000; $60,000–70,000; $70,000.
†Maternal education: 0, less than high school; 1, completed high school; 2, completed 1 y of colleage, no degree; 3, associate's degree (2 y of college); 4, completed college; 5, some graduate school, no degree; 6, completed master's degree or greater.

Fig. 10.1 Demographic Table II. (From Lowe, J. R., Rieger, R. E., Moss, N. C., Yeo, R. A., Winter, S., Patel, S., & Ohls, R. K. (2017).Impact of erythropoiesis-stimulating agents on behavioral measures in children born preterm. *The Journal of Pediatrics, 184*, 75–80, Table II.)

as such will not ask you to evaluate whether the appropriate statistical test was chosen. As you become more expert in critical appraisal and aware of levels of measurement, the same type of statistical test will appear in study after study. For example, in a study or project that measures data at the nominal level (non-numerical and categorical), you would expect that the analysis would only include frequencies and percentages; advanced statistical tests cannot and should not be used to describe the data.

DESCRIPTIVE AND INFERENTIAL CONCEPTS APPLIED TO EVIDENCE-BASED PROJECTS

All research, whether quantitative (Chapters 6, 7, and 8) or qualitative (Chapter 9), collects data in a structured format and requires the investigator to summarize and analyze data in some meaningful way. Some investigators go beyond summarized data and test hypotheses or examine relationships among variables. Statistical analyses can be grouped into two major types: *descriptive* and *inferential*. Descriptive statistical analyses are used to summarize, organize, and display a set of data. Descriptive statistical analyses are used in every research study and evidence-based practice project. Inferential statistics are used to draw conclusions that could be applicable to a population based on information obtained from a sample. They are used to *infer* findings from

a sample onto a population. Some examples of the types of findings that can be produced from inferential statistics include identifying differences and determining the extent and direction of relationships. The following sections describe some specific descriptive and inferential statistical tests common to evidence-based projects.

Descriptive Statistics: Frequencies, Measures of Central Tendency, and Distribution of Data

There are three major elements examined with descriptive statistical analyses: frequencies, measures of central tendency, and distribution of data (i.e., variation of data). Frequency is another name for count. Frequencies are simply the counts of the phenomenon of interest. It is also common to calculate these frequencies as a percentage to give a perspective on the proportion of the sample that had exposure to the specified variable of interest.

Examine Fig. 10.2, which is Table II in Appendix B. In this study, Lowe (2017) describes three groups of preterm infants: one group received the study drug, one group received no drug (placebo), and the third group was a full-term comparison group. The "n" (highlighted in red in the figure) represents the frequency. These numbers can be used to calculate percentages as Lowe did to calculate the primary language and ethnicity of subjects (represented by the green circles in the figure).

The most common descriptive measures utilized are measures of central tendency. These include the mean,

Table II. Demographic data

Factors	Placebo n = 14	ESA n = 35	Term n = 22	Placebo vs ESA	ESA vs term
Gestational age, wk	27.64 (1.52)	27.37 (1.74)	39.05 (1.35)	.40	<.001
Test age, mo	48.79 (3.26)	48.64 (3.69)	45.04 (2.10)	.72	<.001
Income*	4.00 (1.92)	4.59 (2.10)	5.09 (1.68)	.24	.74
Maternal education†	4.50 (1.09)	4.85 (1.20)	5.43 (1.38)	.24	.34
Maternal age, y	24.57 (4.11)	27.92 (6.87)	29.91 (7.62)	.02	.74
Number of family moves	2.29 (1.94)	1.31 (1.28)	1.22 (1.41)	.01	.69
Number of children <6 y of age in home	2.07 (1.39)	1.59 (0.75)	1.65 (0.78)	.11	.19
Primary language				.10	.72
English	100%	83%	86%		
Spanish	0%	17%	14%		
Ethnicity				.92	.05
Hispanic	36%	37%	64%		
Non-Hispanic	64%	63%	36%		

Values shown are mean (SD) or percentiles.
*Income: <$10,000; $10,000–20,000; $20,000–30,000; $30,000–40,000; $40,000–50,000; $50,000–60,000; $60,000–70,000; $70,000.
†Maternal education: 0, less than high school; 1, completed high school; 2, completed 1 y of colleage, no degree; 3, associate's degree (2 y of college); 4, completed college; 5, some graduate school, no degree; 6, completed master's degree or greater.

Fig. 10.2 Demographic Table II. (From Lowe, J. R., Rieger, R. E., Moss, N. C., Yeo, R. A., Winter, S., Patel, S., & Ohls, R. K. (2017). Impact of erythropoiesis-stimulating agents on behavioral measures in children born preterm. *The Journal of Pediatrics, 184*, 75–80, Table II.)

median, and mode. All three are mechanisms to describe the average associated with the specified variable and are widely used to summarize ordinal, interval, and ratio level data. Examine the sample data in Table 10.1—the ages of the people in a fictitious sample. These measures of central tendency are designed to summarize the "typical" value that is found in our sample.

Often, descriptive frequencies, percentages, and means are typically reported in project evaluation work, such as evidence-based practice projects that are not research studies. Commonly, the pre- and post-intervention data are displayed in a table or graph format to assist with evaluation, but no further analysis may be needed if the analysis purpose was to determine whether a clinical improvement was made after implementation of an evidence-based project.

Another important descriptive analysis is to describe the amount of variation that exists in data. Several measures of variation are commonly used in statistical analysis. The most commonly used measure is the standard deviation. The standard deviation (SD) is an indication of how far the variables are spread from the mean. The higher the standard deviation, the higher the variation. The SD also is used in inferential data analyses. The SD formula is very simple: it is the square root of the variance. Use a spreadsheet program or statistical software to calculate the variance and the standard deviation. The standard deviation often is used in conjunction with the mean to summarize continuous, not categorical, data.

A related method to understand variation is describing the range of data. The range is simply the lowest and highest values reported. Ranges are appropriate to use when the data type is interval or ratio. The range would not be appropriate to use for nominal data. Often when ranges are described, the values are accompanied by the standard deviation. With four values of sample size, lowest value, highest value, and standard deviation, we can start to see how spread out the data are, or the extent of the variation.

The variation of the data is directly related to the *distribution* of the data. One of the foundations of inferential statistics is understanding how the data are distributed and whether they are "normally" distributed. Normal distribution is a concept where the mean, median, and mode all align, and the data points follow the classic bell-shaped curve with the same number of data points above and below the mean. Those points are more heavily concentrated around the mean and become more spread out the further one gets from the mean.

The distances from the mean are described in terms of standard deviations from the mean, often represented with the Greek letter *sigma* (σ). When the data are *normally distributed*, 68% of the values will fall within 1 standard deviation from the mean, 95% of values will fall within 2 standard deviations, and 99.7% of values will fall within 3 standard deviations. Keep in mind that these are standard deviations

TABLE 10.1	Sample Data
Data set: ages of individuals in the sample	31, 36, 38, 40, 42, 44, 44, 50, 52, 54, 54, 54, 56
Mean	The average of all the data in a set. To determine the mean, add all of the numbers in the data set and divide by the number of data points. $$\frac{31+36+38+40+42+44+44+50+52+54+54+54+56}{13}=45.77$$
Median	The value in a set that is closest to the middle of a range. To find the median, order the numbers in the data set. The median is the number that appears in the middle of the data set. 31, 36, 38, 40, 42, 44, **44**, 50, 52, 54, 54, 54, 56 44 (6 values appear above the median and 6 below when ranked from lowest to highest)
Mode	The value that occurs most frequently in a data set. 31, 36, 38, 40, 42, 44, 44, 50, 52, **54, 54, 54**, 56 54 (appears 3 times in the data set, more than any other value)

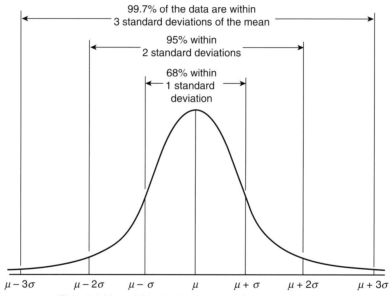

Fig. 10.3 Normal Distribution Including Standard Deviations

above and below the mean and not in only one direction. When the data are normally distributed, they are considered *parametric*. See Fig. 10.3; the classic bell-shaped curve is a graphic representation of data that is normally distributed.

An important consideration in determining whether data are normally distributed is the number in the sample. There is no set sample size to be considered normally distributed but as a general rule, larger is better (review the concept of the central limit theorem in Box 10.1).

CENTRAL LIMIT THEOREM IN PRACTICE

The unexpected appearance of a normal distribution from a population distribution that is skewed, even quite heavily so, has some very important applications in statistical practice. Many practices in statistics, such as those involving hypothesis testing or confidence intervals, make some assumptions concerning the population from which the data were obtained. One assumption initially made in a statistics course is that the populations we work with are distributed normally.

BOX 10.1 The Central Limit Theorem

The central limit theorem can seem quite technical but can be understood if we think through the following steps. We begin with a simple random sample with N individuals from a population of interest. From this sample, we easily can form a sample mean that corresponds to the mean of the measurement we are curious about in our population.

A sampling distribution for the sample mean is produced by repeatedly selecting simple random samples from the same population and of the same size, and then computing the sample mean for each of these samples. The samples are to be thought of as independent of one another. The central limit theorem concerns the sampling distribution of the sample means.

We may ask about the overall shape of the sampling distribution. The central limit theorem says that this sampling distribution is approximately normal, commonly known as a bell curve (see Fig. 10.3). This approximation improves as we increase the size of the simple random samples that are used to produce the sampling distribution. There is a very surprising feature concerning the central limit theorem. The astonishing fact is that this theorem says a normal distribution arises regardless of the initial distribution. Even if our population has a skewed distribution, which occurs when we examine things such as incomes or people's weights, a sampling distribution for a sample with a sufficiently large sample size will be normal.

BOX 10.2 Nonparametric Statistics

When the Author is	Examples of Non-parametric Statistics Found in Studies
Comparing means between two distinct/independent groups	Wilcoxon rank sum test
Comparing two quantitative measurements taken from the same individual	Wilcoxon signed rank test
Comparing means among three or more distinct/independent groups	Kruskal-Wallis test
Estimating the degree of association between two quantitative variables	Spearman's rank correlation
Testing for relationships between two categorical data sets	Chi square

The assumption that data is from a normal distribution simplifies matters but seems a little unrealistic. Just a little work with some real-world data shows that outliers, skewness, multiple peaks, and asymmetry show up quite routinely. We can deal with the problem of data from a population that is not normal. The use of an appropriate sample size and the central limit theorem help us address the problem of data from populations that are not normal.

Thus even though we might not know the shape of the distribution where our data comes from, the central limit theorem states we can treat the sampling distribution as if it were normal. Of course, for the conclusions of the theorem to hold, we do need a sample size that is large enough. Power analysis, the mathematical procedure used to calculate the number or sample size needed in a study to test the hypothesis can help us to determine how large of a sample is necessary for a given situation

(Taylor, 2017). If the sample size is too small, it cannot be assumed that the data are normally distributed; that is following the bell-shaped curve. Another circumstance when the data are not normally distributed is when data are skewed (i.e., concentrated above or below the mean). Another way to think of this is that the mean, median, and mode do not align. Testing for skewness helps the investigator select the appropriate statistic for the data. When the data are not distributed normally, the data are analyzed using *nonparametric* statistics (Box 10.2). When the data are distributed normally, the data are analyzed using parametric statistics (Box 10.3).

Trambert et al. (2016) conducted a randomized control trial to answer the clinical question, "Will the use of aromatherapy tabs in women enhance adaptation to anxiety associated with image-guided breast biopsy?" The investigator compared three groups: Group A received a lavender/sandalwood tab, Group B received an orange/peppermint tab, and Group C received a placebo control tab. Anxiety was measured using the State-Trait Anxiety Inventory. Mild anxiety scores range from 21 to 39, moderate anxiety scores range from 40 to 59, and severe anxiety scores are those greater than 59. If you were performing critical appraisal, at this point, you would identify that the variable (anxiety) is being measured at the interval or ratio level of data. This means that the appropriate

BOX 10.3   Parametric statistics

When the Author is	Examples of Para-metric Statistics Found in Studies
Comparing means between two distinct/independent groups	Two sample *t*-test
Comparing two quantitative measurements taken from the same individual	Paired *t*-test
Comparing means among three or more distinct/independent groups	Analysis of variance (ANOVA)
Estimating the degree of association between two quantitative variables	Pearson coefficient of correlation

statistical test would be a parametric test. If you examine Table 10.2 as discussed later, you will note that the authors compare the differences in the median scores among the three groups. The investigators used a nonparametric test (Kruskal-Wallis test). Why did the authors use a nonparametric test when a parametric test could have been used? The answer lies in determining whether the data are distributed normally.

There are statistical tests that can be used to determine whether or not the data are distributed normally. You should consult a statistical text for tests that determine whether your data are distributed normally.

INFERENTIAL STATISTICS

Descriptive statistics provide us with summary information about the group(s) under study. In other words, when you only use descriptive statistics for your project or investigation, you can only describe your findings as they apply to that group of individuals. You cannot say that your findings apply to similar groups or the entire population of a particular group of patients, or whether your findings merely happened as a result of chance; this is where inferential statistics come in. Regardless of the type of statistic used (see Boxes 10.2 and 10.3), they all have the same purpose: *to tell us the probability that the study findings can be attributed to chance.*

At the heart of inferential statistics is the examination of differences between two groups via the probability value (*p*-value), a numeric value that helps determine

whether the null hypothesis should be rejected or accepted and will be discussed in further detail in the text.

Before arriving at the probability value, data are collected by the researcher on available individuals through a method of selection (see discussion on sampling in Chapter 6). Ideally, we want to examine the entire population for our study. It is impossible or infeasible to examine each member of the population individually, so we choose a representative subset of the population, or a sample. Inferential statistics analyze a statistical sample, and from this analysis, we can say something about the population from which the sample originated. There are two major divisions of inferential statistics: a) tests of significance or a hypothesis testing framework and b) the confidence interval framework.

Testing for Significance or Hypothesis Testing Framework

Tests of statistical significance are ubiquitous in the professional literature. In hypothesis testing, the researcher makes a prediction as to how changes in the experimental variable (independent variable) cause or explain changes in another variable (dependent variable). To perform a test of significance, the researcher assumes that there is no relationship between the two variables; this is a null hypothesis. Testing for significance means that the researcher is assessing the probability that the null hypothesis is true. Through statistical testing (see Boxes 10.2 and 10.3), we either accept or reject the null hypothesis.

You easily can recognize the use of hypothesis testing when researchers report the "*p*-value." This is the probability of an event or outcome occurring in repeated trials under similar conditions. To interpret the *p*-value, the researcher must set a value at which it is considered to be statistically significant, a level known as α. This is the probability at which the observed data are not considered to be consistent with the null hypothesis being true. Thus, if the calculated *p*-value is less than this, it is said to be statistically significant, since it means the data have an even lower probability of being consistent with the null hypothesis. Setting the level of α is a key decision; by convention, it is often set at a level of 0.05.

Because research is not an exact science, there is always a probability that an error can occur in the researcher's conclusion. There are two types of known errors that can occur. The first, a Type I error, is the

TABLE 10.2 Median Baseline Anxiety and Change of Median State Scores

	LAVENDER ($N = 30$)		ORANGE ($N = 30$)		PLACEBO ($N = 27$)		
Variable	Mean	Range	Mean	Range	Mean	Range	p
Baseline state anxiety	48	22–66	43	22–73	43	23–66	.34
Baseline trait anxiety	37	23–61	32	20–64	30	23–59	.30
Change in state anxiety	−11	−35,4	−6	−33,10	−4	−28,23	.050[a]

Note: The change in state score (post/pre) was compared in the three groups using the Kruskal-Wallis test. Pairwise comparisons between groups were made using the Mann-Whitney U test. MDN= mean.
[a]Significant correlation at the $p < .05$ level.

rejection of a true null hypothesis. The second, a **Type II error,** is the failure to reject a false null hypothesis.

A Type I error can occur when the researcher has statistically significant results and, according to the rules of hypothesis testing, rejects the null hypothesis. In other words, the researcher states that the findings are significant when they are not. Why is this serious? When you are using evidence to change practice it can lead to a wrong conclusion and perhaps an inappropriate change in practice (i.e., you believe there are important differences when there really are not) (Guyatt et al., 1995).

The alpha level is the significance level that is the probability of committing the type I error. As discussed, alpha is typically set at 0.05. This means that there is a 5% risk, when there is a significant finding, of rejecting a true null hypothesis. When it is important to have a higher degree of certainty about the difference (for example, when you a study a treatment for a disease), the investigator can reduce alpha, say, to $< .01$, **a priori.** By definition, alpha defines the probability of committing a Type I error; the only way to avoid making a Type I error is by not rejecting the null hypothesis.

A Type II error can occur when the researcher fails to reject the null hypothesis. Plainly speaking, it occurs when we are saying that there is no difference in treatment areas when in truth there is one (Guyatt et al., 1995). When a Type II error occurs, you fail to make an important change in practice because you believe there isn't a need to do so; i.e., the study findings are not significant. In a study, the risk of making a Type II error is often denoted as β. Calculating β is complex and best done with statistical software. The most common reason for making a Type II error relates to an inadequate sample size; small sample sizes make it

difficult to detect a difference. To reduce the probability of committing a Type II error, researchers often conduct a prospective **power analysis.** Statistical power is the probability of correctly rejecting a null hypothesis that is false and thus avoiding a Type II error. It is influenced by sample size, effect size, significance level, and a variety of other factors such as research design. **Effect size** is the magnitude of the difference between groups. During the planning stage of a study, researchers first choose the significance level and then estimate the effect size. To do this, they often ask themselves, "How large of an effect do I want to see on the dependent variable—10%, 20%, 50%?" This is important because at the conclusion of the study, a 10% effect size might be statistically significant but clinically insignificant, whereas a 50% effect size might be both statistically and clinically significant. The chosen effect size often is based on economic or clinical reasons. It is particularly valuable for quantifying the effectiveness of a particular intervention relative to some comparison (see Intervention Studies in Chapter 6). It helps us to move beyond the simplistic question, "Does it work or not?" (statistical significance) to the far more sophisticated question, "How well does it work (clinical meaningfulness)?" It is important to note that effect size and sample size are linked. Detecting small differences requires larger samples, and increasing the effect size reduces sample size requirements. Moreover, by placing the emphasis on the most important aspect of an intervention, the size of the effect, rather than on its statistical significance (which conflates effect size and sample size), it promotes a more scientific approach to the question, "Does it really work?" For these reasons, effect size is an important tool in reporting and interpreting effectiveness and should be reported with intervention studies.

TABLE 10.3   Fall Prevention Interventions by Risk Categories

| Risk-Specific Interventions[c] | BEFORE IMPLEMENTATION (N = 1638 PATIENT DAYS) | | | AFTER IMPLEMENTATION (N = 1606 PATIENT DAYS) | | | |
	Patient Days[a]	Rate per 100 Patient Days[b]	CI	Patient Days	Rate per 100 Patient Days	CI	p Value
History of previous fall	133	0.6	0–1.8	209.7	82	77–87	<0.001
Mobility	1285	31	29–33	1333	88	87–90	<0.001
Toileting/ Elimination	853.7	50	47–53	917.7	66	63–69	<0.001
Cognition/ Mental status	769	2.3	1.3–3.2	531	77	74–80	<0.001
Medication	1525	0.11	0–0.25	1562	0.1	0–0.25	0.981
Risk for injury	1142	66	64–69	1285	88	86–89	<0.001

N = 1638 total patient days before intervention; N = 1606 total patient days after intervention.
[a]Patient days are the number of days of labeled risk (denominator).
[b]Number of times intervention(s) was received per 100 patient days (example: received a mobility intervention 88 times per 100 patient days).
[c]Received fall prevention interventions targeted to patient-specific risk (e.g., based on risk profile).
Not significant finding.
CI, Confidence interval.

Confidence Interval Framework

Null hypothesis significance testing is frequently used in clinical investigations, but this approach to interpreting *p*-values has many challenges that are beyond the scope of this chapter (Riemann & Lininger, 2015), including the arbitrary use of .05 to define the border between concluding *yes* or *no*. Statistical significance should be interpreted as evidence that the likelihood the results could have occurred based on chance is small. Statistical significance does not equate to a clinically meaningful finding. **Clinical meaningfulness** reflects the degree to which the differences and relationships reported in a study are relevant to nursing practice (Riemann & Lininger, 2015). Confidence intervals (CIs) help the clinician provide clinical meaningfulness to study results. A **confidence interval** represents a range of values within which a given population parameter (e.g., a mean, test statistic, or effect size) may be expected to fall. The confidence level (e.g., 95%) describes the chance of the lower and upper bounds of the confidence interval capturing the population value. Typically, investigators record their CI results as a 95% degree of certainty; at times, you also may see the degree of certainty recorded as 99%. More and more professional journals require investigators to include CIs as one of the statistical methods used to interpret study findings. Even when CIs are not

reported, they can be calculated easily from study data. The method for performing these calculations is widely available in statistical texts.

Examine Table 10.3 from the Titler study (Titler et al., 2016), which is located in Appendix C. The study investigators provide confidence intervals to accompany the pre- and post- risk-specific interventions. The rate per 100 patient days is called a point estimate, which is the sample data; in this case, it is the rate of falls. The confidence intervals are considered population parameters and provide the reader with the range of values that might be found in the population for the variable. Let's focus on the post-implementation values, since these are what interest us most.

After the intervention, the adoption of fall prevention interventions increased. For example, collection of history of previous falls increased from 0.6 times per 100 patient days to 82 times per 100 patient days. You know that this is a statistically significant value because the accompanying p <0.001. The investigators also provide you with calculated confidence intervals (via statistical testing—multivariable analysis) to estimate the range of values of rate per 100 days that would be seen in the population. In this case, that value is between 77 times per patient days to 87 times per patient days (α was set at <.05 for all analysis a priori).

Another unique feature of the confidence interval is that it can tell us whether the study results are statistically significant. When an experimental value is obtained indicating there is no difference between the treatment and control groups, we label that value "the value of no effect," or the **null value.** The value of no effect varies according to the outcome measure.

When you are examining a CI, if the interval does not include the null value, the effect is said to be statistically significant. When the CI does contain the null value, the results are said to be nonsignificant because the null value represents the value of no difference; that is, there is no difference between the treatment and control groups. In studies of equivalence (e.g., a study to determine whether two treatments are similar), this is a desired finding, but in studies of superiority or inferiority (e.g., a study to determine whether one treatment is better than the other), this is not the case.

The null value varies depending on the outcome measure. For numerical values determined by proportion or ratio (e.g., relative risk, odds ratio, discussed later in this chapter) the null value is "1." That is, if the CI does not include the value "1," the finding is statistically significant. If the CI does include the value "1," the finding is not statistically significant.

For numerical values determined by a mean difference between the scores in the intervention group and the control group (usually with continuous measures), the null value is "0." In this case, if the CI includes the null value of "0," the result is not statistically significant. If the CI does not include the null value of "0," the result is statistically significant as illustrated in Fig. 10.4 A to D.

If you examine Table 10.3, you will note that for the post-intervention medication variable the confidence interval contains a value of "0," the null value. Because it contains the null value it is considered a nonsignificant funding. This is reinforced by examining the p value for this variable, which is 0.981 and not significant at $\alpha < .05$.

READ, INTERPRET, AND UNDERSTAND EVIDENCE-BASED LITERATURE STATISTICS

Whenever a trial is conducted, there are three possible explanations for the results: (1) the findings are correct (truth), (2) they represent random variation (chance),

or (3) they are influenced by systematic error (bias). Hypothesis testing and confidence intervals help us answer these questions about a study. During the critical appraisal process, we may encounter other types of statistics that not only help determine whether the research evidence is true and free of bias but also provide relevance to our individual patients and groups of patients. The specific statistics you will see in your review of the evidence-based literature depends on the type of clinical question you are asking. Clinical questions are categorized as follows:

1. **Intervention studies:** When you want to answer a question about the effectiveness of a particular treatment or intervention, you will select studies that have the following characteristics:
   - An experimental or quasi-experimental study design (see Chapter 6)
   - An outcome that is known or of probable clinical importance observed over a clinically significant period of time

   When studies are in this category, you use a therapy appraisal tool to evaluate the article. A therapy tool can be accessed at http://www.cebm.net/critical-appraisal/.

2. **Observational studies:** These test treatments retrospectively, cross-sectionally, or prospectively when you are studying cohorts in relation to an outcome of interest when a clinical trial and randomization are not possible. Cohort studies are useful when your clinical question is focused on Diagnosis, Causation *or* Prognosis, and Harm.

   a. **Diagnosis category:** When you want to answer a question about the usefulness, accuracy, selection, or interpretation of a particular measurement instrument or laboratory test, you will select studies that have the following characteristics:
   - Cross-sectional study design (see Chapter 7) with people suspected to have the condition of interest
   - Administration to the patient of both the new instrument or diagnostic test and the accepted "gold standard" measure
   - Comparison of the results of the new instrument or test and the gold standard
   - When studies are in this category, you use a diagnostic test appraisal tool to evaluate the article. A diagnostic tool can be accessed at http://www.cebm.net/critical-appraisal.

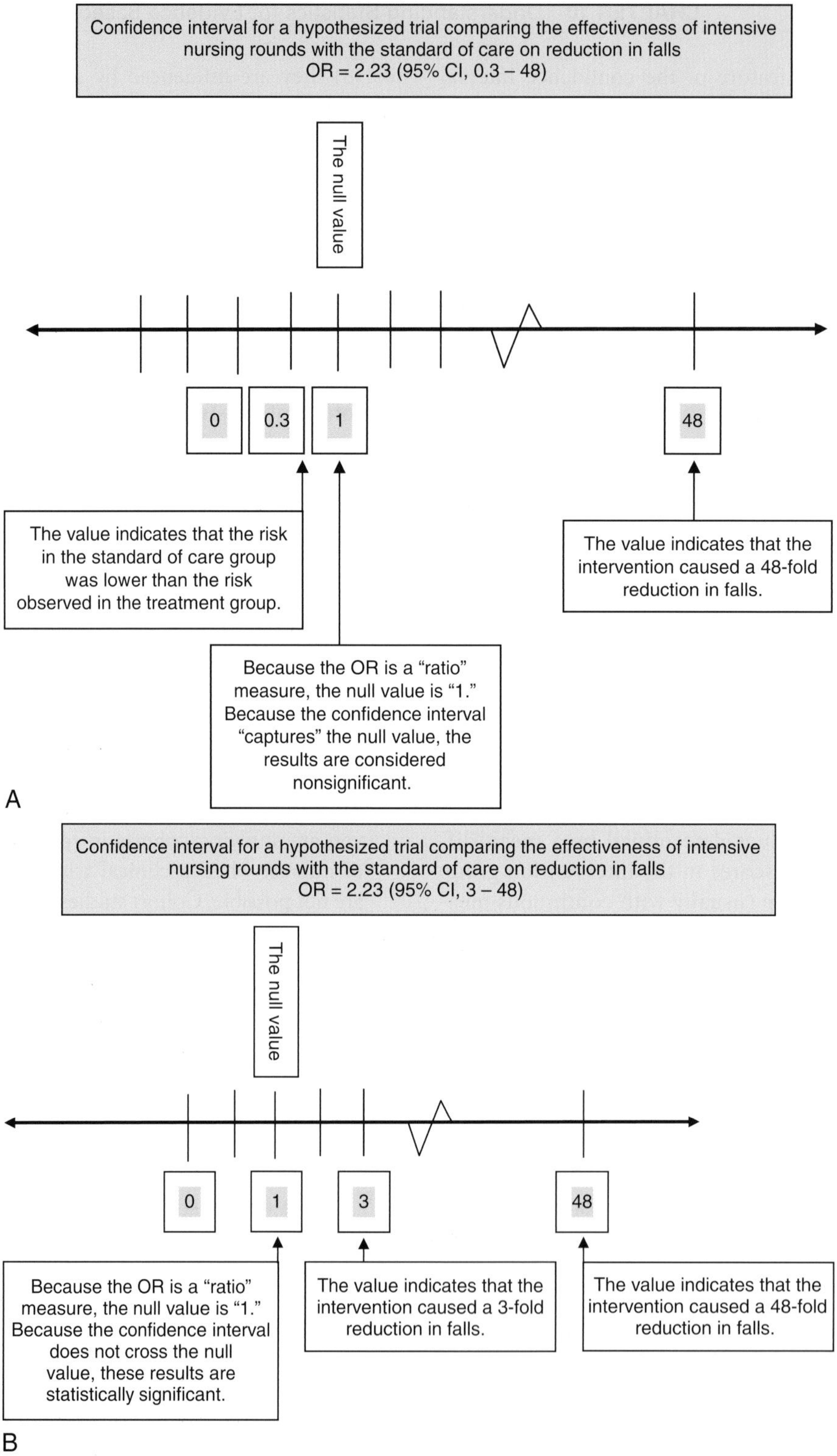

Fig. 10.4 (A) Confidence Interval (nonsignificant) for a hypothesized trial comparing the ratio of events in the experimental group and control group. (B) Confidence Interval (significant) for a hypothesized trial comparing the ratio of events in the experimental group and control group. (C) Confidence Interval (nonsignificant) for a hypothesized control trial comparing the difference between two treatments. (D) Confidence Interval (significant) for a hypothesized control trial comparing the difference between two treatments.

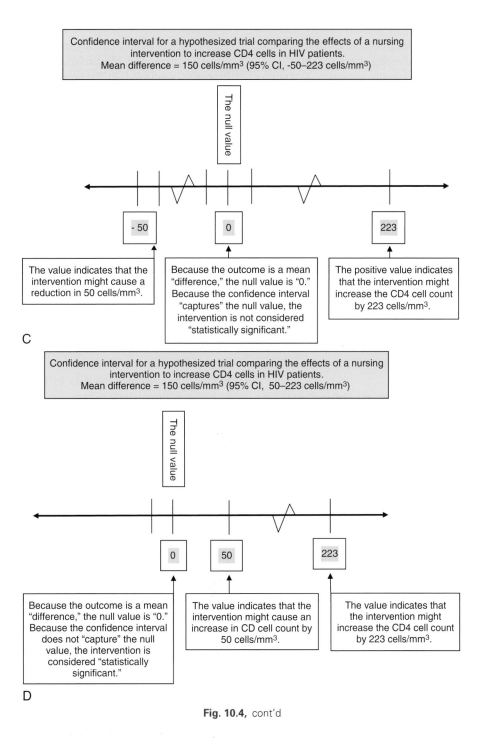

Fig. 10.4, cont'd

b. **Prognosis category:** When you want to answer a question about a patient's likely course for a particular disease state or identify factors that may alter the patient's prognosis, you will select studies that have the following characteristics:

- Nonexperimental, usually longitudinal study of a particular group (cohort) for a particular outcome or disease (see Chapter 7)
- Follow-up for a clinically relevant period (time is the exposure)
- Determination of factors in those who do and do not develop a particular outcome
- When studies are in this category, you use a prognosis appraisal tool (sometimes called a cohort tool) to evaluate the article. A prognosis tool can be accessed at http://www.cebm.net/critical-appraisal/.

c. **Harm category:** When you want to determine whether one variable is related to or caused by another, you will select studies that have the following characteristics:

- Nonexperimental, usually longitudinal or retrospective (ex post facto or case control) study designs over a clinically relevant period of time (see Chapter 7)
- Assessment of whether the patient has been exposed to the independent variable
- When studies are in this category, you use a harm appraisal tool (sometimes called a case-control tool) to evaluate the article. A harm appraisal tool can be accessed at http://www.cebm.net/critical-appraisal/.

3. **Meta-analysis studies**: When you want to answer a focused clinical question through an objective appraisal of carefully synthesized research evidence, you will select studies that have the following characteristics:

- Begins by formulating an important clinical question, identifies eligible studies to answer the question, abstracts study data, performs statistical analysis, and reports results
- Summarizes and analyses a large number of trials and resolves clinical discrepancies raised by these trials (see Chapter 8)

Intervention Studies

Intervention studies, often called randomized controlled (clinical) trials (RCTs), reflect the strongest design type for an individual study, located at Level II on the Evidence Hierarchy (see Chapter 2). This is the most appropriate type of design to answer questions about the effectiveness and efficacy of interventions focused on testing cause and effect relationships (see Chapter 6). Properly conducted RCTs provide essential evidence about the benefits and harms of a therapeutic intervention. To ensure accurate interpretation of study findings EBP leaders should understand the measures of effect and their precision common to intervention studies.

Statistics Common to Intervention Studies

Intervention studies usually contrast data from two or more different groups of subjects. The evidence-based statistics used in an intervention study depends on whether the numerical values of the study variables are **continuous** (a variable that measures a degree of change or a difference on a range, such as blood pressure) or *discrete,* also known as dichotomous (measuring whether an event did or did not occur, such as the number of people diagnosed or not diagnosed with type 2 diabetes).

Continuous outcomes (e.g., mean scores) often are analyzed by a basic statistical test called the *t*-test, a method that assumes the data in the different groups come from populations where the observations have a normal distribution and the same variances (or standard deviations). Similar to a *t*-test, the one-way ANOVA test that can be used to compare the means from three or more groups. There also is the two-way ANOVA that allows you to compare the means of two or more groups in response to two different independent variables. The statistics used depend on the level of measurement, whether your data is normally distributed (parametric vs. nonparametric), and the category of data (see Boxes 10.2 and 10.3, and a statistics textbook).

The goal of most randomized control trials is to measure the effect of an intervention on an outcome. The effect on dichotomous outcomes (measuring whether an event did or did not occur) have common measures that are important to evidence-based practitioners (Mirzazadeh, Malekinejad, & Kahn, 2015). In such trials, we want to know whether the treatment or intervention results in good or bad outcomes and by how much. Investigators use risk calculations to assist EBPs in considering whether to accept or reject a treatment. They are also used to help communication risk-benefit information to patients and/or key stakeholders.

Let's consider that you are concerned about the rate of readmission of older adults with dementia to your facility, and you want to explore an intervention to reduce the rate of readmission. Rubin (2018) used a specialized intervention called *Hospital Elder Life Program* (HELP) with staff on an inpatient unit to reduce hospital readmissions and compared the units that received the HELP training with units that did not receive the training. The study found that patients on HELP units had a readmission rate of 16.9% vs. 18.9% on the control units (Rubin, Bellon, Bilderback, Urda, & Inouye, 2018). Using this data we can describe some of the common risk calculations used in EBP.

Absolute risk reduction. The most basic and simplest measure is absolute risk reduction (ARR), also called risk difference. That is, as a result of using the treatment, is the risk of an event reduced by a clinically meaningful amount? The calculation is the difference between the risk of an event in the control group and the risk of an event in the treated group. Examining the Rubin data we can say that the HELP intervention has a risk difference or ARR of 2%; that is, readmissions were reduced by 2% in the HELP-trained unit. The authors of the study did not report the ARR. If they are reported, confidence intervals should be reported. Recall that a confidence interval that contains zero means that there is no significant difference between the treatment and the placebo in terms of risk.

Number needed to treat. Another useful measure based on ARR is the number needed to treat (NNT), which is defined as the reciprocal of the ARR. The meaning of this measure is the number of patients who need to be treated to get the desired outcome in one patient who would not have benefited otherwise. This number is a great way to communicate the effectiveness of a treatment (or intervention) and is obtained by dividing the absolute risk (or risk difference) into 100.

$$NNT = \frac{100}{Absolute\ Risk}$$

Returning to our Rubin study, the NNT calculation is:

$$50 = \frac{100}{2}$$

On average, 50 patients would have to receive experimental treatment (the HELP intervention) for one additional patient to NOT have a readmission. More effective treatments have lower NNTs. The ideal NNT is 1, which equals everyone benefiting from the treatment but is rarely seen with any treatment or intervention. The clinical meaning of an NNT is subject to interpretation. Without additional knowledge it is difficult to interpret the NNT. In this case, for example, all other readmission interventions might have an NNT of 100, which would make this intervention clinically useful and superior to others. The presentation of an NNT alone without some context (baseline risk, time horizons, and confidence intervals) is ambiguous and less useful for decision making (Mendes, Alves, & Batel-Marques, 2017; Stang, Poole, & Bender, 2010).

Relative risk (RR) and relative risk reduction (RRR). The next two common measures are the relative risk and relative risk reduction. The RR is often used when the study involves comparing the likelihood, or chance, of an event occurring between two groups. **Relative risk** is considered a descriptive statistic, not an inferential one, since it does not determine statistical significance. RR utilizes the probability of an event occurring in one group compared with the probability of an event occurring in the other group. It requires the examination of two dichotomous variables, where one variable measures the event (occurred vs. not occurred) and the other measures the groups (group 1 vs. group 2). When a relative risk value is above 1, it implies that the risk factor(s) increase the probability that the disease will occur. When the relative risk value is below 1, it implies that the probability of developing that disease decreases.

RR is calculated by dividing the probability of an event occurring for group 1 (A) divided by the probability of an event occurring for group 2 (B).

$$Relative\ Risk = \frac{Probability\ of\ the\ disease\ given\ exposure\ (A)}{Probability\ of\ the\ disease\ without\ exposure\ (B)}$$

The relative risk aids in communicating the value of treatment relative to no treatment at all. So how is this information used? Let's return to the Rubin study; we know that the units that did not receive the training on the intervention (control unit) had a readmission rate of 18.9%. The intervention unit had a readmission rate of 16.9%. As we know, the ARR from the vaccine is 2%.

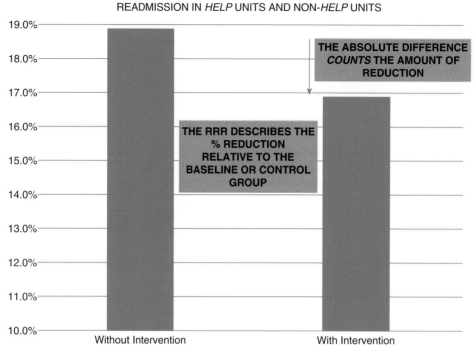

Fig. 10.5 Readmission in *HELP* units and non-*HELP* units

Another way to describe this situation is that 81.1% of older patients will remain at home (not be readmitted) without the intervention while 83.1% will remain at home if they were on the intervention unit. The relative risk is calculated below:

$$0.89 = \frac{0.169}{0.189}$$

Alone, this number is not useful to interpretation, although we know that because it is less than one, readmission is less likely in the experimental group than in the control group (see Evidence-Based Practice Tip box).

EBP TIP

- If the RR (relative risk) = 1 or the CI (confidence interval) = 1, then there is no significant difference between the treatment and control groups.
- If the RR >1 and the CI does not include 1, events are significantly more likely in the treatment group than the control group.
- If the RR <1 and the CI does not include 1, events are significantly less likely in the treatment group than the control group.

We use this ARR to calculate the RRR. It provides information on the percentage reduction of readmissions relative to doing nothing at all (similar to not having any treatment).

Relative Risk Reduction =

$$\frac{ARR}{Probability\ of\ the\ disease}$$
without exposure (B)

The RRR calculation for the Rubin study is:

$$0.105 = \frac{0.02}{0.189}$$

The RRR expresses how much the intervention reduces the risk readmission relative to the natural, untreated risk (readmission without the intervention). It can be interpreted as follows: Receiving the HELP intervention will reduce older adults' readmission risk by 11% relative to the risk of readmission if they have not received the HELP intervention. Fig. 10.5 describes the relationship between the ARR and the RRR.

One use of this statistic is to assist the clinical staff and patients in deciding whether an intervention is beneficial.

TABLE 10.4 Measures of Association for Trials that Report Discrete Outcomes

Measure of Association	Definition	Comment
Control event rate (CER)	Proportion of patients in control group in which an event is observed	The CER is calculated by dividing the number of patients who experienced the outcome of interest by the total number of patients in the control group.
Experimental event rate (EER)	Proportion of patients in experimental treatment groups in which an event is observed	The EER is calculated by dividing the number of patients who experienced the outcome of interest by the total number of patients in the experimental group.
Absolute risk reduction (ARR), also called risk difference or attributable risk reduction	This value tells us the reduction of risk in absolute terms. The ARR is considered the "real" reduction because it is the difference between the risk observed in those who did and did not experience the event.	Arithmetic difference in risk of outcome between patients who have had the event and those who have not had the event, calculated as EER−CER
Relative risk (RR), also called risk ratio	Risk of event after experimental treatment as a percentage of original risk	The RR is calculated by dividing the EER/CER. If CER and EER are the same, the RR = 1 (this means there is no difference between the experimental and control group outcomes). If the risk of the event is reduced in EER compared with CER, RR <1. *The further to the left of 1 the RR is, the greater the event, the less likely the event is to occur.* If the risk of an event is greater in EER compared with CER, RR >1. *The further to the right of 1 the RR is, the more likely the event is to occur.*
Relative risk reduction (RRR)	This value tells us the reduction in risk in relative terms. The RRR is an estimate of the percentage of baseline risk that is removed as a result of the therapy; it is calculated as the ARR between the treatment and control groups divided by the absolute risk among patients in the control group.	Percent reduction in risk that is removed after considering the percent of risk that would occur anyway (the control group's risk), calculated as EER−CER/CER

Other than staff training time, there are few costs associated with the program. From the patient perspective, there is little to no harm or other risk associated with the intervention. From a leadership perspective, the reduction in readmissions seems clinically and perhaps financially significant. It seems the decision to adopt this intervention might benefit clinicians, payers, patients, and the organization.

The RRR statistic is affected by the baseline risk, and this fact makes its interpretation more complex than the ARR statistic. As the baseline risk rises, the RRR also increases but at a much lower rate than the ARR (again, assuming the treated risk is constant). It is clear that at lower baseline risk levels, the RRR is much higher than the ARR, but at higher baseline risk levels, the ARR approaches the RRR. Given the sensitivity of RRR to the baseline risk, it is important for the clinician to consider both the ARR and RRR statistics to understand the amount of risk reduction a drug or other treatment can achieve for a population of patients. It is also important to remember that any individual patient may or may not benefit from a particular intervention. These statistics predict for populations, not individuals.

Table 10.4 summarizes the measures of risk associated with an intervention study with discrete outcomes.

OBSERVATIONAL STUDIES

Observational studies are commonly found in practice-based research. They are so called because the investigator observes individuals without manipulation or intervention. This is in contrast to randomized controlled trials where investigators do intervene and look at the effects of the intervention on an outcome. Although randomized controlled trials are useful in determining causal relationships between treatment and outcome, there are often instances where randomized controlled trials are not appropriate, so observational studies are needed. There are several different types of observational studies; this discussion can be found in detail in Chapter 7. As with intervention studies, there are several statistical measures commonly noted in each of the three types of observational studies seen in clinical queries.

Statistics Common to Diagnosis Studies

In articles that answer clinical questions of diagnosis, investigators study the ability of screening or diagnostic tests, or components of the clinical examination, to detect (or not detect) disease when the patient has (or does not have) the particular disease of interest. All screening and diagnostic tests have the following characteristics:

1. True positive: The patient has the disease and the test is positive.
2. False positive: The patient does not have the disease but the test is positive.
3. True negative: The patient does not have the disease and the test is negative.
4. False negative: The patient has the disease but the test is negative.

The accuracy of a test or technique is measured by its sensitivity and specificity. Sensitivity is the test's ability to correctly designate a subject with the disease as positive. A highly sensitive test means that there are few false negative results; few actual positive cases are missed. Tests with high sensitivity have potential value for screening because they rarely miss subjects with the disease.

Specificity is the test's ability to correctly designate a subject without the disease as negative; a highly specific test means there are few false positive results. Therefore, high-specificity tests perform well for diagnosis because of low false-positive errors. Tests with low specificity have the disadvantage that, among other things, many

TABLE 10.5   Calculating Sensitivity and Specificity

	Disease Present	Disease Absent
Test positive	a (TP)	b(FP)
Test negative	c (FN)	d(TN)
	Sensitivity: a/(a + c)	Specificity: d/(b + d)

FN, False negative; FP, false positive; TN, true negative; TP, true positive.

subjects without the disease will screen positive and potentially receive unnecessary and possibly invasive, risky, or expensive follow-up diagnostic or therapeutic procedures. Table 10.5 shows how investigators calculate the sensitivity and specificity of new tests and interventions. To begin to populate the table, researchers first compare testing information by comparing a new diagnostic test with the gold standard test. The gold standard is the best single test or combination of tests that is considered the current preferred method of diagnosing a particular disease. For example, the gold standard test for diagnosing cancer is the surgical biopsy.

- In cell "a," we enter those in whom the test in question correctly diagnosed the disease as determined by the gold standard. In other words, the test is positive, as is the gold standard. These are the true positives (TPs).
- In cell "b," we enter those who have positive results for the test in question but do not have disease according to the gold standard test. The newer test has wrongly diagnosed the disease. These are false positives (FPs).
- In cell "c," we enter those who have the disease according to the gold standard test but have negative results with the test in question. The test has wrongly labeled a diseased person as "normal." These are false negatives (FNs).
- In cell "d," we enter those who have no disease as determined by the gold standard test and are also negative according to the newer test. These are true negatives (TNs).

Using the data in the table you easily can calculate the sensitivity and specificity of your screening or diagnostic test.

Generally, you will not have to calculate these data. It is often provided in table format to the reader. Frisse et al. (2017) conducted a study to evaluate the validity of women's self-reported history of chlamydia trachomatis (CT) infection compared with chlamydia trachomatis serology, a marker for previous infection (Frisse et al., 2017).

TABLE 10.6 Serological Status by Self-Reported History of CT Infection

	Positive serology (n = 146)	Negative serology (n = 263)
Positive self-report (n = 108)	76	32
Negative self-report (n = 301)	70	231

Sensitivity is 52.1% (95% CI, 43.6–60.4%). Specificity is 87.8% (95% CI, 83.3–91.5%). Positive predictive value is 70.4% (95% CI, 60.8–78.8%). Negative predictive value is 76.7% (95% CI, 71.6–81.4%).
CI, Confidence interval; CT, chlamydia trachomatis.
Frisse et al. (2017). Validity of self-reported CT infection. *American Journal of Obstetrics and Gynecology.*

BOX 10.4 Positive Predictive Value and Negative Predictive Value

Positive predictive value (PPV)	The proportion of people with a positive test who have the target disorder	Formula for positive predictive value: PPV = True Positive/ (True Positive + False Positive)
Negative predictive value (NPV)	The proportion of people with a negative test who do not have the target disorder	Formula for negative predictive value: NPV = True Negative/ (True Negative + False Negative)

They compared participants' survey responses with the question, "Have you ever been told by a health care provider that you had chlamydia?" to serological test results indicating the presence or absence of antibodies to chlamydia trachomatis as assessed by a microimmunofluorescence assay. Prevalence of past infection, sensitivity, and specificity were calculated and are presented in Table 10.6.

Sensitivity of self-report (the new diagnostic test) was 52.1% and the specificity of self-report was 87.8%. The authors concluded, "*When evaluating the validity of self-report in women enrolled in the FACT study, we found self-report to not be a valid marker of past CT infection status. Only 52% of women with positive serology reported a history of CT infection. This low sensitivity indicates a high false-negative rate. Specificity was higher at 88%, indicating a false-positive rate of 12%*" (Frisse, 2017). Sensitivity and specificity, although widely used, are a small part of the story because they describe the specific characteristics of diagnostic tests; these characteristics must be considered along with the prevalence of the disease in the population. The **prevalence** of the disease is the percentage of subjects in the population under study that have the disease. In a population in which a disease is prevalent, a positive test is more meaningful than a positive test in a population in which the disease is very rare.

Predictive values are a measure of accuracy that account for the prevalence of a disease. Predictive values provide information about test *performance*. The **positive predictive value** (PPV) expresses the proportion of those with positive test results who truly have the disease, and a **negative predictive value** (NPV)

expresses the proportion of those with negative test results who truly do not have the disease. To calculate the PPV and NPV you need the sensitivity and specificity. If you refer to Box 10.4, you can see how easy it is to calculate the PPV and NPV; most investigators also provide this information. If you look at Table 10.6 from the Frisse study, you will see that the investigator provides that PPV = 70.4% and NPV is 76.7%. The PPV tells the clinician what percent of those with a positive finding have the disease. The NPV reveals what percent of those with a negative result do not have the disease. The correct interpretation for PPV and NPV for the Frisse study is: "*Our positive and negative predictive values of self-reported CT infection were 70% and 77%, respectively. Thus 30% of participants who reported a history of CT infection did not have a history of infection according to serology, and almost 25% of participants who reported not having a history of CT infection actually had serological evidence of infection*" (Frisse, 2017).

In the process of making a clinical diagnosis, clinicians use diagnostic tests to modify their initial clinical suspicions of disease to make a particular diagnosis more or less likely. The sensitivity or specificity of a particular test may be known, but how does one integrate that information with clinical intuition or pretest probability to determine likelihood of a disease being present, or post-test probability? Fortunately, there is a statistical test that helps the clinician understand how the probability of disease changes once the results of a specific test are known. The statistical tool to aid in obtaining this information is the likelihood ratio. The **likelihood ratio (LR)** expresses the magnitude by which the probability of disease in a specific patient is modified by the result of

BOX 10.5   Positive Likelihood Ratio and Negative Likelihood Ratio

Positive likelihood ratio (LR)	The LR of a positive test tells us how well a positive test result does by comparing its performance when the disease is present to when it is absent. The best test to use for ruling in a disease is the one with the largest likelihood ratio of a positive test.	Formula for positive likelihood ratio: Sensitivity/(1 – Specificity)
Negative likelihood ratio	The LR of a negative test tells us how well a negative test result does by comparing its performance when the disease is absent to when it is present. The better test to use to rule out disease is the one with the smaller likelihood ratio of a negative test.	Formula for negative likelihood ratio: (1 – Sensitivity)/Specificity

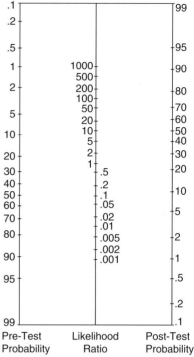

Fig. 10.6 The Likelihood Ratio Nomogram

a test (Deeks & Altman, 2004). Stated another way, the LR can be used to calculate the probability of abnormality. It indicates the degree to which the result increases or decreases the odds of disease from the pre-test odds. The use of odds rather than risks makes the calculation slightly complex, but a nomogram (discussed later) can be used to avoid making conversions between odds and probabilities (Deeks & Altman, 2004).

LRs are not always provided by study authors but where data is dichotomous, the LR can be calculated easily using the simple formula shown in Box 10.5.

In the Frisse study, the authors provide a positive likelihood ratio of 4.28. The practical advantage of the LR is the ability to interpret a particular result in the context of the individual patient and derive a post-test probability for disease. To do this it is necessary to first determine a pretest probability that may be based on clinical assessment, knowledge of local prevalence, other investigations, risk factors, etc. This probability is converted to odds and multiplied by the LR for the test result obtained. The resultant post-test

odds then are converted back to a post-test probability (Empson, 2002).

For example, suppose we take a sexual history on a sexually active female of childbearing age. From epidemiological data, we know that the prevalence of asymptomatic chlamydia infection in the population is about 47% (HEDIS, 2016). This could be our pretest probability; other sources of pretest probability can be based on the patient's history and physical examination. We then apply the diagnostic test with its known likelihood ratio. Multiplying the pretest probability by the likelihood ratio provides the post-test probability. Most EBP practitioners use a likelihood ratio nomogram rather than perform mathematical calculations (Fig. 10.6).

If we note our pretest probability and the test is positive with a known likelihood ratio, the probability that the patient has chlamydia is 70% (Fig. 10.7). With that level of probability, your decision would definitely be to treat the patient. Although the authors of the Frisse study did not provide a negative likelihood ratio, it is calculated easily from sensitivity and specificity (see Box 10.5); the NLR = 0.5. With a pretest probability of 45% and an NLR of 0.5 (and the test is negative), using our

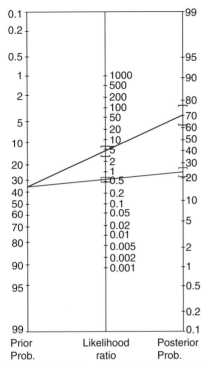

Fig. 10.7 Use of the Likelihood Ratio for Chlamydia Study Data

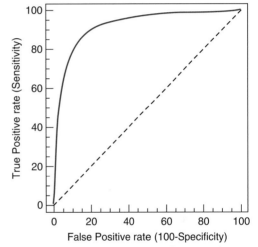

TABLE 10.7   How Much Do Likelihood Ratio Changes Affect Probability of Disease?

Likelihood Ratio Positive	Likelihood Ratio Negative	Probability That Patient Has (LR) or Does Not Have (LR)
LR > 10	LR < 0.1	Large
LR 5–10	LR 0.1–0.2	Moderate
LR 2–5	LR 0.2–0.5	Small
LR < 2	LR > 0.5	Tiny
LR = 1.0		Test provides no useful information

LR, Likelihood ratio.

Fig. 10.8 Example of a Receiver Operating Curve

nomogram, our post-test probability of infection is 23%. Without any other compelling evidence to treat this client, you are less likely to do so given this lowered probability of infection.

As illustrated in Table 10.7, a test with a large positive likelihood ratio (e.g., greater than 10), when applied, provides the clinician with a high degree of certainty that the patient has the suspected disorder. Conversely, tests with a very low positive likelihood ratio (e.g., less than 2), when applied, provide you with little to no change in the degree of certainty that the patient has the suspected disorder. When a test has a likelihood ratio of "1" (the null value), it will not contribute to decision making in any meaningful way and should not be used. A test with a large negative likelihood ratio provides the clinician with a high degree of certainty that the patient does not have the disease. The farther away from "1" the negative LR is, the better the test will be for its use in ruling out disease (i.e., there will be few false negatives). More and more journal articles require authors to provide test LRs; they also may be available in secondary sources.

When a test has only a single threshold or cutpoint value (for instance, positive or negative for disease, such

as a biopsy), likelihood ratios are useful. Tests that yield results on a continuous scale (e.g., Braden Score for pressure ulcer risk) require specification of a test threshold to define positive and negative results. Changing the threshold alters the proportion of false positive and false negative diagnoses.

This change in threshold for a given instrument or diagnostic test can be displayed in a specific type of graph known as the **Receiver Operating Characteristics (ROC) curve**. This graph can be extremely helpful in establishing an acceptable threshold or cutoff point for the instrument or diagnostic test. This graph plots the sensitivity and false positive rate at a given value for the instrument or diagnostic test (Fig. 10.8). The best cutoff has the highest true positive rate together with the lowest false positive rate. Examine Fig. 10.8; the false

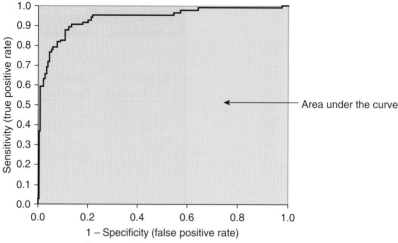

Fig. 10.9 The area under the ROC curve (AUROC)

positive rate is on the X axis and the true positive rate is on the Y axis. All of the cutoff values are determined and plotted on the graph, creating a curve (the blue line in the figure). Thus, every point on the ROC curve represents a chosen cutoff, although you cannot see it. What you can see is the curve of the true positive fraction and the false positive fraction that you will get when you choose this cutoff. The important part of the ROC curve is the area under the curve. The area under the ROC curve (AUROC) of a test can be used as a criterion to measure the test's discriminative ability, i.e., how well the test can discriminate in a given clinical situation (Fig. 10.9).

A perfect test can discriminate between healthy and sick persons with 100% sensitivity and 100% specificity (no such test), and would look like the curve in Fig. 10.10.

When we have a test with no ability to discriminate between those with and without disease, we have a worthless test. A worthless test has a discriminating ability equal to flipping a coin. The ROC curve of the worthless test falls on the diagonal line. It includes the point with 50% sensitivity and 50% specificity (Fig. 10.11). The area under the ROC curve of the worthless test is 0.5.

By examining the graph, the researcher or clinician can better understand the tradeoffs that sometimes have to be made to increase sensitivity or specificity. The closer a ROC curve is to the upper left corner, the more efficient is the test. Computing the area is beyond the scope of this introductory material. Various computer programs can calculate automatically the area under the ROC curve. Use the following guide in Table 10.8 when evaluating a ROC curve.

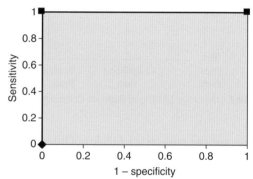

Fig. 10.10 AUROC of Test with 100% Sensitivity and Specificity

In a pediatric study designed to evaluate hospital-acquired pressure injury, investigators constructed a new tool, the Braden QD Scale, which builds on the Braden Q scale that only measures risk for immobility-related pressure ulcer. The Braden QD scale combines immobility-related pressure ulcer and medical device-related pressure injury (MDPI) risk in one scale. The authors' hypothesis was that a new scale would demonstrate sufficient sensitivity and specificity to predict both immobility-related pressure injuries and MDPIs (Curley et al., 2018). Fig. 10.12 is one of several ROCs from this study comparing the AUROC for the original Braden Q with the AUROC for the Braden QD.

You will note that the figure contains *two* ROC curves. In a diagnosis article, it is typical to compare the gold standard test with the new test. In this case, the original Braden Q is compared with the new Braden QD to predict

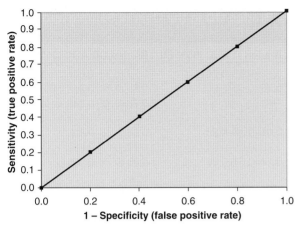

Fig. 10.11 The Area under the ROC Curve (AUROC) for a Worthless Test

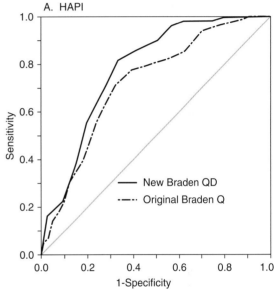

TABLE 10.8	**Guide for Interpreting the Area under the ROC Curve (AUROC)**
AUROC	**Category**
0.69–1.0	Very good
0.8–0.9	Good
0.7–0.8	Fair
0.6–0.7	Poor
0.5–0.6	Fail

ROC, Receiver Operating Characteristics.

Fig. 10.12 AUROC Comparing Original Braden Q with Braden QD

hospital-acquired pressure injuries (HAPI). By examining the area under the curve (AUC), you can tell the scale with the greatest AUC (new Braden QD) has the greatest discrimination to predict pressure injuries. Table 10.9 provides the actual AUC data for this graph, along with many other variables. Here the study authors include confidence intervals for the data. When examining this data, be sure to check that the confidence intervals do not include the null value. If the null value is not included, the results are statistically significant.

Statistics Common to Prognosis Articles

In articles that answer clinical questions of prognosis, investigators conduct studies in which they want to determine the outcome of a particular disease or condition. Prognosis studies often can be identified by their longitudinal cohort designs (see Chapter 7). At the conclusion of a longitudinal study, investigators statistically analyze data to determine which factors are strongly associated with the study outcomes, usually through a technique called multivariate regression analysis or multiple regression. Multivariate analysis examines variables at the interval or ratio level of measurement. We will not examine the complex formulas and calculations used to perform multivariate analysis; there are textbooks written on this subject alone and it is better left to an advanced statistics course or discussion.

Many of the studies you encounter will examine nominal level dependent variables. In these studies, researchers use a type of analysis called logistic regression. A logistic regression analysis produces an equation that predicts the probability of a given category on the dependent variable in light of the values of each independent variable (Persoskie & Ferrer, 2017). The probability is called an **odds ratio.** The odds ratio indicates how much more likely it is that certain independent variables (factors) predict the probability of developing the dependent variable (outcome or disease). Where the relative risk measures the probability of developing the disease, the odds ratio measures the odds that the disease (or other phenomenon) is occurring compared with the disease (or other phenomenon) not occurring. Although the relative risk is the preferable method to describe the chances of a disease occurring in a population, it isn't often feasible to obtain an appropriate sample, and therefore the odds ratio provides an alternative approach that can be applied more readily. The calculation for an odds ratio follows where *P* = probability:

TABLE 10.9 Comparing the AUC for Braden Q vs. Braden QD in the Overall Sample and Stratified by Enrollment Subgroups

Cohort	No. subjects/total	Braden Q AUC (95% CI)	Braden QD AUC (95% CI)
Overall—any HAPI	49/625	0.72 (0.65–0.79)	0.78 (0.73–0.84)
Any immobility-related pressure injury	14/625	0.78 (0.66–0.90)	0.86 (0.78–0.93)
Any MDPI[a]	42/625	—	0.78 (0.72–0.84)
Age category[†]			
Preterm to <1 mo	7/109	0.61 (0.36–0.85)	0.65 (0.45–0.86)
1 mo to 8 y	24/325	0.75 (0.65–0.84)	0.77 (0.69–0.86)
9–21 y	18/191	0.72 (0.61–0.83)	0.83 (0.77–0.90)
Diagnosis at admission[†]			
Medical/surgical diagnosis	22/346	0.81 (0.74–0.87)	0.84 (0.76–0.91)
Cardiovascular diagnosis	27/279	0.67 (0.56–0.77)	0.73 (0.65–0.81)
Endotracheal intubation at enrollment[b]			
Intubated	33/193	0.64 (0.55–0.73)	0.64 (0.54–0.73)
Not intubated	16/432	0.66 (0.53–0.80)	0.77 (0.67–0.87)

[a]The Braden Q Scale was not designed to predict MDPIs; therefore, the AUC was not computed.
[b]AUC for each enrollment subgroup is reported for any HAPI development.
AUC, Area under the curve; *CI,* confidence interval; *HAPI,* hospital-acquired pressure injury; *MDPI,* medical device-related pressure injury.

$$Odds\ Ratio = \frac{P(exposure\backslash diseased)/[1 - P(exposure\backslash diseased)]}{P(exposure\backslash no\ disease)/[1 - P(exposure\backslash no\ disease)]}\ or$$

$$Odds\ Ratio = \frac{P(disease\backslash exposure)/[1 - P(disease\backslash exposure)]}{P(disease\backslash no\ exposure)/[1 - P(disease\backslash no\ exposure)]}$$

The interpretation of the odds ratios is similar to, and interpreted in the same way as, the risk ratio. A higher odds ratio indicates a greater probability of the development of the outcome. An odds ratio of less than 1 indicates that the probability of developing the outcome is reduced. Also recall from our discussion that whenever we are appraising CIs to determine statistical significance, we have to appraise the null value. Because we are evaluating a "ratio," the null value is equal to 1. Thus, any odds ratio confidence internval (CI) that contains a null value of 1 is not a significant finding.

EBP TIP

- If the OR (odds ratio) = 1, or the CI (confidence interval) = 1, exposure does not affect odds of outcome
- If the OR >1, and the CI does not include 1, exposure is associated with higher odds of outcome
- If the RR <1, and the CI does not include 1, exposure is associated with lower odds of outcome

Statistics Common to Harm Articles

In studies that answer clinical questions of harm, investigators want to determine whether an individual has been harmed by being exposed to a particular event. Harm studies can be identified by their case-control design (see Chapter 7). In this type of study, investigators select the outcome they are interested in (e.g., pressure ulcers), and they examine whether any one factor explains those who have and do not have the outcome of interest. The measure of association that best describes the analyzed data in case-control studies is the odds ratio (see information mentioned previously).

Sun, Gerberich, & Ryan (2017) used a case-control study design to investigate the potential relationship between shift work and work-related physical assault (PA). Table 10.10 presents the shift data.

The interpretation of this data is relatively straightforward. You can see from the table that most of the odds ratios are greater than 1 except for staff who worked a combination of rotating day and night shifts. If you were to interpret this data using the odds ratio alone, you would be correct in concluding that the greatest number of assaults occurred on the night shift, followed by rotators to day and evening and then the evening shift staff. If you examine the day and night shifts, you will note that the odds ratio is less than 1. This means that the assaults were less likely to occur

TABLE 10.10   Univariate and Multivariable Analyses of the Relation Between Shift Work and Physical Assault Against Licensed Nurses

Shift type	Unadjusted OR [95%CI]	Unadjusted OR [95%CI]
Day shift	1.0	1.0
Evening shift	2.57 [1.85, 3.57]	1.55 [1.05, 2.27]
Night shift	5.03 [3.46, 7.31]	3.54 [2.31, 5.44]
Day and evening shift	3.86 [1.77, 8.43]	2.88 [1.22, 6.80]
Day and night shift	0.52 [0.16, 1.73]	0.38 [0.10, 1.39]
Other shifts[b]	1.61 [0.51, 5.06]	2.07 [0.55, 7.86]
Shift length		
≤8-hour shift	1.0	1.0
Exactly 10-hour shift	0.64 [0.24, 1.69]	1.09 [0.36, 3.30]
>12-hour shift	1.23 [0.81, 1.88]	1.05 [0.61, 1.81]

[a]Adjusted model controls for confounders for both shift type and shift length, as follows: facility in which they worked the most time, primary population with which they worked, primary professional activity, age, license type, and gender.
[b]Other shifts included the following: evening and night shift; day, evening, and night shift; on call; and other shifts.
CI, Confidence interval; *OR*, odds ratio.

on this shift relative to the day (where the odds ratio is 1). Based on previous discussion you know that the confidence interval indicates how well the study findings can be generalized to the population of registered nurses. A quick review of all of the confidence intervals, except for one, does not include the null value (staff rotating to day and night and other shifts) and, as such, the study findings as they relate to assaults by shift are statistically significant. Does shift matter? If you view the odds ratio alone, you might be quick to assume it does. Examine confidence intervals. All of them contain the null value and therefore none is a significant finding.

Harm data with its measure of probabilities can help you identify factors that may or may not contribute to an adverse or beneficial outcome.

META-ANALYSIS

Meta-analysis statistically combines the results of multiple studies (usually RCTs) to answer a focused clinical question through an objective appraisal of carefully synthesized research evidence. The strength of a meta-analysis lies in its use of statistical analysis to summarize studies.

As discussed in Chapter 8, a meta-analysis has the following characteristics:
- Asks a clinical question that is used to guide the process
- Searches for all relevant studies, published and unpublished, on the question using established inclusion and exclusion criteria to determine which studies are to be used in the meta-analysis
- Uses at least two individuals to independently assess the quality of each study based on established criteria
- Statistically combines the results of individual studies, and presents a balanced and impartial quantitative and narrative evidence summary of the findings that represents a "state-of-the-science" conclusion about the strength, quality, and consistency of evidence supporting benefits and risks of a given health care practice (Cheung & Vijayakumar, 2016; Weatherall, 2017)

Statistics Common to Meta-Analysis

A methodologically sound meta-analysis is more likely than a single intervention study to be successful in identifying the true effect of an intervention because it limits bias. The relative risk or, more commonly, the odds ratio is the statistic of choice for use in a meta-analysis. Meta-analysis also can report on continuous data, and typically the mean difference in outcomes will be reported (see Comparison 1 in Appendix A).

The usual manner of displaying data in a meta-analysis is by a pictorial representation known as a *blobbogram*, accompanied by a summary measure of effect size in relative risk, odds ratio or mean difference. Let us see how blobbograms and relative risk ratios are used to summarize the studies in a systematic review by practicing with the data from the Cochrane Review examining interventions to improve adherence to lipid-lowering medication (see Appendix A). The table "Analysis 1.1" compares intensified patient care vs. usual care at <6 months. In the first column, list all of the studies that examined this phenomenon. The next two columns provide information about the sample size in each of the groups. The first figure is the number of patients in the group that has the outcome, and the second is the overall number of people in each group. In the center of the table, you see a vertical line that represents the null value; you now know that when the statistic is the odds ratio, the null value is "1." When the statistic is the mean difference, the null value is "0."

The findings from each individual study are represented as a blob or square (the measured effect) on the vertical line, as an odds ratio. You also will note that each blob or square is a bit different in size. The size reflects the weight the study has on the overall analysis. This is determined by the sample size and the quality of the study. The width of the horizontal line represents the 95% confidence interval in the individual study. The vertical line is the line of no effect (i.e., the null value). When the confidence interval of the result (horizontal line) touches or crosses the line of no effect (vertical line), we can say that the study findings did not reach statistical significance. If the confidence interval does not cross the vertical line, we can say that the study results reached statistical significance. In the Faulkner, Goswami, and Guthrie study, all either touch or cross the line of no effect. Because the analysis crosses the line of no effect, these studies have statistically insignificant findings (found in Appendix A). To the far right of the blobbogram, the investigators also have provided the numerical equivalent of each blobbogram. You also will notice other important information and additional statistical analyses that may accompany the blobbogram table, such as a test to determine whether the results of each of the individual trials are mathematically compatible (heterogeneity) and a test for overall effect. The reader is referred to a book of advanced research methods for discussion of these topics.

There is a subtotal diamond for the study outcome statistically pooling the results of each of the controlled trials. It shows that these studies, statistically combined, generally favor intensified patient care. Because the total diamond does not touch the line of no effect, the overall interpretation is that intensified patient care improves adherence to lipid-lowering therapy at 6 months.

If this is a methodologically sound review determined through the critical appraisal process, it can be used to support or change practice or specific interventions.

SYNTHESIS-STATISTICAL ANALYSES

Statistical analyses allow us to answer questions about frequencies, relationships, and causation using scientifically rigorous methods. The statistical analysis is an important element of any research study and other rigorous evaluation processes. Whether you are critically appraising a research study or evaluating a quality improvement or EBP project, the statistical analysis must align with the purpose, research or clinical questions, design, and data collection methods to achieve valid results. The specific statistic(s) you encounter depend on the evidence-based question you are trying to answer. The depth of detail you must know about EBP statistics depends on your role. When you are designing or planning evidence-based or QI projects, choosing the appropriate statistics is essential to project rigor and requires a deeper appreciation of both descriptive and inferential methods. Critical appraisal focuses on the application of study results and their influence on practice.

■ KEY POINTS

- A high-quality research study must have alignment among the research question(s), study design, study methods, and statistical analyses.
- It is appropriate to use less-complex statistical analyses like descriptive statistics for quality improvement and EBP projects.
- The statistical analysis used will be driven by the research or project purpose, type and amount of data, and distribution of data.

- Data that normally is distributed utilizes parametric statistical tests, and data that normally is not distributed utilizes nonparametric statistical tests.
- Findings from research studies or quality improvement projects can be clinically significant even though they may not be statistically significant.

REFERENCES

Cheung, M. W. -L., & Vijayakumar, R. (2016). A Guide to Conducting a Meta-Analysis. *Neuropsychology Review*, *26*(2), 121–128.

Curley, M. A. Q., Hasbani, N. R., Quigley, S. M., Stellar, J. J., Pasek, T. A., Shelley, S. S., & Wypij, D. (2018). Predicting pressure injury risk in pediatric patients: the Braden qd scale. *Journal of Pediatrics*, *192*, 189–195.

Deeks, J. J., & Altman, D. G. (2004). Diagnostic tests 4: likelihood ratios. *BMJ (Clinical Research Ed.)*, *329*(7458), 168–169.

Empson, M. B. (2002). Statistics in the pathology laboratory: Diagnostic test interpretation. *Pathology*, *34*(4), 365–369.

Frisse, A. C., Marrazzo, J. M., Tutlam, N. T., Schreiber, C. A., Teal, S. B., Turok, D. K., et al. (2017). Validity of self-reported history of Chlamydia trachomatis infection. *American Journal of Obstetrics and Gynecology*, *216*(4), 393.e1–393.e7. https://doi.org/10.1016/j.ajog.2016.12.005.

Guyatt, G., Jaeschke, R., Heddle, N., Cook, D., Shannon, H., & Walter, S. (1995). Basic statistics for clinicians: 1. Hypothesis testing. *CMAJ: Canadian Medical Association Journal (Journal de l'Association Medicale Canadienne)*, *152*(1), 27–32.

Lowe, J. R., Rieger, R. E., Moss, N. C., Yeo, R. A., Winter, S., Patel, S., & Ohls, R. K. (2017). Impact of erythropoiesis-stimulating agents on behavioral measures in children born preterm. *Journal of Pediatrics*, *184*, 75–80.

Mendes, D., Alves, C., & Batel-Marques, F. (2017). Number needed to treat (NNT) in clinical literature: An appraisal. *BMC Medicine*, *15*(1).

Mirzazadeh, A., Malekinejad, M., & Kahn, J. G. (2015). Relative risk reduction is useful metric to standardize effect size for public heath interventions for translational research. *Journal of Clinical Epidemiology*, *68*(3), 317–323.

Persoskie, A., & Ferrer, R. A. (2017). A Most Odd Ratio. *American Journal of Preventive Medicine*, *52*(2), 224–228.

Riemann, B. L., & Lininger, M. (2015). Statistical primer for athletic trainers: the difference between statistical and clinical meaningfulness. *Journal of Athletic Training*, *50*(12), 1223–1225.

Rubin, F. H., Bellon, J., Bilderback, A., Urda, K., & Inouye, S. K. (2018). Effect of the hospital elder life program on risk of 30-day readmission. *Journal of the American Geriatrics Society*, *66*(1), 145–149.

Stang, A., Poole, C., & Bender, R. (2010). Common problems related to the use of number needed to treat. *Journal of Clinical Epidemiology*, *63*(8), 820–825.

Stevens, S. S. (1946). On the Theory of Scales of Measurement. *Science*, *103*(2684), 677–680.

Sun, S., Gerberich, S. G., & Ryan, A. D. (2017). The relationship between shiftwork and violence against nurses: a case control study. *Workplace Health & Safety*, *65*(12), 603–611.

Taylor, Courtney (2017). Understanding the Importance of the Central Limit Theorem. Retrieved from https://www.thoughtco.com/importance-of-the-central-limit-theorem-3126556.

Titler, M. G., Conlon, P., Reynolds, M. A., Ripley, R., Tsodikov, A., Wilson, D. S., & Montie, M. (2016). The effect of a translating research into practice intervention to promote use of evidence-based fall prevention interventions in hospitalized adults: A prospective pre–post implementation study in the U.S. *Applied Nursing Research*, *31*, 52–59.

Weatherall, M. (2017). Systematic review and meta-analysis: Tools for the information age. *Postgraduate Medical Journal*, *93*(1105), 696–703.

Evidence-Based Approaches for Improving Healthcare Quality

Maja Djukic, Mattia J. Gilmartin

LEARNING OUTCOMES

After reading this chapter, you should be able to do the following:

- Discuss the clinical leader's role in health care quality improvement.
- Apply quality improvement interventions that align with national quality aims, priorities, and initiatives.
- Evaluate the impact of context such as accreditation, payment, and public reporting systems on improvement efforts.
- Select quality measures that best fit your practice to improve care and meet Quality Payment Program requirements.

- Differentiate the characteristics of the major quality improvement (QI) models used in health care.
- Analyze the steps of the improvement process and determine appropriate QI tools to use in each phase of the process.
- Implement evidence-based improvement strategies to optimize success and sustainability of quality improvement interventions.
- Critically appraise a journal article reporting the results of a QI project using the SQUIRE guidelines.

KEY TERMS

Benchmarking
Cause-and-Effect diagrams
Clinical Microsystems
Common cause variation
Control chart
DMAIC Model
Fishbone diagrams
Flowchart

Improvement cycles
Lean
Model for Improvement
Plan-Do-Study-Act (PSDA)
Public reporting
Quality health care
Quality improvement
Root cause analysis (RCA)

Run chart
Six Sigma
Special cause variation
SQUIRE Guidelines
Total Quality Management/
    Continuous Quality
    Improvement

The Institute of Medicine (IOM, 2001), now called the National Academy of Medicine, defines quality health care as care that is safe, effective, patient-centered, timely, efficient, and equitable (Box 11.1). The quality of the health care system was brought to the forefront of national attention in several important reports (IOM, 1999; 2001), including *Crossing the Quality Chasm,* which concluded that "between the health care we have and the care we could have lies not just a gap, but a chasm" (IOM, 2001, p. 1). The report notes that "the performance of the health care system varies considerably. It may be exemplary, but often is not, and millions of Americans fail to receive effective care" (IOM, 2001, p. 3).

Since the IOM (2001) report was published, quality of care has improved for some conditions (Nuti et al., 2015). Based on data from more than 4000 U.S. hospitals, core composite quality process measures for acute myocardial infarction (e.g., aspirin on arrival), heart failure (e.g., smoking cessation advice), and pneumonia (e.g., influenza vaccine) improved from 96% to 99%, 85% to 98%, and 83% to 97% respectively from 2006 to 2011 (Nuti et al., 2015). Also, overall positive improvement trends are noted across more than 200 quality measures, led by 17% reduction of hospital-acquired conditions from 2010 to 2014 (Agency for Healthcare Research and Quality [AHRQ], 2016). Improvements are, however, needed for about 20% of measures in person- and family-centered care, such as receiving care as soon as needed, and for about 40% of measures of healthy living, such as getting prompt smoking cessation help for people trying to quit (AHRQ, 2016). Furthermore, disparities in quality based on earnings, race, and ethnicity continue to persist. For example, "people from poor households compared with those from high-income households received worse care for about 60% of quality measures; Blacks, Hispanics, American Indians, and Alaska Natives compared with Whites received worse care for about 40% of quality measures" (AHRQ, 2016, p. 11). Despite these quality issues, the U.S. spends much more on health care (16% of gross domestic product) compared with other developed nations, but ranks last in health care quality in comparison with 10 other countries (Schneider, Sarnak, Shah, & Doty, 2017).

The purpose of this chapter is to introduce you to the principles of quality improvement (QI) and provide examples of how to apply these principles in your practice so you can effectively contribute to needed health

---

BOX 11.1 Six Dimensions and Definitions of Health Care Quality

1. **Safe:** avoiding injuries to patients from care that is intended to help them
2. **Effective:** providing services based on scientific knowledge to all who could benefit and refraining from providing services to those not likely to benefit
3. **Patient-centered:** providing care that is respectful of and responsive to individual patient preferences, needs, and values, and ensuring that patient values guide all clinical decisions
4. **Timely:** reducing waits and sometimes harmful delays for both those who receive and those who give care
5. **Efficient:** avoiding waste, including waste of equipment, supplies, ideas, and energy
6. **Equitable:** providing care that does not vary in quality because of personal characteristics such as gender, ethnicity, geographical location, and socioeconomic status

From Institute of Medicine. (2001). Crossing the quality chasm: A new health system for the 21st century. Executive summary. Washington, DC: National Academies Press.

---

care improvements. QI "uses data to monitor the outcomes of care processes and improvement methods to design and test changes to continuously improve the quality and safety of health care systems" (Cronenwett et al., 2007, p. 127).

THE CLINICAL LEADER'S ROLE IN HEALTH CARE QUALITY IMPROVEMENT

Florence Nightingale championed QI by systematically documenting high rates of morbidity and mortality resulting from poor sanitary conditions among soldiers serving in the Crimean War of 1854 (Henry et al., 1992). She used statistics to document changes in soldiers' health, including reductions in mortality resulting from a number of nursing interventions such as hand hygiene, instrument sterilization, changing of bed linens, ward sanitation, ventilation, and proper nutrition (Henry et al., 1992). Today, clinical leaders are vital to health system improvement efforts (IOM, 2015). One main initiative developed to bolster graduate nurses' education in health system improvements is the graduate project titled *Quality and Safety Education for Nurses* (QSEN) (Pohl et al., 2009). The overall goal of this project is to

BOX 11.2   National Quality Aims and Priorities

National Quality Aims	National Quality Priorities for Achieving the Aims
• **Better Care:** Improve the overall quality of care by making health care more patient-centered, reliable, accessible, and safe. • **Healthy People/Healthy Communities:** Improve the health of the U.S. population by supporting proven interventions to address behavioral, social, and environmental determinants of health in addition to delivering higher-quality care. • **Affordable Care:** Reduce the cost of quality health care for individuals, families, employers, and government.	• Make care safer by reducing harm caused in the delivery of care. • Ensure each person and family is engaged as a partner in their care. • Promote effective communication and care coordination. • Promote the most effective prevention and treatment practices for the leading causes of mortality, starting with cardiovascular disease. • Work with communities to promote wide use of best practices to enable healthy living. • Make quality care more affordable for individuals, families, employers, and governments by developing and sharing new health care delivery models.

From 2015 National Healthcare Quality and Disparities Report and 5th Anniversary Update on the National Quality Strategy. Rockville, MD: Agency for Healthcare Research and Quality; April 2016. AHRQ Pub. No. 16-0015. http://www.ahrq.gov/research/findings/nhqrdr/nhqdr15/index.html.

support the development of advanced practice nurses' competence in the areas of QI, patient-centered care, teamwork and collaboration, patient safety, informatics, and evidence-based practice (EBP). Other initiatives such as the *Care Innovation and Transformation Program* (American Organization of Nurse Executives, 2016) have been developed to increase engagement in QI. To influence improvements in the work setting effectively and ensure that all patients consistently receive excellent care, it is important to do the following:

• Align national, organizational, and unit level goals for QI
• Recognize external drivers of quality such as accreditation, payment, and performance measurement
• Develop skills to apply QI models and tools

NATIONAL GOALS AND STRATEGIES FOR HEALTH CARE QUALITY IMPROVEMENT

The National Quality Strategy was established by the Affordable Care Act and published in 2011 to pursue the triple health care improvement aims of better care, affordable care, and healthy people/healthy communities (U.S. Department of Health and Human Services [USDHHS], 2016a). It set aims and priorities for QI (Box 11.2). Achieving these national quality targets requires a major redesign of the health care system. One way you, as a clinical leader, can contribute to this redesign is to familiarize yourself with national priorities, corresponding improvement goals, and national initiatives (Table 11.1) and use them to guide improvements in your work setting.

QUALITY STRATEGY LEVERS

QI relies on aligning institutional priorities with several strategy levers that drive it. The National Quality Strategy encourages all members of the health care community, including individuals, family members, payers, providers, and employers, to collaborate in using one or more of the nine strategy levers (USDHHS, 2016a, p. 8). We describe briefly how each lever is used for QI:

• **Measurement and feedback:** Provide performance feedback to plans and providers to improve care. National health care performance standards are developed using a consensus process in which stakeholder groups representing the interests of the public, health professionals, payers, employers, and government identify priorities, measures, and reporting requirements to document and manage the quality of care (National Quality Forum [NQF], 2004). See Box 11.3 for examples of groups responsible for developing measurement standards.
• **Public reporting:** Compare treatment results, costs, and patient experiences. Several major public reporting systems are described in Box 11.4.

TABLE 11.1	National Quality Strategy Priorities, Improvement Goals, and Related Initiatives	
National Quality Strategy Priority	Long-Term Goals	Related National Initiatives
Patient safety	1. Reduce preventable hospital admissions and readmissions. 2. Reduce incidence of adverse health care-associated conditions. 3. Reduce harm from inappropriate or unnecessary care.	Partnership for Patients, Hospital Readmission Reduction Program, Children's Hospital of Pittsburgh of UPMC
Person- and family-centered care	1. Improve patient, family, and caregiver experience of care related to quality, safety, and access across settings. 2. In partnership with patients, families, and caregivers, and using a shared decision-making process, develop culturally sensitive and understandable care plans. 3. Enable patients and their families and caregivers to navigate, coordinate, and manage their care appropriately and effectively.	Consumer Assessment of Healthcare Providers and Systems, National Partnership for Women and Families, Colorado Coalition for the Homeless
Effective communication and care coordination	1. Improve quality of care transitions and communications across care settings. 2. Improve quality of life for patients with chronic illness and disability by following a current care plan that anticipates and addresses pain and symptom management, psychosocial needs, and functional status. 3. Establish shared accountability and integration of communities and health care systems to improve quality of care and reduce health disparities.	Argonaut Project, Boston Children's Hospital Community Asthma Initiative
Prevention and treatment of leading causes of morbidity and mortality	1. Promote cardiovascular health through community interventions that result in improvement of social, economic, and environmental factors. 2. Promote cardiovascular health through interventions that result in adoption of the most important healthy lifestyle behaviors across the lifespan. 3. Promote cardiovascular health through effective clinical preventive services across the lifespan in clinical and community settings.	Million Hearts Campaign, Wind River Reservation
Health and well-being of communities	1. Promote healthy living and well-being through community interventions that result in improvement of social, economic, and environmental factors. 2. Promote healthy living and well-being through interventions that result in adoption of the most important healthy lifestyle behaviors across the lifespan. 3. Promote healthy living and well-being through effective clinical preventive services across the lifespan in clinical and community settings.	Health Leads, Let's Move!
Making quality care more affordable	1. Ensure affordable, accessible, high-quality health care for people, families, employers, and governments. 2. Support and enable communities to ensure accessible, high-quality care while reducing waste and fraud.	Blue Cross Blue Shield Massachusetts Alternative Quality Contract, Medicare Shared Savings Program, Pioneer Accountable Care Organization Model, Arkansas Center for Health Improvement

From the U.S. Department of Health and Human Services. (2016a). *National quality strategy overview.* Retrieved from http://www.ahrq.gov/workingforquality/nqs/overview.pdf.

BOX 11.3   Performance Measurement Standard Setting Groups

Introduction to performance measurement standards

The National Quality Forum (NQF) is a nonprofit organization that seeks to measure and improve the quality of health care in the United States by establishing national health care quality and safety goals and priorities. The NQF's evidence-based measure endorsement process is the gold standard for health care quality measurement. The NQF endorsement process is a transparent, consensus-based model that brings together stakeholders from the private and public sectors to foster quality improvement. Approximately 300 NQF-endorsed measures are used by federal public and private pay-for-performance programs and in private-sector and state health care quality programs.[1]

The Agency for Healthcare Research and Quality, Quality Indicators (AHRQ) are standardized, evidence-based measures of the quality of hospital care that are readily available using hospital administrative data. There are 101 Quality Indicators organized into four main categories: inpatient quality for adult and pediatric patients; preventive quality indicators for ambulatory care; and avoidable complications. Approximately half of the AHRQ quality indicators are endorsed by the National Quality Forum and are used to support hospital quality improvement, health system planning, and pay for performance initiatives.[2]

[1]National Quality Forum. (2015). *National Quality Forum, What We Do*. Retrieved from http://www.qualityforum.org/About_NQF/About_NQF.aspx http://www.qualityforum.org/what_we_do.aspx.
[2]Agency for Healthcare Research and Quality (2015). *About AHRQ Quality Indicators*. Retrieved from: http://qualityindicators.ahrq.gov/FAQs_Support/FAQ_QI_Overview.aspx.

BOX 11.4   Public Reporting Systems

- **Hospital Compare** allows consumers to compare information on hospitals. The database includes performance measures on timely and efficient care; readmissions and deaths; complications; use of medical imaging; survey of patients' experiences; and payment and value of care. For more information, visit www.hospitalcompare.hhs.gov/.
- **Nursing Home Compare** allows consumers to compare information about nursing homes. It contains quality of care information on every Medicare and Medicaid-certified nursing home in the nation. The database includes performance measures on health inspections, staffing, and clinical quality. For more information, visit www.medicare.gov/NursingHomeCompare/.
- **Home Health Compare** has information about the quality of care provided by Medicare-certified home health agencies that meet federal health and safety requirements throughout the nation. For more information, visit www.medicare.gov/homehealthcompare.
- **Hospital Consumer Assessment of Healthcare Providers and Systems (HCAHPS)** is developed by the Agency for Healthcare Research and Quality, and is a standardized survey and data collection method for measuring patients' perspectives on hospital care. The HCAHPS survey contains 32 questions about patient perspectives on care for eight key topics: communication with doctors, communication with nurses,

responsiveness of hospital staff, pain management, communication about medicines, discharge information, cleanliness of the hospital environment and quietness of the hospital environment, post-hospital transitions, admissions through the emergency room, and mental and emotional health. HCAHPS performance is used to calculate incentive payments in the Hospital Value-Based Purchasing program for hospital discharges beginning in October 2012. For more information, visit http://www.hcahpsonline.org http://www.hcahpsonline.org/Files/HCAHPS_Fact_Sheet_June_2015.pdf.
- **Physician Quality Reporting Initiative** is a program administered by CMS that collects performance data at the physician/provider clinical level in the ambulatory and primary care sectors. For more information, visit www.cms.gov/Medicare/Quality-Initiatives-Patient-Assessment-Instruments/PQRS/index.html.
- **The Leapfrog Group** is an initiative of organizations that buy health care and are working to improve the safety, quality, and affordability of health care for Americans. The Leapfrog Group conducts a survey to compare hospitals' performance on the national standards of safety, quality, and efficiency that are most relevant to consumers and purchasers of care. For more information, visit www.leapfroggroup.org/.

BOX 11.5 **QI Accrediting Organizations**

- **Joint Commission:** Responsible for ensuring a minimum standard of structures, processes, and outcomes for patient care. Accreditation by the Joint Commission is voluntary, but it is required to receive reimbursement for patient care services. For more information: www.jointcommission.org/
- **National Committee for Quality Assurance Accreditation for Health Plans (NCQA):** A private not-for-profit organization dedicated to improving health care quality. The NCQA is responsible for accrediting health insurance programs. Accredited health insurance programs are exempt from many or all elements associated with annual state audits. The NCQA developed and maintains the Healthcare Effectiveness Data and Information Set (HEDIS).

- **Healthcare Effectiveness Data and Information Set (HEDIS):** A tool used by the majority of America's health plans to measure performance on important dimensions of care and service. HEDIS allows for comparison of performance across health plans. For more information: http://www.ncqa.org/Programs/Accreditation/HealthPlanHP.aspx http://www.ncqa.org/HEDISQualityMeasurement.aspx
- **American Nurses' Credentialing Center Magnet Recognition Program:** Recognizes health care organizations that provide the very best in nursing care and uphold the tradition of professional nursing practice. For more information: www.nursecredentialing.org/Magnet.aspx

---

- Learning and technical assistance: Foster learning environments that offer training, resources, tools, and guidance to help organizations achieve quality improvement goals.
- Certification, accreditation, regulation: Adopt or adhere to approaches to meet safety and quality standards. Several accrediting bodies are listed in Box 11.5.
- Consumer incentives and benefit designs: Help consumers adopt healthy behaviors and make informed decisions.
- Payment: Incentivize and reward providers who deliver high-quality, patient-centered care. Box 11.6 shows examples of payment incentives.
- Health information technology: Improve communications, transparency, and efficiency for better coordinated health and health care.
- Innovation and diffusion: Foster innovation in health care quality improvement and facilitate rapid adoption within and across organizations and communities.
- Workforce development: Invest in people to prepare the next generation of health care professionals and support lifelong learning for providers.

Measuring Health Care Quality

In alignment with the National Quality Aims for better care, better health, and lower costs, Medicare has initiated several value-based programs (e.g., Alternative Payment Models, Merit-Based Incentive Payment System, Hospital Value-Based Purchasing Program) to reward providers for the quality of care rather than the quantity of care they give to patients (CMS, 2017a). As part of the value-based payment model, Medicare provides incentive payments to clinicians, hospitals, nursing homes, and home health agencies based on how well they perform on each measure or how much they improve their scores on quality measures compared with baseline performance. Therefore, as an advanced practice nurse or clinical leader, you are responsible for knowing which quality measures apply to your practice setting so you can ensure that the care you provide meets appropriate quality standards.

For example, if you are a clinician participating in Medicare Part B, you will be paid for your services through Medicare's Quality Payment Program (CMS, 2017b), the result of the Medicare Access and CHIP Reauthorization Act (MACRA) of 2015. For examples of measures that are part of Medicare's Quality Payment Program see Table 11.2.

QI CHECKPOINT

To identify measures that best apply to your practice and that you can report to the Quality Payment Program, visit https://qpp.cms.gov/mips/quality-measures. Select your specialty practice area and identify the level of reporting priority for the measures to prioritize your improvement efforts.

BOX 11.6   Financial Incentives to Promote Quality in the Health Care Sector

Capitation: A payment arrangement for health care services. Pays a provider (physician or nurse practitioner) or provider group a set amount for each enrolled person assigned to them, per period of time, whether or not that person seeks care. These providers generally are contracted with a type of health maintenance organization (HMO). Payment levels are based on average expected health care use of a particular patient, with greater payment for patients with significant medical histories.[1]

Bundled Payments Initiative: Links payments for multiple services that patients receive during an episode of care. Payments seek to align incentives for hospitals, post-acute care providers, doctors, and other practitioners to improve the patient's care experience during a hospital stay in an acute care hospital through post-discharge recovery.[2]

Pay for Performance: An emerging movement in health insurance where providers are rewarded for meeting pre-established targets for health care delivery services. This model rewards physicians, hospitals, medical groups, and other health care providers for meeting certain performance measures for quality and efficiency.[3]

Value-Based Health Care Purchasing: A project of participating health plans, including the Centers for Medicare and Medicaid Services (CMS), where buyers hold providers of health care accountable for both cost and quality of care. Value-based purchasing brings together information on health care quality, patient outcomes, and health status, with data on dollar outlays going toward health. The focus is on managing health care system use to reduce inappropriate care and to identify and reward the best-performing providers.[4]

Accountable Care Organization (ACO): A payment and care delivery model that seeks to tie provider reimbursements to quality metrics and reductions in the total cost of care for an assigned population of patients. A group of coordinated health care providers forms an ACO, which then provides care to a group of patients. The ACO may use a range of payment models (e.g., capitation, fee-for-service). The ACO is accountable to patients and the third-party payer for the quality, appropriateness, and efficiency of the health care provided.[5]

[1]American Medical Association. (2012). Capitation. Retrieved from http://www.ama-assn.org/ama/pub/physician-resources/practice-management-center/claims-revenue-cycle/managed-care-contracting/evaluating-payment-options/capitation.page http://www.ama-assn.org/ama/pub/advocacy/state-advocacy-arc/state-advocacy-campaigns/private-payer-reform/state-based-payment-reform/evaluating-payment-options/capitation.page.

[2]Centers for Medicare and Medicaid Services. (2016). Bundled payments for care improvement initiative: General information. Retrieved from https://innovation.cms.gov/initiatives/Bundled-Payments/index.html http://www.innovations.cms.gov/initiatives/bundled-payments/index.html.

[3]Integrated Healthcare Association. (2013). National pay for performance issue brief. Retrieved from http://www.iha.org/sites/default/files/resources/issue-brief-value-based-p4p-2013.pdf http://www.iha.org/p4p_national.html.

[4]Damberg, C. L., Sorbero, M. E.; Lovejoy, S. L., Martsolf, G. L., et al. (2014). *Measuring success in health care value-based purchasing programs: Summary and recommendations*. Santa Monica, Calif.: RAND Corporation, RR-306/1-ASPE. Retrieved from http://www.rand.org/pubs/research_reports/RR306z1.html.

[5]American Hospital Association. (2014). Accountable care organizations: Findings from the survey of care systems and payment. Retrieved from http://www.aha.org/content/14/14aug-acocharts.pdf http://www.aha.org/research/cor/accountable/index.shtml.

Benchmarking

Measurement of quality indicators must be done methodically using standardized tools. Standardized measurement allows for **benchmarking**. "Benchmarking is the process of comparing a practice's performance with an external standard. Benchmarking is an important tool that facilitators can use to motivate a practice to engage in improvement work and to help members of a practice understand where their performance falls in comparison to others" (AHRQ, 2013, p.10).

Benchmarking is critical for QI because it helps identify when performance is below an agreed-upon standard, and it signals the need for improvement. For example, when you track a patient population's performance on standard measures defined by HEDIS, such as pneumococcal vaccine coverage for older adults or breast cancer screening, it allows for comparison of your performance to those of providers in other organizations who care for similar patient populations and use the same measures to document provided care. Tracking changes in overall performance on quality measures over time allows you to intervene if the score falls below a set standard. Equally, after you implement needed interventions focused on improving vaccination or cancer screening coverage in your patient population, you can track changes in those measures to determine

TABLE 11.2 The Quality Payment Program Performance Merit-Based Incentive Payment System (MIPS) Measures

Measure Domain	Measures	Description
High-priority, general practice/family medicine and preventive medicine High-priority/pediatrics	1. Care plan 2. Controlling high blood pressure Diabetes: Hb A$_{1c}$ poor control (> 9%) Documentation of current medications in the medical record Osteoarthritis (OA): Function and pain assessment 1. Acute otitis externa (AOE): Systematic antimicrobial therapy – avoidance of inappropriate use 2. Acute otitis externa (AOE): Topical therapy 3. Appropriate testing for children with pharyngitis 4. Appropriate treatment for children with upper respiratory infection (URI) 5. Child and adolescent major depressive disorder (MDD): Suicide Risk Assessment 6. Follow-up after hospitalization for mental illness (FUH) 7. Medication management for people with asthma	1. Percentage of patients aged 65 years and older who have an advance care plan or surrogate decision maker documented in the medical record or documentation that an advance care plan was discussed but the patient did not wish or was not able to name a surrogate decision maker or provide an advance care plan. Percentage of patients 18–85 years of age who had a diagnosis of hypertension and whose blood pressure was adequately controlled (<140/90mm Hg) during the measurement period Percentage of patients 18–75 years of age with diabetes who had hemoglobin A1c > 9.0% during the measurement period Percentage of visits for patients aged 18 years and older for which the eligible professional attests to documenting a list of current medications using all immediate resources available on the date of the encounter. This list must include ALL known prescriptions, over-the-counters, herbals, and vitamin/mineral/dietary (nutritional) supplements AND must contain the medications' names, dosages, frequency, and routes of administration. Percentage of patient visits for patients aged 21 years and older with a diagnosis of osteoarthritis (OA) with assessment for function and pain 1. Percentage of patients aged 2 years and older with a diagnosis of AOE who were not prescribed systemic antimicrobial therapy 2. Percentage of patients aged 2 years and older with a diagnosis of AOE who were prescribed topical preparations 3. Percentage of children 3–18 years of age who were diagnosed with pharyngitis, ordered an antibiotic, and received a group A streptococcus (strep) test for the episode 4. Percentage of children 3 months–18 years of age who were diagnosed with upper respiratory infection (URI) and were not dispensed an antibiotic prescription on the day of or 3 days after the episode 5. Percentage of visits for patients aged 6–17 years with a diagnosis of major depressive disorder with an assessment for suicide risk 6. Percentage of discharges for patients 6 years of age and older who were hospitalized for treatment of selected mental illness diagnoses and who had an outpatient visit, intensive outpatient encounter, or partial hospitalization with a mental health practitioner. Two rates are reported: The percentage of discharges for which the patient received follow up within 30 days of discharge and the percentage of discharges for which the patient received follow up within 7 days of discharge. 7. The percentage of patients 5–64 years of age during the measurement year who were identified as having persistent asthma and were dispensed appropriate medications that they remained on for at least 75% of their treatment period

From the Quality Payment Program MIPS website: https://qpp.cms.gov/mips/quality-measures.

whether the interventions were effective or not. Therefore, standardized measurement can tell you when changes in care are needed and whether implemented interventions have resulted in actual improvement of patient outcomes.

When all clinical practices document care uniformly, it is possible to document patient outcomes across units. These performance data are useful for benchmarking efforts where clinical teams learn from each other how to apply best practices from high-performing practices to the care processes of lower-performing practices. To support the validity of benchmarking, it is essential to ensure that the numerator and denominator for a measure are defined and measured in the same manner across time and among different clinical practices (AHRQ, 2013). For example, when you are trying to understand what percentage of the patients in your practice with a diabetes diagnosis have hemoglobin A1C (HgA1C) values above 8, the numerator should include all patients who have HgA1C values greater than 8 and a diabetes diagnosis, and the denominator should include all patients diagnosed with diabetes with available HgA1C levels. If you include patients with diabetes who do not have HgA1C values available in your denominator, your measure of the percentage of patients with elevated HgA1C levels will be falsely deflated (AHRQ, 2013). To see how your practice compares to others on important quality measures visit one of the public reporting system sites outlined in Box 11.4.

COMMON QUALITY IMPROVEMENT PERSPECTIVES AND MODELS

QI as a management model is both a philosophy of organizational functioning and a set of statistical analysis tools and change techniques to reduce variations in the quality of goods or services that an organization produces (Nelson et al., 2007). The QI model emphasizes customer satisfaction, teams and teamwork, and the continuous improvement of work processes. Other defining features of QI include the use of transformational leadership by leaders at all levels to set performance goals and expectations, use of data to make decisions, and standardization of work processes to reduce variation across providers and service encounters (Nelson et al., 2007). The key principles associated with QI are shown in Table 11.3.

Although QI has its roots in the manufacturing sector, many of the ideas, tools, and techniques used to measure and manage quality have been applied in health care organizations to improve clinical outcomes and reduce waste (McConnell, Lindrooth, Wholey, Maddox, & Bloom, 2016). The major QI models used in health care include the following:
- Total Quality Management/Continuous Quality Improvement (TQM/CQI)
- Six Sigma
- Lean
- Clinical microsystems

The key characteristics of each of these models are described in Table 11.4. Because QI uses a holistic approach, leaders often select one quality model that is used to guide the organization's overarching improvement agenda.

It is important to note that health care organizations have adopted principles and practices associated with the industrial QI approach relatively recently. Historically, the quality of health care was assessed retrospectively using the quality assurance (QA) model. The QA model uses chart audits to compare care against a predetermined standard. Corrective actions associated with QA focus on assigning individual blame and correcting deficiencies in operations. Another model commonly associated with health care QI is the *Structure-Process-Outcome Framework* (Donabedian, 1966). This framework is used to examine the resources that make up health care delivery services, clinicians' work practices, and outcomes associated with the structure and processes. The evolution of key perspectives used to understand and manage QI in health care organizations is summarized in Table 11.5.

QUALITY IMPROVEMENT STEPS AND TOOLS

There are several steps in the QI process used to diagnose, treat, and evaluate health system performance (Massoud et al., 2001):
- Assessing health system performance by collecting and monitoring data
- Analyzing data to identify a problem in need of improvement
- Developing a plan to treat the identified problem
- Testing and implementing the improvement plan

Several tools facilitate each step of the QI process (Table 11.6). You can use these tools to assist with collecting and analyzing data and to identify and test

TABLE 11.3 **Principles of Quality Improvement**	
Improvement Principle	**Key Benefits**
• Principle 1 – Customer focus/patient focus • Health care organizations rely on patients and therefore should understand current and future patient needs, meet patient requirements, and strive to exceed patient expectations.	• Increased customer value • Increased revenue and market share obtained through flexible and fast responses to market opportunities • Increased effectiveness in the organization's resources used to enhance patient satisfaction • Improved patient loyalty leading to repeat business
• Principle 2 – Leadership • Leaders establish unity of purpose and the organization's direction should create and maintain an internal environment in which people can become fully involved in the organization's achievement of objectives.	• People understand and are motivated by the organization's goals and objectives • Activities are evaluated, aligned, and implemented in a unified way • Miscommunication between organization levels is minimized
• Principle 3 – Engagement of people • People at all levels are the essence of an organization and are essential to enhancing organizational capability to create and deliver value.	• Motivated, committed, and involved people within the organization • Innovation and creativity further the organization's objectives • People are accountable for their own performance • Enhanced involvement of people in improvement activities
• Principle 4 – Process approach • Consistent results are achieved more efficiently and effectively when activities are understood and managed as a system of interrelated processes.	• Lower costs and shorter cycle times through effective use of resources • Improved, more consistent, and predictable results through a system of aligned processes • Focused and prioritized improvement opportunities
• Principle 5 – Improvement • Successful organizations have an ongoing focus on improvement. Continual improvement is essential in creating new opportunities.	• Performance advantage through improved organizational capabilities • Focus on root-cause analysis, followed by prevention and corrective action • Consideration of incremental and breakthrough improvements
• Principle 6 – Evidence-based decision making • Effective decisions based on the analysis and evaluation of data and information are more likely to produce desired results.	• Improved decision-making processes • Increased ability to demonstrate effectiveness of past decisions • Increased ability to review, challenge, and change opinions and decisions
• Principle 7 – Relationship management • An organization and its suppliers are interdependent, and a mutually beneficial relationship enhances the ability of both to create value.	• Increased capability to create value for both parties by sharing resources and managing quality-related risks • A well-managed supply chain that provides a stable flow of goods and services • Optimization of costs and resources

TABLE 11.4   Overview of Quality Improvement Models Used in Health Care

Model	Main Characteristics	Related Resources
TQM/CQI (Langley et al., 2009)	• A holistic management approach used to improve organizational performance • Seeks to understand and manage variation in service delivery • Emphasizes customer satisfaction as an important performance measure • Relies on teamwork and collaboration among workers to deliver technically excellent and customer/patient-centered services • Quality management science uses tools and techniques from statistics, engineering, operations research, management, market research, and psychology • TQM/CQI tools and techniques are applied to specific performance problems in the form of improvement projects • The extent to which unit-level QI projects align with larger organizational quality goals is related to their success and sustainability	Institute for Healthcare Improvement: http://www.ihi.org/Pages/default.aspx http://www.ihi.org/resources/Pages/default.aspx
Six Sigma (DelliFraine et al., 2010)	• Developed at Motorola in the 1980s • Takes its name from the statistical notation of sigma (σ) used to measure variation from the mean • Emphasizes meeting customer requirements and eliminating errors or reworking with the goal of reducing process variation • Focuses on tightly controlling variations in production processes with the goal of reducing the number of defects to 3.4 units per 1 million units produced • Process control achieved by applying DMAIC improvement model • **DMAIC** includes: defining, measuring, analyzing, improving, and controlling • Practitioners achieve mastery levels using statistical tools to measure and manage process variation (e.g., yellow belt, green belt, black belt)	AHRQ Innovations Exchange: www.innovations.ahrq.gov https://innovations.ahrq.gov/qualitytools/lean-hospitals-six-sigma-and-lean-healthcare-forms
Lean (DelliFraine et al., 2010)	• Sometimes referred to as the Toyota Quality Model • Focus: eliminating waste from the production system by designing the most efficient and effective system • Production is controlled through standardization and placing the right person and materials at each step of the process • Uses the PDSA improvement cycle • Statistical tools include value stream mapping and Kanban, or a visual cue, used to warn clinicians that there is a process problem • Performance measures vary from project to project and may inform the creation of new performance measures • Uses a master teacher ("Sensei") to spread the practices of Lean through the organizational culture	Institute for Healthcare Improvement: www.ihi.org/knowledge/Pages/IHIWhitePapers/GoingLeaninHealthCare.aspx

TABLE 11.4   Overview of Quality Improvement Models Used in Health Care—cont'd

Model	Main Characteristics	Related Resources
Clinical Microsystems (Nelson et al., 2007)	• Model of service excellence developed specifically for health care • Clinical microsystem is considered the building block of any health care system and is the smallest replicable unit in an organization • Members of a clinical microsystem are interdependent and work together toward a common aim	Clinical Microsystems: www.clinicalmicrosystem.org/

TABLE 11.5   Evolution of Quality Improvement Perspectives in Health Care

Model	Key Features	Quality Monitoring Mechanisms	Representative Research Questions
1920s–1980s QA Used to correct differences between what should be and what actually is (Chassin & Loeb, 2011)	• Uses external standards to guide quality • Quality assessed after the fact • Corrective action is punitive • The focus is on symptoms, individual failures, and compliance with standards	• Accreditation • Chart audit • Morbidity & mortality rounds	What is the effect of the Race program, led by clinical nurse specialists in partnership with nurse leaders to engage front-line staff in process improvement and quality assurance programs to improve nurses' impact on patient safety? Adapted from Tidwell et al. (2016)
1960s–2010s Structure-Process-Outcome Framework examines system components that lead to health care quality (Donabedian, 1966)	• Stresses professional responsibility for evaluating care quality • *Structure* focuses on provider and organizational characteristics; *Process* focuses on how care is delivered • *Outcome* focuses on the end results of medical care	• Accreditation • Work redesign • Benchmarking • Professional education and credentialing	What is the predictive power of measures representing patient characteristics, nurse workload, nurse expertise, and hospital acquired pressure ulcers (HAPU) preventative processes of care on HAPU prevalence? Adapted from Aydin et al. (2015)
1990s–2010s TQM/CQI model used to continually improve services and organizational performance (Bigelow & Arndt, 1995)	• Systems approach to improve efficiency • Incorporates clinical, financial, administrative, and patient satisfaction perspectives • Focuses on meeting actual and unanticipated patient needs • Uses statistical analysis to reduce variation in service processes • Relies on teamwork and data-based decisions	• Accreditation • Benchmarking (HCAHPS) • Clinical practice guidelines • PDSA cycles • Process redesign • Lean • Six Sigma	How do P-D-S-A cycles of change that incorporate peer-reviewed evidence improve patient-centeredness, teamwork, communication, and safety in a 16-bed medical and surgical pediatric intensive care unit? Adapted from Tripathi et al. (2015)

Continued

TABLE 11.5 Evolution of Quality Improvement Perspectives in Health Care—cont'd

Model	Key Features	Quality Monitoring Mechanisms	Representative Research Questions
2000s–2010s Patient Safety Systems approach to reduce harm to patients (Chassin & Loeb, 2011)	• Applies safety science methods to design health care delivery systems • Focuses on reducing or avoiding adverse events • Domains include patients, providers, care routines, system design	• Accreditation • Sentinel event reporting • National Patient Safety Goals • High reliability organization model • Root cause analysis	What is the relationship between employee engagement and the dimensions of patient safety culture in critical care units? Adapted from Collier et al. (2016)

TABLE 11.6 QI Tools and Activities

Basic Tools and Activities	Step 1 Assess	Step 2 Analyze	Step 3 Plan and Implement	Step 4 Test and Evaluate
Data collection	X	X	X	X
Flowcharts	X	X	X	X
Cause-and-effect analysis		X		
Bar and pie charts	X	X		X
Run charts	X	X		X
Control charts	X	X		X
Histograms	X	X		X
Pareto charts	X	X		X
Benchmarking	X			X
Gantt charts		X		X

From Massoud et al. (2001). A modern paradigm for improving healthcare quality. QA Monograph Series 1(1). Bethesda, MD: Published for the U.S. Agency for International Development by the Quality Assurance Project.

improvement ideas. A case example, *Reducing Wait Times in a Pediatric Neurology Outpatient Clinic: A Case Study* (Box 11.7), is presented to introduce the steps of the improvement process and apply several basic QI tools used to measure and manage system performance.

Leading a Quality Improvement Team

QI is inherently an interprofessional team process and requires contributions from various professional perspectives to assess the potential causes of system malfunction and improvement ideas (Nelson et al., 2007). As a leader of a QI team, you should involve representatives from diverse professional groups, support staff, patients, and families. Although all professional staff, support staff, and patients should be involved throughout the improvement process, a smaller number of staff (5–7 members) should be part of a lead QI team responsible for planning, coordinating, implementing, and evaluating improvement efforts. To maintain a productive lead team, it is important to set a meeting schedule and use effective meeting tools such as the following (Nelson et al., 2007):

• Meeting agenda
• Meeting roles
• Ground rules
• Brainstorming
• Multivoting

BOX 11.7 Applying the QI Steps to a Clinical Performance Problem

Reducing Wait Times in a Pediatric Neurology Outpatient Clinic: A Case Study

Background

The follow-up appointment no-show rate at Smithville Health Center's outpatient pediatric neurology clinic was approximately 49%. The high appointment cancellation rate led to much frustration and wasted resources for both the families and the clinic staff. It was clear that something had to be done to manage the system of routine follow-up appointments more effectively.

To this end, the QI team selected the appointment no-show rate as an opportunity for improvement. The team comprised a pediatric nurse practitioner, pediatrician, registered nurse, medical assistant, and administrator, who used the Plan-Do-Study-Act method to learn more about the underlying causes of the high no-show rate and to develop a new system to significantly reduce cancellations. The goal of the improvement project was to align the center's neurology clinic performance on this quality measure with the national average of approximately 10%.

Improvement Step 1: Assessment

The goal of the QI project was to understand and manage the factors that lead to no-shows for follow-up appointments in the pediatric neurology clinic. The QI team began the improvement project by asking broad questions:

- Do we consistently ask families if they are available at the time and day of the scheduled follow-up appointment?
- How do we remind families about their appointments?

The QI team devised a **check sheet** to collect data on the number of appointments offered and the no-shows for a 5-day period. The team also constructed a **fishbone diagram** to cluster data to learn more about the reasons why families were not attending the follow-up appointments.

Improvement Step 2: Analysis

Data from the check sheets and fishbone diagram was tallied and presented in **histograms**. When they graphed the data, a clear pattern emerged. The no-shows were most prevalent Monday through Thursday between 10 am and 2 pm—during school hours. Additionally, the diagram revealed that families were not attending the scheduled clinic appointments because of:

- conflicts with parents' work schedules
- families experiencing financial barriers
- communication barriers for some families whose English was a second language
- frustration with long wait times between appointments

Improvement Step 3: Develop a Plan for Improvement

The QI team worked with the health center librarian to identify relevant studies and develop their improvement plan. The QI team reviewed a number of recent studies and quality improvement projects to identify best practices in managing clinic appointments and wait times. Based on a critical appraisal of the evidence, the QI team decided to try two interventions for the improvement project.

1. Review and verify the follow-up appointment time and date with the parent or caretaker at the time that the appointment is made.
2. Implement a new appointment reminder system by calling families 48 hours before the scheduled follow-up appointment.

The QI team developed a specific aim statement to guide the project:

By the end of the next quarter, reduce the no-show rate for the Pediatric Neurology clinic at Smithville Health Center from 49%–25%.

Improvement Step 4: Test and Implement the Improvement Plan

The QI team tested the two change ideas using PDSA cycles over three successive weeks. The families seen by the seizure service were used as the pilot group for the new appointment verification process. The receptionist offered the family two appointment options between the hours of 7:30 am and 10:00 am or 3:00 pm and 5:00 pm Monday through Friday. The families were asked to verify their availability at the time that the appointment was made. The receptionist collected information from the families to learn more about their preferences and reasons for selecting a given appointment slot. During the testing period, the improvement team reviewed the data at the end of each week to assess for patterns and changes in performance. Based on the barriers identified in the assessment phase, the senior clinicians and managers decided to open an hour earlier and close an hour later each day to accommodate children's school schedules.

At the conclusion of the appointment choice PDSA cycle, the QI team piloted the 48-hour reminder call system for a 3-week period. The nurse practitioner developed a phone script and short training program for the clinic receptionists to convey the necessary information while also protecting patient confidentiality and privacy. The receptionists made reminder phone calls from 4 pm to 5:30 pm each day when families were most likely to be at

Continued

Reducing Wait Times in a Pediatric Neurology Outpatient Clinic: A Case Study

home in the evening to receive the call. Staff feedback was gathered during the PDSA cycle so that the QI team could refine the process further.

Finally, to evaluate the effectiveness of the two-appointment reminder change ideas, the QI team used a **run chart** to track performance on the appointment no-show rates for the 6-week PDSA period. The run chart was annotated to show the days when the two improvement projects were in effect. At the end of the first PDSA cycle, where the receptionists worked with the families to determine a mutually convenient appointment schedule, the no-show rate dropped from 49% to 33% in a 3-week period.

By adding the 48-hour reminder call system, the team was able to reduce the no-show appointment rate among the families followed by the seizure service to the 25% target over 6 weeks. Based on these performance data, the QI team recommended the appointment verification and 48-hour phone call reminder system as the standard of practice for all routine follow-up appointments in the Pediatric Neurology Clinic at Smithville Health Center.

To embed the new appointment scheduling system, the QI team supervised PDSA cycles until the system was in place for all of the Pediatric Neurology services. The run chart data suggested that the appointment scheduling and reminder system was mostly stable on Tuesdays, Wednesdays, and Thursdays, with more cancellations on Mondays and Fridays at the beginning and end of the school week.

Based on the success of the routine follow-up appointment scheduling process, the QI team plans on developing a new scheduling system for the urgent consultation referrals from the Smithville Health Center's emergency department and Pediatric Intensive Care Unit. The team also planned on creating a new system to integrate interpreter services into the appointment scheduling process for families with limited English proficiency. The clinic patients and staff welcomed the improvements in the overall appointment no-show rates.

Adapted from Mohamed, K., Mustafa, S., Tahtamouni, S., Taha E., & Hassan, R. (2016). A quality improvement project to reduce the 'no show' rate in a pediatric neurology clinic. *BMJ Quality Improvement Reports, 5*:u209266.w3789.

Other tools that can help with project management to keep your team and activities organized and focused include action plans and Gantt charts (Nelson et al., 2007). To download templates for meeting agendas, meeting role cards, action plans, and Gantt charts, visit the **Clinical Microsystems** website at https://clinicalmicrosystem.org/ and select the Materials/Worksheets tabs. After the lead team is assembled and processes established, the team can begin assessment of the health system. To access resources on how to best facilitate interprofessional teamwork, visit the National Center for Interprofessional Education and Practice at https://nexusipe.org/.

Improvement Process Step 1: Assessment

In the assessment phase, the first step is to complete a structured assessment to understand more about performance patterns. The improvement team typically begins with a series of broad questions used to guide data collection. Common methods used to collect system performance data include *check sheets* and *data sheets* to understand performance patterns and *surveys, focus groups,* and *interviews* to gather information about patient and staff perceptions of system performance. Commonly collected data elements include information about the following (Nelson et al., 2007):

- Patients: What are the average age, gender, top diagnoses, and satisfaction scores?
- Professionals: What is the level of staff satisfaction? What is their skill set?
- Processes and patterns: What are the processes for admitting and discharging patients?
- Common performance metrics: What are the rates of pressure ulcers and falls with injury?

For useful data collection templates, select the Tools tab at https://clinicalmicrosystem.org/.

Improvement Process Step 2: Analysis

The next phase of the improvement process focuses on data analysis. Because QI uses a team problem-solving approach, data are displayed in graphic form so all team members can see how the system is performing and generate ideas for improvements. Several tools exist to help display and analyze performance data.

Trending Variation in System Performance with Run and Control Charts

If quality health care means that the right care is delivered to the right people in the right way, at the right time, for every person, during each clinical encounter, it is important to learn when criteria are not met and why (IOM, 2001). One method is to track performance over time and understand sources of variation in system performance, which can guide improvement activities to design a better functioning health system. Minimizing performance variation is one of the main goals of QI. There are two main types of system variation (Nelson et al., 2007, p. 346):

- **Common cause variation** occurs at random and is considered a characteristic of the system. For example, you might never leave your house in time for prompt arrival to class. In this case, you must work on better managing multiple random causes of tardiness, such as getting up late or taking too long to shower, dress, and eat, to improve your overall punctuality record.
- **Special cause variation** arises from a special situation that disrupts the causal system beyond what can be accounted for by random variation. An example might be that you usually leave your house on time for prompt arrival to class, but special circumstances such as road construction or a broken elevator delay your arrival. Once these special causes of tardiness are resolved, you will arrive to class on time.

Variations in system performance over time are commonly displayed with run charts and control charts. A **run chart** is a graphical data display that shows trends in a measure of interest; trends reveal what is occurring over time (Nelson et al., 2007). The vertical axis of the run chart depicts the value of measure of interest and the horizontal axis depicts the value of each measure running over time. A run chart shows whether the outcome of interest is running in a targeted area of performance and how much variation there is from point to point and over time. For example, a patient newly diagnosed with diabetes can record her blood glucose levels over a month using a run chart. By regularly charting blood glucose levels, the patient can reveal when blood glucose runs higher or lower than the target level of less than 100 mg/dL for the fasting plasma glucose (FPG) test. The run chart in Fig. 11.1 shows that FPG levels are consistently higher than the target, with a median FPG of 130 mg/dL; the trend of FPG readings in the first 19 days of the month is indicative of common cause variation. These random variations in FPG readings are likely caused by the confluence of several factors such as diet, exercise, and medication adherence. To correct the undesirable variation, the patient can assess what factors might be influencing the higher FPG values and then work with her primary care provider to develop necessary interventions to better control her blood glucose by better managing multiple causal factors. To determine whether interventions are successful, the patient and provider should continue to document blood glucose levels and then compare the median FPG values before and after interventions are implemented.

In addition, special cause variation in FPG is evident on days 19 to 28, where nine consecutive FPG readings are above the median line. It turns out that on these days, the patient had run out of her glucose-lowering medication; this special circumstance caused increased FPG. Although various rules exist for accurately determining the presence of special cause variation, generally special cause variation is present if the following are true (Nelson et al., 2007, p. 349):

- Eight data points in a row are above or below the median or mean
- Six data points in a row are going up
- Six data points in a row are going down

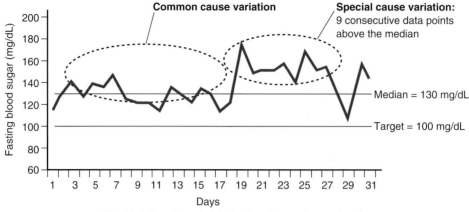

Fig. 11.1 Run chart of daily fasting plasma glucose levels.

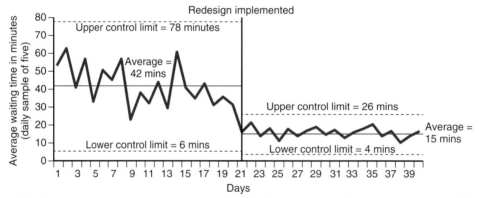

Fig. 11.2 Control chart of average wait time before and after a redesign. (From Massoud et al., 2001. A modern paradigm for improving healthcare quality. QA Monograph Series *1*(1). Bethesda, MD: Published for the U.S. Agency for International Development by the Quality Assurance Project.)

Determining common and special causes of variation is important because treatment strategies for eliminating each type of variation will vary.

A **control chart** (Fig. 11.2) also is used to track system performance over time, but it is a more sophisticated data tool than a run chart (Nelson et al., 2007). A control chart includes information on the average performance level for the system depicted by a center line displaying the system's average performance (the mean value), and the upper and lower limits depicting one to three standard deviations from average performance level. The rules to detect special cause variation are the same for run and control charts, except that for control charts, the upper and lower limits are additional tools used to detect special cause variation. Any point that falls outside the control limit is considered an outlier that merits further examination.

QI CHECKPOINT

Use a run chart in step two of the QI process to analyze causes of variation in fasting plasma glucose (FPG) levels from the target level of 100 mg/dL and in step four of the QI process to evaluate whether changes in diet, exercise, and medication adherence helped the patient achieve the targeted FPG.

Graphs

Graphs commonly used to understand system performance are displayed in Fig. 11.3,and include pie charts, bar charts, and histograms (See chapter 10). Selecting the appropriate chart depends on the type of data collected and the performance pattern the improvement team is trying to understand. A bar chart is used to display categorical-level data. A pareto diagram is a special

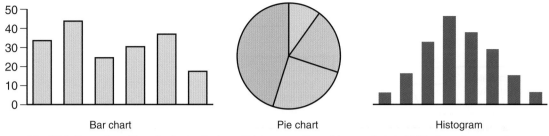

Fig. 11.3 Examples of bar chart, pie chart, and histogram. (From Massoud et al., 2001. A modern paradigm for improving healthcare quality. QA Monograph Series *1*(1). Bethesda, MD: Published for the U.S. Agency for International Development by the Quality Assurance Project.)

type of bar chart used to understand the frequency of factors that contribute to a common effect. It is used to display the Pareto Principle, sometimes referred to as the 80-20 Rule, or the Law of the Few (Massoud et al., 2001), which states that 80% of variation in a problem originates with 20% of cases. In a pareto diagram, the bars are displayed in descending order of frequency. A histogram is another type of bar chart used for continuous-level data to show the distribution of the data around the mean, commonly called the *bell curve* (Massoud et al., 2001).

Cause and Effect Diagrams

More sophisticated visual data displays include **cause and effect diagrams** used to identify and treat the causes of performance problems. Two common tools in this category are the fishbone or Ishikawa diagram and the tree diagram (Massoud et al., 2001). The **fishbone diagram** facilitates brainstorming about potential causes of a problem by grouping causes into the categories of environment, people, materials, and process (Fig. 11.4). Fishbone diagrams can be used proactively to prevent quality defects, including errors, and retrospectively to identify factors that potentially contributed to a quality defect or error that already has occurred. An example of when a fishbone diagram is used retrospectively is during **root cause analyses (RCAs)** to identify system design failures that caused errors.

An RCA is a structured method used to understand sources of system variation that lead to errors or mistakes, including sentinel events, with the goal of learning from mistakes and mitigating hazards that arise as a characteristic of the system design (Zastrow, 2015). An RCA is conducted by a team that includes representatives from nursing, medicine, management, QI, or risk management, and the individual(s) involved in

the incident (sometimes including the patient or family members in the discovery process), and it emphasizes system failures while avoiding individual blame (Zastrow, 2015). An RCA seeks to answer three questions to learn from mistakes:

- What happened?
- Why did it happen?
- What can be done to prevent it from happening again?

Because the RCA is viewed as an opportunity for organizational learning and improvement, the most effective RCAs include a change in practice or work system design to lessen the chances of similar errors occurring in the future.

A tree diagram is particularly useful for identifying the chain of causes with the goal of identifying the root cause of a problem. For example, consider medication errors. The improvement team could use the **Five Whys** method to establish the chain of causes leading to poor glycemic control:

- Question 1: Why did the patient get the incorrect medicine?
  Answer 1: Because the prescription was wrong.
- Question 2: Why was the prescription wrong?
  Answer 2: Because the nurse practitioner had incomplete information when writing the prescription.
- Question 3: Why did the nurse practitioner have incomplete information when writing the prescription?
  Answer 3: Because the patient's chart was incomplete.
- Question 4: Why wasn't the patient's chart complete?
  Answer 4: Because the medical assistant had not entered the latest laboratory report.
- Question 5: Why hadn't the medical assistant charted the latest laboratory report?

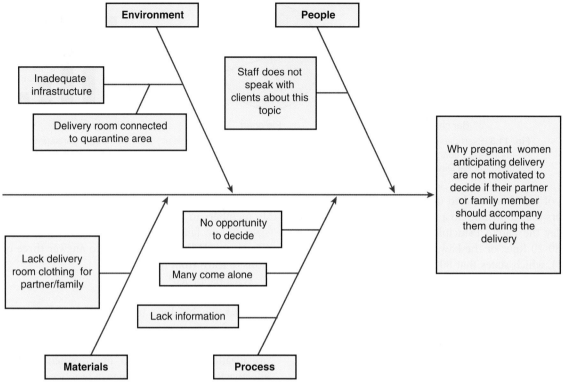

Fig. 11.4 Fishbone diagram. (Adapted from Massoud et al., 2001. A modern paradigm for improving health-care quality. QA Monograph Series *1*(1). Bethesda, MD: Published for the U.S. Agency for International Development by the Quality Assurance Project.)

Answer 5: Because the laboratory technician telephoned the results to the receptionist, who forgot to tell the patient care assistant.

In this case, using the Five Whys technique suggests that a potential solution for avoiding wrong prescriptions in the future might be to develop a system for tracking laboratory reports (Massoud et al., 2001).

Flowcharting

A **flowchart** depicts how a process works, detailing the sequence of steps from the beginning to the end of a process (Massoud et al., 2001). Several types of flowcharts exist, including the simplest (*high level*), a detailed version (*detailed*), and one that also indicates the people involved in the steps (*deployment or matrix*). Fig. 11.5 shows an example of a detailed flowchart. Massoud and colleagues (2001, p. 59) suggest using flowcharts to do the following:

- Understand processes
- Consider ways to simplify processes

- Recognize unnecessary steps in a process
- Determine areas for monitoring or data collection
- Identify who will be involved in or affected by the improvement process
- Formulate questions for further research

When you are flowcharting, it is important to identify beginning and end points of a process and then make a record of the actual, not the ideal, process. To obtain an accurate picture of the process, perform direct observation of the process steps and communicate with people who are directly part of the process to clarify all the steps.

Improvement Process Step 3: Develop a Plan for Improvement

By identifying potential sources of variation, the improvement team can pinpoint problem areas in need of improvement. The next phase is to treat the performance problem. This phase involves developing and testing a plan for improvement. A simple yet powerful

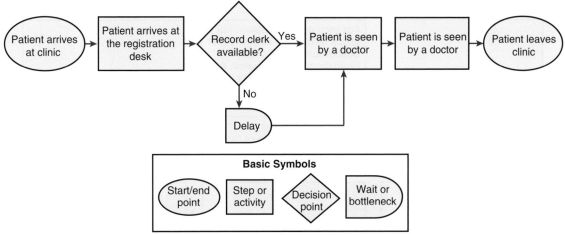

Fig. 11.5 Detailed flow chart of patient registration. (Adapted from Massoud et al., 2001. A modern paradigm for improving healthcare quality. QA Monograph Series *1*(1). Bethesda, MD: Published for the U.S. Agency for International Development by the Quality Assurance Project.)

model for developing and testing improvements is the **Model for Improvement** (Langley et al., 2009). It begins with three questions to guide the change process and focus the improvement work (Langley et al., 2009):

1. **Aim.** What are we trying to accomplish? Set a clear aim with specific measurable targets.
2. **Measures.** How will we know that the change is an improvement? Use qualitative and quantitative measures to support real improvement work to guide change progress toward the stated goal.
3. **Changes.** What changes can we make that will result in an improvement? Develop a statement about what the team believes it can change to cause improvement.

The change ideas reflect the team's hypotheses about what could improve system performance. There are several ways in which change ideas can be generated. These ideas can be identified from the root causes of the performance problems that are evident during cause-and-effect and process analyses using fishbone diagrams, the Five Whys, and flowcharting tools in the Analysis step of the improvement process. Another approach is to select common areas for change associated with the goals and philosophy of QI. Common change topics, also referred to as themes for improvement, include the following (Langley et al., 2009, p. 359):

- Eliminating waste
- Improving work flow
- Optimizing inventory
- Changing the work environment
- Managing time more effectively
- Managing variation
- Designing systems to avoid mistakes
- Focusing on products or services

Change ideas also can come from the evidence provided by your review of the available literature. This is where your EBP skills will be most helpful. You will need to critically appraise research studies and QI studies of interventions that can be applied to remedy the identified problem. To help you decide whether a journal article is a research study or a QI study, see the *critical decision tree* in Fig. 11.6. Because QI studies capture the experiences of an organization or unit, the results of these studies usually are not generalizable. To promote knowledge transfer and learning from others' improvement experiences, the *Standards for Quality Improvement Reporting Excellence,* or SQUIRE Guidelines (Ogrinc, Davies, Goodman, Batalden, Davidoff, & Stevens, 2015), were developed to promote the publication and interpretation of this type of applied research. The SQUIRE Guidelines are presented in Table 11.7; you should use them to evaluate QI studies.

Improvement Process Step 4: Test and Implement the Improvement Plan

Improvement changes identified in the planning phase are tested using the Plan-Do-Study-Act (PDSA) Improvement cycle, which is the last step of the

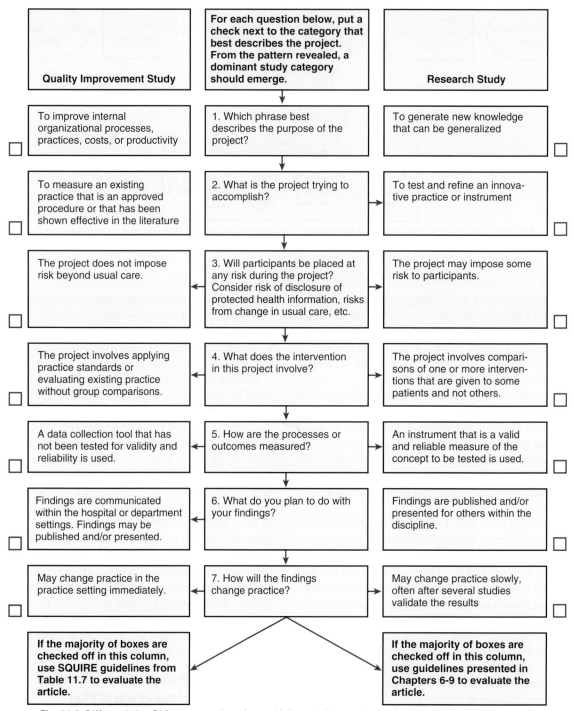

Quality Improvement Study	For each question below, put a check next to the category that best describes the project. From the pattern revealed, a dominant study category should emerge.	Research Study
To improve internal organizational processes, practices, costs, or productivity	1. Which phrase best describes the purpose of the project?	To generate new knowledge that can be generalized
To measure an existing practice that is an approved procedure or that has been shown effective in the literature	2. What is the project trying to accomplish?	To test and refine an innovative practice or instrument
The project does not impose risk beyond usual care.	3. Will participants be placed at any risk during the project? Consider risk of disclosure of protected health information, risks from change in usual care, etc.	The project may impose some risk to participants.
The project involves applying practice standards or evaluating existing practice without group comparisons.	4. What does the intervention in this project involve?	The project involves comparisons of one or more interventions that are given to some patients and not others.
A data collection tool that has not been tested for validity and reliability is used.	5. How are the processes or outcomes measured?	An instrument that is a valid and reliable measure of the concept to be tested is used.
Findings are communicated within the hospital or department settings. Findings may be published and/or presented.	6. What do you plan to do with your findings?	Findings are published and/or presented for others within the discipline.
May change practice in the practice setting immediately.	7. How will the findings change practice?	May change practice slowly, often after several studies validate the results
If the majority of boxes are checked off in this column, use SQUIRE guidelines from Table 11.7 to evaluate the article.		**If the majority of boxes are checked off in this column, use guidelines presented in Chapters 6-9 to evaluate the article.**

Fig. 11.6 Differentiating QI from research projects. (Adapted with permission from King, D.L, 2008. Research and quality improvement: Different processes, different evidence. Medsurg Nursing, 17(3), 167.)

TABLE 11.7 Revised SQUIRE Guidelines Standards for QI Reporting Excellence (SQUIRE 2.0)

Title and Abstract

Title	Indicate that the manuscript concerns an initiative to improve health care (broadly defined to include the quality, safety, effectiveness, patient-centeredness, timeliness, cost, efficiency, and equity of health care).
Abstract	a. Provide adequate information to aid in searching and indexing.
	b. Summarize all key information from various sections of the text using the abstract format of the intended publication or a structured summary, such as background, local problem, methods, interventions, results, or conclusions.

Introduction – Why did you start?

Problem description	Nature and significance of the local problem
Available knowledge	Summary of what is currently known about the problem, including relevant previous studies
Rationale	Informal or formal frameworks, models, concepts, and/or theories used to explain the problem, any reasons or assumptions that were used to develop the intervention(s), and reasons why the intervention(s) was expected to work
Specific aims	Purposes of the project and of this report

Methods – What did you do?

Context	Contextual elements considered important at the outset of the intervention(s)
Intervention(s)	a. Description of the intervention(s) in sufficient detail so that others can reproduce it/them
	b. Specifics of the team involved in the work
Study of intervention(s)	a. Approach chosen for assessing the impact of the intervention(s)
	b. Approach used to establish whether the observed outcomes were due to the intervention(s)
Measures	a. Measures chosen for studying processes and outcomes of the intervention(s), including rationale for choosing them, their operational definitions, and their validity and reliability
	b. Description of the approach to the ongoing assessment of contextual elements that contributed to success, failure, efficiency, and cost
	c. Methods employed for assessing completeness and accuracy of data
Analysis	a. Qualitative and quantitative methods used to draw inferences from the data
	b. Methods for understanding variation within the data, including the effects of time as a variable
Ethical considerations	Ethical aspects of implementing and studying the intervention(s) and how they were addressed, including, but not limited to, formal ethics review and potential conflict(s) of interest

Results – What did you find?

Results	a. Initial steps of the intervention(s) and their evolution over time (e.g., timeline diagram, flow chart, or table), including modifications made to the intervention during the project
	b. Details of the process measures and outcomes
	c. Contextual elements that interacted with the intervention(s)
	d. Observed associations among outcomes, interventions, and relevant contextual elements
	e. Unintended consequences such as unexpected benefits, problems, failures, or costs associated with the intervention(s)
	f. Details about missing data

Discussion – What does it mean?

Summary	a. Key findings, including relevance to the rationale and specific aims
	b. Particular strengths of the project
Interpretation	a. Nature of the association between the intervention(s) and outcomes
	b. Comparison of results with findings from other publications
	c. Impact of the project on people and systems
	d. Reasons for any differences between observed and anticipated outcomes, including the influence of context
	e. Costs and strategic tradeoffs, including opportunity costs

Continued

TABLE 11.7	Revised SQUIRE Guidelines Standards for QI Reporting Excellence (SQUIRE 2.0)—cont'd	
Limitations	a. Limits to the generalizability of the work
	b. Factors that might have limited internal validity, such as confounding, bias, or imprecision in the design, methods, measurement, or analysis
	c. Efforts made to minimize and adjust for limitations
Conclusions	a. Usefulness of the work
	b. Sustainability
	c. Potential for spread to other contexts
	d. Implications for practice and further study in the field
	e. Suggested next steps
Other information	
Funding	Sources of funding that supported this work; role, if any, of the funding organization in the design, implementation, interpretation, and reporting

Reproduced with permission from Ogrinc et al. (2015). SQUIRE 2.0 (Standards for Quality Improvement Reporting Excellence): revised publication guidelines from a detailed consensus process. *BMJ Quality and Safety,* 0, 1-7.
Note: See www.squire-statement.org/ for more information on publishing QI studies.

Improvement Model (Langley et al., 2009; Massoud et al., 2001) depicted in Fig. 11.7. The focus of PDSA is experimentation using small, rapid tests of change. Actions involved in each phase of the PDSA cycle are detailed in Fig. 11.7. In this step, you evaluate the success of the intervention in bringing about improvement. It is important for the team to monitor intended and unintended changes in system performance, patient and staff perceptions of the change, and ideally, cost of the change. Also, in this phase of the improvement process, it is useful to track the stability and sustainability of the new work process by monitoring system performance over time. Results data should be presented in graphic data displays (explained earlier in the chapter) and compared with baseline performance.

To promote successful implementation of your improvement interventions, you should consider using the following evidence-based implementation strategies (Powell et al., 2015, p. 8–10):

- Practice facilitation: A process of interactive problem solving and support that occurs in a context of a recognized need for improvement and a supportive interpersonal relationship
- Educational outreach visit: When a trained person meets with providers in their practice setting to educate them about a clinical innovation with the intent of changing the providers' practices

- Educational meetings and workshops: Meetings targeted toward different stakeholder groups to teach them about a clinical innovation
- Audit and feedback: Collecting and summarizing clinical performance data over a specified time period and giving it to clinicians and administrators to monitor, evaluate, and modify provider behavior
- Reminders: Systems designed to help clinicians recall information and/or prompt them to use the clinical innovation
- Local opinion leaders: Informing providers identified by colleagues as opinion leaders or educationally influential about the clinical innovation in the hope that they will influence colleagues to adopt it

Current primary care evidence suggests that organizational-level strategies such as practice facilitation are consistently effective in promoting compliance with desired practices (Lau et al., 2015). From the strategies targeting individual providers, educational outreach visits demonstrated the largest median change in compliance with desired practice compared with no strategy, followed by educational meetings and workshops, audit and feedback, computerized reminders, printed educational materials, and use of local opinion leaders (Lau et al, 2015). Evidence for use of financial incentives and multiple versus single implementation strategies is currently mixed and inconclusive (Lau et al., 2015).

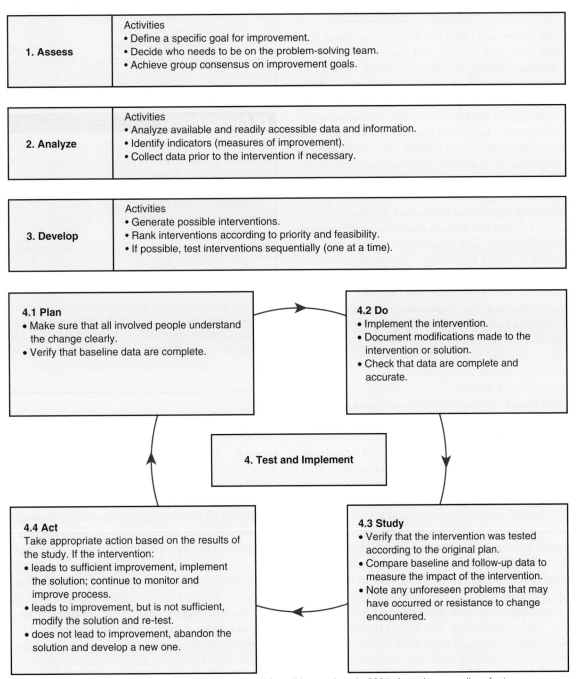

Fig. 11.7 Summary of the QI process. (Adapted from Massoud et al., 2001. A modern paradigm for improving healthcare quality. QA Monograph Series 1(1). Bethesda, MD: Published for the U.S. Agency for International Development by the Quality Assurance Project.)

TAKING ON THE QUALITY IMPROVEMENT CHALLENGE AND LEADING THE WAY

Hospital leaders and other key stakeholders agree that enabling clinicians to lead and participate in QI is vital to strengthening our health system's capacity to provide high-quality patient care (Draper et al., 2008; IOM, 2015). Advanced practice nurses are on the front lines leading care delivery. They offer unique perspectives on the root causes of dysfunctional care and what interventions might work reliably and sustainably in everyday clinical practice to achieve best care. However, there are multiple barriers to the participation of nurse leaders in QI, including insufficient staffing, lack of leadership support and resources for their participation in QI, and not enough educational preparation for knowledgeable and meaningful QI involvement (Draper et al., 2008). For nurse practitioners, midwives, clinical nurse specialists, educators, and administrators to contribute their knowledge and expertise to patient care delivery and the organization's quality enterprise, nursing leadership must engage in the following (Berwick, 2011, p. 326):

- Setting aims and building the will to improve
- Measurement and transparency
- Finding better systems
- Supporting PDSA activities, risk, and change
- Providing resources

Several common elements that make improvement work doable are captured in two bodies of knowledge (Berwick, 2011). One is professional knowledge that includes an understanding of one's discipline, subject matter, and values of the discipline. The other is knowledge of improvement, which includes an understanding of complex systems functioning through dynamic interplay among various technical and human elements; knowledge of how to detect and manage variation in system performance; knowledge of managing group processes through effective conflict resolution and communication; and knowledge of how to gain further understanding by continual experimentation in local settings through rapid tests of change. Linking these two knowledge systems promotes continuous improvement in health care. This chapter provides a starting point for you to develop basic knowledge and skills for the improvement work so you can better meet the leadership challenges embedded in the roles of clinical leaders.

IPE TIP

Remember that important members of the interprofessional QI team are your administrative managers and executives who provide leadership support, including time and resources for your team to implement a QI project.

QI CHECKPOINT

- Discuss the similarities and differences among total quality improvement, Lean, Six Sigma, and Clinical Microsystems models.
- Consider your practice's performance on the HEDIS measures. What suggestions do you have for applying QI principles to improve your practice's score on these key indicators?
- Why is it important to document care outcomes using standardized performance measurement systems? How does performance measurement relate to QI activities?
- What barriers do you see for participating in practice-level quality improvement initiatives? What suggestions do you have for overcoming these barriers?
- In what ways do QI studies differ from research studies? How would you use the results of a QI study to inform a change in practice on your unit?

SYNTHESIS

Leading quality improvement initiatives is proposed to be an important role for advanced practice nurses. Quality improvement initiatives aim to influence improvements in organizational settings and strive to ensure that all patients consistently receive high-quality, cost-effective, and satisfying patient-centered care. Initiatives need to align with organizational priorities that are consistent with national goals and strategies for health care quality improvement. National performance measures, public reporting systems, and accrediting organizations require health care institutions to meet local and national quality and safety standards. Health care organizations also identify those measures that best apply to their practice in acute or primary care settings. Quality improvement models such as TQM/CQI, Six Sigma, Lean, and Clinical Microsystems provide a guide for developing, implementing, and evaluating QI projects. Evidence provided by QI projects, coupled with national quality data, inform clinical decision making.

Teamwork and collaboration across professions is fundamental to success in developing, implementing, and evaluating quality improvement initiatives at the micro, meso, or macrosystem level. Health care leaders agree that involving clinical leaders and clinicians is essential to strengthening our health system's capacity to provide high quality patient care.

KEY POINTS

- There is much room for improvement in the quality of care in the U.S.
- The quality of health care is evaluated in terms of its effectiveness, efficiency, access, safety, timeliness, and patient-centeredness.
- As the largest group of health professionals, nurse leaders play a key role in leading QI efforts in clinical settings.
- Accreditation, payment, and performance measurement are external incentives used to improve the quality of care delivered by hospitals and health professionals. One example of such is the Joint Commission accreditation for health care delivery organizations.
- The Quality Payment Program and HEDIS are sources of standardized measures to assess and improve the quality of care delivered in the U.S.
- Standardized measures such as influenza vaccination rates are used to compare performance across clinical practices and organizations.
- Health care payers use quality performance measures such as 30-day readmission rates as a basis for paying hospitals and providers.
- QI is both a philosophy of organizational functioning and a set of statistical analysis tools and change techniques used to reduce variation.
- The major approaches used to manage quality in health care are Total Quality Management/ Continuous Quality Improvement; Lean; Six Sigma; and the Clinical Microsystems model.
- The defining characteristics of QI are a focus on patients/customers; teams and teamwork to improve work processes; and use of data and statistical analysis tools to understand system variation.
- QI uses benchmarking to compare organizational performance and learn from high-performing organizations.
- QI tools, techniques, and principles are applied to clinical performance problems in the form of improvement projects, such as using a presurgical checklist to prevent wrong-side surgeries, a national patient safety goal.
- Practice-level improvement projects should align with national improvement priorities to promote the sustainability of local projects.
- There are four major steps in the QI process: assessment, analysis, improvement, and evaluation.
- Patient safety focuses on designing systems to remove factors known to cause errors or adverse events.
- Barriers exist that impede the leadership role of nurses in QI, including insufficient staffing, lack of leadership support, and clinical leaders' unfamiliarity with QI principles and practices.

REFERENCES

Agency for Healthcare Research and Quality. (2016). *2015 National healthcare quality and disparities report and 5th anniversary update on the National Quality Strategy.* (AHRQ Pub. No. 16-0015). Retrieved from: http://www.ahrq.gov/sites/default/files/wysiwyg/research/findings/nhqrdr/nhqdr15/2015nhqdr.pdf.

Agency for Healthcare Research and Quality. (2013). *Practice facilitation handbook.* Retrieved from https://www.ahrq.gov/professionals/prevention-chronic-care/improve/system/pfhandbook/mod7.html.

American Organization of Nurse Executives. (2016). *Care innovation and transformation program.* Retrieved from http://www.aone.org/education/cit.shtml.

Aydin, C., Donaldson, N., Stotts, N. A., Fridman, M., & Brown, D. S. (2015). Modeling hospital-acquired pressure ulcer prevalence on medical-surgical units: Nurse workload, expertise, and clinical processes of care. *Health Services Research, 50*(2), 351–373.

Berwick, D. M. (2011). Preparing nurses for participation in and leadership of continual improvement. *Journal of Nursing Education, 50*(6), 322–327.

Bigelow, B., & Arndt, M. (1995). Total quality management: Field of dreams? *Health Care Management Review, 20*(4), 15–25.

Centers for Medicare and Medicaid Services. (2017a). *Value-based Programs.* Retrieved from https://www.cms.gov/Medicare/Quality-Initiatives-Patient-Assessment-Instruments/Value-Based-Programs/Value-Based-Programs.html.

Centers for Medicare and Medicaid Services. (2017b). *The quality payment program.* Retrieved from https://qpp.cms.gov/.

Chassin, M. R., & Loeb, J. M. (2011). The ongoing quality improvement journey: Next stop, high reliability. *Health Affairs, 30*(4), 559–568.

Cronenwett, L., Sherwood, G., Barnsteiner, J., et al. (2007). Quality and safety education for nurses. *Nursing Outlook, 55*(3), 122–131.

DelliFraine, J. L., Langabeer, J. R., II, & Nembhard, I. M. (2010). Assessing the evidence of Six Sigma and Lean in the health care industry. *Quality Management in Health Care, 19*(3), 211–225.

Donabedian, A. (1966). Evaluating the quality of medical care. *The Milbank Memorial Fund Quarterly, 44*(3), 166–206.

Draper, D. A., Felland, L. E., Liebhaber, A., & Melichar, L. (2008). The role of nurses in hospital quality improvement (CSHSC Report no. 3). Retrieved from http://www.hschange.org/CONTENT/972/.

Henry, B., Wood, S., & Nagelkerk, J. (1992). Nightingale's perspective of nursing administration. *Sogo Kango: Comprehensive Nursing Quarterly, 27*, 16–26.

Institute of Medicine. (1999). *To err is human: building a safer health system: executive summary.* Washington, DC: The National Academies Press. Retrieved from http://books.nap.edu/openbook.php?record_id=9728.

Institute of Medicine. (2001). *Crossing the quality chasm: a new health system for the 21st century: executive summary.* Washington, DC: National Academies Press. Retrieved from http://books.nap.edu/catalog/10027.html.

Institute of Medicine. (2015). *Assessing progress on the IOM report The Future of Nursing.* Washington, DC: National Academies Press.

Langley, G. J., Moen, R. D., Nolan, K. M., et al. (2009). *The improvement guide: a practical approach to enhancing organizational performance* (2nd ed.). San Francisco, CA: Jossey-Bass.

Lau, R., Stevenson, F., Ong, B. N., Dziedzic, K., Treweek, S., Eldrige, S., et al. (2015). Achieving change in primary care – effectiveness of strategies for improving implementation of complex interventions: systematic review. *BMJ Open, 5.* https://doi.org/10.1136/bmjopn-2015-009993.

Massoud, R., Askov, K., Reinke, J., et al. (2001). *A modern paradigm for improving healthcare quality. QA Monograph Series 1(1).* Bethseda, MD: Quality Assurance Project.

McConnell, J. K., Lindrooth, R. C., Wholey, D. R., Maddox, T. M., & Bloom, N. (2016). Modern management practices and hospital admissions. *Health Economics, 25*, 470–485.

National Quality Forum. (2004). *National voluntary consensus standard for nursing-sensitive care: an initial performance measure set.* Retrieved from: http://www.qualityforum.org/Publications/2004/10/National_Voluntary_Consensus_Standards_for_Nursing-Sensitive_Care__An_Initial_Performance_Measure_Set.aspx.

Nelson, E. C., Batalden, P. B., & Godfrey, M. M. (2007). *Quality by design: a clinical microsystems approach.* San Francisco, CA: Jossey-Bass.

Nuti, S. V., Wang, Y., Masoudi, F. A., Bratzler, D. W., Bernheim, S. M., et al. (2015). Improvements in the distribution of hospital performance for the care of patients with acute myocardial infarction, heart failure, and pneumonia, 2006–2011. *Medical Care, 53*(6), 485–491.

Ogrinc, G., Davies, L., Goodman, D., Batalden, P., Davidoff, F., & Stevens, D. (2015). SQUIRE 2.0 (Standards for Quality Improvement Reporting Excellence): revised publication guidelines from a detailed consensus process. *BMJ Quality and Safety, 0,* 1–7.

Pohl, J. M., Savrin, C., Fiandt, K., Beauchesne, M., Drayton-Brooks, S., & Werner, K. E. (2009). Quality and safety in graduate nursing education: Cross-mapping QSEN graduate competencies with NONPF's NP core and practice doctorate competencies. *Nursing Outlook, 57*(6), 349–354.

Powell, B. J., Waltz, T. J., Chinman, M. J., Damschroder, L. J., Smith, J. L., Matthieu, M. M., et al. (2015). A refined compilation of implementation strategies: Results from the Expert Recommendations for Implementing Change (ERIC) project. *Implementation Science, 10*(21), 1–14.

Schneider, E. C., Sarnak, D. O., Squires, D., Shah, A., & Doty, M. M. (2017). *Mirror, Mirror 2017: International Comparison Reflects Flaws and Opportunities for Better U.S. Health Care.* The Commonwealth Fund. Retrieved from http://www.commonwealthfund.org/publications/fund-reports/2017/jul/mirror-mirror-international-comparisons-2017.

Tidwell, J., Busby, R., Lewis, B., Falder, K., Langston, A., Allen, S. S., et al. (2016). The race: Quality assurance performance improvement project aimed at achieving superior patient outcomes. *Journal of Nursing Care Quality, 31*(2), 99–104.

Tripathi, S., Arteaga, G., Rohlik, G., Boynton, B., Graner, K., & Ouellette, Y. (2015). Implementation of patient-centered bedside rounds in the pediatric intensive care unit. *Journal of Nursing Care Quality, 30*(2), 160–166.

U. S. Department of Health and Human Services. (2016a). *National quality strategy overview.* Retrieved from http://www.ahrq.gov/workingforquality/nqs/overview.pdf.

U. S. Department of Health and Human Services. (2016b). *Hospital compare.* Retrieved from https://www.medicare.gov/hospitalcompare/search.html.

Zastrow, R. L. (2015). Root cause analysis in infusion nursing: Applying quality improvement tools for adverse events. *Journal of Infusion Nursing, 38*(3), 225–31.

Planning for Success

Marita Titler

LEARNING OUTCOMES

After reading this chapter, you should be able to do the following:

- Apply the Translating Research into Practice Model in implementing evidence-based practices (EBPs).
- Analyze the attributes of an EBP topic that impact adoption.
- Compare and contrast roles of the EBP team in implementation.
- Describe the importance of quality improvement (QI) as a foundation for EBP implementation.

- Apply the implementation principles derived from Rogers's Diffusion of Innovation Theory.
- Apply the principles of organizational functioning to EBP implementation.
- Develop an action plan for implementation of an EBP.
- Analyze three ethical issues in EBP.
- Compare and contrast the definitions, intent, and requirements for Institutional Review Board (IRB) approval for QI, EBP, and research.

KEY TERMS

Action plan
Implementation
Translating research into practice model

INTRODUCTION

Implementation is at the core of evidence-based practice (EBP). It is defined as the processes and strategies used to promote the use of EBPs by clinicians, consumers, and policy makers. Attending to the details of implementation requires attention, without which there is little chance that the EBPs will be used by clinicians and patients. Implementation is messy, iterative, and nonlinear. It requires tenacity, commitment, and relationship building. Furthermore minimal guidance is provided for implementation in many EBP models, including the Iowa Model. Therefore the Implementation portion of this textbook (Section III) is designed for you and your team to be successful in implementing EBPs in your community, organization, and/or primary care site. This chapter provides a model,

principles, and considerations to guide you and your team when planning for implementation. Chapters 13 and 14 provide specific implementation strategies (e.g., audit and feedback) and examples for each. If a practice change is warranted to align health care practices with current evidence recommendations, you and your team will need to develop an action plan to implement the practice changes. An action plan, described in a later section, is a written outline that details the objectives, work to be achieved, person or group responsible for the work, and designated date for completion. Implementation goes beyond writing and disseminating evidence-based standards of practice; it requires interactions among direct care providers to champion and foster evidence adoption, leadership support, and system changes.

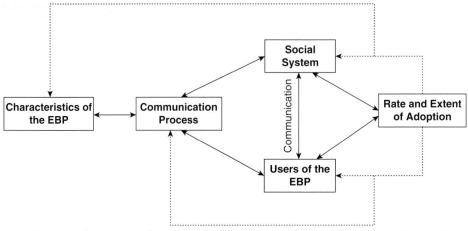

Fig. 12.1 Translating Research into Practice Model. (From Titler, M. G. (2010). Translation science and context. *Research Theory Nursing Practice*, 24(1)).

OVERVIEW OF AN IMPLEMENTATION MODEL

The Translating Research into Practice (TRIP) Model is an implementation model based on Rogers's (2003) seminal work on diffusion of innovations, and is useful in guiding selection of strategies for promoting adoption of EBPs. According to this model (Fig. 12.1), adoption of EBPs is influenced by four key areas:

- The nature of the innovation (e.g., the type and strength of evidence, the clinical topic)
- The manner in which the innovation is communicated to members (clinicians) and the social system (organization, patient care unit)

Successful implementation requires strategies that address these areas within a context of participative, planned change (Titler, 2010; Titler et al., 2016). The TRIP model is used in Chapters 13 and 14 as a guiding framework for your selection of implementation strategies.

> **EBP TIP**
>
> Planning for successful implementation starts with topic selection and continues throughout all steps of the EBP process. If the topic is not a priority for your setting or organization, you will encounter difficulties with implementation no matter how strong the evidence.

THE EVIDENCE-BASED PRACTICE TOPIC

Successful implementation is influenced by the EBP topic. Ideas for your topic may have come from several areas, such as problem- and/or knowledge-focused triggers (see

Chapters 2 and 3). In selecting a topic, it is essential that you and your team consider how the topic fits the priorities of your practice agency (e.g., community setting, health system, primary care practice) to garner support from leaders and necessary resources for successful implementation.

It is imperative that your topic have an evidence base determined by the critical appraisal process and a synthesis of the evidence (see Chapters 2, 4–9). Otherwise, it is not an EBP. All team members should be highly knowledgeable about the strength and quality of the evidence for your topic, the rationale for selecting it, and the quality improvement (QI) data that demonstrate opportunities to improve the quality of care.

Based on your clinical question as outlined in Chapter 3, the purpose of your EBP project will be clear, including the problem, patient population, processes and outcomes of care to be addressed, and setting (e.g., inpatient unit(s), clinic(s), or community setting). It is important to share the purpose statement with all key stakeholders and keep it visible during implementation to prevent "scope creep," or expansion of the project beyond what is realistic and needed for successful implementation.

> **EBP TIP**
>
> **Example of Evidence-Based Practice Purpose Statement**
>
> The purpose of this EBP project is to implement EB fall prevention practices that target patient-specific fall risk factors and thereby reduce fall rates and severity of fall injuries on three adult medical units: 7C, 3W, and 4D. The EB fall prevention practices address mobility, elimination, cognition, medications, and reducing risk for fall injury.

TABLE 12.1 Attributes of EBP Topics and Implementation		
Attributes of EBP Topic	Description	Examples of Implementation Strategies*
Relative Advantage	Degree to which an EBP is perceived as better than the practice it supersedes. Cost and social status motivation aspects of new ideas or EBPs are elements of relative advantage. Early adopters and early majority are more status-motivated than late majority and laggards.	Direct or indirect financial payment incentives may be used to support adoption of an EBP. This strategy is actualized by CMS's value-based payment programs. Performance gap assessment Benchmarking with other organizations
Compatibility	Degree to which an innovation is perceived as consistent with the existing values, norms, past experiences, and needs of potential adopters. If an EBP is compatible with patients' and clinicians' needs, uncertainty will decrease and the rate of adoption will increase.	Naming the EBP is an important part of compatibility. The name should be meaningful to clinicians. Name the EBP project to clearly reflect the focus. Consider adopting an EBP market icon that reflects the EBP.
Complexity	Degree to which an EBP is perceived as relatively difficult to understand and use. Complexity is negatively correlated with the rate of adoption. Excessive complexity is a potential obstacle in its adoption.	Break complex EBP topics into conceptual parts and implement components sequentially rather than simultaneously. Narrow the selected topic so implementation is manageable. Use quick reference guides and decision aids.
Trialability	Degree to which an EBP can be tried on a limited basis. The more an EBP can be tried, the faster its adoption will be. Reinvention–modification of the EBP may occur during the trial and thereby create faster adoption.	Plan for piloting the change in practice as part of implementation (see Iowa Model – Fig. 1.2).
Observability	Degree to which the impact of an EBP is visible to others. Role modeling and peer observation are key.	Audit and feedback Opinion leaders and change champions

*See Chapters 13 and 14 for a discussion of implementation strategies.
CMS, Center for Medicare and Medicaid Services; *EBP*, evidence-based practice.
Data from Rogers, E. M. (2003). *Diffusion of innovations*. New York, NY: The Free Press.

The attributes of the EBP topic that influence implementation are (Table 12.1):

- relative advantage,
- compatibility,
- complexity,
- trialability, and
- observability (Rogers, 2003).

EBPs with more of these attributes, except complexity, will be more readily adopted in practice. Still, adopting a new practice is difficult even when it has these obvious advantages.

EBP TIP

Attributes of the EBP topic as perceived by users and stakeholders are neither stable features nor sure determinants of EBP use.

The Team

EBP work is a team effort requiring representatives from various disciplines, guided by the nature of the EBP topic and clinical question. For example, a team working on evidence-based acute pain management should be interprofessional and include pharmacists, nurses, nurse practitioners, physicians, and psychologists with expertise in pain management. A team working on EBPs for family presence during resuscitation may include a social worker, psychologist, staff nurses, nurse manager, advanced practice nurse, physician(s), and a family member.

Know your team members. Planning for implementation requires that all members participate in some component of the process. Some may be best skilled at teaching their peers about the EBPs to be implemented and the evidence base for each. Others may be best at managing or negotiating organizational system

BOX 12.1 Examples: Rationale for Changing Practice

- The evidence is relevant to our practice with opportunities to improve the quality of care.
- A significant number of studies, evidence-based practice (EBP) guidelines, systematic reviews, and other evidence sources are available.
- Evidence sources reflect or include study subjects and/or study sample characteristics similar to our patient population.
- There is a consistency across evidence sources regarding practices that are supported by research findings and other types of evidence.
- Our current practice is not aligned with the evidence.
- Our quality improvement (QI) data on [insert topic here] suggest we have the opportunity to improve quality of care in this area.
- The benefit for our patient population outweighs the risk of harm.

changes. Still others may be best suited to influence the thinking and actions of their peers using a point-of-care coaching approach. Implementation is about relationships that foster questioning, respect, and trust. Thus, planning for implementation requires that as team members, you know one another's strengths, passions, and biases.

An essential element of planning for successful implementation is your team's clarity about the following:

- Rationale for deciding to change practice (Box 12.1)
- Specific EBPs to be implemented

After evidence synthesis, your team sets forth EBP recommendations with an evidence grade for each (see Chapter 2). These EBP recommendations must be converted into practice statements for your setting. This is so individuals in your setting know the practices are based on evidence and understand the type and evidence grade used in development of the practices.

IPE TIP

Successful implementation of an EBP project is influenced by the cohesiveness of the EBP project team. Their ability to communicate clearly with one another and the degree to which diverse team members understand the value of each member's perspective are important factors in fostering a team culture of respect and safety.

QUALITY IMPROVEMENT AS A FOUNDATION FOR IMPLEMENTATION

QI is an essential foundation for EBP implementation (see Chapter 11). Planning for implementation success requires selecting the following:

- Quality metrics and data sources to evaluate the impact of implementing the EBPs
- Methods for display of quality metrics
- Methods for communicating the quality metrics to staff over time

Selected metrics are collected and analyzed before, during, and upon completion of implementation. These metrics are integrated into the organization's QI program to support and evaluate sustainability of the EBPs and the need for implementation "boosters" over time. For example, if the focus of your EBP project is to implement EB fall prevention practices that mitigate patient-specific fall risk factors, then you would expect fall rates and types of fall injuries to decline over time. Therefore you should track fall rates for 6 to 8 months before implementation, during the implementation process, and after implementation. If fall rates start trending upward after implementation, you will want to understand why and correct the problem, which may be that clinicians have become lax in using the EBPs that were implemented. See Chapter 11 for more information and illustrations of QI.

PRINCIPLES OF IMPLEMENTATION

Implementation is a dynamic, iterative process influenced by all steps of EBP described in Chapter 1 (see Table 1.4). Key principles for implementation (Rogers, 2003) are:

- Decision makers move from knowledge about an innovation (e.g., EBPs) through implementation and confirmation (Fig. 12.2 and Table 12.2).
- Clinicians do not adopt EBPs at the same time.
- Time for implementation varies depending on the nature and complexity of the innovation or EBPs.
- When 30% to 40% of individuals use the new idea (e.g., early adopters), there is a natural take-off (S curve) in the rate of adoption (Fig. 12.3).

You will observe that individuals fall into different adopter categories:

- Innovators
- Early adopters
- Early majority

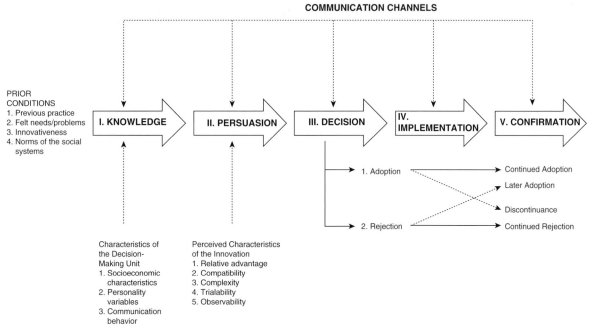

COMMUNICATION CHANNELS

PRIOR CONDITIONS
1. Previous practice
2. Felt needs/problems
3. Innovativeness
4. Norms of the social systems

I. KNOWLEDGE

II. PERSUASION

III. DECISION

IV. IMPLEMENTATION

V. CONFIRMATION

1. Adoption
2. Rejection

Continued Adoption
Later Adoption
Discontinuance
Continued Rejection

Characteristics of the Decision-Making Unit
1. Socioeconomic characteristics
2. Personality variables
3. Communication behavior

Perceived Characteristics of the Innovation
1. Relative advantage
2. Compatibility
3. Complexity
4. Trialability
5. Observability

Fig. 12.2 Stages of the Decision Process. (From Rogers, E. M. (2003). *Diffusion of innovations*. New York, NY: The Free Press.)

- Late majority
- Laggards

In each category, individuals are similar in terms of their innovativeness—the degree to which they are early in adopting new ideas or willing to change their practices compared with others (Fig. 12.4 and Table 12.3).

Time required to adopt EBPs varies by their overall complexity. For example, EBPs that are complex (e.g., implementing fall prevention interventions that target patient-specific fall risks in hospitalized older adults, Innovation III, Fig. 12.3) require a longer time period for implementation compared with simpler ones (e.g., screening for annual flu vaccines for hospitalized older adults, Innovation I, Fig. 12.3). In general, most EBP projects take 12 to 18 months to complete, from formulating the clinical question through evaluation.

Principles of organizational functioning are important considerations when implementing EBPs. Thus, you need to:

- Explain how your EBPs support the mission, vision, strategic agendas, and organizational targets for improving quality of care (e.g., decreasing fall rates, improving patient satisfaction).

- Be strategic in engaging key leaders early in the EBP work and keep them informed of progress. Leaders include the chief nursing officer, chief medical officer, chair of service lines, and/or nurse managers of units where the EBPs will be implemented. In community settings, such as primary care practices, the size and complexity of the primary care medical home (PCMH) will influence who the organizational leader is, ranging from the PCMH director to the PCMH manager.

- Call on the expertise of individuals in your organization, such as QI leaders and advanced practice nurses (APNs). QI leaders can provide guidance on quality metrics needed to evaluate the impact of the EBP. APNs, nurse practitioners, and clinical nurse specialists can provide leadership for many EBP steps, including acquisition and critical appraisal of the evidence, integration of evidence into local practice standards, and communication with key stakeholders.

- Engage organizational and departmental committees in the EBP work. Consider the governance committees you will need to interact with to make changes in practice. Consult with the chairs of these committees throughout the process, and keep them informed of your progress.

TABLE 12.2   Stages of Adoption

Stage of Decision Process	Description	Examples of Implementation Strategies*
Knowledge	Decision makers (individuals or units) are exposed to and gain an understanding of the EBP. Individuals learn about the existence of the evidence for the practice and seek information about the EBP: "What?," "How?," and "Why?"	Educate users about the EBPs, including the strength and evidence grade. Include key stakeholders in evidence appraisal and synthesis.
Persuasion	Decision makers form a favorable or unfavorable attitude toward the EBP. Although the knowledge stage is more cognitive- (knowing) centered, the persuasion stage is more affective- (feeling) centered. The degree of uncertainty about the effectiveness of the EBP and social reinforcement from colleagues and peers affect an individual's opinions and beliefs about the EBP. Close peers' subjective evaluations that reduce uncertainty about the EBP's impact are usually more credible to the individual.	Use opinion leaders and change champions.
Decision	Decision makers engage in activities that lead to a choice to adopt or reject the EBP. If individuals can try the EBP, it usually is adopted more quickly because most want to try applying the EBPs in their own situations and then come to an adoption decision.	Pilot the change on a small scale. Plan for pilot as part of implementation.
Implementation	When an EBP is put into use uncertainty about the impact of the EBP on outcomes still can be a problem at this stage. Assistance from change agents and others to reduce the degree of uncertainty is helpful.	Use opinion leaders and change champions. Use audit and feedback. Use educational outreach and point of care coaching.
Confirmation	Individuals seek reinforcement for the EBP decision that already has been made but may reverse the decision if exposed to conflicting messages. Individuals tend to seek supportive messages that confirm their decisions. Individuals may reject the EBP because they are not satisfied with its performance.	Discuss audit and feedback of process and outcome data.

*See Chapters 13 and 14 for a discussion of implementation strategies.
Data from Rogers, E. M. (2003). *Diffusion of innovations.* New York, NY: The Free Press.

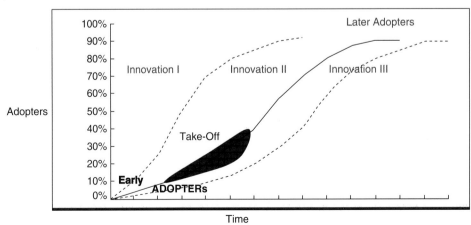

Fig. 12.3 Adoption of EBPs. (From Rogers, E. M. (2003). *Diffusion of innovations.* New York, NY: The Free Press.)

TABLE 12.3 **Description of Adopter Categories**

Adopter Category	Description
Innovators	Innovators are willing to experience new ideas and can cope with uncertainty. They are innovative and bring new ideas into organizations from the outside. They are respected by other members of the social system because of their innovation and close relationships with others outside the organization.
Early Adopters	Compared with innovators, early adopters are more limited to the boundaries of the local setting. Others come to them to get advice or information about the new idea. As role models, their subjective evaluations of the EBPs reach other clinicians through their interpersonal networks. Early adopters put their stamp of approval on a new idea by adopting it and thus decrease uncertainty about it.
Early Majority	Although the early majority have good interaction with other clinicians, they do not have the leadership influence that early adopters have. However, their interpersonal networks are still important in the adoption process. They are deliberate in adopting a new idea and are neither the first nor the last to adopt it. Their adoption of a new idea usually takes longer than for innovators and early adopters. The early majority represents about one-third of all members of a social system.
Late Majority	Late majority adopters wait until most of their peers adopt the innovation before they feel safe to do so. They are skeptical about the new idea and its impact, but peer pressure may lead them to adoption. Interpersonal networks of close peers usually persuade the late majority to adopt the new idea.
Laggards	Laggards hold the traditional view and are more skeptical about new ideas than the late majority. Their interpersonal networks mainly consist of others from the same category. They first want to make sure that an idea works before they adopt it. They tend to make decisions about adoption after seeing whether the idea has been successfully adopted by others. Their process of adopting is relatively long.

Data from Rogers, E. M. (2003). *Diffusion of innovations*. New York, NY: The Free Press.

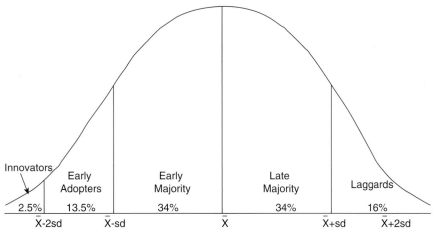

Fig. 12.4 Adopter Categorization. (From Rogers, E. M. (2003). *Diffusion of innovations*. New York, NY: The Free Press.)

- Market messages about the EBP widely across the organization. Content of messages and methods of communication should be customized for types of recipients and will differ according to the EBP steps. For example, if the focus is implementing EBPs to prevent hypothermia in premature infants, your marketing message may be, "It is not 'hot' to be cool." If your project is to improve physical activity of community-dwelling older adults, your message may be, "Mobile for Life."

EBP TIP

Consider the context of implementation when planning. What is the nature of the practice culture with respect to questioning practice, leadership styles, innovativeness, and commitment to quality of care?

TABLE 12.4 Myths and Realities of Implementation

Components of TRIP Model	Myths	Realities and Suggestions for Implementation
Nature of the EBP topic	The evidence is strong, and clinicians will change practice if we show them the evidence. An EBP standard will change practice. Clinicians care about the EBP topic.	• Characteristics of the topic influence adoption: relative advantage, compatibility, complexity, trialability, and observability. • Engage clinicians in topic selection. • Demonstrate improvement opportunities using local QI and bench-marking data. • Explain the relationship with strategic initiatives and QI targets. • Keep discussions patient-centered. • EBP recommendations need localization to fit the practice setting. • Develop local EBP standards. • Engage clinicians in localization of EBP recommendations. • Creation of local EBP standards is essential but alone will not change practice. • Use quick reference guides, decision aids, and clinical reminders.
Communication	Clinicians stay abreast of the latest evidence. Clinicians learn about new evidence by reading journals and other evidence sources. We just need to educate clinicians about the EBP for effective implementation.	• Explosion of evidence makes it difficult to stay abreast of the latest evidence. • Most clinicians learn about the evidence from trusted colleagues. • Education is necessary but not sufficient to change practice. • Interactive education is more effective than didactic education. • Communication factors that influence adoption include interpersonal communication channels, methods of communication, and social networks of users. • There is a simple way to package information so that under the right circumstances, it can be irresistible and spur us to action. • Use opinion leaders, change champions, and educational outreach and display key messages at the site of care delivery.
Users of the EBP	Clinicians will adopt EBPs at about the same pace. "I just need to get those resistors on board." "If I build it, they will come." In other words, "If I tell clinicians about the EBPs, they will implement them." Clinicians have been educated about the EBPs, so they should follow them.	• Clinicians vary in their rates of adoption of EBPs. • Focus on adoption by innovators, early adopters, and early majority. • Implementation of a new practice requires changing how things are done and affects multiple individuals from multiple specialties and their interrelationships. • Implementation requires partnerships and collaboration. • Use performance gap assessment, audit and feedback, and trying the change in practice (pilot).
Social system	"One size fits all." Practice cultures in our organization are similar across units and clinics. Changing practice is the NM's responsibility.	• Context matters. Practice cultures differ within organizations. • Organizational factors affecting adoption include the learning culture, leadership, and capacity to evaluate the impact of the EBP during and after implementation. • Effective implementation needs both a receptive climate and a good fit with intended users' needs and values. • Performance criteria for all professional roles should include EBP. • The governance structure needs to indicate the committees and groups responsible for advancing EBP work. • Human resources professionals with expertise in EBP are necessary (e.g., APNs). • Although unit-level leadership is important, all clinicians are responsible for EBP. • Engage key leaders early and often. • Provide short bulleted updates for key leaders.

APNs, Advanced practice nurses; *EBP*, evidence-based practice; *QI*, quality improvement.

BOX 12.2 **Action Plan**

EBP project purpose statement: The purpose of this EBP project is to implement EB fall prevention practices that target patient-specific fall risk factors and thereby decrease fall rates and severity of fall injuries in 3 adult medical units: 7C, 3W, and 4D. The EB fall prevention practices address mobility, elimination, cognition, medications, and reducing risk for fall injury.

Objective	Action Steps	Responsible Person	Completion Date	Progress
Educate clinicians about the EBP	Decide key educational content.	Jane Smith	June 2018	Completed
	Design educational methods.	Jane Smith		
	Develop educational materials.	Jane Smith		
	Schedule and deliver the education.	Gary Jones		
Develop EBP documents for the units	Select key elements needed at the point of care.	Suzy Jordan Name/group	June 2018	In progress
	Decide on use of QRGs, decision aids, clinical reminders.			
Integrate EBP content into organizational standards	Work with Standards Committee to update fall prevention standards.	Name/group Name/group	Date Date	
	Work with IT personnel to update electronic health record documentation.			
Decide on core outcome measures to evaluate over time	Meet with QI chair to determine available data.	Name/group Name/group	Date Date	
	Note outcomes used from reviewed studies.	EBP team	Date	
	Select outcome metrics.			

EB, Evidence-based; *EBP,* evidence-based practice; *IT,* information technology; *QI,* quality Improvement; *QRG,* quick reference guides. Developed January 15, 2018.

Although there is no one right way to implement a practice change, there are several common myths and realities regarding implementation that warrant consideration (Table 12.4). These are essential to address in planning for success.

ACTION PLANS

An **action plan** assists with EBP implementation. It is a written document developed collectively by the EBP team and other key stakeholders that promotes collective buy-in for the plan. The importance of an action plan is that it:

- provides a good idea of the overall scope of the work and course of action,
- makes the work more intentional,
- breaks the EBP process into actionable steps,
- fosters clear communication about who is responsible for what steps and projected dates of achievement,
- helps to prevent duplication of effort,
- makes it easier to stay focused and make midcourse corrections as needed,
- can be reviewed and updated as EBP processes move forward, and
- can serve as a timeline.

Key components of an action plan are the objectives, action steps, individual(s) responsible for each action item, due date for each item, and progress. The EBP purpose statement is documented in the action plan and used to develop the objectives. Action items are set forth to meet each objective (Box 12.2).

EBP TIP

Include dates in the action plan that show when it was developed and updated.

ETHICAL CONSIDERATIONS FOR EVIDENCE-BASED PRACTICE

Ethical issues are embedded in EBP processes and include:
- critical appraisal and synthesis of the evidence,
- development of EBP recommendations,
- shared decision making, and
- ensuring availability of resources.

Knowledge is ranked and classified in a hierarchical approach. The language of EBP traditionally has mirrored that of empiricism or use of findings from quantitative studies, with evidence from RCTs (Chapter 6) and meta-analyses (Chapter 8) regarded as the most reliable and valid. More recently, experts have argued that qualitative approaches may be more applicable for some health care practices (Rycroft-Malone et al., 2012). Most qualitative research is based on in-depth explorations with smaller, more purposefully selected samples and seeks to understand the meaning that patients and families place on how their problems and health care treatments are experienced (Chapter 9). Practice is complex, and qualitative approaches provide valuable insights for clinicians. In-depth qualitative studies call attention to health care processes that are valuable in helping clinicians deliver practices in real-world situations. Qualitative research findings can provide important insights that quantitative studies may not address. Although not generalizable in the traditional sense, in-depth, qualitative data are referred to in the qualitative literature as "metaphorically generalizable" and are essential for learning about the lived experiences of diverse populations of patients and families (Farley et al., 2009; Furman, 2009; Streubert & Carpenter, 2011). For example, a prospective study used qualitative methods to explore hospitalized older adults' perceptions about their fall risks while hospitalized and discharge instructions for prevention of falls at home. One study finding was that even when designated as a fall risk by clinicians, most patients said they did not believe they were at risk for falling in the hospital. One practice implication from this study is that clinicians should engage patients and family members in understanding why patients are at risk for falling and how they can collaborate with the health care team in preventing falls (Shuman et al., 2016). Thus, in critical appraisal, synthesis of evidence, and development of EBP recommendations, it is essential that we are transparent about (1) methods used to acquire the evidence, (2) types of evidence appraised and synthesized, and (3) inclusiveness of both qualitative and quantitative studies in making practice recommendations (IOM, 2011).

Scientific evidence is central to EBP and may overshadow other important values, such as patient autonomy and choice. If EBP becomes the most important factor in health care delivery, the focus on patient and family empowerment and autonomy may be at risk. For instance, research may show a specific medication or treatment to be most effective, but patients may wish to handle their problems in a manner more consistent with personal values, health beliefs, or strengths. Although EBP does not call for clinicians to ignore the wishes of patients and families, clinicians inadvertently may become overzealous in "pushing" certain interventions. In our zeal to be objective and informed, we may forget that clinical decision making at its core is a patient-centered, ethical matter. For example, patients who experience deep venous thrombosis (DVT) with no specific precipitating factor must decide after the first months of anticoagulant therapy whether to continue taking warfarin or other anticoagulants long term. Even though high-quality RCTs provide evidence that continuing treatment decreases the risk of DVT recurrence, the cost is increased risk of bleeding and inconveniences such as regular laboratory tests. Patients with varying values and preferences will make different choices about continuing treatment. This may affect work with vulnerable and underserved populations, leaving them to feel less empowered and able to participate in decision making (Farley et al., 2009; Furman, 2009). Shared decision making is an important component of EBP (see Chapter 15). We have an ethical obligation to share treatment choices with patients and families in a manner that they can understand and relate to their current situations.

It is incumbent upon organizations and agencies that use EBP to allocate sufficient resources for staff to fully implement all phases of the EBP process. If agencies and the professionals they employ choose to embrace an organizational culture that values EBP, then EBP, in its breadth and complexity, stands to be more fully embraced—especially with respect to elements that may require organizational realignment. By doing so, organizations are providing ethical responsiveness to patients, families, and the communities they serve.

One concern that rises with EBP is the question of IRB approval. EBP does not require IRB approval; it is a type of quality improvement with a definition and intent that differ from research (Table 12.5) (Fitzpatrick, 2016; Hedges, 2009; Hockenberry, 2014; Newhouse et al., 2006; Shirey et al., 2011). However, some organizations recommend submitting EBP projects to the IRB to ensure IRB review is not required. For example, the University of California-San Diego (UCSD) Human Research Protections Program (HRPP) has determined that many projects involving EBP and QI are not likely to meet the definition

TABLE 12.5	**Differentiating QI, EBP, and Conduct of Research**		
	QI	**EBP**	**Conduct of Research**
Definitions	A process by which individuals work together in a specified local setting to improve systems and processes of health care with the intent to improve health outcomes.	Conscientious and judicious use of current best evidence in conjunction with clinical expertise, patient values, and circumstances to guide health care decisions.	A systematic investigation, including research development, testing, and evaluation, designed to develop or contribute to generalizable knowledge.
Intent	Improve health care processes, quality, and safety in a local clinical setting.	Improve quality and safety within the local clinical setting by applying evidence in healthcare decisions.	Contribute to and/or generate new knowledge that can be generalized.
Approaches and Methods	Plan Do Check Act (PDCA) Plan Do Study Act (PDSA) LEAN Six Sigma Continuous Quality Improvement (CQI) Total Quality Management (TQM)	Multiple models for EBP Common steps: Topic selection Team formation Critical appraisal and evidence synthesis Implementation Evaluation: processes and outcomes	Scientific research designs and methods: Quantitative: RCTs, quasi-experimental, observational cohort Qualitative: ethnography, grounded theory, phenomenology
Sample	Convenience sample Size relatively small yet large enough to note change over time	Convenience sample Size relatively small yet large enough to note change over time	Sample varies based on research questions. Size is based on estimates of adequate power (power analysis) or saturation.
Data Analysis	Descriptive statistics, run charts, SPC charts	Descriptive statistics, run charts, SPC charts	Descriptive and inferential statistics to address study aims
Impact	Improved quality and safety in the local setting	Improved quality and safety in the local setting	Generalizable knowledge
Dissemination	In the local setting May publish in clinical or QI journals, but doing so does not indicate this is research.	Within the local setting May publish in clinical or QI journals, but doing so does not indicate this is research.	Expected to publish in peer-reviewed scientific journals and present peer-reviewed papers at scientific meetings.
IRB	Does not meet the definition of research; some organizations require that QI projects be submitted to the IRB to ensure IRB is not required. IRB review varies by organizational IRB expectations.	Does not meet the definition of research; some organizations require that EBP projects be submitted to the IRB to ensure IRB is not required. IRB review varies by organizational IRB expectations.	IRB review and approval are required. The IRB may rule the study is exempt depending on the nature of the study.

EBP, Evidence-based practice; *IRB,* institutional review board; *QI,* quality improvement.

BOX 12.3 Procedures for Submitting EBP and QI Projects to HRPP

University of California, San Diego Human Research Protections Program

Fact Sheet

EBP/QA/QI Projects

The UCSD Human Research Protections Program (HRPP) has determined that many projects involving evidence-based practice (EBP), quality assurance (QA), and quality improvement (QI) are not likely to meet the definition of "research" stated in the Department of Health and Human Services Regulations for the Protection of Human Subjects at 45 CFR Part 46, Subpart A, and would therefore be excluded from IRB review. However, such projects will require review and certification from the HRPP director that the project is not research and no IRB review is required.

These regulations define "research" as "a systematic investigation, including research development, testing and evaluation, designed to develop or contribute to generalizable knowledge."

The UCSD HRPP Standard Operating Policies and Procedures define generalizable knowledge as "activities designed (with intent) to collect information about some individuals to draw general conclusions about other individuals that are predictive of future events and that can be widely applied as expressed in theories, principles, and statements and that enhance scientific or academic understanding."

For a project to be certified as "not research," the following must be true:

1. Implementing the practice outlined in the project will not incur patient harm.

2. The practice change outlined in the project is not new or novel and has been published elsewhere.
3. The practice outlined in the project will be implemented in a project location.
4. All staff and affected patients in the project location will be expected to participate in the project.
5. The project is not testing issues or adding research questions that go beyond common practice.
6. The project will not randomize patients into different intervention groups.
7. The project will not deliberately delay interpretation of data.
8. The project will not deliberately delay or abbreviate feedback to those who would benefit from the findings to enhance likelihood of publication.
9. The project has no funding support from an outside organization with a commercial interest in the results.

To obtain certification, the following procedures must be done:

1. Complete the EBP/QA/QI Project: Standard Application for Review Facesheets (all questions in Section 3 must be answered "Yes").
2. Submit the Facesheets to the HRPP office online.
3. Once the HRPP project number has been obtained, upload the signed Facesheets and the Project Narrative using e-IRB services.
4. If the project is certified as "not research," certification will be e-mailed to the investigator.
5. If the project is determined to be research, a letter will be e-mailed to the investigator noting the determination and providing additional information regarding resubmitting the project for convened IRB or expedited review.

For questions about whether a project constitutes human subject research, please contact the director of the Human Research Protections Program.

Version date: 7/17/15

From the University of California, San Diego.

of "research" stated in the Department of Health and Human Services' Regulations for the Protection of Human Subjects at 45 CFR Part 46, Subpart A. They would therefore be excluded from IRB review. However, such projects require HRPP director review and certification that they are not research and no IRB review is required. Procedures and a form for submitting EBP and QI projects to HRPP are available

and easy to complete (see Box 12.3 and Fig. 12.5). Therefore check with the procedures in your setting to determine what may be expected regarding IRB review.

EBP TIP

Implementation is a process, not an event.

EBP/QA/QI Standard Facesheets
Page 1 of 1 – Complete in full

UCSD Human Research Protections Program
EBP/QA/QI Project: Standard Application for Review

Instructions for submitting

1. Complete this form. **To do this, open the form using your Web Browser** to fill in the form (requires Acrobat Reader or plug-in).

2. Click the **Print button** on below to make a copy for your signature.

3. Click the **Submit button** below to submit the data from the Facesheets to the HRPP Office via the Internet.

4. When you submit the Facesheets, the HRPP system will give you a Temporary Project ID (a "T-number"). Once your information has been imported into the HRPP database, usually within 1-2 working days, the project will receive a HRPP project number. You will then need to log into your "My Protocols at a Glance" through eIRB services. (You must register to create a user ID and password for using e-IRB services if you have not done so previously.) Click on the link for your "new" project and upload your Narrative.

5. Upload the signed Facesheets through eIRB services. If it cannot be uploaded, mail a copy of the signed Facesheets to the HRPP Office.

Section 1: PROJECT TITLE

Section 2: INVESTIGATOR/PROJECT LEADER

Investigator/ Project Leader	Last name		First name		Degree	
	Title		Department		Mail code	
	E-mail		Phone		Fax	
	Investigator is a **nurse affiliated with** UCSD		RCHSD		Investigator is **not a nurse**	

Section 3: DOES PROJECT REQUIRE IRB REVIEW?

Yes	No	
		Requesting review of **EBP/QA/QI** project *(If No, do not use this form)*
		Implementing the practice outlined in the project **will not incur patient harm** *(If No, requires IRB review)*
		The practice change outlined in the project is **not new or novel** and **has been published elsewhere** *(If No, requires IRB review)*
		The practice outlined in the project will be **implemented in a practice location** *(If No, requires IRB review)*
		All staff and affected patients in the project location will be **expected to participate** in the project *(If No, requires IRB review)*
		The project is **not testing issues or adding research questions that go beyond common** practice *(If No, requires IRB review)*
		The project will **not randomize patients** into different intervention groups *(If No, requires IRB review)*
		The project will **not deliberately delay interpretation of data** *(If No, requires IRB review)*
		The project will **not deliberately delay or abbreviate feedback** to those who would benefit from the findings to enhance likelihood of publication *(If No, requires IRB review)*
		The project has **no funding support from an outside organization with a commercial interest in the use of the results** *(If No, requires IRB review)*

By signing below, you certify that the information provided about these activities is accurate to the best of your knowledge, and that you agree to conduct the project in compliance with state and federal regulations.

Section 4: SIGNATURE

| Investigator/ Project Leader | | Date | |

Fig. 12.5 Example of a form to submit evidence-based practice and quality improvement projects to an institutional Human Subjects Protection Program or Institutional Review Board. (From the University of California, San Diego.)

SYNTHESIS

Now that you have been introduced to the principles and considerations of implementation, you and your team will need to plan for implementation. Remember that implementation is a dynamic, iterative process that takes time and commitment from you and your team.

All EBP work is important, but implementation is critical for people, patients, and health care systems to benefit from the work you have invested in setting forth EBP recommendations to improve quality of care and health outcomes. What will you and your team do to plan for success and realize the benefits of promoting EBPs in your setting?

KEY POINTS

- Successful implementation is influenced by the EBP topic.
- Five attributes of the EBP topic influence implementation of the EBP: relative advantage, compatibility, complexity, trialability, and observability.
- Planning for implementation requires that all team members participate in some component of the process.
- Implementation planning necessitates selecting (1) quality metrics and data sources to evaluate the impact of implementing the EBPs, (2) methods for display of quality metrics, and (3) methods for communicating the quality metrics to staff over time.
- Implementation is a dynamic, iterative process.

- Time for implementation varies depending on the nature and complexity of the innovation or EBP.
- Complex EBP topics require a longer time period for implementation compared with simpler topics.
- Principles of organizational functioning are important considerations when implementing EBPs.
- Key components of an implementation action plan are the objectives, action steps, individual(s) responsible for each action item, due date for each action item, and progress.
- EBP is a type of quality improvement with a definition and intent that differ from research and that does not require IRB approval.
- Some organizations require submission of EBP projects to the IRB to ensure IRB review is not required.

REFERENCES

Farley, A. J., Feaster, D., Schapmire, T. J., D'Ambrosio, J. G., Bruce, L. E., Oak, C. S., et al. (2009). The challenges of implementing evidence-based practice: Ethical considerations in practice, education, policy, and research. *Social Work and Society International Online Journal*, 7(2), 246–259.

Fitzpatrick, J. (2016). Distinctions between research, evidence-based practice, and quality improvement. *Applied Nursing Research*, 29, 261.

Furman, R. (2009). Ethical considerations of evidence-based practice. *Social Work*, 54(1), 82–84.

Hedges, C. C. (2009). Putting it all together: QI, EBP, and research. *Nursing Management*, 40(4), 10–12.

Hockenberry, M. (2014). Quality improvement and evidence-based practice change projects and the Institutional Review Board: Is approval necessary? *Worldviews on Evidence-Based Nursing*, 11(4), 217–218.

Institute of Medicine. (2011). *Clinical practice guidelines we can trust*. Washington, D.C: The National Academies Press.

Newhouse, R. P., Pettit, J. C., Poe, S., & Rocco, L. (2006). The slippery slope: Differentiating between quality improvement and research. *Journal of Nursing Administration*, 36(4), 211–219.

Rogers, E. M. (2003). *Diffusion of innovations*. New York, NY: The Free Press.

Rycroft-Malone, J., McCormack, B., Hutchinson, A., DeCorby, K., Bucknall, T., Kent, B., et al. (2012). Realist synthesis: Illustrating the method for implementation research. *Implementation Science*, 7, 1–10.

Shirey, M., Hauck, S. L., Embree, J. L., Kinner, T. J., Schaar, G. L., Phillips, L. A., et al. (2011). Showcasing differences between quality improvement, evidence-based practice, and research. *Journal of Continuing Education in Nursing*, 42(2), 57–68.

Shuman, C. J., Liu, J., Montie, M., Galinato, J. G., Todd, M. A., Hegstad, M., et al. (2016). Patient perception and experiences with falls during hospitalization and after discharge. *Applied Nursing Research*, 31, 79–85.

Streubert, H. J., & Carpenter, D. R. (2011). *Qualitative nursing research: Advancing the humanistic imperative*. Philadelphia, PA: Wolters Klower Health.

Titler, M. G. (2010). Translation science and context. *Research Theory Nursing Practice*, 24(1), 35–55.

Titler, M. G., Conlon, P., Reynolds, M. A., Ripley, R., Tsodikov, A., Wilson, D. S., et al. (2016). The effect of a translating research into practice intervention to promote use of evidence-based fall prevention interventions in hospitalized adults: a prospective pre-post implementation study in the U.S. *Applied Nursing Research*, 31, 52–59.

13

Launching Implementation

Christine Anderson, Marita Titler

LEARNING OUTCOMES

After reading this chapter, you should be able to do the following:

- Describe the translation research model as a guide for implementation.
- Compare and contrast implementation strategies that address the characteristics of the clinical topic and practices to be implemented.

- Compare and contrast implementation strategies that address communication.
- Describe strategies to address sustainability of evidence-based practices.

KEY TERMS

Change champion
Clinical decision support
Diffusion of Innovation

Extent of adoption
Heterophily
Homophily

Opinion leader
Quick reference guides
Rate of adoption

INTRODUCTION

Chapter 12 presented an overview of the *Translating Research into Practice* (TRIP) model (see Fig. 12.1). The components of the model include characteristics, communication process, social system, users, and adoption of the innovation. Communication processes are central connectors among all individual components.

The influence of Rogers's (2003) Diffusion of Innovation (DOI) on the development of the TRIP model also was explained. DOI is a broad framework explaining the adoption of many types of innovations by various groups or populations. TRIP is the application of the broad framework of DOI to the more focused translation of innovative evidence-based practices (EBPs) in health care (Titler & Everett, 2001). The users of EBPs, such as nurses and physicians, are members of social systems in health care organizations of diverse types. Adoption of

EBPs occurs at the individual, unit, and organizational levels. Throughout the stages of adoption defined by Rogers (knowledge, persuasion, decision, implementation, and confirmation), interventions designed to improve the adoption of the EBP and overcome barriers to implementation address the attributes of the EBP topic and communication (see Tables 12.1 and 12.2). The influence of Rogers is observed particularly in that communication is critical for successful implementation in all phases of the process (Rogers, 2003). Likewise, the TRIP model stresses the importance of communication during the implementation stage of an EBP project to sustain the practice change. The focus of this chapter is exploring how implementation strategies that address attributes of the EBP clinical topic and communication affect adoption.

Just as research evidence is used to develop various clinical guidelines, the field of translation science is concerned with research focused on the development and testing of interventions or implementation strategies that affect the rate and extent of EBP adoption. The rate of adoption refers to the speed at which users begin to use the new EBPs. The extent of adoption means the number of users of the EBP after the implementation, compared with before the project (Titler & Everett, 2001). In the last 10 years, the number and quality of research studies on the effectiveness of implementation strategies have grown substantially (Foy et al., 2015). Because of this evidence, leaders involved in clinical EBP projects can apply these findings and increase the likelihood of successful implementation. This chapter focuses on implementation strategies to address the characteristics of the EBP clinical topic and communication. Implementation strategies to address users of the EBP and the social system are presented in Chapter 14.

> **IPE TIP**
>
> Effective communication strategies by interprofessional team members, using targeted messages for specific stakeholder groups at the individual, unit, and organization levels, maximize adoption of an EBP.

IMPLEMENTATION STRATEGIES THAT ADDRESS CHARACTERISTICS OF THE CLINICAL TOPIC

The attributes of the proposed practice change are important considerations leading up to the decision to implement new EBPs. The focus of the TRIP model is implementation in the context of a social system, often an organization. In an organization, the adoption decision may be optional, collective, or authority-driven. (The social system and users of the innovation are further developed in Chapter 14.) Once the decision has been made to adopt a new practice, the characteristics of the EB clinical topic (e.g., complexity) influence adoption, and several implementation strategies are described in the following section to address these characteristics:

- Quick reference guides
- Clinical decision support
- Key messages at the point of care delivery

Quick reference guides. Quick reference guides give targeted, concise information designed to help practitioners perform specific tasks. A variety of quick reference guide formats are helpful, depending on their intended use. For example, laminated checklist cards for

clinicians help ensure that all components of an EBP are addressed. Wallet cards are another example for use by individuals. They can be used to address a number of characteristics of the EBP topic. For example, staff nurses may have some awareness of new evidence but lack knowledge about the relative advantage of a specific practice, or they may be uncertain about the mechanism of action. If the new EBP is complex, quick reference guides can be used to reduce this problem, which often contributes to slow adoption. Quick reference guides are useful when the change is seldom used; for example, if it involves new equipment specific to a certain condition.

The characteristics of good reference guides include clarity, accuracy, and accessibility. Careful editing is needed to distill the necessary information for clinicians. Good reference guides may include tables or graphics and text. For example, one side of the guide may include a table of critical laboratory values, the other an algorithm for EBP treatments. When you are developing these guides, it may be useful to consult with a graphic specialist to ensure proper fonts and that tables, diagrams, and logos are well-placed and easy to read (Grudniewicz, Bhattacharyya, McKibbon, & Straus, 2015; Versloot et al., 2015)

In addition to design considerations, it is also essential that quick reference guides be visible and available at the point of care. The aim is to offer easily accessible information as a supplement to longer policies or references. For example, if the quick reference guide is about medication management, it may be printed on brightly colored paper, laminated, and found in the medication room. Time spent on development and use of special paper, graphics, and lamination may contribute to the cost of quick reference guides, but they are also easy to test during an implementation pilot.

Clinical decision support tools. The use of clinical decision support tools by clinicians and patients is rapidly increasing. Frequently they are used to reduce the complexity of the EBP by offering a visual representation of the processes involved, or to illustrate the compatibility of new practices in the users' context. For example, a clinical decision support tool often is designed in the form of an algorithm that can help illustrate the compatibility of a new practice in the context of the organization, if it is designed with the current clinician workflow in mind. The relative advantage of the practice may be clarified by showing how the EBP reduces uncertainty about clinical decisions. It is important that decision support tools do not add complexity or confusion to an EBP. There are many well-developed clinical decision support tools, tested and available for use, often via toolkits, which is an advantage for organizations planning to implement EBPs.

Good decision support tools are like quick reference guides in that they must be clear, accurate, and to the point. Well-designed aids tested by research are available to clinicians when they are interacting with patients. Decision support tools provide information about evidence supporting the practice and the pros and cons of various options. The clinician may use the tools to confirm his or her own recommendations, influence patients, or converse with them about their preferences and values (Wyatt et al., 2014). Whether used for shared decision making or as a guide to EP treatment algorithms, decision aids should be user-friendly, accessible, and designed to overcome concerns or stress about the perceived time needed for the clinician to effectively use the tool. In the ambulatory setting, pressure associated with appointment lengths must be understood. Likewise, using decision aids in critical care events can reduce errors caused by stress or loss of memory and can overcome team communication problems (Wen & Howard, 2014).

Clinical decision support is a core function of electronic health records (Institute of Medicine, 2003). A variety of tools can be imbedded in the EHR, including alerts, reminders, orders, care plans, and electronic surveillance systems (Lytle, Short, Richesson, & Horvath, 2015; Manaktala & Claypool, 2017). Empirical support for the effectiveness of clinical decision support embedded in electronic health records is mixed (Institute of Medicine, 2011) and research involving nurses and patient outcomes is limited. Electronic clinical decision support has small to modest effects on clinician behavior and appears to be more effective than alerts alone when included as a component of multifaceted implementation strategies (Arditi, Rege-Walther, Wyatt, Durieux, & Burnand, 2012; Kahn et al., 2013).

Two examples from the American Heart Association illustrate diverse types of clinical decision support use. First, the ASCVD risk calculator for cardiovascular disease was developed through multiple research studies related to predicting disease. Based on research evidence, guidelines were developed and the calculator tool was devised. The risk calculator is freely available online for use by clinicians and the public. Based on input parameters, including age and comorbidities such as hypertension

or diabetes, the tool can be used to help patients understand their risk for cardiovascular disease and various options that may reduce that risk. The risk calculator can be embedded in the EHR and is easily accessible at the point of care (American Heart Association, 2017).

On the other hand, guidelines for Advanced Cardiac Life Support (ACLS) include well-designed algorithms used as decision tools in cardiac arrest situations or for treatment of arrhythmias. In these cases, it is helpful if providers can practice using them in simulated experiences ahead of time to avoid treatment delays, for example, when trying to access the tools via cellphone apps (American Heart Association, 2015). Piloting the usefulness of clinical decision support tools is an effective way for organizations to overcome this type of problem. Guidelines, algorithms, and training materials are available online at www.cpr.heart.org.

Key EBP messages at the point-of-care delivery. There are a multitude of ways in which key messages or reminders about an EBP can be delivered at the point of care. Some examples include signs, posters, and infographics. In some cases, they may be built into worksheets used by staff throughout the day. Others can be incorporated into patient education materials. Key messages are useful for reducing complexity. It is not always possible, but distilling the essence of the EBP to a few key points on signs or posters can be very effective when designed correctly. Using posters or infographics to highlight visual displays of progress in process or outcome measures explicitly addresses the relative advantage of the new practice. Selection of key message tools to ease adoption includes consideration of the knowledge of end users, the context in which the tools will be used, and their design and usability. Recently, a form of key message known as the "visual abstract" has been used to disseminate research studies and also may be effective for sharing results of practice changes on patient care units or on organizational websites (Ibrahim, Lillemoe, Klingensmith, & Dimick, 2017). Open source tutorials are available for guidance in developing these tools. For examples, see https://www.surgeryredesign.com/resources/ (Ibrahim, 2017).

EBP TIP

Be creative when designing reference guides and key messages. Consult with colleagues in marketing or graphic design departments to improve usability of these tools.

In summary, EB implementation strategies that address various attributes of the specific EBP being implemented are effective in speeding the rate and extent of adoption. Selection of these implementation strategies to facilitate adoption includes consideration of the users (clinicians) and practice context of the organization.

IMPLEMENTATION STRATEGIES THAT ADDRESS COMMUNICATION

In this section, the focus is on communication strategies to enhance the rate and extent of EBP adoption. The following implementation strategies are discussed in this section:

- Mass media
- Opinion leaders
- Change champions
- Education of clinicians
- Educational outreach (academic detailing)

According to Rogers (2003, p. 5), communication is defined as "a process in which participants create and share information with one another to reach a mutual understanding." Information moves via "channels," including mass media, interpersonal (usually face-to-face), and interactive communication routes such as the Internet and social media. The channels are connectors among the people involved in the project. The transfer of ideas occurs most often among people who are similar or homophilous. Heterophily means the opposite; the individuals have different attributes (e.g., professional groups, education, practice specialties). These concepts are important for implementation because although it is easier to communicate with similar people, unless there is some degree of difference, obtaining current information about innovations is unlikely (Rogers, 2003). The use of various communication channels throughout an implementation project depends on the implementation stage and desired outcomes.

Mass media. Before we get to specifics about interpersonal and interactive communication, it is important to discuss the role of mass media in implementing EBP. The primary outlets of mass media are television, radio, print, and Internet sources. News and information are delivered in a directional message from one to many. The recent and rapid growth of social media platforms such as Facebook and Twitter has led to the increasing use of interactive mass media, where the communication channels are bidirectional but lack the closeness of an interpersonal or face-to-face exchange (Rogers, 2003). Researchers, professional organizations, and government agencies are among the many groups using mass media to send informational messages to stakeholder groups and the public at large. The amount of information available through mass media is staggering and can cause individuals to feel bombarded and to withdraw from media consumption. On the other hand, Rogers (2003) and other diffusion researchers suggest that some individuals are particularly adept at translating knowledge gleaned from mass media into useful practices worthy of adopting to solve problems or make improvements in structures or processes. Often, such individuals are among the first to know about innovations such as new EBP guidelines through their attendance at conferences or by reading journals or following experts on Twitter, for example. People in this category are known as early adopters. They can be both the target of mass media campaigns and active seekers of the latest information.

Opinion leaders. When early adopters are regarded by their peers as credible sources of information, they may have a great deal of influence on the adoption of EBPs. Several attributes contribute to the development of these individuals as opinion leaders. The definition of opinion leadership, according to Rogers (2003), is "the degree to which an individual is able informally to influence other individuals' attitudes or overt behavior in a desired way with relative frequency" (p. 300). Opinion leaders tend to have greater exposure to mass media and bring innovative ideas from the media and other groups to their own social networks (Burt, 1999). They are widely connected with other individuals and groups, and are accessible to their followers, who are usually members of their own peer groups. Opinion leader influence is a balance between being too innovative or heterogeneous and keeping the homophily within the group that leads to credibility and trust in their judgment and evaluation of new clinical practices. Opinion leaders are visible and important for communicating via interpersonal networks that EBP innovations are compatible with community norms. Because of their visibility, opinion leaders also influence adoption by addressing the observability of new EBPs (Rogers, 2003).

The identification and use of opinion leader strategies to influence the speed of adoption of various innovations has been the topic of research for many decades, not only in health care but in sociology, politics, and marketing, to name just a few (Granovetter, 1973; King & Summers, 1970; Rogers & Cartono, 1962). Four methods are useful in identifying opinion leaders. First, the sociometric method involves asking respondents to name people they would go to for advice if they were uncertain about an innovation such as a new EBP. This works best with a high response rate because there are usually few opinion leaders in a group or context. This method has the advantage of obtaining the viewpoint of the followers. A second method for finding opinion leaders is by using key informants or individuals who are knowledgeable about the local context; for example, unit managers, or educators. In the self-designating method, individuals identify themselves as being influential or sources of information for their peers. Finally, the observation method involves collection of observed communication behavior. Although valid, this method is best when employed in small systems and is rarely used because the other methods are similar in validity and more convenient (Rogers, 2003). It is important to be aware that opinion leaders often are identified as such based on their specific knowledge domains and expertise. Because opinion leaders emerge in a changing local context, it is possible that their ability to influence others may change over time (Doumit, Wright, Graham, Smith, & Grimshaw, 2011).

Opinion leader influence is primarily achieved via word of mouth and interpersonal communication through extensive personal networks (Thompson, Estabrooks, & Degner, 2006; Valente, 1996; Valente & Davis, 1999). Recruiting opinion leaders for specific implementation projects should include knowledge about their expertise on a given topic and the extent to which they favor a given practice change. Obtaining opinion leaders' buy-in is essential; they must be willing to take part in the project. Opinion leaders often influence their peers by being role models for new practices, visibly demonstrating compatibility of the EBP with local norms. Opportunities for interpersonal communication between opinion leaders and their peers can take many forms, including several of the education strategies discussed in the following section.

Change champions. The term champion is often used interchangeably with opinion leader, but there are conceptual differences. According to Thompson et al. (2006), there also are several similarities. These include

the fact that they are both individual, informal social influence roles that are internal to an organization or system and rely upon ongoing relationships. Neither opinion leaders nor champions need to be specifically trained or chosen for the role; they may instead emerge within a context based on the needs of the local organization. Opinion leaders evaluate new practices and are influential based on their expertise relative to their domains, such as a patient care unit or specialty practice. Their innovativeness may be slightly greater than that of their peers, but it still is within boundaries relative to the group. Champions, however, actively advocate for practice change. Their influence is based on persuasion within their personal and organizational networks and is often project-specific (Thompson et al., 2006).

Similarly, Rogers (2003) contends that the role of a champion in organizational change is like that of the opinion leader except that the opinion leader is more effective in less complex or optional adoption situations. Although organizations may allow some degree of individual innovation decisions, often such choices are collective or authority-driven. His definition of a champion is "a charismatic individual who throws his or her weight behind an innovation, thus overcoming indifference or resistance that the new idea may provoke in an organization" (p. 414). Champions can come from all levels of an organization. Important qualities include being in key linking positions (for example, middle managers); understanding the various interests of stakeholders; and finally, having interpersonal communication and negotiation skills. Change champions often have a role in organizing and brokering change because of their advocacy and personal network relationships (Rogers, 2003).

Ploeg et al. (2010) studied the role of nursing practice champions in the diffusion of guidelines. The purpose of the study was to learn what strategies were used by champions (nursing staff, educators, administrators) in a variety of practice settings. The researchers found that the three main approaches were dissemination of information, persuasive practice leadership, and tailoring implementation strategies to the organizational context. Among the activities associated with these strategies were the offering of education and mentoring, committee and interdisciplinary teamwork and leadership, auditing and monitoring best practices, and making changes in organizational documentation to incorporate the best practice recommendations (Ploeg et al., 2010).

Education. Education of clinicians about the EBPs is necessary but not sufficient to change practice, and didactic continuing education alone does little to change practice behaviors (Flodgren et al., 2013; Forsetlund et al., 2009; Giguere et al., 2012). It is essential, however, that clinicians delivering the EBPs have the knowledge and skills, including the evidence base regarding the EBPs to be implemented. In some cases, if the change is not overly complex and fits the current workflow well, a mass media-style announcement, lecture, or self-study module may be appropriate as an educational approach. For larger projects involving meaningful change, it is more likely that a formal gap analysis or audit of current practice should be conducted to address the knowledge and skills required to understand the evidence, overcome barriers, and perform the required practice. Opinion leaders and champions may need to devise individual or committee education as a means of obtaining buy-in from organizational leadership, not only for the implementation decision, but also so that adequate resources are included in the planning and execution of the change. Involving stakeholders, including potential opinion leaders and champions, in educational material development, resources, and point-of-care tools may be initially costly but will pay off later as part of a "train the trainer" approach, where early learners can go on to teach others in classroom settings or in the practice area. Individual mentoring and coaching are useful educational strategies in ongoing development of staff skills. Many of the interventions that address the characteristics of the innovation, mentioned previously, are useful adjuncts for learning in addition to printed materials, training videos, and slide presentations (Gagliardi, Marshall, Huckson, James, & Moore, 2015). The Centers for Disease Control and Prevention (CDC) developed multiple bundled strategies in the form of "toolkits" that enable implementation of their evidence-based guidelines. One comprehensive example is the CDC Guideline for Prescribing Opioids for Chronic Pain (Dowell, Haegerich, & Chou, 2016). The agency used mass and social media to announce the release of the guideline. A website devoted to promoting the adoption of the guidelines includes a wide variety of tip sheets, key messaging materials, infographics, pocket guides, and mobile apps, along with training materials such as slide presentations and videos (CDC, 2017).

> ### EBP TIP
>
> Explore government agency and professional organization websites for comprehensive toolkits that provide bundled resources useful for strategies addressing the characteristics of clinical topics as well as communication strategies.

Educational outreach/academic detailing. Multiple studies have demonstrated the effectiveness of educational outreach, also known as academic detailing, in improving the practice behaviors of clinicians (Avorn, 2010; Institute of Medicine, 2011; Wilson et al., 2016). Educational outreach involves interactive face-to-face education of individual practitioners in their practice settings by an individual (usually a clinician) with expertise in a particular topic (e.g., cancer pain management). Academic detailers can explain the research foundations of the EBP recommendations and respond convincingly to specific questions, concerns, or challenges that a practitioner might raise. An academic detailer also might deliver feedback on provider or team performance with respect to a selected EBP recommendation (e.g., frequency of pain assessment). In planning for implementation, you should identify the individual who will perform the educational outreach and the frequency with which this will be done. For example, with implementation of patient-specific fall prevention practices, an expert on fall prevention rounded every five to six weeks on each of the patient care units that were implementing this practice. Rounding was done in conjunction with the opinion leaders and change champions to identify areas of improvement and address questions and issues they encountered while implementing the EBPs (Titler et al., 2016; Wilson et al., 2016).

In summary, traditional mass media communication, interactive media, and interpersonal communication are all extremely important when implementing EBPs. Opinion leaders and champions facilitate the translation of new ideas to members of their peer groups and organizational leaders through their social network connections, enthusiasm, expertise, and credibility. Once the implementation decision is made, individuals in these roles encourage and support the engagement of key stakeholders, including staff, organizational leadership, and interdisciplinary practice partners. As credible experts, opinion leaders and champions are important resources in developing educational materials, modeling new EBPs, and providing effective feedback to peers.

SUSTAINABILITY

Guided by the TRIP model, implementation planners should consider sustainability of the EBP from the very beginning of the project. Building the evidence base for sustainability is currently a high priority for implementation scientists (Chambers, Glasgow, & Stange, 2013; Moore, Mascarenhas, Bain, & Straus, 2017; Proctor et al., 2015; Wiltsey Stirman et al., 2012). In a recent review, Moore and colleagues (2017) arrived at a "definition of sustainability that includes five constructs: (1) after a defined period of time, (2) the program, clinical intervention, and/or implementation strategies continue to be delivered and/or (3) individual behavior change (i.e., clinician, patient) is maintained; (4) the program and individual behavior change may evolve or adapt while (5) continuing to produce benefits for individuals/

systems" (p. 7). Among the potential influences on sustainability are the innovation characteristics, context, capacity, and processes such as education and integration with organizational governance structures (Wiltsey Stirman et al., 2012).

SYNTHESIS

Remember that when planning your EBP implementation project, it is important to consider the characteristics of the clinical topic so you can select effective strategies that align with your goals. Is the new practice a minor adjustment to a clinical guideline? If so, your plan may include an email announcement and a new point of care message in an EHR. On the other hand, if the EBP change is complex, or potentially controversial, involving influential clinicians who can function as opinion leaders or change champions may contribute greatly to the success of implementing and sustaining EBP.

KEY POINTS

- The implementation phase of EBP projects is difficult. Translation Science and the Diffusion of Innovations model aid in designing and implementing projects that have an increased likelihood of sustainability.
- The characteristic of an innovation accounts for up to 87% of the variance in the rate of adoption and is therefore most important in ensuring successful implementation.

- Quick reference guides, clinical decision support tools, and key messaging are strategies that address the characteristics of the EBP.
- Interpersonal communication strategies require additional resources but are unquestionably more effective than the use of mass media.
- Opinion leaders and change champions help translate EBPs into the local context through advocacy, persuasion, and extensive personal relationship networks.

REFERENCES

American Heart Association. (2015). American Heart Association Guidelines for Cardiopulmonary Resuscitation and Emergency Cardiovascular Care: Part 7, Adult Advanced Cardiac Life Support. Retrieved from https://eccguide-lines.heart.org/index.php/circulation/cpr-ecc-guide-lines-2/part-7-adult-advanced-cardiovascular-life-support/.

American Heart Association. (2017). ASCVD Risk Calculator. Retrieved from http://static.heart.org/riskcalc/app/index.html#!/baseline-risk.

Arditi, C., Rege-Walther, M., Wyatt, J. C., Durieux, P., & Burnand, B. (2012). Computer-generated reminders delivered

on paper to healthcare professionals; effects on professional practice and health care outcomes. *Cochrane Database of Systematic Reviews*, 12, CD001175.

Avorn, J. (2010). Transforming trial results into practice change: The final translational hurdle: comment on impact of the allhat/jnc7 dissemination project on thiazide-type diuretic use. *Archives of Internal Medicine*, 170(10), 858–860.

Burt, R. S. (1999). The social capital of opinion leaders. *Annals of the American Academy of Political and Social Science*, 566, 37–54.

CDC. (2017). CDC Guideline for Prescribing Opioids for Chronic Pain. Retrieved from https://www.cdc.gov/drugoverdose/prescribing/guideline.html.

Chambers, D. A., Glasgow, R. E., & Stange, K. C. (2013). The dynamic sustainability framework: addressing the paradox of sustainment amid ongoing change. *Implementation Science, 8,* 117.

Doumit, G., Wright, F. C., Graham, I. D., Smith, A., & Grimshaw, J. (2011). Opinion leaders and changes over time: a survey. *Implementation Science, 6,* 117.

Dowell, D., Haegerich, T. M., & Chou, R. (2016). CDC Guideline for Prescribing Opioids for Chronic Pain - United States, 2016. *MMWR Recommendations and Reports, 65*(1), 1–49.

Flodgren, G., Conterno, L. O., Mayhew, A., Omar, O., Pereira, C. R., & Shepperd, S. (2013). Interventions to improve professional adherence to guidelines for prevention of device-related infections. *Cochrane Database of Systematic Reviews* (3), CD006559.

Forsetlund, L., Bjorndal, A., Rashidian, A., Jamtvedt, G., O'Brien, M. A., Wolf, F., et al. (2009). Continuing education meetings and workshops: effects on professional practice and health care outcomes. *Cochrane Database of Systematic Reviews* (2), CD003030.

Foy, R., Sales, A., Wensing, M., Aarons, G. A., Flottorp, S., Kent, B., et al. (2015). Implementation science: a reappraisal of our journal mission and scope. *Implementation Science, 10,* 51.

Gagliardi, A. R., Marshall, C., Huckson, S., James, R., & Moore, V. (2015). Developing a checklist for guideline implementation planning: review and synthesis of guideline development and implementation advice. *Implementation Science, 10*(1), 19.

Giguere, A., Legare, F., Grimshaw, J., Turcotte, S., Fiander, M., Grudniewicz, A., et al. (2012). Printed educational materials: effects on professional practice and healthcare outcomes. *Cochrane Database of Systematic Reviews, 10,* Cd004398.

Granovetter, M. S. (1973). The Strength of weak ties. *American Journal of Sociology, 78*(6), 1360–1380.

Grudniewicz, A., Bhattacharyya, O., McKibbon, K. A., & Straus, S. E. (2015). Redesigning printed educational materials for primary care physicians: design improvements increase usability. *Implementation Science, 10,* 156.

Ibrahim, A. M. (2017). Visual Abstract Open Source Primer. Retrieved from https://www.surgeryredesign.com/.

Ibrahim, A. M., Lillemoe, K. D., Klingensmith, M. E., & Dimick, J. B. (2017). Visual abstracts to disseminate research on social media: A prospective, case-control crossover study. *Annals of Surgery, 266*(6), e46–e48.

Institute of Medicine. (2003). *Key Capabilities of an Electronic Health Record System: Letter Report.* Washington, DC: National Academies Press.

Institute of Medicine. (2011). *Clinical Practice Guidelines We Can Trust.* Washington, DC: National Academies Press. Retrieved from https://www.nap.edu/catalog/13058/clinical-practice-guidelines-we-can-trust.

Kahn, S. R., Morrison, D. R., Cohen, J. M., Emed, J., Tagalakis, V., Roussin, A., et al. (2013). Interventions for implementation of thromboprophylaxis in hospitalized medical and surgical patients at risk for venous thromboembolism. *Cochrane Database of Systematic Reviews* (7), CD008201.

King, C. W., & Summers, J. O. (1970). Overlap of opinion leadership across consumer product categories. *Journal of Marketing Research, 7*(1), 43–50.

Lytle, K. S., Short, N. M., Richesson, R. L., & Horvath, M. M. (2015). Clinical decision support for nurses: A fall risk and prevention example. *CIN: Computers, Informatics,. Nursing, 33*(12), 530–537 quiz E531.

Manaktala, S., & Claypool, S. R. (2017). Evaluating the impact of a computerized surveillance algorithm and decision support system on sepsis mortality. *Journal of the American Medical Informatics Association, 24*(1), 88–95.

Moore, J. E., Mascarenhas, A., Bain, J., & Straus, S. E. (2017). Developing a comprehensive definition of sustainability. *Implement Science, 12*(1), 110.

Ploeg, J., Skelly, J., Rowan, M., Edwards, N., Davies, B., Grinspun, D., et al. (2010). The role of nursing best practice champions in diffusing practice guidelines: A mixed methods study. *Worldviews on Evidence-Based Nursing, 7*(4), 238–251.

Proctor, E., Luke, D., Calhoun, A., McMillen, C., Brownson, R., McCrary, S., & Padek, M. (2015). Sustainability of evidence-based healthcare: research agenda, methodological advances, and infrastructure support. *Implementation Science, 10*(1), 88.

Rogers, E. M. (2003). *Diffusion of innovations* (5th ed.). New York: Free Press.

Rogers, E. M., & Cartono, D. G. (1962). Methods of measuring opinion leadership. *Public Opinion Quarterly, 26*(3), 435–441.

Thompson, G. N., Estabrooks, C. A., & Degner, L. F. (2006). Clarifying the concepts in knowledge transfer: a literature review. *Journal of Advanced Nursing, 53*(6), 691–701.

Titler, M. G., Conlon, P., Reynolds, M. A., Ripley, R., Tsodikov, A., Wilson, D. S., & Montie, M. (2016). The effect of a translating research into practice intervention to promote use of evidence-based fall prevention interventions in hospitalized adults: A prospective pre-post implementation study in the U.S. *Applied Nursing Research, 31,* 52–59.

Titler, M. G., & Everett, L. Q. (2001). Translating research into practice. Considerations for critical care investigators. *Critical Care Nursing Clinics of North America, 13*(4), 587–604.

Valente, T. W. (1996). Social network thresholds in the diffusion of innovations. *Social Networks, 18*(1), 69–89.

Valente, T. W., & Davis, R. L. (1999). Accelerating the diffusion of innovations using opinion leaders. *Annals of the American Academy of Political and Social Science, 566,* 55–67.

Versloot, J., Grudniewicz, A., Chatterjee, A., Hayden, L., Kastner, M., & Bhattacharyya, O. (2015). Format guidelines to make them vivid, intuitive, and visual: use simple formatting rules to optimize usability and accessibility of clinical practice guidelines. *International Journal of Evidence-Based Healthcare*, *13*(2), 52–57.

Wen, L. Y., & Howard, S. K. (2014). Value of expert systems, quick reference guides and other cognitive aids. *Current Opinion in Anaesthesiology*, *27*(6), 643–648.

Wilson, D. S., Montie, M., Conlon, P., Reynolds, M., Ripley, R., & Titler, M. G. (2016). Nurses' Perceptions of Implementing Fall Prevention Interventions to Mitigate Patient-Specific Fall Risk Factors. *Western Journal of Nursing Research*, *38*(8), 1012–1034.

Wiltsey Stirman, S., Kimberly, J., Cook, N., Calloway, A., Castro, F., & Charns, M. (2012). The sustainability of new programs and innovations: a review of the empirical literature and recommendations for future research. *Implementation Science*, *7*, 17.

Wyatt, K. D., Branda, M. E., Anderson, R. T., Pencille, L. J., Montori, V. M., Hess, E. P., et al. (2014). Peering into the black box: a meta-analysis of how clinicians use decision aids during clinical encounters. *Implementation Science*, *9*, 26.

Implementation Strategies for Stakeholders

Marita Titler, Christine Anderson

LEARNING OUTCOMES

After reading this chapter, you should be able to do the following:

- Apply performance gap assessment, audit, and feedback as implementation strategies.
- Develop action steps for piloting evidence-based practice (EBP).
- Describe the use of meetings as an implementation strategy.
- Analyze the influence of the practice context on implementation of EBPs.
- Analyze the role of leaders in EBP implementation.

- Describe the purposes of conducting an environmental scan as an implementation strategy.
- Apply tools to assess various components of the practice context.
- Prioritize essential elements of meetings with key leadership stakeholders.
- Describe the importance of revisions in standards of practice and documentation systems as part of implementation.
- Identify examples of recognitions and rewards for EBP implementation and their importance.

KEY TERMS

Audit and feedback
Climate for evidence-based
  practice implementation
Context
Environmental scan

Leadership behaviors for
  evidence-based practice
  (EBP) implementation
Performance gap assessment
Pilot

Recognition
Reward
Social system
Users of EBPs

Implementing evidence-based practice (EBP) is a complex, iterative process that involves multiple disciplines and their relationships in the provision of care based on evidence. Implementation is a nonlinear process and takes time, depending on the complexity of the EBPs being implemented. Merely increasing staff knowledge about an EBP and using passive dissemination strategies will not work. In Chapter 13, you learned about implementation strategies that address the *nature of the EBPs* (e.g., fall prevention, acute pain management in older adults) and *communication* with key clinicians. In this chapter, you will learn about implementation strategies that address users of EBPs and the social system where they work (see Fig. 12.1, Chapter 12). Implementation strategies are described, and methods for actualizing them are addressed.

USERS OF EVIDENCE-BASED PRACTICE

Potential users of EBP, also called members of a social system (e.g., nurses, physicians, clerical staff), influence how quickly and widely EBPs are adopted (Rogers, 2003; Valente, 2012). Implementation strategies targeted

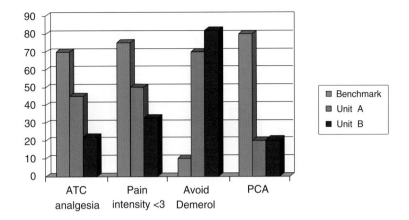

ATC = around-the-clock adminstration of analgesic; PCA = patient controlled analgesic

Fig. 14.1 Example of Performance Gap Assessment: Four Performance Indicators for Improving Acute Pain Management of Hospitalized Older Adults.

at users include the following (Greenhalgh et al., 2005; Titler et al., 2016):

- Audit and feedback
- Performance gap assessment
- Trying the evidence-based practice
- Eliciting patient values and preferences
- Regular meetings among the implementation team members to address challenges and recognize successes

Performance Gap Assessment

Performance gap assessment (PGA) is defined as the baseline practice performance that provides information on the state of current practices at the beginning of a practice change. This implementation strategy engages clinicians in discussions about practice issues and formulation of strategies to promote alignment of their practices with EBP recommendations. Specific practice indicators selected for PGA are derived from EBP recommendations for the specified topic, such as pain assessment every 4 hours for acute pain management (Titler et al., 2009). Studies have demonstrated improvements in performance when PGA is part of multifaceted implementation strategies (Titler et al., 2009; Titler et al., 2016). The following steps are a guide for using performance gap assessment:

- Select the practice performance indicators to use (e.g., acute pain assessment every 4 hours).

- Illustrate the current state of practice using these indicators.
- Select a venue for discussing the gap between the current practice indicators and recommendations based on evidence.
- Engage clinicians in a dialogue about improving practices to align with the evidence.

Fig. 14.1 illustrates an example of a performance gap assessment for improving acute pain management in hospitalized older adults. Four indicators were selected to illustrate the performance gap based on evidence-based guidelines for acute pain management of hospitalized older adults (Titler et al., 2009):

- Process indicators of:
  - administering analgesics around the clock on a scheduled basis (e.g., every 4–6 hours) rather than PRN,
  - avoiding the use of Demerol,
  - use of patient-controlled analgesic administration, and
- an outcome indicator of pain intensity less than 3 on a 0 to 10 scale.

The purpose of this graph was to stimulate discussion and engage clinicians to improve acute pain management practices. The discussion included critical decision making for around-the-clock administration of an analgesic, which necessitates assessing pain every 4 hours and within 30 to 60 minutes after analgesic

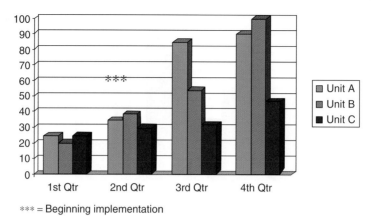

*** = Beginning implementation

Fig. 14.2 Example of Audit and Feedback for Every-Four-Hour Pain Assessment of Older Adults 48 Hours Following Hip Replacement.

administration as well as assessing analgesic side effects (e.g., respiratory rate). When order sets for older adults included Demerol, the team decided to exclude Demerol from physician orders.

Audit and Feedback

Audit and feedback is ongoing auditing of performance indicators, aggregating data into reports, and discussing the findings with practitioners on a regular basis *during the practice change* (Ivers et al., 2012; Hysong, 2009; Hysong et al., 2012). This strategy helps staff see how their efforts to improve care and patient outcomes are progressing throughout the implementation process (Ivers et al., 2014). Action steps to consider include the following:

- Selection of the performance indicators to audit
- Selection of the data source (e.g., medical records, observation, patients, and family members) and methods for auditing (frequency, selection of records, or observation time points)
- Deciding who will do the audits
- Designing methods for data displays
- Deciding who will receive the reports
- Deciding on frequency and methods for dissemination of reports (e.g., paper or electronic such as website or e-mail)
- Determining how feedback reports will be shared with staff (e.g., verbally, display in the practice setting, monthly staff meetings)

Fig. 14.2 illustrates an example of audit and feedback for improving 4-hour pain assessment of hospitalized older adults after hip replacement surgery—a process

indicator. Evidence recommends pain assessment every 4 hours, which is imperative to improve pain management. Data are presented for each quarter over a year; one may choose to report data by month or by week. Other considerations include displaying this indicator by time of day (night, evening, day) or day of the week (weekday versus weekend). Fig. 14.3 illustrates fall rates—an outcome indicator reported for each unit by month.

> ### EBP TIP
>
> Audit and feedback reports are more effective when they are disseminated regularly and are used to discuss practice with staff rather than passive dissemination to selected individuals.

Piloting the Change

Clinicians who will be using an EBP usually try the practice for a period of time (pilot) before adopting it in their practices (Greenhalgh et al., 2005; Rogers, 2003). When an EBP is piloted as part of implementation, users have an opportunity to use it, provide feedback to those in charge of implementation, and modify the practice if necessary. Action steps for piloting an EBP include the following:

- Selecting the time frame for the pilot
- Selecting the unit for the pilot if the EBP is targeted to multiple units in a health system
- Selecting implementation strategies for the pilot
- Selecting performance measures for evaluation
- Eliciting feedback from clinicians who implemented and used the EBP

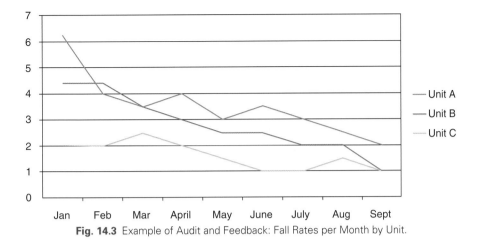

Fig. 14.3 Example of Audit and Feedback: Fall Rates per Month by Unit.

- Revising the implementation plan based on the pilot

For example, before adopting system-wide changes in practice for assessment of nasogastric tube placement, the change was piloted on three units, which revealed the difficulties and challenges in carrying out these practices as part of day-to-day care delivery. Based on the pilot, a decision was made not to adopt the practices from research (Rakel et al., 1994).

Meetings

Regular meetings among opinion leaders, change champions, and leaders of the EBP project are essential to track the process of implementation, provide guidance, address questions that arise, solve ongoing challenges, and share implementation strategies that are working (Titler et al., 2009; Titler et al., 2016). You should (1) decide who will participate in these meetings, (2) select a regular meeting time and date (e.g., first Tuesday of the month at 1 p.m.), (3) determine the length and location of the meeting (we recommend 60 minutes), and (4) set forth and distribute a meeting agenda, such as:
- progress in meeting action items in the action plan (see Chapter 12),
- what is working well,
- what issues have arisen,
- questions about the EBPs or implementation approaches,
- report on action items from the previous meeting,
- plan for follow-up of action items from the current meeting, and
- verbal summary of the meeting.

As the leader of an EBP project, you will need to ensure that each individual participates in meetings and has a voice at the table. Meeting minutes and accountability for actions after the meeting are important to engage participants and move the project forward. For example, monthly meetings to implement fall prevention practices and mitigate patient-specific fall risk factors addressed challenges in education of nursing assistants, strategies to make each patient's fall prevention interventions visible, and strategies to modify prescribed medications to avoid use of high-risk drugs that contribute to falls. Participants shared the approaches they used to meet these challenges, such as a structured education session for nursing assistants, use of white boards in patients' rooms to list their specific fall prevention interventions, review of medications by a clinical nurse leader, and discussions with physicians to modify medication orders.

> **EBP TIP**
>
> As recipients of health care practices, patients and families should be incorporated into the implementation processes. Patient-centered EBP is discussed in Chapter 15.

SOCIAL SYSTEM (CONTEXT)

Overview

Clearly, the social system or context of care delivery matters when implementing EBPs (Squires et al., 2015; Titler, 2010; Jacobs et al., 2014). For example, investigators demonstrated the effectiveness of a prompted voiding intervention to address urinary incontinence in nursing home residents, but sustaining the intervention in day-to-day practice was limited when the responsibility of carrying out the intervention was shifted to nursing home staff rather than the investigative team, and required staffing levels higher than those found in a majority of nursing home settings (Engberg, Kincade, & Thompson, 2004). This illustrates the importance of embedding EBP interventions into ongoing care processes.

Context for EBP implementation traditionally has been defined as the physical setting, with little attention paid to the dynamics of the practice environment (Chambers, Glasgow, & Stange, 2013; May, Johnson, & Finch, 2016). Context refers to the characteristics of the physical setting of implementation and the dynamic practice factors in which implementation processes occur (May et al., 2016; Squires et al., 2015). Contextual factors that impact implementation include the following:
- Organizational capacity for EBP (Doran et al., 2012; Everett & Sitterding, 2011; French et al., 2009; Kajermo et al., 2010; Kueny et al., 2015; Stetler et al., 2009; Yamanda et al., 2017)
- Leadership support (Aarons, Ehrhart, Farahnak, & Sklar, 2014; Birken et al., 2016; Jun, Kovner, & Stimpfel, 2016; Hauck, Winsett, & Kuric, 2012; Richter et al., 2016; Wong & Giallonardo, 2013)
- Practice climates for use of EBPs (Jacobs, Weiner, & Bunger, 2014; Yamanda et al., 2017)
- EBP competencies of staff and nurse managers (Gifford, Davies, Edwards, Griffin, & Lybanon, 2007; Melnyk, Gallagher-Ford, Long, & Fineoult-Overholt, 2014; Shuman et al., 2018; Stevens, 2009).

Organizational Capacity

Organizational capacity is important in building an EBP culture (Everett & Sitterding, 2011; Stetler et al., 2009). Components of organizational capacity for EBP include the following:
- Strong leadership
- Clear strategic vision
- Good managerial relations
- Visionary staff in key positions
- A climate conducive to experimentation and risk-taking
- Effective data-capture systems

An organization may be generally amenable to innovations but not ready or willing to assimilate a particular EBP. Elements of system readiness include the following (French et al., 2009; Litaker, Ruhe, Weyer, & Stange, 2008):
- Tension for change
- EBP and system fit
- Implications of using the EBP
- Support and advocacy for the EBP
- Dedicated time and resources
- Capacity to evaluate the impact of the EBP during and after implementation

Leadership

Leadership support is critical for promoting use of EBPs. It is expressed verbally and by providing necessary resources, materials, and time to fulfill responsibilities (Everett & Sitterding, 2011; French et al., 2009; Sandstrom et al., 2011; Stetler et al., 2009). Senior leadership needs to:
- create an organizational mission, vision, and strategic plan that incorporate EBP,
- implement performance expectations for staff that include the work of EBP,
- integrate the work of EBP into the governance structure of the health care system,
- demonstrate the value of EBPs through administrative behaviors, and
- establish explicit expectations that nurse leaders will create microsystems that value and support clinical inquiry.

EBP TIP

Practice environments matter because clinical settings for implementation are dynamic and each setting carries its own set of contextual factors, such as practice climate and leadership behaviors that influence implementation and sustainability of EBPs.

Implementation Strategies to Address the Social System/Practice Context

Implementation strategies to address the social system are based on the following principles:
- Building relationships among and across disciplines
- Garnering initial and ongoing support of key senior leaders and middle managers
- Providing rewards and recognition for staff who align practices with the evidence
- Ensuring that organizational practice standards and documentation systems support the ongoing use of the EBPs

These principles are essential for ongoing sustainability of the practice change after implementation. Implementation strategies that target the social system are the following:

- Conducting an environmental scan
- Meeting with key leadership stakeholders
- Revising practice standards and documentation systems
- Providing recognition and rewards

Environmental Scan

An **environmental scan** is a process that assesses internal strengths and challenges for a specific topic; in this case, implementation of EBPs. Environmental scans include the structure and function of the organization, or how things get done. The scan incorporates assessment of factors such as organizational climate for implementation and conversations with informal leaders and staff.

Two purposes of an environmental scan are to understand the organization's mission, vision, and values and to articulate how the EBP project contributes to meeting these organizational goals. For example, the mission of a local health system in southeast Michigan is to provide compassionate, extraordinary care every day. Its vision is to be the leading high-value health care network focused on extraordinary outcomes through education, innovation, and compassion. Its values are Compassion, Respect, Integrity, Teamwork, and Excellence. If you are focusing on fall reduction, you should be able to articulate how your improvements contribute to extraordinary care through patient safety and implementation of the EBP. They should go beyond generic fall prevention interventions to implementation of interventions that target patient-specific fall risk factors (innovation) and address teamwork, excellence, and integrity.

Another purpose of an environmental scan is to review the governance structure and identify senior leaders in various disciplines whom you will need to interact with for implementation. Specifically, you will want to understand the functions and roles of the various committees or councils that compose the governance structure and evaluate which ones you need to work with for implementation. For example, the department of nursing governance may include a Nursing Quality Committee, a Standards Committee, and a Research Committee (see Fig. 14.4 for an example). You will want to meet with the chairs of each to engage their expertise and seek guidance on what processes may be required to institutionalize the work of your team. The Standards Committee can guide the team on revising existing standards to align with the evidence base and understanding the steps necessary to have the revised standards approved. The Nursing Quality Committee can assist with quality performance indicators for performance gap assessment, audit and feedback, and evaluation. The Research Committee may have members with expertise regarding EBPs that are the focus of your project and thus may serve as consultants.

> **IPE TIP**
>
> EBP project leaders need to cultivate a non-judgmental culture where team members from different professions feel respected and valued when they provide feedback about challenges of sustaining implementation of an EBP and offer suggestions for modifying the implementation plan.

Context assessment. Your environmental scan may include assessment of key context factors that impact implementation, such as unit climate and leadership behaviors for EBP implementation. A variety of tools with good reliability and validity are available for assessment and are summarized in Table 14.1. Two scales are discussed for illustrative purposes: the Implementation Climate Scale and the Implementation Leadership Scale. Findings from context assessments provide insights for tailoring implementation strategies such as educational approaches and fostering leadership behaviors that promote EBP.

The **unit climate for EBP implementation** is staff's "shared perceptions of the practices, policies, procedures, and clinical behaviors that are rewarded, supported, and expected in order to facilitate effective implementation of evidence-based practices" (Ehrhart et al., 2014). The Implementation Climate Scale (ICS) is a reliable and valid instrument to measure the unit climate for EBP implementation (Ehrhart et al., 2014). It is short (18 items) and evaluates the extent (1 = slight to 4 = very great) to which the unit or setting prioritizes and values EBP in six areas:

- Focus on EBP
- Educational support for EBP
- Recognition for EBP
- Rewards for EBP
- Selection of staff for EBP knowledge and experience
- Selection of staff for openness (flexible, adaptable, open to new interventions)

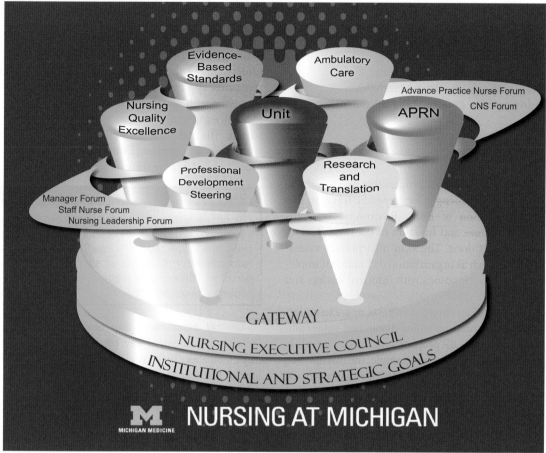

Fig. 14.4 Department of Nursing Governance Structure at the University of Michigan Health System. Committees are depicted by cones (e.g., Nursing Quality Excellence Committee). (From the University of Michigan Health System.)

All items are anchored to a specific unit or practice setting as a point of reference.

Leadership behaviors for EBP implementation are behaviors enacted by organization and unit leaders that facilitate evidence-based practice implementation and foster an evidence-based practice climate (Aarons et al., 2014; Birken et al., 2012; Hauck et al., 2012). These behaviors can be assessed using the Implementation Leadership Scale (ILS). This is a 12-item scale that measures the extent to which leaders enact behaviors that support EBP implementation (0 = not at all to 4 = great extent) (Aarons et al., 2014; Torres et al., 2018). There are two versions of the ILS, one for staff to report their perceptions of supervisors' leadership and another for supervisors and leaders to assess themselves. The leadership characteristics are the following:

- Proactive
- Knowledgeable
- Supportive
- Perseverant

> **EBP TIP**
>
> Consider using the ILS to assess leadership behaviors of nurse managers, clinical nurse leaders, directors of clinical services, and/or advanced practice nurses.

Performing a context assessment. When performing a context assessment, you will need to do the following:

- Select concepts that you believe will impact implementation and that are important to assess (e.g., climate, leadership, competencies).

TABLE 14.1 Examples of EBP Assessment Tools

Name of Tool	What it Measures	Number of Items	Scores	References
Implementation Climate Scale (ICS)	Staff perceptions of the extent to which a unit or practice setting prioritizes and values EBP	18 items Likert scale: 0 = not at all to 4 = very great extent	Total score and 6 subscale scores: Focus; Educational Support; Recognition; Rewards; EBP Selection; Openness	Ehrhart et al., 2014
Work Environment for EBP Scale	Staff perceptions of the values and resources available to support EBP	8 items Likert scale: Strongly agree to strongly disagree	Total score No subscales	Pryse, McDaniel, & Schafer, 2014
Absorptive and Receptive Capacity Scale (ARCS)	Staff's perception about organizational processes to use knowledge (evidence) in practice	14 items. Likert scale: 1 = lack of routine processes to 5 = good processes in place	Total score and 5 subscale scores: Questioning culture; Acquiring new knowledge; Knowledge sharing; Knowledge use; Vision, Culture, & Leadership	Burton, 2017
Implementation Leadership Scale (ILS)	Staff perceptions regarding the extent to which leaders enact behaviors that support EBP implementation	12 items. Likert scale 0 = not at all to 4 = great extent	Total score and 4 subscale scores: Proactive, Knowledgeable, Supportive, Perseverant Leadership	Aarons, Ehrhart, & Farahnak, 2014; Torres et al., 2018
Nursing Leadership for EBP Scale	Staff perceptions about the behaviors of their managers who support EBP	10 items. Likert scale: Strongly agree to strongly disagree	Total score No subscales	Pryse, McDaniel, & Schafer, 2014
Implementation Citizenship Behavior Scale (ICBS)	Behaviors employees perform that exceed their expected job tasks to support implementation of EBPs	6 items Likert scale: 0 = not at all to 4 = frequently if not always	Total score and 2 subscale scores: Helping others Keeping informed	Ehrhart et al., 2015
Nurse Manager EBP Competency Scale	Self-assessment of level of competency for EBP knowledge and skills	16 items. Likert scale: 0 = not competent to 3 = expertly competent	Total score and 2 subscale scores: EBP Knowledge, EBP Activity	Shuman et al., 2018
RNs EBP Competency Scale	Assessment of RNs' abilities in selected aspects of EBP	13 items	Total score No subscale scores	Melnyk et al., 2014
APN EBP Competency Scale	Assessment of APNs' abilities in all aspects of EBP	24 items	Total score No subscale score	Melnyk et al., 2014
Organizational Readiness for Implementing Change (ORIC) Instrument	Assessment of an organization's readiness for implementing change	12 items. Likert scale: 1 = disagree to 5 = agree	Total score and 2 subscale scores: Change Commitment, Change Efficacy	Shea et al., 2014

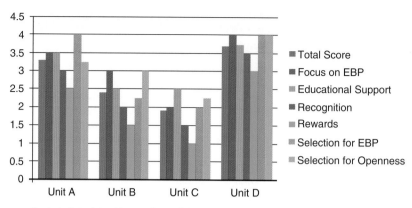

Scale is 0 to 4.0 = Not at all; 1 = Slight extent; 2 = Moderate extent;
3 = Great extent; 4 = Very great extent

Fig. 14.5 Implementation Climate Scores by Unit.

- Select tools that are aligned with the concepts.
- Be thoughtful about how the results of the assessment will be incorporated into implementation.
- Select methods for sharing the results of the assessment and deciding who will receive them.

You should treat individual responses as confidential, and results should be aggregated for reporting. Comparing certain assessment measures (e.g., ILS, ICS) across units is helpful to guide implementation, but units should be blinded. For example, ICS for units can be reported (Fig. 14.5) and when discussing EBP implementation with a specific unit, staff would be informed which one is their unit (A, B, C, or D). Fig. 14.5 suggests that the unit climate for EBP implementation in unit D is quite positive, whereas the climate of unit C is not as positive. You should consider how these results can guide the tailoring of implementation.

> **EBP TIP**
>
> Be selective when choosing assessment tools, refrain from measuring all concepts, and consider the length of the tool.

Meetings with Key Leadership Stakeholders

As a leader of the EBP project, you and your selected team members will want to initially meet with the chief nurse executive (CNE) to describe the project and overall goals related to quality and safety. This initial meeting should include a discussion of the current practice, the gap in alignment with EBPs, and practice sites for implementation. You will want to include data about current practice indicators and a beginning synthesis of the evidence to illustrate EBPs that need to be modified. You should also articulate how this work aligns with the organization's mission, vision, and strategic agenda. The purpose of this meeting is to garner support to proceed with the project and the overall implementation plan. The CNE is likely to provide recommendations for involvement of key stakeholders, additional members to consider for the implementation team, units for implementation, and individuals to serve as opinion leaders. A subsequent meeting(s) with the CNE may be warranted to provide follow-up information. Ongoing methods of communication with the CNE should be established (e.g., e-mail updates, face-to-face meetings, quarterly reports).

Conversely, the EBP project may be driven by the CNE to address a quality of care issue. It is still important to meet with the CNE to understand his or her perspective and be clear about the focus of the project.

Other disciplines. After meeting with the CNE, you and your EBP team will need to meet with key leaders from other disciplines who will be impacted by the EBP changes. It is helpful to have the CNE attend these meetings to illustrate his or her support for the project. They can be structured as one gathering of all senior leaders or individual meetings with each senior leader. The meetings should include the following:

- Data that illustrate opportunity for improvement such as the performance gap assessment report

- A summary of the EBPs to be implemented, including references
- The role of each discipline in promoting and facilitating implementation of the EBPs
- Planned implementation strategies
- The evaluation plan
- Summary of the implementation timeline and action plan
- Opportunity for discussion and eliciting any additional implementation strategies they recommend

For example, when implementing EB fall prevention practices targeted to patient-specific fall risk factors, consider meeting with the CNE, the chief medical officer (CMO), directors of pharmacy and physical therapy services, and the director of quality improvement.

Nurse managers. Nurse managers (NMs) of practice sites (e.g., ambulatory care clinic, patient care unit) where EBPs will be implemented are key to success (Birken et al., 2012; Wilkinson, Nutley, & Davies, 2011). These individuals have different titles depending on the site of implementation, but they are characterized as licensed registered nurses who are direct supervisors of staff nurses on the unit or in a clinical practice, and who have responsibility and accountability for unit-level or practice operations, including budget, resource allocation, staffing, and quality of care. Engaging with NMs early in the planning and implementation process is essential to ensure their support for implementation. One strategy to engage with NMs is an organizational meeting to discuss:

- an overview of the project,
- the EBPs,
- timeline and rationale for the practice change,
- commitment to implementation, and
- the role of NMs in implementation.

NMs can foster implementation by role modeling the EBPs, providing visible feedback and support to staff who are aligning their practices with the evidence base, providing resources such as time for change champions to attend meetings and do EBP work, including EBP as part of staff evaluations, and creating enthusiasm among staff for improving care based on evidence. These meetings usually take 60 to 90 minutes, depending on the group size. Meeting as a collective group of NMs provides opportunities for rich dialogue and discussion.

Standards of Practice and Documentation Systems

It is important that written standards of practice (e.g., policies, procedures, clinical pathways) and documentation systems support the use of EBPs (Titler, 2010). Clinical information systems may need revision to support practice changes; documentation systems that fail to readily support the new practice thwart change (see Chapter 13). For example, if staff members are expected to reassess and document pain intensity within 30 minutes after administration of an analgesic, documentation systems must reflect this practice standard. It is the role of leadership to ensure that organizational documents and systems are flexible and supportive of EBPs.

Recognition and Rewards

As you plan for implementation, you will need to decide how staff will be recognized and rewarded for their work. Recognition and rewards are important to acknowledge staff's investment in delivery of EB care. Recognition can be achieved through organizational publications such as newsletters, personal thank-you notes from the nurse manager and EBP team, highlighting the work at system-level quality improvement meetings, and nominating individuals or teams for practice excellence awards offered by the health system, the clinical practice, or professional organizations.

Many health systems have recognition programs for nurses through events such as an annual recognition day or celebration dinner. For example, you may want to solicit nominations for an Annual EBP Nurse of the Year Award for individuals who exemplify excellence in nursing practice through implementing EBPs to improve quality of care.

Recognition also can be achieved by nominations for awards offered by professional organizations. For example, the Association for Pediatric Hematology/Oncology Nurses presents an annual EBP Excellence Award to an APOHN member who demonstrates high-quality contributions to EBP in the nursing care of children and their families. The recipient of this award receives a $250 honorarium, recognition at the annual conference awards luncheon and through a press release, and an announcement sent to the recipient's employer. The Center for Nursing at the Foundation of the New York State Nurses Board of Trustees recognizes excellence in implementing nursing research in the practice setting through an Evidence-Based Practice Award. It is given to an individual or group using research-based evidence to make a practice change that results in demonstrated improvement in outcomes for patients, families, staff, community, or the organization. The Eastern Nursing Research Society (ENRS) has an EBP

Award for an individual or group using research-based evidence to make a practice change that results in demonstrated improvement in health outcomes.

Rewards can be achieved through bonus payments, salary increases, and educational funds to be used at the discretion of the individual, team, or unit. For example, an individual or team who has been instrumental in implementing EBPs may receive financial support to attend a regional or national conference to present their work.

Successful implementation requires strategies that address the context or social system of implementation, including an environmental scan, engagement with leadership stakeholders, alignment of practice standards and documentation systems with the evidence, and provision of recognition and rewards.

SYNTHESIS

Now that you are informed about multiple implementation strategies, you and your team can decide which strategies to use and formulate a reasonable timeline for implementation. Use the action plan (see Chapter 12) to guide your work, the time frame for each implementation strategy, and the individual(s) who will take the lead in enacting each implementation strategy. Be creative in imparting information to others, and consider how you and your team can continuously engage staff at all levels of the organization. Implementation is perhaps the most fun and rewarding component of EBP. Enjoy the journey, and keep a journal of lessons learned to use in your future work.

■ KEY POINTS

- Performance Gap Assessment is used at the beginning of implementation to engage clinicians in discussions about the EBPs EPS.
- Audit and Feedback requires decisions about performance indicators, methods of data display, and frequency and methods for distributing reports to clinicians.
- Use audit and feedback reports during implementation to discuss practices with clinicians.

- Piloting the EBPs as a part of implementation has a positive effect on adoption.
- Perform an environmental scan to assess strengths and challenges.
- Engage senior leaders in implementation.
- Know your governance structure and how you will interact with each committee or group.
- Plan for recognition and rewards.

REFERENCES

Aarons, G. A., Ehrhart, M. G., & Farahnak, L. R. (2014). The Implementation Leadership Scale (ILS): Development of a brief measure of unit level implementation leadership. *Implementation Science, 9*(1), 45.

Aarons, G. A., Ehrhart, M. G., Farahnak, L. R., & Sklar, M. (2014). Aligning leadership across systems and organizations to develop a strategic climate for evidence-based practice implementation. *Annual Review of Public Health, 35*, 255–274.

Birken, S. A., DiMartino, L. D., Kirk, M. A., Lee, S. Y., McClelland, M., & Albert, N. M. (2016). Elaborating on theory with middle managers' experience implementing healthcare innovations in practice. *Implementation Science, 11*(1), 2.

Birken, S. A., Lee, S. Y.D., & Weiner, B. J. (2012). Uncovering middle managers' role in healthcare innovation implementation. *Implementation Science, 7*(4), 28.

Burton, C. (2017, March). *The Absorptive and Receptive Capacity Scale (ARCS) [personal correspondence with Burton, C.]*.

Chambers, D. A., Glasgow, R. E., & Stange, K. C. (2013). The dynamic sustainability framework: Addressing the paradox of sustainment amid ongoing change. *Implementation Science, 8*(1), 117.

Doran, D., Haynes, B. R., Estabrooks, C. A., Kushniruk, A., Dubrowski, A., Bajnok, I., et al. (2012). The role of organizational context and individual nurse characteristics in explaining variation in use of information technologies in evidence based practice. *Implementation Science, 7*(122).

Ehrhart, M. G., Aarons, G. A., & Farahnak, L. R. (2014). Assessing the organizational context for EBP implementation: The development and validity testing of the Implementation Climate Scale (ICS). *Implementation Science, 9*(1), 157.

Ehrhart, M. G., Aarons, G. A., & Farahnak, L. R. (2015). Going above and beyond for implementation: The development and validity testing of the Implementation Citizenship Behavior Scale (ICBS). *Implementation Science, 10*, 65–54.

Engberg, S., Kincade, J., & Thompson, D. (2004). Future directions for incontinence research with frail elders. *Nursing Research, 53*(Suppl 6), S22–S29.

Everett, L. Q., & Sitterding, M. C. (2011). Transformational leadership required to design and sustain evidence-based practice: A system exemplar. *Western Journal of Nursing Research, 33*(3), 398–426.

French, B., Thomas, L. H., Baker, P., Burton, C. R., Pennington, L., & Roddam, H. (2009). What can management theories offer evidence-based practice? A comparative analysis of measurement tools for organisational context. *Implementation Science, 4*(28).

Gifford, W., Davies, B., Edwards, N., Griffin, P., & Lybanon, V. (2007). Managerial leadership for nurses' use of research evidence: an integrative review of the literature. *Worldviews on Evidence-Based Nursing, 4*(3), 126–145.

Greenhalgh, T., Robert, G., Bate, P., Macfarlane, F., & Kyriakidou, O. (2005). *Diffusion of innovations in health service organisations: A systematic literature review.* Massachusetts: Blackwell Publishing Ltd. https://doi.org/10.1002/9780470987407.

Hauck, S., Winsett, R. P., & Kuric, J. (2012). Leadership facilitation strategies to establish evidence-based practice in an acute care hospital. *Journal of Advanced Nursing, 69*(3), 664–674.

Hysong, S. J. (2009). Meta-analysis: Audit and feedback features impact effectiveness on care quality. *Medical Care, 47*(3), 356–363.

Hysong, S. J., Teal, C. R., Khan, M. J., & Haidet, P. (2012). Improving quality of care through improved audit and feedback. *Implementation Science, 7*, 45.

Ivers, N., Jamtvedt, G., Flottorp, S., Young, J. M., Odgaard-Jensen, J., French, S. D., et al. (2012). Audit and feedback: Effects on professional practice and healthcare outcomes. *Cochrane Database of Systematic Reviews, 6*, Article No. CD000259.

Ivers, N. M., Sales, A., Colquhoun, H., Michie, S., Foy, R., Francis, J. J., et al. (2014). No more "business as usual" with audit and feedback interventions: Towards an agenda for a reinvigorated intervention. *Implementation Science, 9*, 14.

Jacobs, S. R., Weiner, B. J., & Bunger, A. C. (2014). Context matters: Measuring implementation climate among individuals and groups. *Implementation Science, 9*(1), 46.

Jun, J., Kovner, C. T., & Stimpfel, A. W. (2016). Barriers and facilitators of nurses' use of clinical practice guidelines: An integrative review. *International Journal of Nursing Studies, 60*, 54–68.

Kajermo, K. N., Boström, A. M., Thompson, D. S., Hutchinson, A. M., Estabrooks, C. A., & Wallin, L. (2010). The BARRIERS scale–the barriers to research utilization scale: A systematic review. *Implementation Science, 5*(1), 32.

Kueny, A., Shever, L., Lehan Mackin, M., & Titler, M. G. (2015). Facilitating the implementation of evidence-based practice through contextual support for nursing leadership. *Journal of Healthcare Leadership, 7*, 29–39.

Litaker, D., Ruhe, M., Weyer, S., & Stange, K. C. (2008). Association of intervention outcomes with practice capacity for change: Subgroup analysis from a group randomized trial. *Implementation Science, 3*, 25.

May, C. R., Johnson, M., & Finch, T. (2016). Implementation, context and complexity. *Implementation Science, 11*(1), 141.

Melnyk, B. M., Gallagher-Ford, L., Long, L. E., & Fineout-Overholt, E. (2014). Practice competencies for practicing registered nurses and advanced practice nurses in real-world clinical settings: proficiencies to improve healthcare quality, reliability, patient outcomes, and costs. *Worldviews on Evidence-Based Nursing, 11*(1), 5–15.

Pryse, Y., McDaniel, A., & Schafer, J. (2014). Psychometric analysis of two new scales: the evidence-based practice nursing leadership and work environment scales. *Worldviews on Evidence-Based Nursing, 11*(4), 240–247.

Rakel, B. A., Titler, M. G., Goode, C., Barry-Walker, J., Budreau, G., & Buckwalter, K. C. (1994). Nasogastric and nasointestinal feeding tube placement: an integrative review of research. *AACN Advanced Critical Care, 5*(2), 194–206. PMID: 7767814.

Rogers, E. M. (2003). *Diffusion of innovations* (5th ed.). New York, NY: The Free Press.

Richter, A., von Thiele Schwarz, U., Lornudd, C., Lundmark, R., Mosson, R., & Hasson, H. (2016). iLead—A transformational leadership intervention to train healthcare managers' implementation leadership. *Implementation Science, 11*(1), 108.

Sandstrom, B., Borglin, G., Nilsson, R., & Willman, A. (2011). Promoting the implementation of evidence-based practice: A literature review focusing on the role of nursing leadership. *Worldviews on Evidence-Based Nursing, 8*(4), 212–223.

Shea, C. M., Jacobs, S. R., Esserman, D. A., Bruce, K., & Weiner, B. J. (2014). Organizational readiness for implementing change: a psychometric assessment of a new measure. *Implementation Science, 9*, 7–22.

Shuman, C. J., Ploutz-Snyder, R., & Titler, M. G. (2018). Development and testing of the NM EBP Competency Scale. *Western Journal of Nursing Research, 40*(2), 175–190.

Squires, J. E., Graham, I. D., Hutchinson, A. M., Michie, S., Francis, J. J., Sales, A., et al. (2015). Identifying the domains of context important to implementation science: a study protocol. *Implementation Science, 10*(1), 135.

Stetler, C. B., Ritchie, J. A., Rycroft-Malone, J., Schultz, A. A., & Charns, M. P. (2009). Institutionalizing evidence-based practice: An organizational case study using a model of strategic change. *Implementation Science, 4*(1), 78.

Stevens, K. R. (2009). *Essential competencies for evidence-based practice in nursing.* San Antonio, TX: Academic Center for Evidence-Based Practice, University of Texas Health Science Center at San Antonio.

Titler, M. G. (2010). Translation science and context. *Research and Theory for Nursing Practice, 24*(1), 35–55.

Titler, M. G., Conlon, P., Reynolds, M. A., Ripley, R., Tsodikov, A., Wilson, D. S., et al. (2016). The effect of translating research into practice intervention to promote use of evidence-based fall prevention interventions in hospitalized adults: a prospective pre-post implementation study in the U.S. *Applied Nursing Research, 31*, 52–59.

Titler, M. G., Herr, K., Brooks, J. M., Xie, X. J., Ardery, G., Schilling, M. L., et al. (2009). Translating research into practice intervention improves management of acute pain in older hip fracture patients. *Health Services Research, 44*(1), 264–287.

Torres, E. M., Ehrhart, M. G., Beidas, R. S., Farahnak, L. R., Finn, N. K., & Aarons, G. A. (2018). Validation of the Implementation Leadership Scale (ILS) with supervisors self-ratings. *Community Mental Health Journal, 54*(1), 49–53.

Valente, T. W. (2012). Network interventions. *Science, 337*(49), 49–53.

Wilkinson, J. E., Nutley, S. M., & Davies, H. T. O. (2011). An exploration of the roles of nurse managers in evidence-based practice implementation. *Worldviews on Evidence-Based Nursing, 8*(4), 236–246.

Wong, C. A., & Giallonardo, L. M. (2013). Authentic leadership and nurse-assessed adverse patient outcomes. *Journal of Nursing Management, 21*(5), 740–752.

Yamada, J., Squires, J. E., Estabrooks, C. A., Victor, C., & Stevens, B. (2017). The role of organizational context in moderating the effect of research use on pain outcomes in hospitalized children: A cross sectional study. *BMC Health Services Research, 17*(1), 68.

Patient-Centered Evidence-Based Practices

Amy L. Msowoya, Sheila M. Gephart

LEARNING OUTCOMES

After reading this chapter, you should be able to do the following:

- Apply principles of evidence-based practice to patient-centered care.
- Discuss the evidence about the value of shared decision making.
- Discuss the principles and assessment of patient activation.

- Compare patient activation and real-world strategies to activate patients across levels of health literacy and numeracy.
- Describe evidence-based shared decision making and identify strategies to engage individuals, families, and communities in the process.
- Identify real-world strategies to incorporate shared decision making into practice.

KEY TERMS

Contextual barriers	Patient activation	Shared decision making
Health literacy	Patient portal	Shared decision-making aids
Health numeracy		

INTRODUCTION

Putting the patient, family, and community at the center of all care decisions is at the core of evidence-based practice (EBP). In the EBP process, it is essential to address patients' values, characteristics, and contextual factors that are important to them. If patients' concerns are ignored or not addressed, how will they be able to experience their best outcomes? Although this is important at the individual and family levels, it is also valuable when considering the health of communities or organizations. For administrators, educators, and policy-leading clinicians, this topic is of vital importance because it impacts resource utilization, provider satisfaction, and clinical and financial outcomes for which they are accountable, such as satisfaction and readmission

rates. By keeping EBP patient-centric, the filter for interpreting and applying evidence is the contextual world in which that patient lives to achieve health. It means that strategies to engage patients in their care are applied with awareness of evidence that supports such strategies. For example, the rich science supported for decades by the National Institute of Nursing Research (NINR) to study self-management, caregiver supports, and strategies to engage in effective behavior change can inform all efforts to engage patients. Matching strategies for engagement that address individuals of all levels of health understanding and that target how involved they want to (or believe they can) be in their care becomes necessary when behavior change or self-management is the goal. This chapter builds on content in previous chapters that addresses the "doing" of EBP by emphasizing considerations for applying that evidence *with* individual patients and groups, not *to* them. Evidence-based strategies to address patient characteristics that impact understanding, ways to engage them deeper in their care, and the evidence-based methods that are necessary to create tools to promote working *with* patients are addressed in this chapter.

CLINICAL SCENARIO

Try to imagine the following scenario: You're a patient sitting in a hospital bed, and you've just been told that you have cancer. Provider A walks into your room, and after saying hello, starts rattling off a description of the latest treatment options available for your condition. You can only comprehend the word "cancer," yet this provider keeps talking at you. Too afraid to ask questions of someone you perceive is much smarter than yourself, you sit there, silently overwhelmed by the amount of information being discussed, and feel even more out of control of your situation and health as the conversation ends and Provider A asks you to make a choice as to which treatment you want to undertake. Do you think this doesn't happen? Guess again.

Let's look at an alternative approach to this same situation. You're there, sitting in your hospital bed, and Provider B has just told you that you have cancer. Seeing that you are visibly shaken by this information, Provider B asks what is most important to you with regard to your future health. The provider asks if you have any questions right now and recommends that you reach out to anyone you want to share this news with before having to make a treatment decision. Provider B also leaves you with a piece of paper called a shared decision-making aid, with a link to your patient portal website, and tells you that the clinical team will be available to answer any questions you may have, and to help you make a decision about treatment when you're ready.

Which provider would you feel has *you* at the center of his or her mindset? Odds are you'd say Provider B because that person has just shown you an example of patient-centered care. Patient centricity and involvement in health care guides nurse practitioners to provide evidence-based care based on outcomes that patients and their families feel matter. In giving up their own centricity, providers can feel more professionally fulfilled by managing patient health instead of patient flow. Patient engagement has been deemed a potential

"blockbuster drug" but also has been historically one of the most underutilized resources in health care (Higgins, Larson, & Schnall, 2016). Why?

PATIENT EMPOWERMENT THROUGH SHARED DECISION MAKING

Patients need to fully understand their treatment options and evaluate their own preferences and beliefs to make informed decisions and truly engage in their health decision making. This is a task easier said than done. Emotional forces, lack of knowledge, organizational constraints, autonomy, family forces, and cultural beliefs, among other factors, all can influence patient decision making (Street, Volk, Lowenstein, & Fordis, 2017). This puts health care providers in a difficult position, namely how to provide guidance and direction in questioning patients without exercising paternalistic control, in a way that makes decisions *with* patients instead of *for* them.

Shared decision making is defined as a process by which patients and clinicians partner to make informed health decisions that benefit the patient. It encourages patients to evaluate their own knowledge and beliefs about treatment options before talking to their providers (Rose, Rosewilliam, & Soundy, 2016). Similarly, it requires providers to clarify patient values and concerns as they talk *with* their patients, not simply *to* them. This fosters effective, open dialogue between the patient and provider and keeps the focus on the patient. The risk of not engaging the patient is too great, since it puts clinicians at risk of making a "silent misdiagnosis" by not addressing a patient's preferences for care (Street et al., 2017). Given that patients must implement many health care decisions and deal with the financial, emotional, and quality of life implications of those decisions on their own (such as whether to fill prescriptions, attend follow-up visits, or monitor blood pressures), shared decision making between the patient and provider should be the norm rather than the exception. Although barriers do exist to implementing shared decision making, the information presented here is intended to reduce the impact of those barriers and support you in implementing patient-centered EBPs in real time within the constraints of actual clinical practice.

EVIDENCE TO SUPPORT SHARED DECISION MAKING

Shared decision making gained traction in the health care industry with shifts in payment models from a fee-for-service payment structure to a pay-for-performance structure based on value. In the emerging value-based delivery system, there is increased focus on providing quality care at low cost for populations. Proper utilization of shared decision-making interventions has the potential to decrease overall health care costs while increasing the quality of health care delivered—all reasons why federal support for shared decision making has grown in recent years (Higgins et al., 2016). When the United States Congress authorized creation of the Patient-Centered Outcomes Research Institute (PCORI), a non-governmental, nonprofit, independent organization in 2010, its mission was to sponsor high-quality research that addressed the questions that concerned stakeholders (e.g., patients, caregivers, clinicians, policymakers). Quickly, the goal of helping consumers make informed health decisions was followed by funding streams to promote the study of methods, instrumentation, and decision making models (Patient-Centered Outcomes Research Institute, 2012). One of the national priorities for research within this institute is to empower health consumers to ask for and use health information to support shared decision making between patients and their providers. In the reimbursement schema of today and tomorrow, clinicians are incentivized to share health care information with patients and with each other, and to promote shared decision making and patient engagement (Higgins et al., 2016). As the saying goes, "Money talks," and right now the "money" being paid to health care providers is incentivized by providing care that is deemed valuable to the patient.

Although some organizations state that value is determined through subjective goals stated by the patient, others argue that solid research must support the value of an intervention for use in a clinical situation. Patient-centered shared decision making bridges these two extremes by including patients as partners so that the best evidence-based treatment plans for their lifestyles and clinical situations is created *with* them and not *for* them.

SHARED DECISION-MAKING AIDS

Many Americans are familiar with remaining components of the Affordable Care Act (ACA), such as the creation of health insurance exchanges, but few realize the benefit of some of the more minor provisions. One such provision that was explicitly written into the ACA was the promotion of shared decision making and the use of patient decision support interventions such as decision aids to improve patient knowledge (Alston et al., 2014). Shared decision-making aids are defined as evidence-based documents or tools that portray health care options; give information about risks, benefits, and outcomes for the options; assist patients in clarifying their values; and incorporate clinical judgment and counseling (Kijewski, 2016). A variety of decision-making tools are available to primary care clinicians in both online and print formats, such as the exemplar discussed in the patient scenario at the beginning of this chapter. Unfortunately, even after proof of the efficacy of such tools has been shown, few clinicians and patients utilize existing decision-making tools such as patient decision aids, citing a lack of access to these resources (Alston et al., 2014). More than 500 evidence-based decision aids are currently available on the Internet, but they are scattered across dozens of websites and not well advertised. The IT Resources box provides examples of free-to-use decision aids that may be accessed from the Internet.

IT RESOURCES

Shared Decision-Making Aids

- Mayo Clinic Shared Decision Making National Resource Center at http://shareddecisions.mayoclinic.org/
- Agency for Healthcare Research and Quality: Effective Healthcare Program at https://effectivehealthcare.ahrq.gov/index.cfm/tools-and-resources/patient-decision-aids/
- OptionGrid™ program – Dartmouth College at http://optiongrid.org/
- Ottawa Hospital Research Institute at https://decision-aid.ohri.ca/index.html

EVIDENCE-BASED METHODS TO DEVELOP PATIENT ENGAGEMENT TOOLS

One example of a method used to create an evidence-based tool for patient engagement is Oral Health Patient Facts (see EBP Exemplar). The Oral Health Nursing Education and Practice (OHNEP) Program and the American College of Physicians (ACP) collaborated on this evidence-based project to develop a set of four user-friendly oral health literacy handouts: Oral Health and HPV; Oral Health and You; Oral Health and Older Adults; and Oral Health and Diabetes. To create and validate these tools, the EBP project team conducted a search and critical appraisal of the literature to find the best available evidence that provided a base for developing the content. Consumer focus groups were conducted for each of the target populations to identify their knowledge gaps and concerns. Based on the literature review and qualitative data from the focus groups, drafts of the four Oral Health Patient Facts handouts were developed in

EBP EXEMPLAR

Oral Health Patients Facts

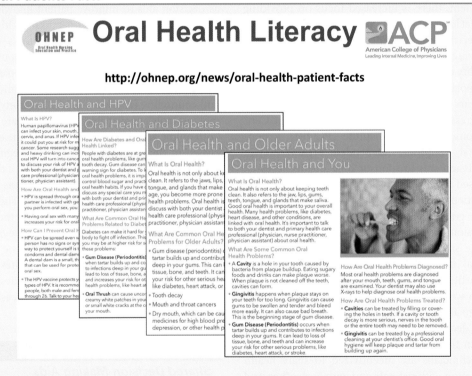

Oral Health Patient Facts, an evidence-based oral health literacy product, was developed to address a problem-focused trigger (see Chapter 3). Clinicians had difficulty integrating oral health promotion into overall health care for their primary care patients. There was a lack of consumer-friendly, evidence-based oral health literacy products targeting specific patient populations at high risk for oral health comorbidities. For example, preteens, adolescents, and young adults not yet or currently sexually active often do not realize that if they contract human papillomavirus (HPV), they are at risk for oropharyngeal cancer. Immunization with Gardasil protects this population and decreases risk of HPV and its negative sequelae, oral cancer. Another population, those with type 2 diabetes, is at high risk for periodontal disease with potential infection and tooth loss. Effective glycemic control and education about the importance of oral hygiene in primary care practices is significantly correlated with decreasing risk for periodontal disease. Similarly, collaboration with and referral to dental colleagues for treatment of gum disease is associated with improvement of glycemic status. More information and direct download of the tools are available at http://ohnep.org/news/oral-health-patient-facts.

English and Spanish and written at a sixth-grade reading level. Handouts were reviewed by an interprofessional panel of health professional judges with content and clinical expertise in each of the target areas. Once the content validity was established, the Oral Health Patient Facts handouts were reviewed by another panel of consumers for face validity, readability, and relevance to their health issues. Feedback from content judges and consumer panelists was used by the EBP team to revise the drafts and finalize the Oral Health Patient Facts for pilot testing. The pilot study included a sample of primary care clinicians, physicians, nurse practitioners, and physician assistants, who introduced the health literacy handouts to patients in their primary care settings. They used each with the appropriate patient populations to test their comfort as professionals using the Oral Health Patient Facts to engage patients in promoting shared decision making and effective self-management. Qualitative data from the pilot study showed that the tools were viewed positively. Targeted dissemination was done via a press release, email blasts, and posting on the ACP and OHNEP websites.

PATIENT ACTIVATION

To truly implement patient-centered EBPs, one must "meet patients where they are," tailoring strategies that address their strengths and challenges. Patient activation is defined as the knowledge, confidence, and skills that a patient possesses and is willing to use to make decisions about health. By assessing level of patient activation, a clinician can better understand the knowledge, confidence, and skill level patients have to engage in shared decision making about their care (Hibbard, 2016). Activation is a dynamic state, not a static one, meaning that patients can progress and regress between levels of activation at various points in their lives. Patient expectations for involvement in decision making vary based on clinical setting and patient characteristics, and a good provider needs to be able to tailor shared decision-making interventions based on a patient's activation level and the type of support individuals at that activation level need.

The most common tool used to assess a patient's activation level is the Patient Activation Measure (PAM). The PAM is a validated assessment tool that objectively measures an individual's mindset about managing their own health using a 13-item scale (Hibbard, 2016). The literature supports that the PAM score is a predictor of many health behaviors, such as costly service utilization of the emergency department, adherence to medication regimens, health maintenance behaviors, and self-management of chronic conditions (Cohen, 2017; Hibbard, 2016). Individuals are classified by levels 1 to 4. Level 1 identifies low-activated individuals and Level 4 identifies the most activated patients. See Fig. 15.1 for a further description of the levels of patient activation described in the PAM.

Level 1	Level 2	Level 3	Level 4
Disengaged and overwhelmed	**Becoming aware, but still struggling**	**Taking action**	**Maintaining behaviors and pushing further**
Individuals are passive and lack confidence. Knowledge is low, goal-orientation is weak, and adherence is poor. Their perspective: "My doctor is in charge of my health."	Individuals have some knowledge, but large gaps remain. They believe health is largely out of their control, but can set simple goals. Their perspective: "I could be doing more."	Individuals have the key facts and are building self-management skills. They strive for best practice behaviors, and are goal-oriented. Their perspective: "I'm part of my health care team."	Individuals have adopted new behaviors, but may struggle in times of stress or change. Maintaining a healthy lifestyle is a key focus. Their perspective: "I'm my own advocate."

Increasing Levels of Activation

Fig. 15.1 Patient Characteristics Based on and Description of Patient Activation Measure (PAM) Scores. (Adapted from Insignia Health (2016). Patient Activation Measure® (PAM®) Survey Levels. Retrieved from http://www.insigniahealth.com/products/pam-survey.)

Over time, it has been shown that highly activated individuals (PAM Levels 3 and 4) are more likely to seek and use information to be advocates for their own health (Hibbard, 2016). They are also more likely to participate in wellness activities like regular exercise, maintaining a healthy diet, and adhering to medical regimens because they consider themselves partners in their own health promotion. Individuals with lower PAM scores (Levels 1 and 2) are more likely to have low confidence in their ability to self-manage and tend to take a more passive approach to their health (Hibbard, 2016). PAM Level 1 and 2 patients are less likely to embrace patient support resources even when offered, and they are more likely to be overwhelmed by stressful situations due to limited problem-solving agility. It's important to remember that individuals can move between levels depending on clinical context, life situations, and efforts made to engage and empower them by the clinical team (McCormack, Thomas, Lewis, & Rudd, 2016).

HEALTH LITERACY AND NUMERACY

Individuals with limited activation in their own care (PAM Level 1 and 2) may struggle more to participate in care decisions because they can't comprehend or use the information being discussed, not because they don't desire to do so. Health literacy is defined as an individual's ability to access, interpret, and understand qualitative data about their health (i.e., delivered without numbers, typically as words or pictures). Conversely, health numeracy is defined as an individual's ability to access, interpret, and understand quantitative data about their health (i.e., delivered with numbers or portraying numbers). Clinicians can gain insight into an individual's problem-solving ability and potential for activation by assessing the person's health literacy and health numeracy levels (Smith, Curtis, O'Conor, Federman, & Wolf, 2015). Health literacy and numeracy, while related, are not interchangeable concepts. When assessing an individual's health *literacy* level, one evaluates a person's ability to access, interpret, and understand qualitative data (i.e., written text) to improve health. Much health information is delivered as numbers (e.g., prescription dosing recommendations, appropriate laboratory values, or target carbohydrate limits for a person with diabetes). Health *numeracy* becomes important when information is given in nontextual formats such as graphs, tables, or raw numbers. Box 15.1 highlights

---

> **BOX 15.1**   **Assessing Health Literacy and Health Numeracy**
>
> Clinicians can gain insight into an individual's problem-solving ability and potential for activation by assessing his or her **health literacy** and **health numeracy** levels. Health literacy and numeracy, while related, are not interchangeable concepts.
> - When assessing an individual's health *literacy* level, a clinician is looking at that person's ability to access, interpret, and understand qualitative data (i.e., written text) to improve health. Health numeracy is therefore that individual's ability to access, interpret, and understand quantitative data (i.e., nontext formats, computational data, graphs, tables).

---

assessment of health literacy and health numeracy. One way of addressing individuals with low health numeracy is to provide infographics that break down numbers and display them as pictures. Examples can be found in the March of Dimes campaign "Healthy Babies Are Worth the Wait," which educates the public about preventing premature birth (see https://www.marchofdimes.org/glue/images/HBWW-Infographic.jpg).

To judge health literacy and numeracy objectively, the Organization for Economic Cooperation and Development created the Program for the International Assessment of Adult Competencies (PIAAC) with the goal of developing a tool to assess and compare the basic literacy and numeracy skills of individuals across the globe (Rampey et al., 2016). Individuals in 24 participating countries were surveyed in 2012, and another nine countries were surveyed in 2014. The PIAAC survey built and expanded upon previous international adult assessments such as the International Adult Literacy Survey and the Adult Literacy and Life Skills Survey (Rampey et al., 2016). The United States participated in data collection during the initial field test of the PIAAC survey in 2010, then began a second round of data collection from 2013 to 2014. A third round of data collection was planned for late 2017. Results from the first two rounds of data collection offer a sobering picture of the health literacy and numeracy of the average American adult.

Participants are scored in the PIAAC survey with "proficiency levels" of 1 to 5, with "below level 1" as the lowest level of problem solving/proficiency, and "level 5" as the highest. In the first two rounds of data collection, only 13% of adults in the United States scored at level

5 for health literacy, with another 13% scoring at level 1 to 4 and 5% scoring "below level 1" (Rampey et al., 2016). Evaluation of health numeracy provides an even more sobering view of patient activation. Only 10% of U.S. adults scored at level 5 for health numeracy, 19% scored at level 1, and 8% scored "below level 1" (Rampey et al., 2016). (See Figs. 15.2 and 15.3 for a more detailed breakdown of the health literacy and numeracy proficiency levels of adults in the United States, respectively.)

STRATEGIES TO IMPROVE HEALTH LITERACY AND NUMERACY

Even adults with limited skills can increase engagement and have better health outcomes if their environment supports the health literacy and numeracy skills that they *do* have. Individuals may be skilled in one, both, or neither of these areas, and different strategies may need to be implemented to support a person across numerous levels of influence. Clinicians and patients can both affect change at the individual, interpersonal, organizational, community, and macro levels of influence (Cohen, 2017). Strategies to address barriers across levels of health literacy and engagement are described in Table 15.1 along with effective and evidence-based exemplars.

At the individual level, factors such as a lack of knowledge of health information and a low value placed on engagement can make it difficult to improve health literacy or numeracy. Using plain language, with no medical jargon, when communicating and offering personalized health education sessions is one type of intervention to address these challenges (McCormack et al., 2016). Interpersonal barriers such as poor communication skills and lack of social support can be addressed with teach-back methods and patient and family support groups. One example of a family support resource is the network of 30 advocacy groups affiliated with the Preemie Parent Alliance (http://www.preemie-parentalliance.org/). They offer evidence-based education, in-person peer support, and navigation help during transitions when fragile infants are discharged from neonatal intensive care units. Another example is provided by an advocacy group to end rare diseases that affect fragile infants such as necrotizing enterocolitis (NEC), one of the 10 leading causes of infant death in the United States (www.necsociety.org, www.morgansfund.com). Evidence reveals that risk for NEC can be reduced significantly by feeding at-risk preemies with breast milk (Herrmann and Carroll, 2014). Groups that are organized around and promote EBPs can vet their information by engaging with clinical and research

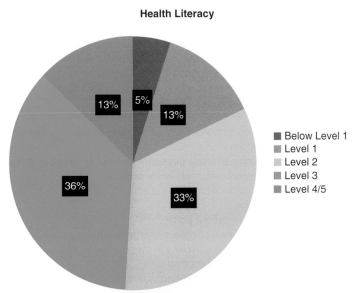

Fig. 15.2 Percentage of Adults at Each Health Literacy Proficiency Level. (Adapted from Centers for Disease Control and Prevention (2016). Understanding literacy & numeracy. Retrieved from https://www.cdc.gov/healthliteracy/learn/understandingliteracy.html.)

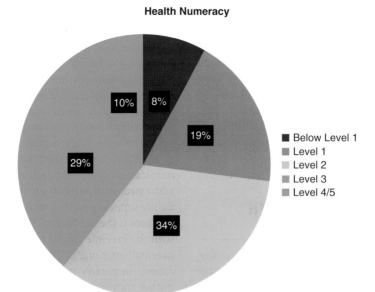

Health Numeracy

- Below Level 1
- Level 1
- Level 2
- Level 3
- Level 4/5

8%
19%
10%
29%
34%

Fig. 15.3 Percentage of Adults at Each Health Numeracy Proficiency Level.

TABLE 15.1	Barriers Against and Strategies for Patient Engagement
Barriers to Engagement	**Strategies That Address Engagement Barrier**
Low health literacy or health numeracy	• Ask patients what they understand about their health. • Educational materials should be understandable at the sixth-grade reading level. • Ask patients to "teach back" what you have taught them. • Ensure decision aids and shared decision-making tools have been shown to be effective in individuals with limited health literacy or numeracy.
Language	• Communicate via certified medical interpreters. • Ensure that educational materials in the patient's own language convey the appropriate meaning after translation.
Values and cultural beliefs	• Ask patients what role they want to play in decision making. If they don't decide or don't want to decide, work with family and those who are perceived to decide to make sure they all understand the health education or condition. • Encourage patients to express their values and cultural beliefs and ask questions. • Education with evaluation in cross-cultural care. • Involve family.
Time constraints	• Include patient-reported outcomes and other measures of engagement in surveys they complete when arriving at the office. • Provide time, opportunity, and safe places for patients to reflect on information and ask questions. • Reduce the need for quick decisions when possible. • Provide evidence-based decision aids and educational materials for them to take home and consider before deciding.
Clinical workflow	• Embed decision aids into patient portal. • Use electronic patient portals to collect information before appointments. • Embed decision guidance for clinicians in their clinical workflow to assist patients in making decisions and learning about their health. • Engage patients after diagnosis, prognosis, and available treatment options have been clarified by the clinical team.
Organizational priority	• Payment models that incentivize shared decision making. • Leadership commitment to patient engagement.

Adapted from Blumenthal-Barby, J. S. (2016). "That's the doctor's job": Overcoming patient reluctance to be involved in medical decision making. *Patient Education and Counseling, 100*(1), 15.

advisory board members, as is the case with the NEC Society. Table 15.2 provides examples of multilevel strategies to improve health literacy and numeracy.

The physical layout of a building and signage, although seemingly unimportant, can have a great effect on the organizational factors of system integration and infrastructure planning and implementation to support health outcomes. Social marketing campaigns can support integration of public health concerns and health care systems when addressing community factors. Finally, macroenvironmental initiatives address adjustments that need to be made in public policy and legal regulations to support improved health literacy and numeracy, such as ongoing health care reforms through the Centers for Medicare and Medicaid Services (Cohen, 2017; Rathert, Mittler, Banerjee, & McDaniel, 2016).

PATIENT ENGAGEMENT STRATEGIES FOR CLINICAL PRACTICE

Health care in the United States today is marked by constant evolution and increasing complexity. No longer is it acceptable to say, "That's how we've always done it." Health care teams are engaged in evidence-based practice and quality improvement initiatives that consistently seek improved methods of caring for patients and optimizing health outcomes. Using a patient activation "lens," we as clinicians need to be able to look at an intervention and ask ourselves:

- Who is the intervention reaching?
- Who is the intervention helping?
- What is the evidence base for this intervention for this population?

The answers to these questions allow practitioners to remain patient-centered, but often unveil barriers that exist and must be addressed before an engagement strategy can be implemented in clinical practice. Barriers to patient engagement are multifactorial in nature, so strategies to overcome them should address this complexity (Rose et al., 2016). For further details on these barriers and strategies to address them, see Table 15.1.

Patient portals are web-based platforms that compile various evidence-based resources for patient engagement, such as decision-making aids, educational materials, and communication applications. They are typically connected to the Electronic Health Record (EHR) used by their providers to communicate health care data to the patient. They are designed to promote patient engagement and self-care. Patient portals can be tailored to the individual needs of a clinical setting and patient population (Kijewski, 2016). Clinics and hospitals may choose to design a patient portal companion website, or can contract for stand-alone portal access. EHRs also may include a patient portal to provide secure messaging and educational information such as the athenaCommunicator feature of the athenaNet electronic health record. Incorporating patient portal access allows primary care practices to achieve patient engagement core measures that are required to meet Stage 2 of Meaningful Use for implementing EHRs (Blumenthal & Tavenner, 2010). Omitting these features can place clinicians at risk for not meeting benchmarks in the Merit-Based Incentive Payment System, a Centers for Medicare and Medicaid Services initiative that became mandatory in early 2017. Additional virtualist skills will be required by interprofessional clinical teams as they increasingly communicate with patients in non–face-to-face encounters. Fickenscher, Kvedar, and Nichols (2018) remind us about the importance of effective collaboration, information sharing across the professions that will require a team model of care delivery.

INDIVIDUAL BARRIERS AGAINST PATIENT ENGAGEMENT

Individual barriers are those that pertain to the intrinsic characteristics and values of the patient or provider. These barriers tie closely to personal traits that determine an individual's activation level, as discussed earlier in this chapter. Barriers such as low health literacy and lack of education can be countered by clinicians with direct patient-provider interactions (McCormack et al., 2016; Smith et al., 2015). Asking patients what they already know and understand, and using teach-back methods to assess that understanding allows patients and providers to enter into conversations with a more-equal knowledge base. Language barriers can be mitigated by using trained interpreters and ensuring that materials are available in a patient's language of preference. Translation also can occur over the phone or be mediated with smartphone- or tablet-based applications such as *MediBabble* (NiteFloat, Inc). Training in cross-cultural care to ensure that providers understand a patient's cultural values and encouraging patients to express those values can illuminate many otherwise missed value discussions (Hibbard, 2016).

TABLE 15.2 Multilevel Strategies to Improve Health Literacy and Numeracy

Level of Influence	Influential Factors	Interventions to Address Limitations	Exemplars
Individual	Health-related knowledge; attitudes/health beliefs; values/preferences for levels of engagement; health literacy skills	• Use of plain language, best practices, and clear communication in written communications • Data visualization to communicate health information (infographics) • Clarify values by asking, "What are you concerned about today?"	U.S. "Safe Sleep" campaign to prevent Sudden Infant Death Syndrome uses the "A-B-C" metaphor to remind all caregivers how to prevent SIDS when they put a baby to sleep: A = alone B = [on the] back C = [in a] crib
Interpersonal	Promote communication skills and leverage social support	• Patient-centered communication • Active listening and teach back • Group health visits, patient and family support groups • Community health workers • Shared decision making	March of Dimes promotes group prenatal care courses to prevent premature birth, especially in states and populations with high premature birth rates. The Mayo Clinic has a well-validated, evidence-based suite of decision aids that are freely available to support shared decision making on topics such as selecting medications for diabetes, hypertension, and cancer treatment.
Organizational	Infrastructure planning and implementation; system integration and coordination	• Staff training, workforce enhancement • Team-based care with care coordination • Physical environment, layout, and signage • Electronic health records that integrate decision support into patient education or shared decision making • Pay-for-performance systems that value prevention and support self-management	Intermountain Healthcare in Utah links patient portals to the electronic and billing systems making patient information visible in one place Kaiser Healthcare locates all services a patient will need in one place to support ease of access. The National Health Service in the U.K. is adapting the PAM to make care more patient-centered and holistic. Based on level of activation, patients are enrolled in different intensities of coaching for prevention and disease management.
Community	Community-based programs; integration of public health and health care systems	• Leverage virtual and physical social networks using targeted marketing campaigns • E-health communication (i.e., applications, patient portals) • Community-based participatory research to adapt patient engagement approach to meet the needs of the target community	MedlinePlus is hosted and curated by the National Library of Medicine to provide evidence-based health information to consumers on a wide variety of topics. Regional library affiliates of the National Library of Medicine are working together to teach professional and lay people about available resources and how to use them.
Macro	Public policy; regulation; legal regulations and initiatives; accountability; reliance on evidence-based policies	• National legislation to promote reimbursement models for Medicare and Medicaid that value quality of care, outcomes, and population-based care. Clinical guidelines are vetted by professional organizations and include specific recommendations.	The Choosing Wisely campaign engages clinicians and consumers to select the best evidence-supported treatments and avoid those that have been shown to be harmful or ineffective. A clearinghouse of active guidelines is available at www. guidelines.gov.

PAM, Patient Activation Measure; *SIDS,* sudden infant death syndrome.
Adapted from McCormack, L., Thomas, V., Lewis, M., & Rudd, R. (2016). Improving low health literacy and patient engagement: A social ecological approach. *Patient Education and Counseling, 100*(1), 10.

CONTEXTUAL BARRIERS AGAINST PATIENT ENGAGEMENT

Contextual barriers are defined as challenges in the environment, health care system, clinical workflow, administrative, and patient care contexts that make engagement more difficult to accomplish (Blumenthal-Barby, 2016). These barriers are often more related to system constraints and, as such, require more resources to resolve them than the individual patient and provider. One barrier cited repeatedly in the literature is a lack of time for patient-provider interactions (Blumenthal-Barby, 2016; Cohen, 2017). Providing adequate time and safe places for patients to reflect on information, such as the time that Provider B gave our patient in the opening chapter scenario, is vital to ensuring that a patient feels like a valued partner in the clinical team. Clinical workflow can be a barrier to patient engagement, if we insist that patients make quick clinical decisions and we don't engage patients throughout the clinical progression, from diagnosis and prognosis to treatment options. Finally, institutional attitudes such as payment models that support shared decision-making interventions can encourage a continued culture of patient-centered care (Blumenthal-Barby, 2016).

SYNTHESIS

Patient-centered care will continue to be a buzzword in the health care industry, encompassing the view that patients should be allowed to decide their own treatment courses with the support of a team of educated and invested health care providers. Proper utilization of evidence-based shared decision-making interventions has the potential to decrease overall health care costs while increasing the quality of health care delivered, which is why federal and organizational support for these programs has grown in recent years. By assessing levels of patient activation and health literacy and numeracy, clinical leaders like you are better able to meet patients "where they are" and engage in productive shared decision making. Using tools such as shared decision-making aids and patient portals can decrease some of the workload of shared decision making for individual clinicians, making it easier to incorporate EBPs into existing clinical settings and patient workflows. What are some areas in your own clinical settings where you can implement some of these practices? What new and novel ways are there to implement patient-centered, evidence-based care in your own clinical practice?

▌ KEY POINTS

- Putting patients at the center of health care decisions is the core of EBP.
- Patient-centered EBP practices are important considerations for clinicians, administrators, educators, and policy leading nurses because of the impact on clinical outcomes, resource utilization, provider and patient satisfaction, and policy.
- Shared decision making is a process by which patients and clinicians partner to make informed decisions to benefit the patient, whether the patient is an individual, family, or community.
- Evidence supports the use of shared decision-making aids that are patient engagement tools.

- Patient engagement tools should reflect the appropriate level of health literacy and health numeracy tailored to meet the needs of a specific patient or patient population.
- Level of patient activation needs to be assessed using tools like the Patient Activation Measure (PAM) to measure an individual's mindset toward being a manager of his or her own health.
- Patient portals aim to be an online strategy to promote patient engagement and self-care.
- Individual and contextual barriers can mitigate against patient engagement and activation, and need to be addressed by clinical leaders and teams through tailored evidence-based strategies that are relevant to a specific patient population.

REFERENCES

Alston, C., Berger, Z., Brownlee, S., Elwyn, G., Jr., F. J. F., Hall, L. K., & Henderson, D. (2014). Shared decision-making strategies for best care: patient decision aids. *IOM Roundtable on Value & Science-Driven Health Care: Learning Health System Series*. Retrieved from http://www.iom.edu/Global/Perspectives/2014/SDM-forBestCare.aspx?utm_source=Hootsuite&utm_medium=Dashboard&utm_campaign=SentviaHootsuite.

Blumenthal, D., & Tavenner, M. (2010). The "Meaningful Use" regulation for Electronic Health Records. *New England Journal of Medicine*, 363(6), 501–504.

Blumenthal-Barby, J. S. (2016). "That's the doctors job": Overcoming patient reluctance to be involved in medical decision making. *Patient Education & Counseling*, 100(1), 14–17.

Cohen, M. D. (2017). Engaging patients in understanding and using evidence to inform shared decision making. *Patient Education & Counseling*, 100(1), 2–3.

Fickenscher, K., Kvedar, J., & Nichols, J. (2018). Beyond the: Creating capability in the health care team. *Health Affairs Blog*, 1–12.

Herrmann, K., & Carroll, K. (2014). An exclusively human milk diet reduces necrotizing enterocolitis. *Breastfeeding Medicine*, 9(4), 184–190.

Hibbard, J. H. (2016). Patient activation and the use of information to support informed health decisions. *Patient Education & Counseling*, 100(1), 5–7.

Higgins, T., Larson, E., & Schnall, R. (2016). Unraveling the meaning of patient engagement: A concept analysis. *Patient Education & Counseling*, 100(1), 30–36.

Kijewski, A. (2016). *Dissemination of patient decision-making aids via a web-based platform* (Doctor of Nursing Practice) Tucson: University of Arizona. Retrieved from http://arizona.openrepository.com/arizona/bitstream/10150/621453/1/azu_etd_14868_sip1_m.pdf.

McCormack, L., Thomas, V., Lewis, M. A., & Rudd, R. (2016). Improving low health literacy and patient engagement: A social ecological approach. *Patient Education & Counseling*, 100(1), 8–13.

Patient-Centered Outcomes Research Institute. (2012). National priorities for research and research agenda [Press release]. Retrieved from http://www.pcori.org/sites/default/files/PCORI-National-Priorities-and-Research-Agenda.pdf.

Rampey, B. D., Finnegan, R., Goodman, M., Mohadjer, L., Krenzke, T., Hogan, J., et al. (2016). *Skills of U.S. Unemployed, Young, and Older Adults in Sharper Focus: Results from the Program for the International Assessment of Adult Competencies (PIAAC) 2012/2014: First Look* (NCES 2016039REV). National Center for Education Statistics. Retrieved from https://nces.ed.gov/pubsearch/pubsinfo.asp?pubid=2016039rev.

Rathert, C., Mittler, J. N., Banerjee, S., & McDaniel, J. (2016). Patient-centered communication in the era of electronic health records: What does the evidence say? *Patient Education & Counseling*, 100(1), 50–64.

Rose, A., Rosewilliam, S., & Soundy, A. (2016). Shared decision making within goal setting in rehabilitation settings: A systematic review. *Patient Education & Counseling*, 100(1), 65–75.

Smith, S. G., Curtis, L. M., O'Conor, R., Federman, A. D., & Wolf, M. S. (2015). ABCs or 123s? The independent contributions of literacy and numeracy skills on health task performance among older adults. *Patient Education & Counseling*, 98(8), 991–997.

Street, R. L., Jr., Volk, R. J., Lowenstein, L., & Michael Fordis, C., Jr. (2017). Engaging patients in the uptake, understanding, and use of evidence: Addressing barriers and facilitators of successful engagement. *Patient Education & Counseling*, 100(1), 4.

Evaluation of Evidence-Based Practice

Marita G. Titler, Barbara R. Medvec

LEARNING OUTCOMES

After reading this chapter, you should be able to do the following:

- Summarize the purpose of evaluating the impact of implementing evidence-based practices (EBPs).
- Select process and outcome measures to use in evaluation.
- Describe the common method used for evaluation.

- Summarize approaches to evaluate the impact of EBP implementation on cost.
- Apply principles of quality improvement (see Chapter 11) in the collection, analysis, and display of evaluation data.
- Synthesize key elements of evaluation summaries designed for key stakeholders.

KEY TERMS

Evaluation

Fiscal outcomes

Outcome measures

Process measures

INTRODUCTION

As illustrated in the Iowa Model (see Fig. 1.2), evaluation of implementing evidence-based practices (EBPs) is essential to illustrate the impact on processes and outcomes of care (see Chapter 2). **Evaluation** is a structured approach to evaluating the impact of EBPs when implemented in practice. Evaluation should be included as a key part of piloting the changes in practice (see Chapter 14) and when the EBPs are being extended to additional patient care areas. The purpose of evaluation is to collect and analyze data from the practice setting to determine whether the EBPs should be retained, modified, or eliminated. Evaluation is essential because

outcomes achieved in a controlled environment when an investigator is implementing a study protocol with a homogenous sample of subjects (conduct of research efficacy) may not result in similar outcomes (implementation effectiveness) when the EBPs are implemented in a practice setting by multiple clinicians for a heterogenous patient population (see Chapter 6). The key to effective evaluation is to demonstrate that the EBPs that are implemented improve the quality of care and do not bring harm to the patients. The steps of evaluation are summarized in Box 16.1. You will want to have a good understanding of quality improvement (QI) (see Chapter 11) as a basis for evaluation.

BOX 16.1 Steps of Evaluation for Evidence-Based Practice

1. Identify process and outcome variables of interest.
   Example: Process variable—Patients will have a fall risk assessment every 12 hours.
   Outcome variables—Fall rates, fall injury rates, severity of fall injuries
2. Determine methods and frequency of data collection.
   Example: Process variable—Chart audit of all patients on [name unit] 1 day a month.
   Outcome variable—Calculated by month by quality improvement program
3. Determine number of baseline and follow-up patients needed for each measure as appropriate.
4. Design data collection forms.
   Example: Process chart audit abstraction form for fall risk assessment
   Risk or incident reports standardized in the organization for adverse events such as falls
5. Establish content validity of data collection forms.
6. Train data collectors.
7. Assess interrater reliability of data collectors.
8. Collect data at specified intervals.
9. Provide staff regular feedback of measures (e.g., every 3 months) to illustrate progress in achieving the practice change.
10. Use data to assist staff in modifying or integrating the evidence-based practice change.
11. Provide final evaluation to staff and senior executives.
12. Write final evaluation report.

EBP TIP

EBP evaluation is a type of quality improvement, not conduct of research. Refrain from turning the evaluation of EBPs into a study (conduct of research). It is not necessary to have a simultaneous comparison group, calculate a sample size, or randomly select subjects; all are research methods used in the conduct of research but not necessary in EBP evaluation.

METHODS FOR EVALUATION

A common approach used for evaluation is a prospective pre-post implementation design. For example, Leavitt (2017) (see Appendix D) used a pre-post implementation approach to evaluate improvements in exercise prescribing in a free health clinic. It is important that baseline measures be collected before implementation to compare with the same measures at post-implementation (Titler et al., 2016). Depending on the size of the practice(s)

and length of implementation, you also may want to collect and analyze evaluation data during implementation to share with staff who are implementing the practice change(s). To promote sustainability of the EBPs, you also should plan to evaluate at strategic time points after implementation (e.g., every 3 months) and include selected evaluation metrics in your QI program.

WHAT TO MEASURE

Evaluation must include process and outcome measures. Process measures are derived from the "I" component of PICO, the EBP intervention (see Chapters 3 and 6). Process of care measures are designed to evaluate staff's use of the EBPs as detailed in the local EBP standard. They measure whether the EBPs demonstrated to benefit patients are followed correctly. Examples of process measures are:

- Percent of patient days in which fall risk was assessed every 12 hours (Titler et al., 2016)
- Use of nonpharmacologic pain management interventions (DeVore et al., 2017)
- Delivery of an educational brochure to parents of 11- and 12-year-old girls regarding human papillomavirus (HPV) and HPV vaccine (Cassidy et al., 2014)
- Application of a polyethylene bag for thermal management (decrease in heat loss) of very low birth weight infants immediately after birth (Godfrey et al., 2013)

QI CHECKPOINT
Process Measures

When selecting process measures, think about the EBP recommendations, what practices should be changing, and the key EBPs that need to be followed to obtain the desired outcomes. Were clinicians correctly carrying out the EBPs that are embedded in the practice standard?

Outcome measures are those projected to change as a result of implementing the EBPs, the "O" component of the PICO (see Chapters 3 and 6). Outcome measures are used to evaluate whether implementation of the selected EBPs is resulting in improvements in health outcomes, such as decreasing falls with injuries. Outcome measures do not reflect care processes but the actual results of care delivered on patient outcomes (see Chapter 11). Outcome measures may include not only patient outcomes, but also clinician outcomes such as improvement in staff knowledge (Leung et al., 2014), and fiscal outcomes such as cost reductions (Stenger et al., 2009). Examples of outcome measures are:

- Fall rates and severity of fall injuries (Titler et al., 2016)
- Patient satisfaction with pain management (Devore et al., 2017)
- Completion of the 3-dose series of HPV vaccine (Cassidy et al., 2014)
- Neotnatal intensive care unit admission rectal temperatures of premature infants (Godfrey et al., 2013)
- Improvement in knowledge regarding breastfeeding practices (Ullman & Fisher, 2017).

QI CHECKPOINT

Outcome Measures

Measuring outcomes is essential to evaluating whether the implementation of the EBPs results in outcomes similar to those in the studies that formed the basis of your EBP standard. A note of caution, however, is that measuring outcomes alone without also measuring process of care is not recommended. Improving outcomes requires improvement of care processes. When outcomes do not improve, there is a tendency to jump to the conclusion that EBPs are not "working" (achieving the desired outcomes). In reality, there may be too much variability in implementation of the EBPs (process measures) and thus the impact on outcomes may be limited. You will not know this if you do not measure both processes of care and outcomes.

All measures, both process and outcomes, require clear conceptual and operational definitions for calculations of the measures. Examples are provided in Table 16.1 (Godfrey et al., 2013; Titler et al., 2016).

A question often raised with evaluation of EBPs is how much data will be needed to evaluate the practice change. There is no one right answer. The preferred number of patients (N), patient days, or ambulatory visits is somewhat dependent on:

- Nature of the practice setting
- Type of EBP being implemented
- Size of the patient population affected by the practice change

For example, in evaluating HPV vaccine rates (outcome measure), the number of pediatric visits of 11- and 12-year-old girls may be 250 per year (about 21 per month). You will need to decide how many visits to assess, pre- and post-implementation. You may decide to evaluate about half of the 21 visits per month for 3 months pre- and 3 months post-implementation. This should provide a reasonable number to examine changes in trends over time for this outcome measure. This is not a research study, therefore you do not need to conduct a power calculation or do random assignment. Evaluation of EBPs examines clinically meaningful changes in process and outcomes. Ullman et al. (2017) used a convenience sample of 24 nurses to assess improvements in knowledge about breastfeeding and self-reported comfort level in delivering breastfeeding practices (see Appendix E). Leavitt (2017) audited 52 patient records pre-implementation and 42 records post-implementation to evaluate improvements in provider exercise prescribing practices for patients seen in a free health clinic (see Appendix D).

FISCAL OUTCOMES

Fiscal outcomes are estimated health care costs that may be affected by implementing EBPs. Fiscal outcomes can be addressed in three ways. The first is evaluating the potential cost savings of an EBP using selected outcome measures such as additional costs of care delivery associated with adverse events (e.g., fall injuries). For example, the average cost of a nonfatal fall injury during hospitalization is estimated at $29,562 (Burns et al., 2016). The annual cost savings of implementing evidence-based fall prevention interventions can be calculated by multiplying the number of reductions in fall injuries (n = 9/year) by $29,562 for an estimated cost savings of $266,058 annually. Furthermore, injuries associated with adverse events such as falls are not reimbursed by the Centers for Medicare & Medicaid Services (CMS). This provides an additional cost savings depending on the nature of the injury.

A second approach focuses on cost reductions with use of EBPs. Cost reductions focus on actual reduction in delivery of care. For example, the average direct cost of implementing EB acute pain management practices for older adults hospitalized with a hip fracture was $17,714 (Brooks et al., 2009; Titler et al., 2009). Use of the EB acute pain management practices reduced the cost of an average inpatient stay by about $1500/patient. Given this estimated cost reduction, it would only take the treatment of 12 patients with acute pain for the EB acute pain management practices to reduce hospital costs. Therefore, a hospital treating 100 older adults with acute hip fracture could expect an overall *net* cost reduction of $132,286 [$150,000 – $17,714] from implementing the EB acute pain management practices (Brooks et al., 2009)

TABLE 16.1	**Examples of Process and Outcome Measures**		
Outcome Measures	**Conceptual Definition**	**Operational Definition**	**Calculation**
Fall rates	Number of patient falls, defined as unplanned descent to the floor, on a designated unit	Number of falls per 1000 patient days	Number of falls X 1000 divided by number of inpatient days
Severity of fall injury	Minor, moderate, major or death	Minor: Needs application of dressing, ice, cleaning of wound, limb elevation or topical medicine. Moderate: Results in suturing, steri-strips, fracture or splinting. Major: results in surgery, casting, or traction. Death: Death as a result of fall.	For fall events, proportion in each category represented as a percent
NICU admission temperature	Number of NICU admissions with hypothermic, normothermic, and hyperthermic rectal temperatures	Normal temperature 36.5–37.5; Hypothermic <36.5; Hyperthermic >37.5. Proportion of NICU admissions with normothermia, hypothermia, hyperthermia.	Number of normothermic infants upon admission to NICU divided by total number of NICU admissions
Nurses' knowledge regarding pain management	Pre- and post-test scores on knowledge assessment test regarding pain management via an educational test	Number/percent of correct answers	For each nurse, the number of correct responses divided by the number of test items
Process Measures	**Conceptual Definition**	**Operational Definition**	**Calculation**
Delivery of fall prevention interventions targeted to patient-specific risk factor	Frequency and type of fall prevention interventions implemented to mitigate a patient-specific fall risk factor	Delivery of a fall prevention intervention targeted to a specified type of risk factor (e.g., mobility, elimination) for each patient day in which the risk factor was present	Rate per 100 patient days: Number of times per 100 patient days when a fall prevention intervention was implemented to mitigate a specific type of risk. Example: Of the 1333 patient days of mobility risk factors, fall prevention interventions targeted to mobility were delivered 88/100 patient days.
Rate of applying the polyethylene bag for thermal management (decrease heat loss) to very low birth weight infants immediately after birth	For each premature birth, the number of times the polyethylene bag for thermal management is applied	Application of the polyethylene bag for thermal management for each premature delivery	Number of infants with application of the polyethylene bag divided by the number of premature births. Example: Out of 50 premature deliveries, the polyethylene bag was applied 44 times. 44/50 = .88

NICU, Neonatal intensive care unit.

Cost benefit is evaluating the benefits of an EB intervention on outcomes in relation to the cost of delivering the EB intervention. This requires that the cost of delivering the EBPs is compared with the overall benefits in the face of no cost savings or cost reductions. For example, the FOCUS Program is an EB, dyadic, psycho-educational intervention that improves outcomes of cancer patients and their caregivers (Dockham et al., 2016; Titler et al., 2017). The average estimated costs for oversight and delivery of the FOCUS program in Cancer Support Communities (CSCs) were $669.45 for one-five session program (Titler et al., 2017). Because FOCUS is delivered in a group format of 3 to 4 dyads per group, estimated cost per dyad was $168.00, assuming 4 dyads per group. Delivery of FOCUS in a group format at CSC sites improved overall quality of life, emotional and functional well being, emotional distress, perceived benefits of experiencing cancer, and level of confidence in managing it (Dockham et al., 2016; Titler et al., 2017). Caregivers and patients were highly satisfied with the program and more than 85% reported that the program did not duplicate services provided at their cancer treatment centers. More than 90% of the patients and caregivers reported that they would recommend the program to others facing cancer (Titler et al., 2017). Thus, in this example of cost-benefit analysis, directors of CSC affiliate sites will need to consider whether the benefits of the FOCUS program outweigh the costs before offering the FOCUS program in their communities.

> **IPE TIP**
>
> When evaluating the cost benefit of making a practice change, you, as a team leader, need to think "out of the box." That kind of decision often involves team members who are from the finance department of your organization. If the practice change involves supplies or equipment, representatives from the purchasing department also may need to be included in evaluating the cost benefit of making a practice change.

DATA SOURCES

Sources for process and outcome data can include staff and/or patient self-reports, medical records, or clinical observations. When collecting data from these sources, it is important that the data collection tools are user-friendly, short, concise, and easy to complete, and have content validity. The focus must be on collecting the most-essential data. Those responsible for collecting evaluative data must be trained on data collection methods and be assessed for interrater reliability to ensure consistency and fidelity to the data collection methods (see Chapter 11). It is our experience that individuals who have participated in implementing the protocol can be very helpful in evaluation by collecting data, providing timely feedback to staff, and helping staff overcome barriers encountered when implementing the changes in practice.

Other data sources to consider are those available as part of the QI or infection control programs in your practice setting for both ambulatory and acute care. For example, if you are implementing EBPs to decrease catheter-associated urinary tract infections (CAUTIs), you will want to work with your Infection Control Department to determine whether they collect measures you can use for your project. Most health care organizations have data available on patient satisfaction, falls, fall risk assessment, infection rates, medication errors, unplanned readmissions, and visits to the emergency room. Other data commonly available particularly for ambulatory care include blood pressure control, body mass index, and vaccination rates (e.g., flu and pneumococcal vaccines). Also consider using core measures associated with the CMS value-based purchasing programs. For example, the CMS core measures for primary care include breast and colorectal cancer screening, comprehensive diabetes care (e.g., HgbA1c, foot examination), and medication reconciliation. We recommend that as part of your action planning (see Chapter 12), you meet early in the planning process with individuals responsible for these data to determine what data are available and how you might use them in your evaluation.

> **EBP TIP**
>
> Health care organizations have multiple measures that are routinely used to improve quality of care. You can gain efficiencies in evaluation by meeting with members of the health care system responsible for the variety of measures. For example, you will want to meet with the person(s) responsible for core measures required by Centers for Medicare & Medicaid Services and determine which measures may be useful for your evaluation. If your organization contributes to national quality improvement (QI) data sets such as the National Database of Nursing Quality Indicators, it is important to understand the QI measures your organization reports and their data definitions.

ANALYSIS AND DISPLAY OF DATA

Evaluation measures are analyzed by comparing measures from pre- to post-implementation. Descriptive statistics such as frequencies, means, and rates commonly are used in the analyses. Depending on the type of data you use, tests of differences such as *t*-tests or chi-square can be employed to examine differences from pre- to post-implementation (Chapter 10). When evaluation measures are collected at multiple time points before, during, and after implementation, use of statistical process control charts may be most useful to examine trends over time (see Chapter 11).

An important component of evaluation is deciding how to display measures to illustrate impact on quality of care and cost. You will need to decide:

1) How data will be aggregated in relation to the frequency of data collection
2) The time period for display of evaluation measures (e.g., every week, month, or quarter)
3) How data will be displayed (e.g., numbers, bar charts, statistical process control charts).

For example, you may be reviewing 10 medical records per week to evaluate whether fall risk assessments are done at least every 12 hours (process measure = percent of patients with fall risk completed every 12 hours). The data may be aggregated to 1 month for data display using run charts or statistical process control charts (Carey & Lloyd, 2001) (see Chapter 11). Similarly, the QI program may standardize reporting of fall rates to every quarter, but you are interested in displaying fall rates by month for your project. Discuss this with your QI department personnel; it is likely they will be able to supply fall rates per month.

Selection of methods for display of your evaluation data is important to 1) understand if there is a wide variation in the processes or outcomes of care, and 2) determine whether the measures are moving care in the desired direction over time. Achieving the desired outcomes requires decreasing variability in processes and shifting the process in the desired direction (changing the mean or median) (see Chapter 11). For example,

are all staff nurses on the designated units consistently implementing the EBPs for prevention of catheter associated urinary track infections (CAUTIs) in adult patients with indwelling urinary catheters? If the answer is yes, the decreased variability should be associated with a decrease in CAUTIs in this patient population. The EBP Evaluation Form in Table 16.2 and the associated guideline in Box 16.2 can be used to facilitate evaluation activities.

You and your team will want to decide on methods and frequency for sharing with your clinicians the reports of process and outcome measures. Discussing these reports with your clinicians will support an understanding of how well their efforts to improve care and patient outcomes are progressing throughout the implementation process (Ivers et al., 2014). Discussions provide a forum for recognizing clinicians' efforts to improve care based on evidence and address challenges encountered with implementation. These reports also should be shared with your organizational leaders and other key stakeholder groups every 3 to 6 months.

EVALUATION SUMMARY FOR KEY STAKEHOLDERS

A summary report of your EBP work should be written for your executive leaders and QI program. Essential elements of the report include:

- Project team members and team leader
- Purpose of the EBP project
- Synthesis of the evidence with practice recommendations
- EB practice standard that was implemented
- Units, clinics, or practices in which the EBPs were implemented
- Strategies used for implementation
- Impact on quality of care (processes of care, outcomes)
- Lessons learned

The report should be brief—about 2 to 3 pages. Impact on quality of care can be appended to the report to illustrate improvements using statistical process control charts (see Chapter 11). A template for reporting is in Fig. 16.1.

TABLE 16.2   Evaluation of Evidence-Based Practice Form

Purpose of the EBP project:

Evaluation Focus:

Measures/ metrics (Process, Outcome, Knowledge, Fiscal)	Operational Definition	Data Source	Frequency of Data Collection	Aggregate Data Every _____ by time (e.g., month) _____ variable (e.g., unit; clinic; patient population)	Data Feedback to _____ (who) every _____ (frequency)	Modifications in Practice	Other Actions	Frequency of Submission to Quality Improvement
Process:								
Patient Outcomes:								
Clinician Knowledge:								
Fiscal Outcomes:								

BOX 16.2   Guidelines for the EBP Evaluation Form in Table 16.2

- Measures/metrics—This column should include process, outcome, and knowledge measures. Serious consideration also should be given to including fiscal outcomes. Be selective of the indicators you choose. Group indicators into categories: Process, Outcome, Knowledge, and Cost.
- Be clear about the operational definition of each metric—how will you measure each. If you are using a rate (e.g., fall rate), define the numerator and denominator. See Table 16.1 for examples.
- Define the data source for each indicator. If you need to collect data, the form should include directions specific enough for each individual collecting information to do so in the same manner.

- Define how frequently each indicator will be collected. Examples are daily for 1 week per month or one day per month for 6 months. Include dates.
- Define how data will be aggregated. For example, data collected daily for 1 week per month could be aggregated by day (e.g., Monday, Tuesday, Wednesday...) over 3 months for each unit.
- Define who will receive the data and frequency.
- Define what modifications are needed in practice, if any, and what additional actions are needed. This should include continuing to monitor specified indicators over time.
- Define frequency of time submitting a report to quality improvement program (e.g., annually; every 6 months).

Directions: The following template is a guide to assist you with the report of your EBP work. It should be customized to your project.

Title of the Project Here
Date of the Report Here

Purpose of the EBP project: [Describe the purpose of the EBP project guided by your PICO]

Rationale: [Describe the rationale for this work. What is the clinical problem to be addressed by this work? Include QI data to support the work if available]

Team Leader(s): [Names, credentials and titles of the leader or co-leaders of the project]

Team Member(s) [Names, credentials, and titles of the team members]

Patient Population: [Describe the nature of the patient population that is the focus of your project]

Practice Sites: [Name the units, clinics, or other practice sites that were the focus of the project. Names, and credentials of the nurse managers of practice sites]

Disciplines involved in the practice change: [Types of clinicians involved in the EBP project such as physicians, nurses, respiratory therapists etc.]

Time Frame: Summarize the time frame for the project. [May include critique and synthesis of the evidence (dates); formulation and approval of EBP standard (dates); implementation (dates); evaluation (dates)]

Synthesis of the Evidence and Practice Recommendations: [Describe in one to two paragraphs the synthesis of the evidence that supported the project. Set forth practice recommendations used to formulate the EBP standard. Evidence tables can be appended to this report]

EBP Standard and Approval Process: [Describe the EBP standard that was implemented and the governance committee(s) that approved the standard. The EBP standard can be appended to this report]

Implementation Strategies: [List and briefly describe the strategies used for implementation. Some are listed under this section as prompts. Only include those that you used for implementation]

Fig. 16.1 Template for Reporting an EBP Project to Key Stakeholders

- Education of clinicians – [describe who was educated, the educational methods used, and the focus of the education.]

- Performance gap assessment – [describe the baseline data that illustrated a gap between the practice and the evidence. Describe how these data were shared with clinicians]

- Clinical decision support such as quick reference guides, pocket cards, or algorithms. Include any decision support or reminders added to the EHR [briefly describe each, may append copies of each]

- Key reminders or messages at the point of care delivery such as posters or infographics

- Opinion leadership – [Names of opinion leaders and their role]

- Change champions – [Names and their role]

- Educational outreach (academic detailing) – [Describe how this was done and by who (e.g. rounds made on units every two weeks by the NAME)]

- Audit and feedback – [Describe what practices were audited, how the data were shared with clinicians (e.g., posters, etc.), and how often it was shared (e.g., every 6 weeks over 6 months).

- Piloting – [If the change in practice was piloted, describe the practice site and length of the pilot as well as lessons learned and any revisions made in the EBP standard and/or implementation strategies]

- Meetings – [Describe frequency of meetings of the team]

- Engagement of key leaders – [Describe the names and roles of key organizational leaders who you met with to garner initial support and methods used to keep them appraised of your work. Address the involvement and support of nurse managers of the practice sites where the EBPs were implemented]

- Modification of documentation systems – [Describe any modifications made to the clinical documentation system. If no changes were made but you have recommendations for modification of the documentation system, include them here]

- Recognition and rewards – [Describe activities used to recognize and reward staff]

Evaluation: [List the process and outcome measures used for evaluation. Include the definitions of each. Summarize the impact on each measure from pre- to post-implementation. Append data displays (e.g., statistical process control charts, run charts) and indicate the beginning and end of the implementation phase.]

Sustainability: [Indicate what measures will be integrated into QI program and what measures are taken to assure sustained improvements in practice]

Lessons Learned: [Briefly describe the lessons learned and how these lessons may be applied to future implementation of EBPs]

Plans for Dissemination: [Describe plans for presentations at conferences and/or publications. List any presentations that have occurred to date]

Reference List: [Provide a list of references as an appendix]

Fig. 16.1, cont'd

SYNTHESIS

Evaluation is essential to demonstrate the impact of EBP implementation on processes of care and patient outcomes. It is imperative that you use both process and outcome measures in the evaluation. Standardizing data definitions of measures is required to compare measures over time and across different units of practice. You should include fiscal outcomes as part of evaluation when possible. Most evaluation data are analyzed using descriptive statistics. A summary of evaluation

is warranted and should be designed based on the key stakeholder groups who will receive the report.

EBP TIP

Evaluation demonstrates the impact of your work on improving quality of care. It is essential to illustrate how your work improves patient outcomes, addresses cost, and supports strategic initiatives such as meeting national benchmarks and Centers for Medicare & Medicaid Services core measures.

■ KEY POINTS

- Evaluation is a structured approach to evaluate the impact of implementing EBPs on process and outcomes.
- A common approach used for evaluation is a prospective pre-post implementation design.
- Evaluation must include both process and outcome measures.
- Process measures reflect staff's use of the EBPs and whether the EBPs demonstrated to benefit patients are followed correctly.
- When selecting process measures, think about the EBP recommendations, what practices should be changing, and the key EBPs that need to be followed to get the desired outcomes.
- Outcome measures are used to evaluate whether use of the selected EBPs results in improvements in patient outcomes.

- Outcome measures also may include clinician outcomes such as improvement in knowledge, and fiscal outcomes such as cost reductions.
- Fiscal outcomes may include cost savings, cost reductions, and cost-benefit.
- Data sources for evaluation measures include staff and/or patient self-reports, medical records, clinical observations, and those available in your QI program (e.g., fall rates, patient satisfaction).
- Descriptive statistics such as frequencies, means, or rates are commonly used in the analyses.
- An important component of evaluation is deciding how to display measures to illustrate impact on processes and outcomes.
- An evaluation summary report is important to share with key stakeholders.

REFERENCES

Brooks, J., Titler, M. G., Ardery, G., & Herr, K. (2009). The effect of evidence-based acute pain management practices on inpatient costs. *Health Services Research, 44*(1), 245–263.

Burns, E. R., Stevens, J. A., & Lee, R. (2016). The direct costs of fatal and non-fatal falls among older adults – United States. *Journal of Safety Research, 58*, 99–103.

Cassidy, B., Braxter, B., Charron-Prochownik, D., & Schlenk, E. (2014). A quality improvement initiative to increase HPV vaccine rates using and educational and reminder strategy with parents of preteen girls. *Journal of Pediatric Health Care, 28*(2), 155–164.

DeVore, J., Clontz, A., Ren, D., Cairns, L., & Beach, M. (2017). Improving patient satisfaction with better pain management in hospitalized patients. *The Journal of Nurse Practitioners, 13*(1), 23–27.

Dockham, B., Schafenacker, A., Yoon, H., Ronis, D. L., Kershaw, T., Titler, M. G., et al. (2016). Implementation of a psychoeducational program for cancer survivors and family caregivers at a cancer support community affiliate: a pilot effectiveness study. *Cancer Nursing, 39*(3), 169–180.

Godfrey, K., Nativio, D., Bender, C. V., & Schlenk, E. A. (2013). Occlusive bags to prevent hypothermia in premature infants. *Advances in Neonatal Care, 13*(5), 311–316.

Ivers, N. M., Sales, A., Colquhoun, H., Michie, S., Foy, R., Francis, J. J., et al. (2014). No more business as usual with audit and feedback interventions: towards an agenda for a reinvigorated intervention. *Implementation Science, 9*, 14–22.

Leavitt, P. T. (2017). Improving exercise prescribing in rural New England free clinic. *Journal for Nurse Practitioners, 13*(1), 29–33.

Leung, L., Trevena, L., & Waters, D. (2014). Systematic review of instruments for measuring nurses' knowledge, skill and attitudes for evidence-based practice. *Journal of Advanced Nursing, 70*, 2181–2195.

Stenger, K., Montgomery, L. A., & Briesemeister, E. (2009). Creating a culture of change through implementation of a safe patient handling program. *Critical Care Clinics Of North America, 21*(4), 595.

Titler, M. G., Conlon, P., Reynolds, M. A., Ripley, R., Tsodikov, A., Wilson, D. S., et al. (2016). The effect of a translating research into practice intervention to promote use of evidence-based fall prevention interventions in hospitalized adults: a prospective pre-post implementation study in the U.S. *Applied Nursing Research, 31*, 52–59.

Titler, M. G., Herr, K., Brooks, J., Xie, X.-J., Ardery, G., Schilling, M., et al. (2009). Translating research into practice intervention improves management of acute pain in older hip fracture patients. *Health Services Research, 44*(1), 264–287.

Titler, M. G., Visovatti, M., Shuman, C., Ellis, K. R., Banerjee, T., Dockham, B., et al. (2017). Effectiveness of implementing a dyadic psychoeducational intervention for cancer patients and family caregivers. *Supportive Care in Cancer, 25*(11), 3395–3406.

Ullman, F. M., & Fisher, M. (2017). Application of the EBP process: maximizing lactation support with minimal education. *Journal of Pediatric Nursing, 33*, 97–100.

17

Dissemination

Carl Kirton

LEARNING OUTCOMES

After reading this chapter, you should be able to do the following:

- Apply the principles of dissemination in sharing evidence-based practice projects.
- Compare and contrast types of dissemination and advantages of each type.

- Differentiate between traditional and nontraditional dissemination methods.
- Use the RE-AIM framework to guide inclusion of essential components in dissemination reports.

KEY TERMS

Active dissemination

Dissemination

Implementation fidelity

Passive dissemination

Sustainability

INTRODUCTION

Communicating and disseminating the results of an evidence-based practice (EBP) change is an important phase of the Iowa Model of EBP (see Chapters 1 and 2). As a clinical leader, you may have to disseminate your results to the staff nurses on a nursing unit or interprofessional colleagues on a Quality Improvement Council. You may be asked to present your findings at a local or national conference or prepare your findings for journal publication. The purpose of this chapter is to apply principles of dissemination for sharing your EBP project with the professional community and internal stakeholder groups.

Dissemination is the act of widely spreading information or ideas to many individuals. In health care, dissemination is the purposive distribution of information and intervention materials to a specific public health or clinical practice audience. The intent is to spread information and the associated evidence-based interventions (Marín-González, Malmusi, Camprubí, & Borrell, 2016). Dissemination is defined for our

purposes as the spreading of the methods and results of an EBP project to potential relevant audiences such as the nursing staff, interprofessional clinical team, academic community, patients, or policymakers. The intent is to spread the EBPs, the methods for implementation, and the impact on care delivery—both process and outcomes. Communicating the results of your work is an important part of EBP. Widespread dissemination of your EBP project can assist others in considering whether to use all or part of your project in their practice settings. Sharing your work engages others to help advance clinical practice and optimize patient care. You will want to incorporate dissemination into your action plan (see Chapter 12) and your key stakeholder summary (see Chapter 16, Fig. 16.1). Research on dissemination provides insights on how to package, transmit, and share your EBP work with other professionals nationally and with key stakeholders locally (U.S. Dept. of Health and Human Services Program announcement number PAR-10–038. Retrieved from http://grants.nih.gov/grants/guide/pa-files/PAR-10–038.html. 2017, n.d.)

PRINCIPLES OF DISSEMINATION

Principles of dissemination are important to guiding your plans for sharing your EBP project. These include considering the following:

- The intended audience
- The primary objective(s) of dissemination
- Types of dissemination

INTENDED AUDIENCE

As you analyze your evaluation data (see Chapter 16), you will want to reflect on who needs to be informed about your work—both internal and external audiences. For example, internal audiences include clinicians (nurses, physicians, clinical pharmacists, social workers) where the EBPs were implemented; leaders such as nurse managers, chairs of service lines, chief nurse executives, chief medical officers, chief executive officers; and selected governance councils or committees such as the organization and nursing department Quality Improvement Committee. External audiences to consider are clinicians within your geographical region, members of national professional societies, and public policymakers. Examples include professional societies (e.g., Sigma Theta Tau International), specialty organizations (e.g., Oncology Nursing Society), interdisciplinary meetings (e.g., American Geriatric Society Annual Conference), and regional research meetings (e.g., Midwestern Nursing Research Society [MNRS] annual conference). It is important to identify the intended audience because objectives, methods, and venues for dissemination need to be tailored to the intended audience. For example, busy clinical leaders in your organization are more likely to read short two-page executive summaries with details appended rather than a 15-page project report.

PRIMARY OBJECTIVE(S) OF DISSEMINATION

After identification of the intended audience, you and your team will want to determine the primary objectives for disseminating information to the group. For example, objectives for dissemination to staff nurses on the unit where the EBPs are implemented may be to illustrate how their contributions have improved processes of care delivery and outcomes, and to discuss strategies for ongoing sustainability of the EB practice improvements. In contrast, an objective for dissemination

to key senior leaders may be to illustrate improvements in both quality and cost. In considering your audience, identify the one or two key messages and lessons learned that you want to convey. It is important for you and your team to discuss the primary objectives(s) for dissemination to each specified audience, as this will guide the key messages that you want to convey. Essential elements to consider in your EBP project reports are discussed in a subsequent section of this chapter.

TYPES OF DISSEMINATION

Dissemination methods have conceptually been categorized as passive and active. Passive dissemination is a one-way communication process such as publishing or posting information with the expectation that the intended audience will access and use the information. Passive dissemination is not as effective as active dissemination, which is real-time interaction with the intended audience to impart key messages or information (Grimshaw et al., 2001; Grimshaw et al., 2004). In active dissemination, bidirectional communication and multiple conversations are used to discuss EBPs and rationale for their use.

Passive dissemination is popular and generally inexpensive in terms of material cost and requires a minimal amount of labor, expense, and effort. This strategy is generally a one-way process of communication using a top-down approach (e.g., clinical leader to staff). For example, Underwood (2015) implemented a unit-based protocol aimed at reducing the number of catheter-associated urinary tract infections (CAUTIs) in a neurosurgical and neurological intensive care unit. The staff received didactic education on the proper maintenance and care of urinary catheters. At the end of the training session, each staff member signed a document indicating awareness of the EBPs and agreed to the principles to prevent CAUTIs. Posters were placed in the unit to remind staff of urinary catheter removal practices. These are examples of passive dissemination strategies. As you plan for dissemination, consider the effectiveness of reaching staff nurses and interprofessional team members about the results of the EBP project by sending them an email with an attached report, putting up a poster in the unit, or rounding in the unit at various times of day and days of the week with the intent of interacting with the staff to illustrate in a graph the results of the project and thanking them for their contributions. Which method do you believe would be more effective?

DISSEMINATION VENUES

As you reflect on the methods and impact of your EBP project, you will want to consider the various venues for dissemination. These include traditional methods and social media.

TRADITIONAL METHODS

Traditional methods for disseminating your EBP work include the following:

- Poster presentations
- Oral presentations
- Publications

Poster presentations. A poster presentation is a story board of key information. Posters generally are prepared for scientific meetings. Posters are displayed throughout the meeting or at designated times. Conference organizers will inform you of attendance requirements, but it is advantageous to have one or more members of the EB team present to showcase your work. Because it is a summary of your work, conference participants will have questions about specific components. Presenting a poster is a social and interactive experience. The design and layout of your poster is important, since this will draw people to your work. There are many excellent tutorials that will help you create effective and appealing posters.

IT RESOURCES

Online resources and tutorials for creating effective poster presentations:

https://www.youtube.com/watch?v = k6FzrwW3oKQ;
https://www.youtube.com/watch?v = twcKWdZ6oEg
https://projects.ncsu.edu/project/posters/
https://www.csun.edu/plunk/documents/poster_
    presentation.pdf
http://colinpurrington.com/tips/poster-design

Oral presentation. An oral presentation requires you to present your work in front of a live (or virtual) audience; sometimes it is referred to as presenting a "paper." The hardest part of doing an oral presentation is anticipating your audience and tailoring your presentation to that audience. Does your audience consist of individuals who know nothing about your topic or subject matter and have some level of curiosity or is your audience individuals who know a great deal about the subject matter and

---

BOX 17.1   Template for Presenting EBP Projects

Description of the problem, patient population, and clinical setting
Evidence-based practice (EBP) purpose statement
Synthesis of the evidence on the clinical topic being implemented
EBPs to be implemented
Implementation strategies
Evaluation (process and outcome measures)
Lessons learned

---

are interested in your perspective on the subject matter? Is your audience interprofessional or solely nursing?

Oral presentations are always timed, generally for about 15 to 20 minutes. Always tailor your talk so that the audience has 5 minutes to critique or ask questions about your work. Use of PowerPoint slides to accompany your talk is the expectation today. Because of the limited time frame and the number of presentations to be heard in a day, the audience generally wants the speaker to get to the point. Don't burden your talk with conceptually or methodically complex discussions. In preparation for your talk, define your central message and do your best to develop a summary of your work and its impact that you can state in 25 words or less (your "elevator speech"), preferably in words that your intended audience will understand. You should practice your presentation, being mindful of the time allocation for your talk. If you are new to presenting, this tutorial will walk you through the do and don'ts of effective presentations: https://www.youtube.com/watch?v=gF3FWu56dc8.

As you develop your presentation, think about the template you will use for your presentation. Some templates that are available may overwhelm the information you wish to present, so feel free to modify them. For example, templates designed for reporting conduct of research are not likely to be useful for presenting an EBP project. Box 17.1 is an example of a template for presentations on EBP projects. The font you use in your presentation should be easy to read. One recommendation is for the font to be at least 30 pt. (Delvin, 2018).

Publishing. Preparing your work for publication is time-consuming and can be a tedious process. Publishing in a peer-reviewed journal adds a high level of credibility to your work and makes it available to a larger audience than oral or poster presentations can reach. Your work will be indexed in a large database, searchable by anyone with access to it (see Chapter 4). Every journal has "information for authors" listed on its website or in the journal. It is essential that you follow these submission requirements to ensure that you meet the journal's technical requirements for publication. Your manuscript should be reviewed by those with expertise in publishing before submission to the journal. It is likely that your manuscript will undergo multiple revisions before it is ready for submission.

With publication, having subject matter experts review and comment on your work is a cornerstone of the peer review process. Once these comments are sent to you, it is important to respond to each one in a collegial, nondefensive manner. Providing corrections and clarifications moves your manuscript one step closer to publication. Having your work published is an enormous professional accomplishment, because you will have contributed to the body of work in your professional discipline.

Publication is also an important vehicle for promoting replication of your project. Success in reaching your goals or targets may happen in one unit or department, but you may not be able to achieve the same results in other practice settings. Because EBP projects are not controlled experiments, many variables can be at play and affect results. However, encouraging replication of your work through publication or presentation helps to confirm that the findings of your original work are accurate, applicable in different situations, and can serve as a resource to others who may be experiencing the same or similar issues.

SOCIAL MEDIA

Social media are potentially novel ways of enabling teams to communicate and disseminate their EBP findings. The use of social media is growing rapidly and gaining popularity. Social media are not simply a one-way avenue for a stream of information, but a two-way engaging process that allows for feedback, criticism, and conversation (Ferguson, 2013).

Twitter is a popular online social network that enables users to send short messages called tweets. Twitter can allow you to connect directly, rapidly, and inexpensively with communities; disseminate information; and promote translation of research into practice and policy (Archibald & Clark, 2014).

SlideShare is the world's largest community for sharing online presentations and other documents (reports, videos, and infographics). This platform allows practitioners to reach a worldwide audience, amplifying the impact of work beyond conferences, congresses, or lectures. Founded in 2006 and acquired by LinkedIn in 2012, SlideShare is one of the top 100 most-visited websites in the world with more than 18 million uploads in 40 content categories (Esposito, 2016).

YouTube and Vimeo are two popular video-sharing websites where users can upload, share, and view videos. Online video has become a major platform for dissemination of multimedia information. These tools can be effective dissemination tools for evidence-based findings.

Web 2.0 refers to a collection of Web-based applications and technologies that "facilitate interactive information sharing, interoperability, user-centered design, and collaboration. What differentiates Web 1.0 from Web 2.0? Web 1.0 is limited to passive dissemination of content, whereas Web 2.0 and the related application are a media space where clinicians create and interact with information content and with each other; active dissemination" (Bernhardt, Mays, & Kreuter, 2011). Many Web 2.0 products can be used to rapidly increase awareness of new evidence. Many peer-reviewed scientific journals have entered the Web 2.0 space to disseminate publications (*JANAC, Journal of the Association of Nurse in AIDS Care, New England Journal of Medicine, AORN Journal, AACN, Association of Critical Care Nurses*) (Fig. 16.6). Federal agencies such as the Centers for Disease Control and Prevention, the Agency for Healthcare Research and Quality, and the National Institutes of Health have made use of Web 2.0 channels including Facebook, Twitter, buttons/badges (graphics with embedded links for more information), widgets/gadgets (online applications built by one website that can be displayed on another), bookmarking, sharing, RSS feeds, mobile websites, text messaging, and blogs (Bernhardt et al., 2011).

Using social media for dissemination can virally share success stories that increase awareness of evidence-based products and influence others. They also allow practitioners to collect and analyze social media data. Closely analyzing data can provide a much deeper knowledge of end users' information needs that could then be targeted via strategic dissemination efforts (Bernhardt et al., 2011). The value and possibility of these social media tools and platforms is that they not only provide possibilities for local dissemination but have the potential for dissemination of information to global communities (Smith & Milnes, 2016). Information technology and the Internet have revolutionized communication to such an extent that humans now can communicate with colleagues anywhere at any time using social media platforms (Rolls et al., 2016).

Evidence is beginning to appear in the literature on the impact of Web 2.0 tools in research dissemination. Archambault (2012) says that health care workers were in favor of the use of wikis as knowledge translation tools that could help health professionals implement best practices in trauma care.

> **IPE TIP**
>
> Remember that disseminating your EBP project requires collaboration among your EBP team members. Review the IPEC Competencies in Appendix G for a guide to effective interprofessional collaborative competencies.

ESSENTIAL ELEMENTS IN DISSEMINATION OF EVIDENCE-BASED PRACTICE PROJECTS

There are essential elements you should include in dissemination of your work to internal (see Fig. 16.1, Chapter 16) and external audiences. The RE-AIM framework, illustrated in Fig. 17.1, provides a guide for these essential elements. It originally was designed to plan and evaluate implementation of public health EB programs or interventions (Glasgow et al., 1999; Gaglio et al., 2013). Today, RE-AIM is used in the planning stages for implementation in diverse areas of health care (e.g., health promotion, disease prevention, disease management) and settings (e.g., communities, hospitals, primary care, schools) as well as *reporting* results of implementing EBPs (Gaglio et al., 2013). RE-AIM focuses on five RE-AIM dimensions:

* Reach
* Effectiveness
* Adoption
* Implementation
* Maintenance (Gaglio, 2013)

Table 17.1 defines each of the RE-AIM dimensions and important elements to include in your EBP project presentation or publication. Table 17.2 provides a description of sections to consider in publications and presentations of EBP projects with linkages to the RE-AIM framework dimensions.

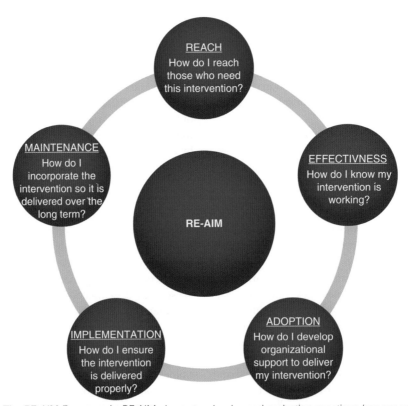

Fig. 17.1 The RE-AIM Framework. RE-AIM elements: planning and evaluating questions (see www.reaim.org for more information).

TABLE 17.1	RE-AIM Dimensions to Consider When Preparing Presentations or Publications		
RE-AIM Dimension	**Definition**	**Questions to Consider**	**Examples from Ullman & Fisher (2017) (see Appendix)**
Reach	Participants or intended users of the EB practice change (e.g., staff nurses). This should include the number and representativeness of those participating in the EBP change and the setting. (see Chapters 12 & 14)	Who were the users (e.g., types of clinicians) of the EBPs? Did the users include multiple disciplines? What were the characteristics of the users? What settings were targeted for implementation?	NICU bedside nursing staff Tertiary care NICU
Effectiveness	Impact of EBPs on outcomes. Effectiveness can be measured at the individual, unit, or organizational level. (see Chapters 11 & 16)	Did implementation of the EBPs improve outcomes? What outcomes were improved? Were there any negative effects of implementing the EBPs? If so, what were they?	Improved NICU staff knowledge about breastfeeding [Note: No patient outcomes were measured.]
Adoption	Uptake or participation rate of using the new EBPs Fidelity to the EBPs or interventions Proportion of patients who received the EBPs **Fidelity** is the degree to which the EBPs are delivered as intended. (see Chapter 16)	Were EBPs adopted by the end users? What were the processes of care measures that reflect adoption? Were the EBPs being carried out as intended (fidelity to the clinical intervention), or were some components of the EBPs not followed?	NICU staff nurses' comfort level in five areas: assist mother with breastfeeding issues; provide accurate information; initiate a conversation about breastfeeding; provide directions on use of breast pump; assist other staff with a breastfeeding issue that a patient's mother is experiencing. [Note: No data were reported on actual use of these practices or fidelity.]
Implementation	Strategies used to promote adoption of the EBPs (e.g., education, audit, and feedback)** Strategies used to ensure ongoing use of the EBPs (e.g., modification of documentation systems) (see Chapters 13 & 14)	What implementation strategies were used to promote use of the EBPs? When were they done? If done repeatedly, how often (e.g., every 4 weeks for 6 months)? How long was the implementation phase (e.g., 6 months)?	Education session of 2 hours – content of education detailed in the article.
Maintenance	Sustainability - Continued use of the EBPs after implementation. Sustained use of the EBPs for 6 months after implementation (see Chapter 13)	What process and outcome measures were sustained after implementation? What strategies were used to promote sustained use and integration of the EBPs into routine care? Are practices now embedded into daily workflow?	No data included about maintenance of process or outcomes Education program continues to be offered. Education session is being incorporated into a three-tiered lactation support program.

**Modified from RE-AIM

EBP, Evidence-based practice; *NICU,* neonatal intensive care unit.

TABLE 17.2   Sections to Consider in Publications and Presentations of EBP Projects

Section of Paper or Presentation	Description	Relationship to RE-AIM Dimensions
Background & rationale	Description of the clinical topic, why it is important, rationale for using an EBP approach	
Purpose of the EBP project	Formulated from PICO. Describes project's purpose, including problem and patient population, EB intervention, and the outcomes to be achieved	Reach Effectiveness
Synthesis of the evidence base	Describes the synthesized evidence used to formulate the EBP intervention, program, or standard	
Description of the EBPs to be implemented (clinical intervention)	Detailed description of the EB clinical intervention that was implemented, including each of the component parts	Adoption
Setting	Where the EBPs were implemented	Reach
Users of the EBPs	Principal users of the EBP implemented	Reach
Design	The design used to compare the impact of implementing the EBPs	
What was measured and when (include process and outcomes)	Description of process measures, outcome measures, calculation of each measure, data sources, and when they were measured during the project	Effectiveness Adoption Maintenance (if measures are collected at time points after implementation)
Description of the users of the EBPs (characteristics, number, etc.)	Description of the clinicians who used the EBPs; description of the patient population who were recipients of the EBPs.	Reach
How the EBPS were implemented; implementation strategies used; length of time for implementation	Describe specific strategies used for EBP implementation, how often each was done, and when completed (e.g., beginning of implementation, during implementation, etc.); describe or illustrate tools used for implementation such as decision-support algorithms, etc.	Implementation
Results	Describe the impact of EBP implementation on outcomes and processes before and at the end of implementation and at follow-up time periods after implementation is completed.	Effectiveness Adoption Maintenance
Discussion	Discuss how your results compare to the synthesized evidence base mentioned previously and to other EBP projects.	
Lessons learned	Description of what you learned during this project considering what went well, what challenges you encountered, and what you would recommend for others interested in implementing similar EBPs.	

EBP, Evidence-based practice.

IPE TIP

Disseminating the findings of your team's EBP or QI project to internal and external audiences involves collaboration with other departments in your organization to develop targeted messaging for each stakeholder group to maximize adoption and sustainability of the initiative.

SYNTHESIS

As coordinators of interprofessional health care teams, clinical leaders like yourself use evidence to achieve positive patient and health system outcomes. Nurses in all roles are important consumers and generators of evidence. Effective dissemination of EBP work by leaders in clinical, education, or administrative roles provides an opportunity to promote the visibility of clinical leaders and the nursing profession overall. EBP innovators like you lead their communities and health care organizations to make significant and replicable evidence-based contributions to improving population health and quality of care, cost-effective health care delivery, and satisfying patient experiences.

▌ KEY POINTS

- Dissemination is the purposive distribution of information and intervention materials to a specific public health or clinical practice audience.
- Principles of dissemination include considering the intended audience, primary objectives of dissemination, and types of dissemination.
- Passive dissemination is a one-way communication process such as publishing or posting information with the expectation that the intended audience will access and use it.
- Active dissemination fosters bidirectional communication with the intended audience.
- Traditional methods of dissemination include poster presentations, oral presentations, and publication.
- Nontraditional methods of communication include use of social media such as Twitter, Slideshare, and Web 2.0 tools.
- The RE-AIM framework provides a structured approach to reporting results of implementing EBPs and addresses the five dimensions: Reach, Effectiveness, Adoption, Implementation, and Maintenance.

- Reach is the intended audience or users of the EBP change.
- Effectiveness is the impact of the EBPs on outcomes and can be measured at the individual, unit, or organizational level.
- Adoption is the uptake or use of the EBPs by the intended clinicians and/or patients and is usually reflected in the process of care measures that are part of evaluation.
- Implementation is how the EBPs were put into practice—the strategies used to promote adoption of the EBPs (e.g., education, audit, and feedback) and their sustainability.
- Maintenance is the sustained use of the EBPs after implementation.
- Implementation fidelity measures the degree to which participants carry out the EBPs as intended.
- Sustainability occurs when a new practice becomes embedded into daily workflow.

REFERENCES

Archambault, P. M., Bilodeau, A., Gagnon, M. P., Aubin, K., Lavoie, A., Lapointe, J., et al. (2012). Health care professionals' beliefs about using wiki-based reminders to promote best practices in trauma care. *Journal of Medical Internet Research, 14*(2), e49. http://dx.doi.org/10.2196/jmir.1983.

Archibald, M. M., & Clark, A. M. (2014). Twitter and nursing research: How diffusion of innovation theory can help uptake. *Journal of Advanced Nursing, 70*(3), e3–e5. https://doi.org/10.1111/jan.12343.

Bernhardt, J. M., Mays, D., & Kreuter, M. W. (2011). Dissemination 2.0: Closing the gap between knowledge and practice with new media and marketing. *Journal of Health Communication, 16*, 32–44.

Delvin, A. S. (2018). *The research experience*. Thousand Oaks, CA: Sage.

Esposito, A. (2016). *Research 2.0 and the impact of digital technologies on scholarly inquiry*. Hershey, PA: IGI Global.

Ferguson, C. (2013). It's time for the nursing profession to leverage social media. *Journal of Advanced Nursing, 69*(4), 745–747.

Gaglio, B., Shoup, J. A., & Glasgow, R. E. (2013). The RE-AIM framework: A systematic review of use over time. *American Journal of Public Health, 103*(6), 38–46.

Grimshaw, J. M., Shirran, L., Thomas, R., Mowatt, G., Fraser, C., Bero, L., et al. (2001). Changing provider behavior: An overview of systematic reviews of interventions. *Medical Care, 39*(8 Suppl 2), II2–45. Retrieved from http://www.jstor.org/stable/3767642.

Grimshaw, J. M., Thomas, R. E., MacLennan, G., Fraser, C., Ramsay, C. R., Vale, L., et al. (2004). Effectiveness and efficiency of guideline dissemination and implementation strategies. *International Journey of Technology Assessment in Healthcare, 21*(1), 49.

Marín-González, E., Malmusi, D., Camprubí, L., & Borrell, C. (2016). The role of dissemination as a fundamental part of a research project. *International Journal of Health Services, 47*(2), 258–276.

Rolls, K., Hansen, M., Jackson, D., & Elliott, D. (2016). How health care professionals use social media to create virtual communities: An integrative review. *Journal of Medical Internet Research, 18*(6), e166. https://doi.org/10.2196/jmir.5312.

Smith, J., & Milnes, L. J. (2016). Social media: The relevance for research. *Evidence-Based Nursing, 19*(4).

Underwood, L. (2015). The effect of implementing a comprehensive unit-based safety program on urinary catheter use. *Urologic Nursing, 35*(6), 271–279.

[Intervention Review]

Interventions to improve adherence to lipid-lowering medication

Mieke L van Driel[1,2], Michael D Morledge[3], Robin Ulep[3], Johnathon P Shaffer[3], Philippa Davies[4], Richard Deichmann[5]

[1]Discipline of General Practice, School of Medicine, The University of Queensland, Brisbane, Australia. [2]Department of Family Medicine and Primary Health Care, Ghent University, Ghent, Belgium. [3]Ochsner Clinical School, School of Medicine, The University of Queensland, New Orleans, USA. [4]School of Social and Community Medicine, University of Bristol, Bristol, UK. [5]Department of Internal Medicine, Ochsner Health System, New Orleans, USA

Contact address: Mieke L van Driel, Discipline of General Practice, School of Medicine, The University of Queensland, Brisbane, Queensland, 4029, Australia. m.vandriel@uq.edu.au, mieke.vandriel@ugent.be.

Editorial group: Cochrane Heart Group.
Publication status and date: New search for studies and content updated (conclusions changed), published in Issue 12, 2016.
Review content assessed as up-to-date: 3 February 2016.

Citation: van Driel ML, Morledge MD, Ulep R, Shaffer JP, Davies P, Deichmann R. Interventions to improve adherence to lipid-lowering medication. *Cochrane Database of Systematic Reviews* 2016, Issue 12. Art. No.: CD004371. DOI: 10.1002/14651858.CD004371.pub4.

ABSTRACT

Background

Lipid-lowering drugs are widely underused, despite strong evidence indicating they improve cardiovascular end points. Poor patient adherence to a medication regimen can affect the success of lipid-lowering treatment.

Objectives

To assess the effects of interventions aimed at improving adherence to lipid-lowering drugs, focusing on measures of adherence and clinical outcomes.

Search methods

We searched the Cochrane Central Register of Controlled Trials (CENTRAL), MEDLINE, Embase, PsycINFO and CINAHL up to 3 February 2016, and clinical trials registers (ANZCTR and ClinicalTrials.gov) up to 27 July 2016. We applied no language restrictions.

Selection criteria

We evaluated randomised controlled trials of adherence-enhancing interventions for lipid-lowering medication in adults in an ambulatory setting with a variety of measurable outcomes, such as adherence to treatment and changes to serum lipid levels. Two teams of review authors independently selected the studies.

Data collection and analysis

Three review authors extracted and assessed data, following criteria outlined by the *Cochrane Handbook for Systematic Reviews of Interventions*. We assessed the quality of the evidence using GRADEPro.

Main results

For this updated review, we added 24 new studies meeting the eligibility criteria to the 11 studies from prior updates. We have therefore included 35 studies, randomising 925,171 participants. Seven studies including 11,204 individuals compared adherence rates of those in an intensification of a patient care intervention (e.g. electronic reminders, pharmacist-led interventions, healthcare professional education of patients) versus usual care over the short term (six months or less), and were pooled in a meta-analysis. Participants in the intervention group had better adherence than those receiving usual care (odds ratio (OR) 1.93, 95% confidence interval (CI) 1.29 to 2.88; 7 studies; 11,204 participants; moderate-quality evidence). A separate analysis also showed improvements in long-term adherence rates (more than six months) using intensification of care (OR 2.87, 95% CI 1.91 to 4.29; 3 studies; 663 participants; high-quality evidence). Analyses of the effect on total cholesterol and LDL-cholesterol levels also showed a positive effect of intensified interventions over both short- and long-term follow-up. Over the short term, total cholesterol decreased by a mean of 17.15 mg/dL (95% CI 1.17 to 33.14; 4 studies; 430 participants; low-quality evidence) and LDL-cholesterol decreased by a mean of 19.51 mg/dL (95% CI 8.51 to 30.51; 3 studies; 333 participants; moderate-quality evidence). Over the long term (more than six months) total cholesterol decreased by a mean of 17.57 mg/dL (95% CI 14.95 to 20.19; 2 studies; 127 participants; high-quality evidence). Included studies did not report usable data for health outcome indications, adverse effects or costs/resource use, so we could not pool these outcomes. We assessed each included study for bias using methods described in the Cochrane Handbook for Systematic Reviews of Interventions. In general, the risk of bias assessment revealed a low risk of selection bias, attrition bias, and reporting bias. There was unclear risk of bias relating to blinding for most studies.

Authors' conclusions

The evidence in our review demonstrates that intensification of patient care interventions improves short- and long-term medication adherence, as well as total cholesterol and LDL-cholesterol levels. Healthcare systems which can implement team-based intensification of patient care interventions may be successful in improving patient adherence rates to lipid-lowering medicines.

PLAIN LANGUAGE SUMMARY

Interventions to improve people's drug-taking behaviour with lipid-lowering drugs

Review question

Which interventions help improve people's ability to take lipid-lowering medications more regularly?

Background

Lipid-lowering therapy has been shown to decrease the risk of both heart attacks and strokes. However, taking these medications as prescribed has not been as high as one would wish. In the past, several methods have been tried to improve the rate at which people take these lipid-lowering treatments. Previous Cochrane Reviews have not shown a clear benefit of any particular method. We have updated our review to see if any new methods in this digital age have been tested as ways of improving these rates.

Search

Our search included the 11 studies identified from previous versions in 2004 and 2010. We conducted an updated search of the same electronic databases on 3 February 2016, and we searched clinical trials registers up to 27 July 2016.

Study characteristics

The people included in the studies were adults over 18 years of age in outpatient settings, for whom lipid-lowering therapy was recommended. We now include 35 studies covering 925,171 participants in this review.

Key results

Of the 35 included studies, 16 compared interventions categorised as 'intensified patient care' versus usual care. These interventions included electronic reminders, pharmacist-led interventions, and healthcare professional education to help people better remember to take their medications. These types of interventions when compared to standard care demonstrated significantly better adherence rates both over the short term (up to and including six months) as well as the long term (longer than six months). Additionally, cholesterol levels were better over both long- and short-term periods in those offered the intervention, compared to those receiving usual care.

Quality of the evidence

We considered only randomised controlled trials for this review. Given the nature of the interventions, it was not possible to keep participants unaware of which group they were in. However, analysis of other forms of bias indicated that generally the studies were at low risk of bias. We assessed the evidence for the outcomes using the GRADE system, and rated it as high quality for long-term adherence (more than six months) and for reduction in total cholesterol, and moderate quality for short-term medication adherence (up to six months) and for LDL-cholesterol levels. For the outcome total cholesterol levels at less than six months follow-up, we downgraded the evidence to low quality.

SUMMARY OF FINDINGS FOR THE MAIN COMPARISON [Explanation]

Intensified patient care vs usual care

Patient or population: People receiving lipid-lowering medications
Setting: Ambulatory
Intervention: Intensified patient care
Comparison: Usual care

Outcomes	Anticipated absolute effects* (95% CI)		Relative effect (95% CI)	№ of participants (studies)	Quality of the evidence (GRADE)
	Risk with usual care	Risk with Intensified patient care			
Medication adherence at ≤ 6 months	Study population		OR 1.93 (1.29 to 2.88)	11,204 (7 RCTs)	⊕⊕⊕◯ MODERATE [1]
	456 per 1,000	618 per 1,000 (519 to 707)			
Medication adherence at > 6 months	Study population		OR 2.87 (1.91 to 4.29)	663 (3 RCTs)	⊕⊕⊕⊕ HIGH
	705 per 1,000	873 per 1,000 (820 to 911)			
Reduction in LDL-C at ≤ 6 months (mg/dL)	The mean reduction in LDL-C at ≤ 6 months (mg/dL) was 0	The mean reduction in LDL-C at ≤ 6 months (mg/dL) in the intervention group was 19.51 greater (8.51 greater to 30.51 greater)	-	333 (3 RCTs)	⊕⊕⊕◯ MODERATE [1]
Reduction in total serum cholesterol at ≤ 6 months (mg/dL)	The mean reduction in total serum cholesterol at ≤ 6 mos (mg/dL) was 0	The mean reduction in total serum cholesterol at ≤ 6 months (mg/dL) in the intervention group was 17.15 greater (1.17 greater to 33.14 greater)	-	430 (4 RCTs)	⊕⊕◯◯ LOW [1,2]

Reduction in total serum cholesterol at > 6 mos (mg/ dL)	The mean reduction in to-tal serum cholesterol at > 6 months (mg/dL) was 0	The mean reduction in to-tal serum cholesterol at > 6 months (mg/dL) in the in-tervention group was 17.57 greater (14.95 greater to 20. 19 greater)	127 (2 RCTs)

⊕⊕⊕⊕
HIGH

*The risk in the intervention group (and its 95% confidence interval) is based on the assumed risk in the comparison group and the relative effect of the intervention (and its 95% CI).

CI: Confidence interval; OR: Odds ratio;

GRADE Working Group grades of evidence
High quality: We are very confident that the true effect lies close to that of the estimate of the effect
Moderate quality: We are moderately confident in the effect estimate: The true effect is likely to be close to the estimate of the effect, but there is a possibility that it is substantially different
Low quality: Our confidence in the effect estimate is limited: The true effect may be substantially different from the estimate of the effect
Very low quality: We have very little confidence in the effect estimate: The true effect is likely to be substantially different from the estimate of effect

[1] Downgraded due to heterogeneity
[2] Downgraded due to wide confidence interval

5

BACKGROUND

Despite compelling evidence about the effectiveness of lipid-lowering drugs and the introduction of clear guidelines, lipid-lowering therapy is still underused (Rosenson 2015). Recent recommendations by the American College of Cardiology/American Heart Association are expected to significantly increase the number of individuals for whom statin therapy is indicated (ACC/AHA Guidelines 2013). Lack of adherence and high rates of discontinuation have been shown to be important factors in failing treatment when looking both at high cholesterol levels and at morbidity in terms of recurrent myocardial infarction (Blackburn 2005; Cheng 2004; Wei 2002).

Description of the condition

High cholesterol is one of the top 10 risk factors that account for more than one-third of all deaths worldwide (WHO Report 2002). It is an important risk factor for cardiovascular disease (CVD), estimated to cause 18% of CVD and 56% of ischaemic heart disease (WHO Report 2002). There is compelling evidence for the effectiveness of lipid-lowering drugs in reducing both lipid levels and the risk of heart attacks and strokes (Baigent 2005). Elevated serum concentrations of total cholesterol (TC), low-density lipoprotein (LDL) and total triglycerides (TRG) are associated with increased risk of coronary heart disease (CHD), whereas high-density lipoproteins (HDL) or a low TC to HDL ratio appear to be protective. Lipid-lowering medications (hypolipidaemics) for the treatment of hyperlipidaemia include statins, fibrates and anion-exchange resins. Statins, in particular, have been shown in large randomised controlled trials to be effective in preventing CHD events and in reducing overall mortality (4S 1994; Athyros 2002a; Downs 1998; LIPID 1998; MRC/BHF 2002; Sacks 1996; Shepherd 1995). Fibrates and anion-exchange resins achieved reductions in CHD events, but showed a non-significant increase in non-coronary mortality (Downs 1998). Statins are therefore recommended as first-line therapy, whereas fibrates and anion-exchange resins can be considered as second-line therapy and also in combination with statins (SIGN 2007).

Recommendations about drug treatments vary from country to country. In the UK, treatment with statins for secondary prevention is indicated in people with clinical evidence of CVD to reduce further ischaemic events. For primary prevention of CVD, lipid-lowering medication is recommended in asymptomatic adults who have a 20% or greater risk of developing CVD in the next 10 years (NICE 2014; SIGN 2007). A combination of statins, blood pressure-lowering drugs and low-dose aspirin is recommended by the World Health Report (WHO Report 2002) for secondary prevention of CVD, as this could cut death and disability rates from CVD by more than 50%. A meta-analysis confirmed an approximately linear relationship between the absolute reduction in LDL-cholesterol and the proportional reductions in the incidence of coronary and major vascular events (Baigent 2005). Statin therapy resulted in a 19% proportional reduction in CHD deaths per mmol/L LDL-cholesterol reduction. It can safely reduce the five-year incidence of cardiovascular events largely irrespective of the initial lipid profile, relating the absolute benefit mainly to an individual's absolute risk of such events and the absolute reduction in LDL-cholesterol achieved (Baigent 2005). In England, 7000 myocardial infarctions and 2500 strokes could be avoided each year if individuals at high risk, who are not taking medication, received lipid-lowering treatment (Primatesta 2000). These figures show the impact of lipid-lowering drugs on public health and thus the importance of the acceptance of and adherence to medication by the public.

Description of the intervention

Adherence is defined as the extent to which people take medication as prescribed. Since the landmark publication by Sackett 1976, it has been the focus of research over the last three decades (Vermeire 2001). Adherence can either be intentional or non-intentional, and is determined by a variety of factors such as lack of knowledge, denial, adverse effects, poor memory and adverse attitudes to treatment. Reliable indicators of adherent behaviour have not been found to date and demographic factors such as age, sex or social class have been shown to be poor predictors of adherence (Vermeire 2001). The importance of the person's agreement (Lewis 2003) and the significance of their role within the doctor-patient relationship have been emphasised, which has led to replacing the term 'compliance' with more patient-centred synonyms such as 'adherence' and 'concordance' (Lewis 2003; Marinker 1997; Mullen 1997). The treatment of a symptomless condition such as hyperlipidaemia signifies a particular challenge to both doctor and patient. It has been difficult to identify the scope of the problem, as adherence rates from hyperlipidaemia trials show considerable variation, ranging from 37% to 80%, depending on factors such as study population, background morbidity, classes of drugs, duration of follow-up and adherence-measuring methods (Tsuyuki 2001). Epidemiological data show that target cholesterol concentrations are achieved in fewer than 50% of people receiving cholesterol-lowering drugs and that only one in four people continue taking medication in the long term (Benner 2002; Primatesta 2000). Not surprisingly, primary prevention trials appear to have higher discontinuation rates than secondary prevention trials, which indicates a relationship between adherence and awareness of illness (Tsuyuki 2001). This was confirmed in a population-based study involving elderly people, where 60% of people prescribed a statin for acute coronary syndrome gave up treatment within two years, compared to 75% of those without coronary disease (Jackevicius 2002).

A wide range of interventions to improve adherence to medication have been studied (Brown 2011; Costa 2015). They can focus on the person, the drug regimen, the physician or the health system (delivery of medication). Patient education and empowerment is important, as people adhere less to drugs or treatments if they do not understand why they need to take them (Brown 2011). Simplification of the drug regimen may assist, as adherence is inversely related to the number of drugs the person is taking (Pasina 2014), and especially complex dosing schedules are at risk. Interventions focused on physicians advocate good communication and a patient-centred approach (Brown 2011), which could include appropriate follow-up and support. System-based approaches could include pharmacist involvement and (automated) patient reminder systems.

How the intervention might work

A number of systematic reviews looking at adherence-enhancing interventions have been published in the Cochrane Library. Nieuwlaat 2014 identified effective ways to improve medication adherence for a variety of medical conditions in widely differing populations. Adherence to short-term drug treatment was improved by written information, personal phone calls and counselling. For long-term treatments, no simple intervention and only some complex ones led to some improvement in health outcomes (Nieuwlaat 2014). Schroeder 2004 focused on medications for controlling blood pressure and reported enhanced adherence by reducing the number of daily doses. Patient support and education interventions improved adherence to antiretroviral therapy when targeting practical medication management skills aimed at individuals rather than groups (Rueda 2006). In the treatment of type 2 diabetes, it was concluded that nurse-led interventions, home aids, diabetes education and pharmacy-led interventions do not show significant effects (Vermeire 2005). Another review concluded that reminder packaging increased the proportion of people taking their medications, but the effect was not large (Mahtani 2011).

Why it is important to do this review

The indication for prescribing lipid-lowering drugs has changed substantially over the last 20 years (ACC/AHA Guidelines 2013; Baigent 2005). With evidence to suggest that effectiveness of statins occurs irrespective of initial lipid level, greater numbers of people are being actively prescribed lipid-lowering agents. Observational studies have shown that adherence to lipid-lowering drugs is poor, with people taking their medication only 60% of the time in a one-year period (Avorn 1998). There is strong evidence that adherence diminishes over time in people who are being treated as part of a primary or secondary prevention strategy (Benner 2002; Jackevicius 2002). The consequence of inadequate adherence to lipid-lowering therapy is substantial. In secondary prevention, inadequate adherence is associated with an increase in recurrent myocardial infarction and all-cause mortality (Wei

2002). For these reasons, it is important that clinically effective and cost-effective strategies to improve adherence are found for primary and secondary prevention of cardiovascular disease in the community. The findings of our review can be integrated into clinical practice guidelines and assist clinicians in making a difference to patient outcomes. This update of previous reviews, published in 2004 and updated in 2010 (Schedlbauer 2004; Schedlbauer 2010), assessed interventions designed to help people take their lipid-lowering medication in an ambulatory care setting, taking into account new and emerging evidence.

OBJECTIVES

To assess the effects of interventions aimed at improving adherence to lipid-lowering drugs, focusing on measures of adherence and clinical outcomes.

METHODS

Criteria for considering studies for this review

Types of studies

Randomised controlled trials (RCTs), of parallel-group or crossover design, that used individual or cluster randomisation.

Types of participants

All adults (over 18 years of age) who were prescribed lipid-lowering medication for primary or secondary prevention of cardiovascular disease in ambulatory care settings.

Types of interventions

Interventions of any type intended to increase adherence to self-administered lipid-lowering medication versus usual care or no intervention.
This included, but was not exclusive to, interventions such as:
1. simplification of drug regimen;
2. patient education and information;
3. intensified patient care (increased follow-up, sending out reminders, etc.);
4. complex behavioural approaches (increasing motivation by arranging group sessions, giving out rewards, etc.);
5. decision support systems (computer-based information systems aimed at support of decision-making);
6. administrative improvements (audit, documentation, computers, co-payments);
7. large-scale pharmacy-led automated telephone intervention.

Types of outcome measures

Primary outcomes

Methods of measuring adherence continue to be widely variable and remain controversial. We identify three categories of adherence assessment, and have included them in this review:

1. Indirect measures of adherence (e.g. pill count, prescription refill rate, electronic monitoring);

2. Subjective measures of adherence (e.g. person's self-report in diaries, interviews);

3. Direct measures of adherence (tracer substances in blood or urine).

Secondary outcomes

We have also included the following outcome measures, in addition to adherence measures:

1. Physiological indicators (e.g. total cholesterol);

2. Health outcome indications (e.g. quality of life, morbidity, mortality);

3. Adverse effects;

4. Implications for costs (impact of intervention on economic outcomes, economic evaluation).

In the literature, physiological indicators, health outcomes and adverse effects have been used as proxy measures for adherence. We included these studies only if those indicators were reported in association with adherence outcomes (see Characteristics of included studies).

Search methods for identification of studies

Electronic searches

Previous searches

The 2010 version of this review included searches of the Cochrane Central Register of Controlled Trials (CENTRAL) (the Cochrane Library 2008, Issue 1), MEDLINE (January 2000 to March 2008), Embase (January 1998 to March 2008), PsycINFO (1972 to March 2008) and CINAHL (January 1982 to March 2008). CENTRAL incorporates all controlled trials from Embase and MEDLINE, except in the most recent years. We used an appropriate RCT filter for MEDLINE (Dickersin 1994) and Embase (Lefebvre 1996). Details of the previous search strategies are in Appendix 1 and Appendix 2.

Latest Searches

For this updated review we included the studies from the previously published review (Schedlbauer 2010; search date 31 March 2008). We updated the search terms to increase the sensitivity of the searches. We applied these changes and reran the searches from database inception. We subsequently applied limits to entry dates or equivalent to all databases except CENTRAL, to identify only those records which had been added to the databases since the last search in 2008.

We ran the most recent database search on 3 February 2016 and included the following databases:

- CENTRAL in the Cochrane Library (Issue 1, 2016)
- MEDLINE (Ovid, 1946 to January Week 3 2016)
- Embase (Ovid, 1980 to Week 5 2016)
- PsycINFO (Ovid, 1806 to January Week 4 2016)
- CINAHL Plus with Full Text (EBSCO, 1937 to 3 February 2016).

We also searched clinical trials registers (www.anzctr.org.au/ and ClinicalTrials.gov) up to 27 July 2016, using the following search terms: "statin", "adherence", "compliance", "intervention". We updated the RCT filters for MEDLINE and Embase according to the latest recommendations in the *Cochrane Handbook* (Lefebvre 2011), and applied adaptations of it to the other databases, except for CENTRAL. Details of the latest search strategies are in Appendix 3. We applied no language restrictions.

Searching other resources

We sought additional studies through scrutinising the reference lists of identified eligible studies.

Data collection and analysis

Selection of studies

Three review authors (JS, MM, and RU) selected studies independently by assessing titles and abstracts. We obtained full-text articles of potentially relevant studies. Following this initial screening, the three review authors (JS, MM, RU) selected trials independently by applying predetermined inclusion criteria. We included a trial if it met all of our inclusion criteria. The review authors discussed disagreements and resolved them, with recourse to MVD and RD when necessary. We used a spreadsheet to identify and extract studies in duplicate.

Data extraction and management

We extracted study outcome data using a predefined data collection tool that had been developed by one of the review authors (MVD). The form had been developed and piloted on a random sample of three studies and refined appropriately. For this updated version of the review, we conducted the 'Risk of bias' assessment for all included studies with Review Manager 5. Three review authors (JS, MM, and RU) extracted data from the newly-selected studies, with a second author checking the extracted data for accuracy.

Assessment of risk of bias in included studies

We performed 'Risk of bias' assessment using the Cochrane 'Risk of bias' tool in the Cochrane Handbook of Systematic Reviews of Interventions (Higgins 2011). We assessed the following 'Risk of bias' categories:

• **selection bias** (by assessing the method of random number generation and the process of allocation concealment);

• **performance and detection bias** (blinding of participants, providers and outcomes assessors);

• **attrition bias** (by assessing how incomplete data were managed); and

• **reporting bias** (by assessing whether all intended outcomes were reported).

See Risk of bias in included studies. We rated each of the studies as 'high risk', 'low risk' or 'unclear risk' for each of these risk of bias domains. We also took into consideration the method used to measure adherence, as some methods are more likely to be biased than others (see Characteristics of included studies). For instance, medication refill data are likely to measure adherence more objectively than manual pill counts, even if outcome assessors are not blinded to group allocation. We applied a judgement of 'unclear risk' to blinding where participant and physician were not blinded. We applied a judgement of 'unclear risk' to blinding where outcome assessors were not blinded. We also applied a judgement of 'unclear risk' to any risk assessment when information was not provided or if there was insufficient information to permit a judgement.

Measures of treatment effect

For dichotomous data, we reported the results as odds ratios (ORs) with 95% confidence intervals (CIs). For continuous data, we reported the mean difference (MD) with standard deviation (SD) of pre- and post-measurements. For serum cholesterol, we report values in mg/dL. We converted cholesterol values reported as mmol/L to mg/dL, using the formula: 1 mmol/l = 38.66976 mg/dL.

Unit of analysis issues

The unit of analysis in our meta-analysis was the participant; however, if this was not the case, such as in cluster-randomised trials, we planned to make adjustment for clustering in the pooled analysis following the guidelines in the *Cochrane Handbook* (Higgins 2011).

Dealing with missing data

If data for analysis were missing, we attempted to obtain information from authors. If no additional data were provided by the authors we used available-case analysis, which includes analysis of the available data only (thus ignoring the missing data), assuming that the data were missing at random.

Assessment of heterogeneity

We used the data analysis tools in Review Manager 5 for the assessment of heterogeneity, which is indicated in the forest plots measuring the treatment effect. We assessed heterogeneity by first assessing the comparability of the included studies in terms of population, setting and outcomes (face value or "clinical" heterogeneity). We considered pooling only studies that were sufficiently similar from a clinical perspective. We assessed statistical heterogeneity by calculating the Chi^2 statistic (with P value < 0.10 as level of significance) and the I^2 statistic.

We used I^2 thresholds as described in the *Cochrane Handbook* as a rough guide to interpretation as follows (Higgins 2011), and used 40% as a cut-off value for important heterogeneity, which means that we considered an I^2 under 40% heterogeneity as low:

• 0% to 40%: might not be important;

• 30% to 60%: may represent moderate heterogeneity;

• 50% to 90%: may represent substantial heterogeneity;

• 75% to 100%: considerable heterogeneity.

Assessment of reporting biases

If we suspected reporting bias, we contacted the authors to request missing data. As the number of studies available for meta-analysis was fewer than 10 we did not investigate publication bias by means of a funnel plot.

Data synthesis

We grouped the studies according to the type of intervention. In the absence of an existing standard classification for such interventions, the review authors agreed upon a classification based on the pragmatic focus of the intervention. For instance, we considered interventions related to the medication regimen separate from the behavioural approaches involving doctors or other healthcare professionals. We identified seven types of interventions and reported them separately:

1. Simplification of drug regimen;
2. Patient education and information;
3. Intensified patient care;
4. Complex behavioural approaches;
5. Decision support systems;
6. Administrative improvements; and
7. Pharmacy-led interventions.

'Usual care' was not defined as a separate intervention. We compared outcomes for each comparison independently, and performed pooling of data and meta-analysis where possible. We chose a per-protocol analysis, as intention-to-treat analysis would yield misleading results in many of these studies due to the pragmatic nature of the study designs. We pooled data by using the random-effects model. We also performed a fixed-effect model analysis if we assessed statistical heterogeneity as low (I^2 < 40%). We used dichotomous outcomes for analysis of medication adherence, and continuous outcomes for analysis of clinical markers.

We included the cross-over trial (Brown 1997) from the previous version of this review. However, we classified this study as a simplification of drug regimen intervention and could not perform pooling of data and meta-analysis. Thus, we did not include it in our meta-analysis for intensified patient care versus usual care.

Subgroup analysis and investigation of heterogeneity

We did not plan any subgroup analyses for this review.

Sensitivity analysis

We performed sensitivity analysis for the pooled results by removing the studies that contributed to heterogeneity and comparing the overall outcome estimate. We also compared the results of pooling with a random-effects model to those using a fixed-effect model when statistical heterogeneity was low ($I^2 < 40\%$, see Assessment of heterogeneity), in order to assess the robustness of the effect estimate. We performed sensitivity analysis for the impact of high attrition on the overall study outcome by removing the studies with high attrition (> 20%).

Summary of findings table

We created a Summary of findings table using the following outcomes - medication adherence, reduction in LDL-C and reduction in total serum cholesterol. We used the five GRADE considerations (study limitations, consistency of effect, imprecision, indirectness and publication bias) to assess the quality of a body of evidence as it relates to the studies which contribute data to the meta-analyses for the prespecified outcomes (Guyatt 2008). We used methods and recommendations described in Section 8.5 and Chapter 12 of the Cochrane Handbook for Systematic Reviews of Interventions (Higgins 2011) using GRADEpro software (https://gradepro.org/). We justified all decisions to downgrade the quality of studies using footnotes.

RESULTS

Description of studies

Results of the search

The search for the original 2004 review of this topic retrieved 2380 articles from all sources (Schedlbauer 2004). Eight studies met all inclusion criteria and were analysed. The search for the first update in 2010 (Schedlbauer 2010) identified three additional studies from the 4227 screened records.

The updated search in January 2015 retrieved 6785 articles from all sources. After de-duplication, we reviewed 5768 titles. Of these references, we excluded 5734 studies by identifying titles and abstracts which did not meet the study criteria for inclusion. We added 16 new studies to the 2010 review. The updated search in February 2016 retrieved 6719 articles from all sources. We reviewed these articles and excluded those which, on the basis of title and abstracts, did not meet the study criteria for inclusion. We added five new studies. One study that was previously excluded was reconsidered and included (Choudhry 2011). We reviewed three other studies also identified in previous searches and originally excluded, and these are awaiting classification (Johnson 2006; Harrison 2015; Lee 2006).

The search in the clinical trials registers retrieved eight references. We identified and included two additional studies (Gujral 2014; PILL 2011) and included two others as ongoing studies (ACTRN12616000422426; ACTRN12616000233426). We identified the protocol of another ongoing study in the 2016 search (Thom 2014).

We summarise the search results in Figure 1.

Figure 1. Study flow diagram.

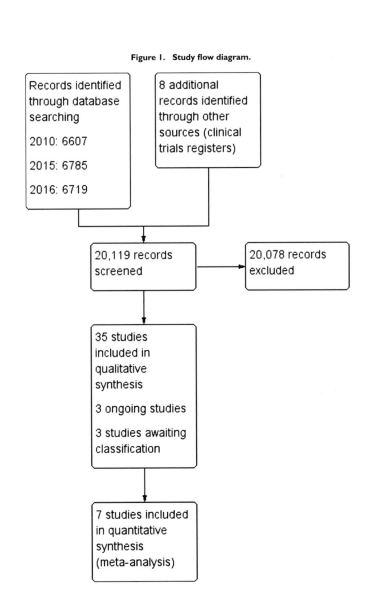

Included studies

This review includes 35 references to 35 studies. The study sizes varied from 30 (Faulkner 2000) to 861,894 (Fischer 2014) with a total of 919,316 participants included in the review. Most trials included both men and women. Two trials included only men (Brown 1997; Schectman 1994). Mean age ranged from 49 to 76.5 years and was not reported in three studies (Fang 2015; Poston 1998; Powell 1995). There was great variation in the types of participants, setting, medication, interventions used and outcomes measured. This is described in more detail in the Characteristics of included studies table. Among the included studies, one study (Brown 1997) was identified as a cross-over trial and five studies (Aslani 2010; Choudhry 2011; Poston 1998; Tamblyn 2009; Vrijens 2006) as cluster-RCTs.

See Characteristics of included studies.

Interventions

We stratified interventions into groups on pragmatic grounds, as generally accepted categories do not exist. We identified seven main groups:

1. Drug regimen simplification (Brown 1997; Castellano 2014; Patel 2015; PILL 2011; Selak 2014; Sweeney 1991; Thom 2013);
2. Patient education and information (Gujral 2014; Park 2013; Poston 1998; Powell 1995; Willich 2009);
3. Intensified patient care with reminders via mail, telephone and hand-held pill devices (Aslani 2010; Derose 2012; Eussen 2010; Fang 2015; Faulkner 2000; Goswami 2013; Guthrie 2001; Ho 2014; Kardas 2013; Ma 2010; Márquez 2004; Márquez 2007; Nieuwkerk 2012; Schectman 1994; Vrijens 2006; Wald 2014);
4. Complex behavioural approaches, group sessions (Márquez 1998; Pladevall 2014);
5. Decision support systems (Kooy 2013);
6. Administrative improvements (Choudhry 2011; Tamblyn 2009);
7. Large-scale pharmacy-led automated telephone intervention (Fischer 2014; Vollmer 2014).

Drug regimen simplification was described as using a formulation (e.g. slow release) that could be given twice rather than four times a day (Brown 1997; Sweeney 1991), or a fixed dose formulation such as a 'polypill' or other (Castellano 2014; Patel 2015; PILL 2011; Selak 2014; Thom 2013).

Patient education and information was in the form of educative text messages delivered to participants (Park 2013), a 'Program Kit', including a videotape, information booklet, and newsletter (Poston 1998), videotapes mailed to participants (Powell 1995), or

a pack containing a videotape, an educational leaflet, details of the free phone patient helpline and website, and labels with a reminder to take study medication, in addition to regular personalised letters and phone calls (Willich 2009). In Gujral 2014 the community pharmacist reviewed the participant monthly when they collected their prescriptions, and at three and six months the pharmacist had a longer discussion with the participant, tailored to their assessed medication beliefs.

Intensified patient care was delivered by different healthcare providers. Interventions involving pharmacists included counselling visits at the pharmacy (Eussen 2010), phone calls by a pharmacist (Faulkner 2000), pharmacist-led voice messaging (educational and medication refill reminder calls) (Ho 2014), a computer-based tracking system and a series of co-ordinated patient-centred pharmacist-delivered telephone counselling contacts (Ma 2010), and review by the participants' pharmacist and a 'beep-card' to remind the participant of the dosing time (Vrijens 2006). Nurses were involved in two studies: counselling from a nurse and an adherence tip sheet (Goswami 2013), and multifactorial risk-factor counselling by a nurse practitioner (Nieuwkerk 2012). Doctor-led counselling was delivered in two studies as counselling and advice about the disease, medicine, medicine use, adherence and lifestyle measures (Aslani 2010), counselling every eight weeks (Kardas 2013). Other interventions included automated telephone calls followed by letters (Derose 2012), telephone reminders and reminder postcards (Guthrie 2001), telephone call reminders (Márquez 2004), a calendar reminder (Márquez 2007), telephone calls (Schectman 1994), and text messages using an automated computer programme (Wald 2014) or sent live (Fang 2015).

Complex behavioural approaches were used by Márquez 1998 and consisted of a group session of 90 minutes for a maximum of 15 participants at a time, educating them about hypercholesterolaemia, followed by monthly letters written by the same clinician who delivered the group sessions with reinforcing messages. Pladevall 2014 used medication adherence information given by physicians and motivational interviewing by trained staff (nurses, pharmacists).

Decision support systems consisted of an electronic reminder device (ERD) that started beeping every day at the same time until the participant switched it off (Kooy 2013).

Administrative improvements: in Tamblyn 2009 the physician was provided with the participant's drug profile which included the total costs of medications dispensed each month, the amount of out-of-pocket expenditure paid by the participant, a graphic representation of unfilled prescriptions, and days of drug supply for each medication. Then at each visit the participant's adherence was calculated and if treatment adherence was less than 80%, the physician received an alert to check with the participant. In Choudhry

2011 medication co-payments for participants in the intervention group were waived at the point of care (i.e. pharmacy), whereas participants in the control group continued to pay their usual co-payments when refilling their prescriptions.

Large-scale pharmacy-led automated telephone intervention was delivered entirely by the pharmacy in Fischer 2014. In the first intervention, the 'automated intervention' participants received automated phone calls on days three and seven to remind them that their prescription was ready for them to pick up if the prescription had been processed by the pharmacy but the participant had not collected it. In the subsequent 'live intervention' a pharmacist or technician called participants who had not collected their prescription despite the reminders. The calls aimed to better understand why participants were not taking their medication and to counsel them regarding appropriate medication use. Vollmer 2014 used automated *Interactive Voice Recognition (IVR) Calls* to participants when they were due or overdue for a refill. Speech-recognition technology was used in these calls to educate participants about their medications.

Medication

The lipid-lowering medications used to treat hyperlipidaemia in most trials were statins (3-hydroxy-3-methyl-glutaryl-coenzyme A (HMG-CoA) reductase inhibitors) (Castellano 2014; Choudhry 2011; Derose 2012; Eussen 2010; Fang 2015; Faulkner 2000; Fischer 2014; Goswami 2013; Gujral 2014 Guthrie 2001; Ho 2014; Kardas 2013; Kooy 2013; Ma 2010; Márquez 1998; Márquez 2004; Márquez 2007; Nieuwkerk 2012; Park 2013; Patel 2015; PILL 2011; Pladevall 2014; Poston 1998; Powell 1995; Selak 2014; Tamblyn 2009; Thom 2013; Vollmer 2014; Vrijens 2006; Wald 2014; Willich 2009). Anion-exchange resins or bile acid sequestrants were used in five trials (Faulkner 2000; Pladevall 2014; Schectman 1994; Sweeney 1991; Wald 2014). Niacin or nicotinic acid were used in three trials (Brown 1997; Pladevall 2014; Schectman 1994). Two trials used a combined medication regimen (Faulkner 2000; Schectman 1994), and two trials did not specify a lipid-lowering medication (Aslani 2010; Tamblyn 2009). Drug therapy was most commonly started after study allocation; only eight studies included participants who were already taking lipid-lowering medication (Castellano 2014; Fischer 2014; Pladevall 2014; Poston 1998; Powell 1995; Selak 2014; Vollmer 2014; Wald 2014).

Cardiovascular risk

Most studies included in this review enrolled participants at high risk of suffering a cardiovascular event, where lipid-lowering medication was used for primary prevention, whether or not serum cholesterol levels were high (Aslani 2010; Brown 1997; Choudhry 2011; Derose 2012; Eussen 2010; Goswami 2013; Guthrie 2001; Kardas 2013; Kooy 2013; Márquez 1998; Márquez 2004; Márquez 2007; PILL 2011; Selak 2014; Sweeney 1991; Tamblyn 2009; Wald 2014). Nine trials included participants with pre-existing cardiovascular pathology, thus taking medication for secondary prevention (Castellano 2014; Choudhry 2011; Fang 2015; Faulkner 2000; Gujral 2014; Ho 2014; Ma 2010; Park 2013; Vollmer 2014). The remaining studies looked at people on medication for both primary and secondary prevention (Nieuwkerk 2012; Patel 2015; Pladevall 2014; Poston 1998; Powell 1995; Schectman 1994; Thom 2013; Vrijens 2006; Willich 2009). One study (Fischer 2014) identified people at a community pharmacy and did not indicate whether the medication was for primary or secondary prevention.

Settings

Twelve of the included trials took place in primary care (Castellano 2014; Guthrie 2001; Kardas 2013; Márquez 1998; Márquez 2004; Márquez 2007; Patel 2015; PILL 2011; Selak 2014; Tamblyn 2009; Wald 2014; Willich 2009). In six studies participants were followed up in secondary care (Brown 1997; Fang 2015; Faulkner 2000; Goswami 2013; Nieuwkerk 2012; Park 2013), and three studies took place in both settings (Ma 2010; Sweeney 1991; Thom 2013). Other settings were community pharmacies (Aslani 2010; Eussen 2010; Fischer 2014; Gujral 2014; Kooy 2013; Poston 1998; Vrijens 2006), healthcare system (Derose 2012; Pladevall 2014), health maintenance organisation (Choudhry 2011; Powell 1995; Vollmer 2014), and Veterans Affairs medical centres (Ho 2014; Schectman 1994). Trials were set geographically in the USA (15 trials), Netherlands (four trials), Australia (three trials), Spain (three trials), Canada (two trials), England (two trials), Poland (one trial), New Zealand (one trial), India (one trial), China (one trial), Ireland (one trial), and Belgium (one trial). The FOCUS, ORBITAL and PILL trials were conducted across several countries. FOCUS: Argentina, Paraguay, Italy, Spain (Castellano 2014); ORBITAL: Germany, Denmark, Switzerland, and Greece (Willich 2009); PILL: Australia, Brazil, India, Netherlands, New Zealand, United Kingdom, United States (PILL 2011).

Follow-up

Follow-up times ranged from no follow-up to 24 months of follow-up. Most studies achieved their end point outcomes at nine months beginning at three-month intervals. The frequency of the intervention varied, ranging from one single contact up to 12 (see Characteristics of included studies table).

Outcome measures

The methods used to measure adherence included self-report, Medication Adherence Report Scale (MARS), time to discontinuation, medication possession ratio (MPR), proportion of days covered (PDC), continuous multiple interval (CMI), Medication

Event Monitoring System (MEMS), drug profile review, prescription refill rate, prescription abandonment, and pill count. Self-report was assessed by asking participants if they had taken their medication as prescribed and how many doses they missed over a given time period (Choudhry 2011; Guthrie 2001, Nieuwkerk 2012; Patel 2015; Poston 1998; Selak 2014; Wald 2014). The MARS questionnaire was used in two studies (Aslani 2010; Gujral 2014). Time to discontinuation of lipid-lowering medication was used by three studies (Eussen 2010; Kooy 2013; Schectman 1994). MPR is defined as the number of days on medication after study enrolment divided by the number of days between the first fill and the last refill plus the day's supply of last refill. MPR was used in six studies (Eussen 2010; Goswami 2013; Gujral 2014; Kardas 2013; Poston 1998; Powell 1995). PDC was used in three studies (Goswami 2013; Ho 2014; Vollmer 2014). CMI, the ratio of days supply obtained to total days between refill records, was based on pharmacy records from one study (Ma 2010). MEMS is an electronic system of standard pill bottles with microprocessors in the cap that record the timing and frequency of bottle openings, providing detailed and reliable outcome measures at low risk of bias. MEMS was used in three trials (Márquez 2007; Park 2013; Vrijens 2006). Drug profile review by a physician on each visit with study participants was used in one study (Tamblyn 2009). Prescription refill rates were used by seven studies, where refill information was obtained from pharmacies (Derose 2012; Faulkner 2000; Kooy 2013; Pladevall 2014; Poston 1998; Powell 1995; Schectman 1994). Prescription abandonment was used in one study (Fischer 2014). Manual pill counting was performed in seven trials (Brown 1997; Castellano 2014; Faulkner 2000; Márquez 1998; Márquez 2004; PILL 2011; Sweeney 1991). Counting pills is a measure vulnerable to participant manipulation, and one author attempted to increase the reliability of this method by performing unexpected visits to participants' homes for pill counts (Márquez 1998). In another study, pills were not counted in the participant's view in order to avoid influencing their subsequent adherent behaviour (Faulkner 2000). The different methods of measuring adherence was one of the main obstacles in comparing results from the studies, which was further complicated by the fact that some authors used more than one method to measure adherence during their trials.

The report of percentage of mean compliance was considered as the most valid description of compliant behaviour and is reported in the tables of included studies as a main outcome measure, providing the opportunity of comparison between the studies. Other outcome measures reported were: thresholds to define compliant behaviour, i.e. the proportion of participants taking more than 80% of the prescribed medication; discontinuation rates; absolute risk reduction; relative risk reduction; and number needed to intervene in order to save one non-adherent behaviour (see Characteristics of included studies table).

Serum lipids consisting of total cholesterol, HDL, LDL and triglycerides are physiological indicators of participant compliance that were the most frequently reported outcome in the following trials: Aslani 2010; Brown 1997; Castellano 2014; Eussen 2010; Faulkner 2000; Ho 2014; Ma 2010; Márquez 1998; Márquez 2004; Márquez 2007; Nieuwkerk 2012; Patel 2015; PILL 2011; Pladevall 2014; Selak 2014; Sweeney 1991; Thom 2013; Vollmer 2014; Wald 2014; Willich 2009. Some trials began with a 'start-up' phase where participants were either taking medication (Brown 1997) or following a diet (Sweeney 1991) before baseline blood samples were taken; the majority of the trials took baseline blood samples immediately after recruitment. Other reported outcome measures included side effects experienced (Brown 1997; Castellano 2014; Márquez 1998; Patel 2015; PILL 2011; Schectman 1994; Thom 2013; Willich 2009), participant satisfaction (Park 2013), and self-reported lifestyle measures (Aslani 2010; Guthrie 2001; Nieuwkerk 2012; Sweeney 1991). None of the studies provided data on morbidity or mortality as additional outcome measures.

Commercial sponsorship

Authors declared some form of funding by drug companies in Brown 1997; Derose 2012; Eussen 2010; Goswami 2013; Gujral 2014; Guthrie 2001; Nieuwkerk 2012; Patel 2015; PILL 2011; Poston 1998; Powell 1995; Schectman 1994; Sweeney 1991; Vrijens 2006; Wald 2014; Willich 2009.

Excluded studies

We excluded 62 studies after review (see Characteristics of excluded studies). The most common reason for exclusion was that the study was not aimed at improving adherence. One article was a study description without any outcomes and appeared to be the same as Thom 2013, which we included for analysis; however, the two studies had different trial registration numbers.

Risk of bias in included studies

The results of the 'Risk of bias' analysis are shown in Figure 2; Figure 3.

Figure 2.   Methodological quality summary: review authors' judgements about each methodological quality item for each included study.

Figure 3.   Risk of bias graph: review authors' judgements about each risk of bias item presented as percentages across all included studies.

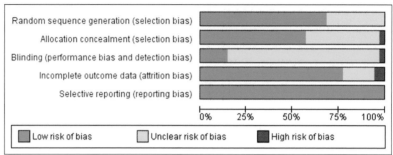

Allocation

We rated 11 studies at 'unclear risk' for random sequence generation, as they did not provide sufficient information to make a judgement (Aslani 2010; Brown 1997; Gujral 2014; Guthrie 2001; Kardas 2013; Márquez 1998; Poston 1998; Powell 1995; Schectman 1994; Sweeney 1991; Vrijens 2006). We assessed 24 studies at 'low risk' for random sequence generation, as they reported using a computer-generated allocation process, telephone allocation, or allocation by a statistician who was not involved in conducting the study (Castellano 2014; Choudhry 2011; Derose 2012; Eussen 2010; Fang 2015; Faulkner 2000; Fischer 2014; Goswami 2013; Ho 2014; Kooy 2013; Ma 2010; Márquez 2004; Márquez 2007; Nieuwkerk 2012; Park 2013; Patel 2015; PILL 2011; Pladevall 2014; Selak 2014; Tamblyn 2009; Thom 2013; Vollmer 2014; Wald 2014; Willich 2009). We rated none of the studies at 'high risk' for random sequence generation.

We assessed 14 studies at 'unclear risk' for allocation concealment, as they did not report sufficient information to allow judgement. (Aslani 2010; Brown 1997; Choudhry 2011; Faulkner 2000; Goswami 2013; Guthrie 2001; Kardas 2013; PILL 2011; Poston 1998; Powell 1995; Schectman 1994; Sweeney 1991; Vrijens 2006; Wald 2014) We rated 20 studies at 'low risk' for allocation concealment as this was adequately described and deemed appropriate (Castellano 2014; Derose 2012; Eussen 2010; Fang 2015; Fischer 2014; Ho 2014; Kooy 2013; Ma 2010; Márquez 1998; Márquez 2004; Márquez 2007; Nieuwkerk 2012; Park 2013; Patel 2015; Pladevall 2014; Selak 2014; Tamblyn 2009; Thom 2013; Vollmer 2014; Willich 2009). In Gujral 2014 allocation

was not concealed as reported in the protocol of the study (AC-TRN12611000322932), so we judged this to be at 'high risk' for allocation concealment.

Blinding

One study (Tamblyn 2009) had a single-blinded study design and was rated as 'high risk'. Physicians and participants were blind to the outcome assessed, but not to the intervention in this study. We assessed 28 studies as being at 'unclear risk', as they had an unblinded, open-label study design or did not report open-label design (Aslani 2010; Brown 1997; Castellano 2014; Choudhry 2011; Eussen 2010; Fang 2015; Faulkner 2000; Fischer 2014; Goswami 2013; Gujral 2014; Guthrie 2001; Ho 2014; Kardas 2013; Kooy 2013; Ma 2010; Márquez 2004; Márquez 2007; Nieuwkerk 2012; Park 2013; Patel 2015; Pladevall 2014; Poston 1998; Selak 2014; Sweeney 1991; Thom 2013; Vollmer 2014; Vrijens 2006; Wald 2014). Five studies at low risk stated a method where investigators and participants were blind to the outcome and intervention (Derose 2012; Márquez 1998; PILL 2011; Powell 1995; Schectman 1994). Blinding participants to the intervention they were receiving and blinding key study personnel including physicians was often not possible, given the nature of the intervention. Most trials did not report blinding of those assessing the outcome 'adherence'.

Incomplete outcome data

We judged two studies (Gujral 2014; Guthrie 2001) as being at 'high risk' for attrition bias, due to a high rate of attrition in return of a survey tool (Guthrie 2001) or high attrition (31.5%) at the primary end point after 12 months follow-up (Gujral 2014). We rated six studies as being at 'unclear risk' due to variable rates of study attrition (Brown 1997; Goswami 2013; Márquez 1998; Pladevall 2014; Tamblyn 2009) or not reporting on attrition (Derose 2012). We judged the other studies as being at 'low risk', as they reported minimal to no loss to follow-up.

Selective reporting

All included studies reported on all intended outcomes, as assessed by comparing the Methods section with the Results section or with the available protocol.

Effects of interventions

See: **Summary of findings for the main comparison** Summary of findings table for the comparison of 'intensified patient care' vs 'usual care'

Types of interventions

The trials in this review aimed to increase adherence to lipid-lowering medication by applying one of the following seven intervention categories. In order to determine study similarities, we created a grid into which we placed studies with similar interventions and comparators. We then further grouped those studies which we found to have both similar interventions and comparators, according to similar outcome measures. In grouping the studies in this manner, we found that there were sufficient studies to conduct a meta-analysis among those studies comparing such interventions with usual care (see Table 1).

1. Drug regimen simplification vs usual care

Seven studies attempted to simplify the drug regimen (Brown 1997; Castellano 2014; Patel 2015; PILL 2011; Selak 2014; Sweeney 1991; Thom 2013). Two studies (Brown 1997; Sweeney 1991) used a regimen with reduction of daily dosing, whereas the other five studies used a fixed-dose combination or 'polypill' regimen (Castellano 2014; Patel 2015; PILL 2011; Selak 2014; Thom 2013).

We were unable to pool data, as the study publications provided insufficient data, so we describe the results for each of the individual studies below.

Medication adherence - Reducing medication intake from four times to twice daily improved mean medication intake by 11% (96% in the intervention group vs 85% in the control group; P = 0.01; n = 29) (Brown 1997). Drug modification, by administering colestyramine bars instead of powder to make intake easier, did not decrease the adherence rate (91.8% in the intervention group vs 94.8% in the control group; P > 0.05; n = 83) (Sweeney 1991). In the five studies that used a fixed-dose combination (FDC) or polypill, four out of five studies showed better adherence with the polypill compared with the separate dosing regimens.

In Castellano 2014, the polypill group showed improved adherence compared with the group receiving separate medications after nine months of follow-up: 50.8% vs 41%; P = 0.019 (for the intention-to-treat population) and 65.7% vs 55.7%; P = 0.012 (for the per-protocol population); n = 458 (per-protocol population). In Patel 2015 participants in the polypill-based strategy showed greater use of treatment compared to those receiving separate medications after a median of 18 months (70% vs 47%; risk ratio (RR) 1.49, 95% confidence interval (CI) 1.30 to 1.72; P < 0.0001; number needed to treat for an additional beneficial outcome (NNTB) 4 (95% CI 3 to 7); n = 623).

In the PILL 2011 study, discontinuation rates were 23% in the polypill group vs 18% in the placebo group (RR 1.33, 95% CI 0.89 to 2.00; P = 0.2; n = 373).

In Selak 2014 (n = 513) adherence was greater with the FDC than with usual care at 12 months (81% vs 46%; RR 1.75, 95% CI 1.52 to 2.03; P < 0.001; NNTB 3, 95% CI 2 to 4). Adherence specifically for the statins was not different in the FDC group (94% vs 89%; P = 0.06).

In Thom 2013 using FDC improved adherence vs usual care (86% vs 65%; RR 1.33, 95% CI 1.26 to 1.41; P < 0.001; n = 1921).

Total serum cholesterol - Brown 1997 demonstrated low-/high-density lipoprotein (LDL/HDL) change from means of 215/46 mg/dl at baseline, to 94/59 mg/dl after run-in, to 85/52 mg/dl after eight months of controlled-release niacin, and to 98/56 mg/dl after eight months of regular niacin (regular niacin vs controlled-release niacin, P < 0.005/ < 0.05). The target of LDL < 100 mg/dl was achieved at eight months by 83% of these participants with controlled-release niacin and by 52% with regular niacin (P < 0.01).

In Sweeney 1991, total cholesterol decreased by 16% in the bar group and 17% in the powder group (P < 0.01). LDL-cholesterol decreased by 28% and 29% in the bar and powder groups respectively (P < 0.01). There was no change in HDL cholesterol. Triglycerides increased in both groups, by 29% in the bar group and by 25% in the powder group. There was no difference between bar and powder in the effect on blood lipids.

In the five studies that used a FDC or polypill, two out of five studies found a reduction in LDL-cholesterol levels with the polypill as compared with the separate dosing regimens (PILL 2011; Thom 2013).

Castellano 2014 did not find a difference in mean low-density lipoprotein cholesterol levels (89.9 mg/dl vs 91.7 mg/dl) between the groups receiving the polypill or the three drugs administered separately.

In Patel 2015 there was no difference in total cholesterol levels in the polypill-based strategy compared to those receiving separate medications after a median of 18 months (0.08 mmol/l, 95% CI 0.06 to 0.22; P = 0.26).

The PILL 2011 study found a reduction in LDL-cholesterol of 0.8 mmol/L, 95% CI 0.6 to 0.9 in favour of the group that was given the polypill.

Selak 2014 did not find any difference in LDL-cholesterol levels between the FDC group and the control group (difference −0.05 mmol/L (−0.20 vs −0.15, 95% CI −0.17 to 0.08; P = 0.46)).

Thom 2013 found a difference in LDL-cholesterol in favour of the FDC group (difference −4.2 mg/dL, 95% CI −6.6 to −1.9 mg/dL; P < 0.001) at the end of the study.

Blood pressure - In the studies that used a FDC or polypill, three out of five studies found a reduction in systolic blood pressure (SBP) with the intervention groups as compared with the separate dosing regimens (PILL 2011; Selak 2014; Thom 2013). Brown 1997 and Sweeney 1991 do not report effects on blood pressure. Castellano 2014 did not find a difference in mean SBP (129.6 mmHg vs 128.6 mm Hg) between the groups receiving the polypill or the three drugs administered separately.

In Patel 2015 there was no difference in SBP in the polypill-based strategy compared to those receiving separate medications after a median of 18 months (1.5 mmHg, 95% CI 4.0 to 1.0; P = 0.24).

The PILL 2011 study found a reduction in SBP of 9.9 mmHg, 95% CI 7.7 to 12.1 in favour of the group that was given the polypill.

Selak 2014 showed reductions in SBP (−2.6 mmHg, 95% CI −4.0 to −1.1 mmHg; P < 0.001) in the FDC group vs the usual care group.

Thom 2013 showed reduction of SBP (−2.6 mmHg, 95% CI −4.0 to −1.1 mmHg) in the FDC group compared with the usual care group at the end of the study.

Adverse events -
Castellano 2014 did not find a difference in number of adverse events between the groups receiving the polypill or the three drugs administered separately (35.4% vs 32.5%, respectively). There were 21 reported serious adverse events (6.0%) in the polypill group vs 23 (6.6% in the control group). There was 1 death in each group (0.3% vs 0.3%).

In Patel 2015 there was at least one serious adverse event reported in 46.3% of participants in the polypill group vs 40.7% in the usual care group (P = 0.16).

The PILL 2011 study 58% in the polypill group reported adverse events compared with 42% in the control group (P = 0.001) The authors report that the side effects were known side effects of the medication contained in the polypill. Four serious adverse events were reported in each group (polypill group: chest pain, newly diagnosed Type 2 diabetes, removal of wisdom teeth, syncope; placebo group: syncope,

depression, transient ischaemic attack, hip fracture). No deaths, major vascular events, major bleeds or episodes of gastrointestinal ulceration were reported.

In Selak 2014 the number of participants with serious adverse events was not different between groups (fixed dose combination 99 vs usual care 93, P = 0.56). Four deaths occurred in the group with fixed dose combination and 6 in the usual care group (P = 0.75).

Thom 2013 showed no significant differences in serious adverse events (5% in the foxed dose combination group and 3.5% in the usual care group (P = 0.09) between the groups. Seventeen deaths occurred in the fixed dose combination group vs 15 in the usual care group (P = 0.72).

2. Patient education and information vs usual care

Five studies including 8116 participants intended to improve medication adherence by improving patient information and eduction. No consistent improvement was found (Gujral 2014; Park 2013; Poston 1998; Powell 1995; Willich 2009).

Medication adherence - Pharmacist-mediated information and postal backups, where videotapes, booklets and newspapers were handed out by the local pharmacist followed by educational newsletters sent by post, successfully improved adherence in people who had started taking statins within 60 days before recruitment into the study, but did not improve adherence in those who had been taking statins for more than 60 days before recruitment into the study (Poston 1998). In participants who had started taking statins within 60 days before recruitment into the study, the increase in adherence was 13% (92% in intervention group vs 79% in control group; P ≤ 0.005). In participants who had been taking statins for more than 60 days before recruitment into the study, adherence to long-term therapy was not improved (92% vs 91%; P value reported as non-significant but not based on a correct interaction test).

Another study applied a less personal approach, by sending out videotapes to members of a health maintenance organisation who were known to have a pharmacy claim for statins (Powell 1995), not increasing adherence rates (73% in intervention group vs 70% in control group; P > 0.05; n = 568).

Medication Event Monitoring Systems (MEMS) revealed that those who received text messages for antiplatelets had a higher percentage of correct doses taken (t(36) = 2.5; P = 0.02), percentage number of doses taken (t(31) = 2.8; P = 0.01), and percentage of prescribed doses taken on schedule (t(37) = 2.6; P = 0.01; n = 84). Text message response rates were higher for antiplatelets (M = 90.2%; SD = 9) than statins (M = 83.4%; SD = 15.8) (t(26) = 3.1; P = 0.005). Self-reported adherence revealed no differences among groups (Park 2013).

In another study, participants received a starter pack containing a videotape, an educational leaflet, details of the free-phone patient helpline and website, and labels with a reminder to take study medication. Participants also received regular personalised letters and phone calls throughout the study. The compliance-enhancing programme was only effective in statin-naïve participants at three and six months, but had no overall effect over 12 months (80%

vs 76% and 78% vs 73%; P < 0.01; n = 6872) (Willich 2009).
In Gujral 2014 participants in the intervention group received education from the pharmacists tailored to identified misconceptions and beliefs about their medication. However, at the end of the study (after 12 months) there was no difference in adherence: 29% of the participants in the intervention group were non-adherent compared with 25% in the control group (P = 0.605; n = 137).

Total serum cholesterol - Willich 2009 reports that at month 12, 2231 (68.2%) of participants on rosuvastatin plus compliance initiatives and rosuvastatin alone - 2152 (68.4%) were reported as achieving LDL-cholesterol < 115 mg/dl (P = 0.97), and 1894 (57.6%) of participants on rosuvastatin plus compliance initiatives and 1837 (57.9%) on rosuvastatin alone reported achieving total cholesterol < 190 mg/dl; P = 0.8732; n = 6872.

3. Intensified patient care vs usual care

Sixteen studies randomising 22,785 participants and reporting outcomes on 13,602 participants, investigated the effect of intensified patient care. Reinforcing people to take their medication in the form of written postal material, telephone or other reminders was associated with improved adherence in 10 studies, with results from eight trials reaching statistical significance. There was a positive trend towards improvement in lipid levels in two studies (Márquez 2004; Márquez 2007).

Pooling of data for medication adherence at up to six months included Derose 2012; Eussen 2010; Faulkner 2000; Goswami 2013; Guthrie 2001; Márquez 2004; Márquez 2007. Pooling of data for medication adherence at more than six months included Faulkner 2000; Ho 2014; Vrijens 2006.

Of the 16 RCTs with an intensified patient care intervention, five studies used continuous instead of dichotomous outcomes or cumulative results, and could not be included in the pooled data for medication adherence (Aslani 2010; Fang 2015; Kardas 2013; Ma 2010; Nieuwkerk 2012). For Aslani 2010, low recruitment and high drop-out rate had a significant impact on the study power (reducing it to 44%) to detect changes in adherence levels but study had sufficient power to detect a statistically and clinically significant difference in total cholesterol levels.

We could not include Schectman 1994 in the pooled data for medication adherence, as this study was very different from the other studies; the medications used, niacin and bile acid salts, had very low adherence due to side effects. In Faulkner 2000, for medication adherence at more than six months, outcome adherence with colestipol was much lower than with lovastatin, due to side effects, so we used lovastatin adherence for pooling of data. Wald 2014 could not be included in the pooled data as outcome measures included combined data from blood pressure and lipid-lowering medications.

Medication adherence

Sixteen studies report medication adherence for intensified vs usual

care interventions (see Table 2); seven provided data for pooling of short-term adherence and three studies for long-term adherence. We describe the pooled results below, and report results for the studies that could not be pooled here.

In Aslani 2010 (n = 97), Medication Adherence Report Scales showed no changes in medicine adherence scores, although intervention participants were less likely to take less than the prescribed dose after the first-time interval (main effect $F_{2,178}$ = 4.3; P < 0.05; contrast $F_{1,89}$ = 5.7; P < 0.05), and the intervention group reported that compared with the control group they were more liable to alter the dose of their medicine at the third reading compared to the second reading ($F_{1,89}$ = 4.97; P < 0.05).

In Kardas 2013, the intervention group received educational counselling at each visit (i.e. every eight weeks) and were also asked to adopt a routine evening activity of their choice for a reminder. Study arms differed in their level of adherence: mean ± SD MPR was 95.4% ± 53.7% and 81.7% ± 31.0%, for intervention and control groups respectively (P < 0.05; n = 196).

Participants in the intervention group of Ma 2010 (n = 559) received five pharmacist-delivered telephone counselling calls posthospital discharge. The continuous multiple interval (CMI) for statin medication use was 0.88 (SD 0.3) in the pharmacy-delivered intervention (PI) (referring to the participant being 88% adherent to their statins medication), and 0.90 (SD 0.3) in the usual care condition (P = 0.51), leading to the conclusion that a pharmacist-delivered intervention aimed only at improving participant adherence is unlikely to positively affect outcomes.

Nieuwkerk 2012 (n = 181) demonstrated that statin adherence was higher (P < 0.01) and anxiety was lower (P < 0.01) in the intervention group, which received nurse-led cardiovascular risk-factor counselling than in the routine-care group.

In Fang 2015 (n = 271) participants who were randomised to the short message service (SMS) and those in the SMS + Micro Letter group had better cumulative adherence (lower Morisky Medication Adherence Scale scores) after six months than the phone group. The SMS + Micro Letter group had better cumulative adherence (lower Morisky Medication Adherence Scale scores) than the SMS-alone group.

Pooling of the results

We grouped the results into long-term adherence and short-term outcomes. We defined short-term results as those outcomes measured at up to six months, and long-term outcomes as measured at more than six months. We then pooled results according to long-term or short-term outcomes. When it was not provided, we estimated the SD for the difference between means using the formula $\sigma_d = \mathrm{sqrt}\,(\,\sigma_1{}^2\,/\,n_1 + \sigma_2{}^2\,/\,n_2\,)$. We estimated the SDs for Aslani 2010 and Faulkner 2000.

The forest plots in Analysis 1.1 and Analysis 1.2 both show pooled treatment effects of the intensification of patient care category of interventions when compared with usual care and using adherence measures as an outcome in both short-term and long-term measures. Forest plots in Analysis 1.4 show the pooled effect estimate for total cholesterol level over both short- and long-term follow-up.

We did not adjust the Aslani 2010 data for clustering as the expected clustering effect of patients within pharmacies in Australia is very low (Armour 2007).

Medication adherence at ≤ 6 months

Pooling of data for medication adherence at up to six months using per-protocol analysis of dichotomous outcomes included seven studies involving 11,204 participants. There was considerable heterogeneity (I^2 = 88%). Meta-analysis using a random-effects model estimated an odds ratio of 1.93 (95% CI 1.29 to 2.88; 7 studies; 11,204 participants; moderate-quality evidence), favouring the intervention (Analysis 1.1). Removing the three studies with less intensive interventions that contributed to the heterogeneity (as is also apparent from the forest plot) from the pooled analysis (Derose 2012; Márquez 2004; Márquez 2007) resulted in an of OR 1.19 (95% CI 1.02 to 1.39; I^2 = 0%), favouring the intervention. All but one study (Guthrie 2001) had low attrition rates. A sensitivity analysis excluding Guthrie 2001, which had very high attrition (only 35% of surveys were returned to the investigators), resulted in an OR 2.22, 95% CI 1.41 to 3.49 (Analysis 1.7). The conclusions remained unaltered (Summary of findings for the main comparison).

Medication adherence at > 6 months

Pooling of data for medication adherence at more than six months using per-protocol analysis of dichotomous outcomes included three studies involving 663 participants. The studies were homogeneous (I^2 = 0%). Meta-analysis using a random-effects model estimated an odds ratio of 2.87 (95% CI 1.91 to 4.29; 3 studies; 663 participants; high-quality evidence), favouring the intervention (Analysis 1.2). Using a fixed-effect model did not alter the estimate (OR = 2.87, 95% CI 1.92 to 4.30) nor the conclusions. Although Vrijens 2006 contributes 59% of the weighting, the estimate remains robust if this study is removed: the result is OR 3.82, 95% CI 2.03 to 7.18; I^2 = 0%, favouring the intervention, and hence the overall conclusion remained unchanged (Summary of findings for the main comparison).

Total serum cholesterol and low-density lipoprotein cholesterol - From the 16 RCTs that used intensified patient care, five studies (Derose 2012; Goswami 2013; Guthrie 2001; Schectman 1994; Vrijens 2006) did not use lipid levels as an outcome measure.

Eussen 2010 reported adjusted levels of total cholesterol at three months, but did not report the raw data for inclusion in the meta-analysis. Kardas 2013 also reported a decrease in total cholesterol, LDL, and triglycerides with constant HDL, but it did not include any raw data except for baseline measures. Ma 2010 did not

provide baseline or change scores and cholesterol data included participants not receiving lipid-lowering medications. However, no other studies reported the same time point for comparison. Nieuwkerk 2012 was not included, as the lipid level data were compiled as an average of three time points: three months, nine months, and 18 months. Ho 2014 could not be included in the pooled data as cholesterol data included participants not taking lipid-lowering medications. Means and SD were pooled and compared for Aslani 2010; Faulkner 2000; Márquez 2004; Márquez 2007 at up to six-month time points. Additionally, the means and SD were compared for Aslani 2010 and Faulkner 2000 at more than six months.

The studies that we could not pool are described here.

Eussen 2010 reported a significant decline in mean total cholesterol and LDL-cholesterol levels in those receiving pharmaceutical care. Total cholesterol and LDL-cholesterol decreased by a mean of 17.2 mg/dL, 95% CI 12.3 to 22.0, and 9.47 mg/dL, 95% CI 5.02 to 13.9 respectively. Three months after initiating statin therapy 65% of participants achieved a target LDL-cholesterol level of ≤ 115 mg/dL. The intervention appeared to have a sustained effect, given the fact that at six and 12 months after treatment, these percentages were 72% and 77% respectively.

Kardas 2013 reported that both the control and intervention groups had decreases in total cholesterol, LDL-cholesterol, and triglycerides, with a relatively constant level of HDL-cholesterol. At the end of the 48-week follow-up period, the two groups showed no differences in these lipid parameters.

In a study of 689 individuals, Ma 2010 found no differences in those receiving the pharmacist-delivered intervention versus usual care. Sixty-five per cent of individuals achieved a goal LDL-cholesterol of < 100 mg/dl in the intervention group versus 65% (P = 0.29). After 12 months there were no differences in total cholesterol, LDL-cholesterol, HDL-cholesterol, or triglycerides between the two groups.

Nieuwkerk 2012 found that the LDL-cholesterol was lower in the intensified patient care group when compared to the routine-care group during follow-up in primary prevention participants, but not in secondary prevention participants.

Wald 2014 found no differences in serum cholesterol (4.20 mmol/L versus 4.21 mmol/L total cholesterol and 2.29 mmol/L versus 2.22 mmol/L LDL-cholesterol) between the Text and No-text groups respectively.

Pooling of the results

Reduction in total serum cholesterol (mg/dL) at ≤ 6 months: Pooling of data for total serum cholesterol at up to six months using per-protocol analysis of continuous outcomes included four studies with 430 participants. There was considerable heterogeneity (I^2 = 89%). Meta-analysis using a random-effects model produced a mean difference (MD) of 17.15, 95% CI 1.17 to 33.14; 4 studies; 430 participants; low-quality evidence, favouring the intervention (Analysis 1.3). Removing the studies that contributed most to the heterogeneity from the pooled analysis resulted in MD 3.79, 95% CI -2.42 to 10.00; I^2 = 18%, favouring the intervention but not reaching statistical significance. The smaller reductions in the Aslani 2010 study may have been related to the fact that participants were being treated for hyperlipidaemia at the time and were already on therapy, whereas in Márquez 2004; Márquez 2007; Faulkner 2000, participants were relatively statin-naïve and either had therapy initiated or intensified, which would account for a greater initial decline in lipid levels. We used mean difference here as it has a more direct clinical meaning and is easier to interpret compared to the standardised mean difference (SMD). Also, using SMD did not change the conclusion of the analysis (Summary of findings for the main comparison)

Reduction in total serum cholesterol (mg/dL) at > 6 months: Pooling of data for total serum cholesterol at up to six months using per-protocol analysis of continuous outcomes included two studies with 127 participants. The studies were homogeneous (I^2 = 0%). Meta-analysis using a random-effects model produced an MD of 17.57, 95% CI 14.95 to 20.19; 2 studies; 127 participants; high-quality evidence, favouring the intervention (Analysis 1.4). Using a fixed-effect model did not change the overall estimate (Summary of findings for the main comparison).

Reduction in LDL-cholesterol (mg/dL) at ≤ 6 months: Pooling of data for low-density lipoprotein cholesterol at up to six months using per-protocol analysis of continuous outcomes included three studies with 333 participants. There was moderate heterogeneity (I^2 = 53%). Meta-analysis using a random-effects model produced a MD of 19.51, 95% CI 8.51 to 30.51; 3 studies; 333 participants; moderate-quality evidence, favouring the intervention (Analysis 1.5). Removing the studies that contributed to the heterogeneity from the pooled analysis resulted in MD 9.00, 95% CI -3.57 to 21.57, favouring the intervention, but not reaching statistical significance (Summary of findings for the main comparison).

Reduction in LDL-cholesterol (mg/dL) at > 6 months: Pooling of data for LDL-cholesterol at more than six months using per-protocol analysis of continuous outcomes included one study with 30 participants. Meta-analysis using a random-effects model estimated a MD of 18.00, 95% CI 5.12 to 30.88, favouring the intervention (Analysis 1.6) (Summary of findings for the main comparison).

4. Complex behavioural approaches vs usual care

Medication adherence - Only one trial (Márquez 1998) used a group behavioural approach, where participants initially attended small-group training followed by postal information. The adherence in the intervention group was no different from the control group (88.5% in intervention group versus 83.8% in control group, P > 0.05; n = 108).

Total serum cholesterol - There were differences between inter-vention and control groups for TC, LDL and HDL. Compared final mean differences in the intervention groups vs the control groups were: 7.5 mg/dl reduction in mean TC (P > 0.05); 5.2 mg/dl reduction in mean LDL (P > 0.05), 2.1 mg/dl increase in mean HDL (P > 0.05), and 30 mg/dl reduction in mean triglyceride levels (TRG) (P < 0.05).

5. Decision support systems vs complex behavioural approaches

Medication adherence - In Kooy 2013 (n = 108) the median PDC360 (25th - 75th percentile) was 90.0% (76.75 - 98.25) in the counselling/ERD group, 91.0% (76.00 - 99.00) in the ERD group and 87.5% (75.00 - 99.00) in the control group (ITT analysis). We found no differences in the median refill adherence. In Pladevall 2014 (n = 1692) there was no difference between participants in the study arms that received adherence information and motivational interviewing when compared with usual care.

Total serum cholesterol - This outcome was not reported in Kooy 2013. In Pladevall 2014 there were no differences in LDL-cholesterol levels between the different groups (P = 0.084).

6. Administrative improvements vs usual care

Medication adherence - In Tamblyn 2009 (n = 2293) participants in the intervention group were more likely to have their drug profile reviewed compared to those in the control group (44.5% vs 35.5%; OR 1.46; P < 0.001). Overall, however, there was no difference in the magnitude of the decline in adherence between the intervention and control group (mean -6.2 (intervention) vs -6.4 (control); P = 0.90). In Choudhry 2011 (n = 5855) rates of full adherence (defined as having a supply of medications available on at least 80% of days during follow-up) for statins were 41.9% in the usual care group and 49.3% in the full-coverage group (increase by 6.2 percentage points, 95% CI 3.9 to 8.5); OR 1.36, 95% CI 1.18 to 1.56; P < 0.001 . Rates of adherence to other medications for which copayments remained the same were no different between the two study groups.

Total serum cholesterol - This outcome was not reported in Choudhry 2011 or Tamblyn 2009.

Costs - Choudhry 2011 evaluated costs related to the intervention and found that elimination of co-payments in the intervention group did not increase total spending for the health system (USD 66,008 for the full-coverage group and USD 71,778 for the usual-coverage group; relative spending 0.89, 95% CI 0.50 to 1.56; P = 0.68). Participants in the intervention group paid less for drugs and other services (relative spending 0.74, 95% CI 0.68 to 0.80; P < 0.001).

7. Large-scale pharmacy-led automated telephone intervention vs usual care

Fischer 2014 (n = 861,894) included two interventions on nearly a million participants, initiated by a commercial pharmacy dispensing medications. One intervention consisted of automated phone calls to participants on the third and seventh days after a prescription was processed but remained unpurchased. The other intervention was a live intervention which used calls from a pharmacist or technician to participants who still had not picked up their prescriptions after eight days. Data for analysis were obtained following the interventions being commercially conducted. Data were not recorded on whether pharmacists or technicians left a message or actually spoke with participants, or on the content of conversations. In Vollmer 2014 the intervention consisted of automated phone reminders using interactive voice recognition to participants when they were due or overdue for a refill. Participants in the enhanced study arm also received a letter if they were 60 to 89 days overdue. This study randomised 16,280 participants.

Medication adherence - Fischer 2014: For the automated intervention, the proportion of abandoned prescriptions was 4.2% in the intervention group and 4.5% in the control group (P = 0.23). For antihypertensives, the proportion of abandoned prescriptions was 3.7% in the intervention group and 4.1% in the control group (P = 0.06), whereas for antihyperlipidaemics the proportions were the same (6.0%).

For the live intervention, the proportion of abandoned prescriptions was 36.9% in the intervention group and 41.7% in the control group, a difference of 4.8% (P < 0.0001). The difference for antihypertensives was 6.9% (P < 0.0001) but for antihyperlipidaemics was only 1.4 (P = 0.25)

In Vollmer 2014 (n = 16,366) statin adherence increased for both intervention groups compared with usual care, but adherence was no different between the phone group and the enhance phone group. On average, adherence among the group that only received the phone calls was 2.2 percentage points higher than for usual care (95% CI 1.1 to 3.4), while the difference was 3.0, 95% CI 1.9 to 4.2 percentage points for the group that also received a reminder letter.

Total serum cholesterol - This outcome was not reported in Fischer 2014. In Vollmer 2014 a reduction in LDL-cholesterol levels was found among the participants receiving phone calls and a letter, compared to usual care (mean difference -1.5, 95% CI -2.7 to -0.2 mg/dL; P = 0.019).

DISCUSSION

Summary of main results

This updated systematic review identified new evidence to suggest that patient interventions which we grouped as intensified patient adherence to lipid-lowering therapy when compared to usual care may improve patient adherence to lipid-lowering therapy when compared to usual care. These types of interventions took the form of telephone reminders, calendar reminders, integrated multidisciplinary educational activities and pharmacist-led interventions. The interventions appeared to be effective in improving medication adherence, both over the short term (up to six months) and the long term (more than six months). Physiologic outcome data in the form of cholesterol levels also demonstrated significant improvement over short-term and long-term periods. The effectiveness of these types of interventions was sustained even when we removed studies contributing to heterogeneity from the analysis.

Other types of interventions which we grouped as drug regimen simplification, complex behavioural approaches, decision support systems, administrative improvements, and a large-scale pharmacy-led automated telephone intervention did not consistently show an overall improvement in adherence rates or other physiologic measures of adherence. Some outcomes were not measured in all studies and comparisons were made only where possible.

Overall completeness and applicability of evidence

The significant increase in research activity in this field has yielded more robust data from which to draw conclusions. In the studies classified as intensification of patient care, enough high-quality studies exist with similar outcomes where we noted significant trends favouring the interventions. The types of studies in this category included large groups of outpatients and would seem to be generalisable to other outpatient cohorts. Studies in the other categories could address the objectives of our meta-analysis, but given the relatively small number of comparable studies with similar interventions and outcome measures, no clear trends emerged. The interventions in the intensified patient care group are of a type which is applicable to current practice. Many large healthcare systems are evaluating methods to improve the health of large populations of patients. Large-scale structural interventions noted in the intensified patient care group of interventions are generally feasible for these types of systems.

Quality of the evidence

The studies in this review investigate the impact of a wide range of interventions on adherence to lipid-lowering treatments. The nature of the majority of interventions implies that blinding of participants was not possible (e.g. interventions such as reminder phone calls or education sessions). As this is acceptable in a pragmatic context, we have not downgraded the evidence for lack of blinding. Studies demonstrating a fixed dose combination or 'polypill' placebo comparison are feasible, but we could not pool them in our review.

We assessed the quality of the pooled evidence using the GRADE classification for five pooled outcomes in the comparison of intensification of patient care vs usual care. We graded the evidence for the outcomes of long-term adherence (more than six months) and reduction in total cholesterol as being of high quality. We rated the short-term outcomes (up to six months) of patient adherence and LDL-cholesterol as being of moderate quality. We downgraded these outcomes by one level because of heterogeneity of the pooled data. We downgraded the short-term outcome of total serum cholesterol to low quality, due to heterogeneity and a wide confidence interval (imprecision).

The review authors independently reviewed data at various checkpoints, ensuring the selection of a series of rigorous studies. The review authors believe that systematic error did not threaten the validity of the results of the studies included in this review (see Risk of bias in included studies).

Potential biases in the review process

We have searched in several different databases, including trials registers, and we have handsearched reference lists in order to identify eligible studies. It is nevertheless still possible that we have missed relevant material. In addition, two review authors selected studies independently, thus minimising the risk of overlooking any. The updated searches in 2015 and 2016 retrieved a considerable number of new studies for inclusion, indicating that the topic is still being actively researched. In order to maintain the relevance of this review, we will therefore attempt to update our searches regularly. The evidence is quite consistent and robust and it may therefore be unlikely that a missed study could have changed our conclusions.

The diverse nature of the studied interventions and absence of a standard classification of interventions to improve medication adherence means that studies can be grouped in different ways. We have grouped the studies from the perspective of the health system/ provider, as this has relevance to implementation strategies.

In the pooled analysis Analysis 1.3 the Aslani 2010 study was a clustered RCT, however we did not adjust for clustering as in Australia pharmacies do not serve specific populations. Patients generally purchase their medication from a number of different pharmacies. A study in a similar setting found a clustering effect of -0.006, which justifies using uni-level analysis. It is possible that we have overestimated the effect of the intervention, however, it is unlikely that this will have influenced the conclusion.

Agreements and disagreements with other studies or reviews

The two previous versions of this review concluded that there were no reliable interventions that have been shown to improve adherence rates to lipid-lowering medications (Schedlbauer 2004; Schedlbauer 2010). However, this updated review which includes 24 additional studies indicates that interventions classified as intensification of patient care could improve both short-term and long-term adherence rates when compared to usual care.

An earlier systematic review (Muller-Nordhorn 2005), including 10 RCTs, found that interventions (ranging from postal reminders to coaching, delivered by nurses, pharmacists or physicians) was associated with a significant increase in patient adherence to statin therapy compared with the control group in four of the 10 RCTs. The remaining six RCTs found no significant difference in adherence. The authors conclude that "given the inconsistency of the findings and the limitations of certain study designs, RCTs with a large sample size are needed to further investigate the effectiveness of adherence-increasing interventions in patients with statin therapy." The most recent systematic review by Rash 2016, which includes 29 RCTs, pooled data for interventions labelled as 'simplification of drug regimen', 'provision of education', and 'multi-faceted interventions'. They conclude that all these types of interventions had a small positive effect on statin adherence, but that additional methodologically rigorous trials are needed.

AUTHORS' CONCLUSIONS

Implications for practice

High-quality evidence shows that intensification of patient care interventions improves long-term medication adherence and total cholesterol. Moderate-quality evidence shows that intensification of patient care interventions improves short-term medication adherence and LDL-cholesterol. The evidence for total cholesterol reduction in the short term is of low quality. Given the importance of statin therapy in both primary and secondary prevention, strategies to improve adherence rates should have significant benefit in those people for whom statin therapy is recommended. The interventions which were identified as successful in the intensification of patient care interventions typically involved strategies beyond what a single clinician could provide. Instead, healthcare delivery systems might be better equipped to deliver the types of interventions which have been shown to best improve adherence rates. Health system-related interventions which showed benefit involved strategies such as pharmacist-led interventions, multidisciplinary educational or counselling sessions, and automated reminders of various types. A combination of all of these types of interventions, along with an added focus on teamwork with the primary physician, also proved to be effective (Ho 2014). In these studies, effectiveness was generally demonstrated by improvements in both adherence rates and in lipid levels. The effect appeared durable and was significant over both short-term and long-term time periods. Healthcare systems which are able to involve teams of healthcare professionals in the implementation of such interventions may well be successful in decreasing the burden of cardiovascular disease in the populations whom they serve through improved adherence to statin medications.

The results of our meta-analysis must, however, be seen in the context of the healthcare system in which they were trialled. For instance, the pharmacy-led interventions are applicable in systems with a strong and well-structured medication delivery system through pharmacies, but will not be feasible in, for instance, low-income countries where drug dispensing is much less controlled or integrated into the healthcare system. Cultural and social context will also play a role and the impact of automated reminders delivered as text messages, for instance, will be less effective if patients' beliefs regarding their medicines have not been addressed.

it is important to acknowledge the wide diversity of control interventions that we have grouped as 'usual care', which is different in each setting. For instance, pharmacy usual care can include patient education in some settings but none at all in others. Likewise, usual care in the context of physician-delivered interventions can also vary extensively. The results of our comparisons therefore need to be interpreted with caution.

Implications for research

Exploration of additional factors which influence adherence to drug therapy may help in identifying other targets for interventions. These additional factors include knowledge, health beliefs, risk perception, memory, side effects of medication, costs of medication and inconvenience (Ebrahim 1998). The phenomenon of adherence is complex and it would seem reasonable for interventions to address this complexity with a more patient-centred approach. People's beliefs and preferences need to be acknowledged and incorporated into adherence-enhancing interventions

(Marinker 1997). A combination of strategies including information, reminding, adherence reinforcement and emphasis on the person's perspective might lead to more effective strategies. In terms of the lipid-lowering drug class, the main focus should be on statins, as they have been shown to be the most potent lipid-lowering drugs (ACC/AHA Guidelines 2013; Baigent 2005). Other important aspects for future studies include valid methods for measuring adherence and assessing the effects on serum lipid levels. Long-term follow-up, of 12 months and more, will reveal a more realistic picture of adherence to life-long treatment and allow for the evaluation of morbidity and costs. Finally, studies evaluating these types of interventions on other outcomes such as morbidity, mortality, quality of life and cost effectiveness would be very useful. Data relating to which interventions were the most cost-effective can provide guidance to healthcare systems.

ACKNOWLEDGEMENTS

We would like to acknowledge the important contributions by Knut Schroeder and Tim Peters, who were co-authors of the original review. Knut Schroeder conceived the original review and contributed to the screening of search results, data extraction and interpretation of data. Tim Peters was involved with the analysis of data and provided general advice on interpreting the data. Thanks to the authors of the original studies (BG Brown, E Bruckert, M Faulkner, E de Klerk, E Lesaffre, E Marquez-Contreras) and the updates (A Shedlbauer, P Davies, T Fahey) for their work which was included in this update.

We would like to thank the Cochrane Heart Group for the support they gave for the update of this review; Margaret Burke, Liz Bickerdike, and Nicole Martin in particular for their help with the literature search, and Zulian Liu from PenTAG for her help with the abstract selection.

REFERENCES

References to studies included in this review

Aslani 2010 *{published data only}*
Aslani P, Rose G, Chen TF, Whitehead PA, Krass I. A community pharmacist delivered adherence support service for dyslipidaemia. *European Journal of Public Health* 2010; **21**(5):567–72. [3224075]

Brown 1997 *{published data only}*
Brown BG, Bardsley J, Poulin D, Hillger LA, Dowdy A, Maher VM, et al. Moderate dose, three-drug therapy with niacin, lovastatin, and colestipol to reduce low-density lipoprotein cholesterol <100 mg/dl in patients with hyperlipidemia and coronary artery disease. *American Journal of Cardiology* 1997;**80**(2):111–15. [3224077]

Castellano 2014 *{published data only}*
Castellano JM, Gines S, Penalvo JL, Bansilal S, Fernandez-Ortiz A, Alvarez L, et al. A polypill strategy to improve adherence: results from the FOCUS Project. *Journal of the American College of Cardiology* 2014;**64**(20):2071–82. [4491277; DOI: 10.1016/j.jacc.2014.08.021]

Choudhry 2011 *{published data only}*
Choudhry NK, Avorn J, Glynn RJ, Antman EM, Schneeweiss S, Toscano M, et al. Full coverage for preventive medications after myocardial infarction. *New England Journal of Medicine* 2011;**365**(22):2088–97. [4491279]

Derose 2012 *{published data only}*
Derose SF, Green K, Marrett E, Tunceli K, Cheetham TC,

Chiu VY, et al. Automated outreach to increase primary adherence to cholesterol-lowering medications. *JAMA Internal Medicine* 2013;**173**(1):38–43. [4491280; DOI: 10.1001/2013.jamainternmed.717]

Eussen 2010 *{published data only}*

Eussen SR, Van der Elst ME, Klungel OH, Rompelberg CJ, Garssen J, Oosterveld MH, et al. A pharmaceutical care program to improve adherence to statin therapy: a randomized controlled trial. *Annals of Pharmacotherapy* 2010;**44**(12):1905–13. [4491281]

Fang 2015 *{published data only}*

Fang R, Li X. Electronic messaging support service programs improve adherence to lipid-lowering therapy among outpatients with coronary artery disease: an exploratory randomised control study. *Journal of Clinical Nursing* 2015; **25**(5-6):664–71. [4491283; DOI: 10.1111/jocn.12988]

Faulkner 2000 *{published data only}*

Faulkner MA, Wadibia EC, Lucas BD, Hilleman DE. Impact of pharmacy counseling on compliance and effectiveness of combination lipid-lowering therapy in patients undergoing coronary artery revascularization: a randomized, controlled trial. *Pharmacotherapy* 2000;**20**(4): 410–6. [4491284]

Fischer 2014 *{published data only}*

Fischer MA, Choudhry NK, Bykov K, Brill G, Bopp G, Wurst AM, et al. Pharmacy-based interventions to reduce primary medication nonadherence to cardiovascular medications. *Medical Care* 2014;**52**(12):1050–4. [4491285]

Goswami 2013 *{published data only}*

Goswami NJ, Dekoven M, Kuznik A, Mardekian J, Krukas MR, Liu LZ, et al. Impact of an integrated intervention program on atorvastatin adherence: a randomized controlled trial. *International Journal of General Medicine* 2013;**6**:647–55. [4491286; DOI: 10.2147/IJGM.S47518]

Gujral 2014 *{published data only}*

Gujral G, Winckel K, Nissen LM, Cottrell WN. Impact of community pharmacist intervention discussing patients' beliefs to improve medication adherence. *International Journal of Clinical Pharmacy* 2014;**36**(5):1048–58. [4491288]

Guthrie 2001 *{published data only}*

Guthrie RM. The effects of postal and telephone reminders on compliance with pravastatin therapy in a national registry: results of the first myocardial infarction risk reduction program. *Clinical Therapeutics* 2001;**23**(6): 970–80. [3224089]

Ho 2014 *{published data only}*

Ho PM, Lambert-Kerzner A, Carey EP, Fahdi IE, Bryson CL, Melnyk SD, et al. Multifaceted intervention to improve medication adherence and secondary prevention measures after acute coronary syndrome hospital discharge: a randomized clinical trial. *JAMA Internal Medicine* 2014; **174**(2):186–93. [4491289]

Kardas 2013 *{published data only}*

Kardas P. An education-behavioural intervention improves adherence to statins. *Central European Journal of Medicine* 2013;**8**(5):580–5. [4491290]

Kooy 2013 *{published data only}*

Kooy MJ, Van Wijk BL, Heerdink ER, De Boer A, Bouvy ML. Does the use of an electronic reminder device with or without counseling improve adherence to lipid-lowering treatment? The results of a randomized controlled trial. *Frontiers in Pharmacology* 2013;**4**:69. [4491291]

Ma 2010 *{published data only}*

Ma YS, Ockene IS, Rosal MC, Merriam PA, Ockene JK, Gandhi PJ. Randomized trial of a pharmacist-delivered intervention for improving lipid-lowering medication adherence among patients with coronary heart disease. *Cholesterol* 2010;**2010**:383281. [3224097; DOI: 10.1155/2010/383281]

Márquez 1998 *{published data only}*

Márquez Contreras E, Casado Martínez JJ, López de Andrés M, Corés Prieto E, López Zamorano JM, Moreno García JP, et al. Therapeutic compliance in dyslipidemias. A trial of the efficacy of health education. *Atencion Primaria* 1998; **22**(2):79–84. [4491293]

Márquez 2004 *{published data only}*

Márquez Contreras E, Casado Martínez JJ, Corchado Albalat Y, Chaves Gonzalez R, Grandio A, Losada Velasco C, et al. Efficacy of an intervention to improve therapy compliance in lipaemia cases. *Atencion Primaria* 2004;**33** (8):15. [4491295]

Márquez 2007 *{published data only}*

Márquez Contreras E, Casado Martínez JJ, Motero Carrasco J, Martín de Pablos JL, Chaves Gonzales R, Losada Ruiz C, et al. Therapy compliance in cases of hyperlipaemia, as measured through electronic monitors. Is a reminder calendar to avoid forgetfulness effective?. *Atencion Primaria* 2007;**39**(12):661–8. [4491297]

Nieuwkerk 2012 *{published data only}*

Nieuwkerk PT, Nierman MC, Vissers MN, Locadia M, Greggers-Peusch P, Knape LPM, et al. Intervention to improve adherence to lipid-lowering medication and lipid-levels in patients with an increased cardiovascular risk. *American Journal of Cardiology* 2012;**110**(5):666–72. [4491298]

Park 2013 *{published data only}*

Park LG, Howie-Esquivel J, Chung ML, Dracup K. A text messaging intervention to promote medication adherence for patients with coronary heart disease: A randomized controlled trial. *Patient Education and Counseling* 2013;**94** (2):261–8. [4491299]

Patel 2015 *{published data only}*

Patel A, Cass A, Peiris D, Usherwood T, Brown A, Jan S, et al. A pragmatic randomized trial of a polypill-based strategy to improve use of indicated preventive treatments in people at high cardiovascular disease risk. *European Journal of Preventive Cardiology* 2015;**22**(7):920–30. [4491301]

PILL 2011 *{published data only}*

PILL Collaborative Group. An international randomised placebo-controlled trial of a four-component combination pill ("Polypill") in people with raised cardiovascular risk. *PLOS One* 2011;**6**(5):e19857. [4491303]

Pladevall 2014 *{published data only}*

Pladevall M, Divine G, Wells KE, Resnicow K, Williams LK. A randomized controlled trial to provide adherence information and motivational interviewing to improve diabetes and lipid control. *Diabetes Educator* 2015;**41**(1): 136–46. [4491305]

Poston 1998 *{published data only}*

Poston J, Loh E, Dunham W. The medication use study. *Canadian Pharmaceutical Journal* 1998;**131**(10):31–8. [4491306]

Powell 1995 *{published data only}*

Powell KM, Edgren B. Failure of educational videotapes to improve medication compliance in a health maintenance organization. *American Journal of Health-System Pharmacy* 1995;**52**(20):2196–9. [3224111]

Schectman 1994 *{published data only}*

Schectman G, Hiatt J, Hartz A. Telephone contacts do not improve adherence to niacin or bile acid sequestrant therapy. *Annals of Pharmacotherapy* 1994;**28**(1):29–35. [3224113]

Selak 2014 *{published data only}*

Selak V, Elley CR, Bullen C, Crengle S, Wadham A, Rafter N, et al. Effect of fixed dose combination treatment on adherence and risk factor control among patients at high risk of cardiovascular disease: randomised controlled trial in primary care. *BMJ* 2014;**348**:g3318. [4491307]

Sweeney 1991 *{published data only}*

Sweeney ME, Fletcher BJ, Rice CR, Berra KA, Rudd CM, Fletcher GF, et al. Efficacy and compliance with cholestyramine bar versus powder in the treatment of hyperlipidemia. *American Journal of Medicine* 1991;**90**(4): 469–73. [3224117]

Tamblyn 2009 *{published data only}*

Tamblyn R, Reidel K, Huang A, Taylor L, Winslade N, Bartlett G, et al. Increasing the detection and response to adherence problems with cardiovascular medication in primary care through computerized drug management systems: a randomized controlled trial. *Medical Decision Making* 2009;**30**(2):176–88. [4491308]

Thom 2013 *{published data only}*

Thom S, Poulter N, Field J, Patel A, Prabhakaran D, Stanton A, et al. Effects of a fixed-dose combination strategy on adherence and risk factors in patients with or at high risk of CVD (UMPIRE). *JAMA* 2013;**310**(9):918–29. [4491309]

Vollmer 2014 *{published data only}*

Vollmer WM, Owen-Smith AA, Tom JO, Laws R, Ditmer DG, Smith DH, et al. Improving adherence to cardiovascular disease medications with information technology. *American Journal of Managed Care* 2014;**20**(11 Spec No. 17):SP502–10. [4491311]

Vrijens 2006 *{published data only}*

Vrijens B, Belmans A, Matthys K, De Klerke E, Lesaffre E. Effect of intervention through a pharmaceutical care program on patient adherence with prescribed once-daily atorvastatin. *Pharmacoepidemiology and Drug Safety* 2006; **15**(2):115–21. [4491312]

Wald 2014 *{published data only}*

Wald DS, Bestwick JP, Raiman L, Brendell R, Wald NJ. Randomised trial of text messaging on adherence to cardiovascular preventive treatment (INTERACT Trial). *PLoS ONE* 2014;**9**(12):e114268. [4491313]

Willich 2009 *{published data only}*

Willich SN, Englert H, Sonntag F, Voller H, Meyer-Sabellek W, Wegscheider K, et al. Impact of a compliance program on cholesterol control: results of the randomized ORBITAL study in 8108 patients treated with rosuvastatin. *European Journal of Cardiovascular Prevention and Rehabilitation* 2009;**16**(2):180–7. [4491314]

References to studies excluded from this review

Allen 2000 *{published data only}*

Allen JK. Cholesterol management: an opportunity for nurse case managers. *Journal of Cardiovascular Nursing* 2000;**14**(2):50–8. [3224129]

Anon 2002 *{published data only}*

Anonymous. Is alternate day dosing more cost-effective?. *Pharmaceutical Journal* 2002;**269**(7224):706. [3224131]

Athyros 2002b *{published data only}*

Athyros VG, Mikhailidis DP, Papageorgiou AA, Mercouris BR, Athyrou VV, Symeonidis AN, et al. Attaining United Kingdom-European Atherosclerosis Society low-density lipoprotein cholesterol guideline target values in the GREek Atorvastatin and Coronary-heart-disease Evaluation (GREACE) study. *Current Medical Research and Opinion* 2002;**18**(8):499–502. [3224133]

Becker 1998 *{published data only}*

Becker DM, Raqueno JV, Yook RM, Kral BG, Blumenthal RS, Moy TF, et al. Nurse-mediated cholesterol management compared with enhanced primary care in siblings of individuals with premature coronary disease. *Archives of Internal Medicine* 1998;**158**(14):1533–9. [4491315]

Bogden 1997 *{published data only}*

Bogden PE, Koontz LM, Williamson P, Abbott RD. The physician and pharmacist team. An effective approach to cholesterol reduction. *Journal of General Internal Medicine* 1997;**12**(3):158–64. [3224137; MEDLINE: 9100140]

Bruckert 1999 *{published data only}*

Bruckert E, Simonetta C, Giral P. Compliance with fluvastatin treatment characterization of the noncompliant population within a population of 3845 patients with hyperlipidemia: CREOLE Study Team. *Journal of Clinical Epidemiology* 1999;**52**(6):589–94. [3224139]

Burkett 1990 *{published data only}*

Burkett PA, Southard DR, Herbert WG, Walberg J. Frequent cholesterol feedback as an aid in lowering cholesterol levels. *Journal of Cardiopulmonary Rehabilitation* 1990;**10**(4):141–6. [4491316; EMBASE: 1990218703]

Casebeer 1999 *{published data only}*
Casebeer LL, Klapow JC, Centor RM, Stafford MA, Renkl LA, Mallinger AP, et al. An intervention to increase physicians' use of adherence-enhancing strategies in managing hypercholesterolemic patients. *Academic Medicine* 1999;**74**(12):1334–9. [4491317]

Coates 1982 *{published data only}*
Coates TJ, Jeffery RW, Slinkard LA. Frequency of contact and monetary reward in weight loss, lipid change, and blood pressure reduction with adolescents. *Behavior Therapy* 1982;**13**(2):175–85. [3224147]

DeBusk 1994 *{published data only}*
DeBusk RF, Miller NH, Superko HR, Dennis CA, Thomas RJ, Lew HT, et al. A case-management system for coronary risk factor modification after acute myocardial infarction. *Annals of Internal Medicine* 1994;**120**(9):721–9. [3224149]

Diabetes 2000 *{published data only}*
Diabetes Prevention Program Research Group. The Diabetes Prevention Program: baseline characteristics of the randomized cohort. *Diabetes Care* 2000;**23**(11):1619–29. [4491318]

Diwan 1995 *{published data only}*
Diwan VK, Wahlstrom R, Tomson G, Beermann B, Sterky G, Eriksson B. Effects of "group detailing" on the prescribing of lipid-lowering drugs: a randomized controlled trial in Swedish primary care. *Journal of Clinical Epidemiology* 1995;**48**(5):705–11. [3224153]

Dobs 1994 *{published data only}*
Dobs AS, Masters RB, Rajaram L, Stillman FA, Wilder LB, Margolis S, et al. A comparison of education methods and their impact on behavioral change in patients with hyperlipidemia. *Patient Education and Counseling* 1994;**24** (2):157–64. [3224155]

Dunham 2000 *{published data only}*
Dunham DM, Stewart RD, Laucka PV. Low-density-lipoprotein cholesterol in patients treated by a lipid clinic versus a primary care clinic. *American Journal of Health-System Pharmacy* 2000;**57**(24):2285–6. [3224157]

Ellis 2000 *{published data only}*
Ellis SL, Carter BL, Malone DC, Billups SJ, Okano GJ, Valuck RJ, et al. Clinical and economic impact of ambulatory care clinical pharmacists in management of dyslipidemia in older adults: the IMPROVE study. Impact of Managed Pharmaceutical Care on Resource Utilization and Outcomes in Veterans Affairs Medical Centers. *Pharmacotherapy* 2000;**20**(12):1508–16. [3224159]

Eriksson 1998 *{published data only}*
* Eriksson M, Hadell K, Holme I, Walldius G, Kjellstrom T. Compliance with and efficacy of treatment with pravastatin and cholestyramine: A randomized study on lipid-lowering in primary care. *Journal of Internal Medicine* 1998;**243**(5): 373–80. [3224161]
Eriksson M, Hadell K, Holme I, Walldius G, Kjellstrom T. Compliance with and efficacy of treatment with pravastatin

and cholestyramine: a randomized study on lipid-lowering in primary care. *Athereosclerosis* 1997;**134**:55. [3224162]

Frances 2001 *{published data only}*
Frances CD, Alperin P, Adler JS, Grady D. Does a fixed physician reminder system improve the care of patients with coronary artery disease? A randomized controlled trial. *Western Journal of Medicine* 2001;**175**(3):165–6. [4491319]

Fretheim 2006 *{published data only}*
Fretheim A, Oxman AD, Havelsrud K, Treweek S, Kristoffersen DT, Bjorndal A. Rational prescribing in primary care (RaPP): a cluster randomized trial of a tailored intervention. *PLoS Medicine / Public Library of Science* 2006;**3**(6):e134. [3224166]

Friedman 1998 *{published data only}*
Friedman RH. Automated telephone conversations to assess health behavior and deliver behavioral interventions. *Journal of Medical Systems* 1998;**22**(2):95–102. [3224168]

Gaede 1999 *{published data only}*
Gaede P, Vedel P, Parving HH, Pedersen O. Intensified multifactorial intervention in patients with type 2 diabetes mellitus and microalbuminuria: the Steno type 2 randomised study. *Lancet* 1999;**353**(9153):617–22. [3224170]

Gaede 2003 *{published data only}*
Gaede P, Vedel P, Larsen N, Jensen GV, Parving HH, Pedersen O. Multifactorial intervention and cardiovascular disease in patients with type 2 diabetes. *New England Journal of Medicine* 2003;**348**(5):383–93. [3224172]

Hae 2007 *{published data only}*
Hae MC. Impact of patient financial incentives on participation and outcomes in a statin pill-splitting program. *American Journal of Managed Care* 2007;**13**(6): 298–304. [4491320]

Ives 1993 *{published data only}*
Ives DG, Kuller LH, Traven ND. Use and outcomes of a cholesterol-lowering intervention for rural elderly subjects. *American Journal of Preventive Medicine* 1993;**9**(5):274–81. [3224176; MEDLINE: 94079785]

Jafari 2003 *{published data only}*
Jafari M, Ebrahimi R, Ahmadi-Kashani M, Balian H, Bashir M. Efficacy of alternate-day dosing versus daily dosing of atorvastatin. *Journal of Cardiovascular Pharmacology and Therapeutics* 2003;**8**(2):123–6. [4491321]

Jiang 2007 *{published data only}*
Jiang X, Sit JW, Wong TK. A nurse-led cardiac rehabilitation programme improves health behaviours and cardiac physiological risk parameters: evidence from Chengdu, China. *Journal of Clinical Nursing* 2007;**16**(10):1886–97. [3224180]

Johannesson 1996 *{published data only}*
Johannesson M, Borgquist L, Jonsson B, Lindholm LH. The cost effectiveness of lipid lowering in Swedish primary health care. The CELL Study Group. *Journal of Internal Medicine* 1996;**240**(1):23–9. [3224182]

Jolly 1998 *{published data only}*

Jolly K, Bradley F, Sharp S, Smith H, Mant D. Follow-up care in general practice of patients with myocardial infarction or angina pectoris: initial results of the SHIP trial. Southampton Heart Integrated Care Project. *Family Practice* 1998;**15**(6):548–55. [3224186; MEDLINE: 99176682]

Keyserling 1997 *{published data only}*

Keyserling TC, Ammerman AS, Davis CE, Mok MC, Garrett J, Simpson R Jr. A randomized controlled trial of a physician-directed treatment program for low-income patients with high blood cholesterol: the Southeast Cholesterol Project. *Archives of Family Medicine* 1997;**6**(2): 135–45. [4491322; MEDLINE: 97229885]

Kirkman 1994 *{published data only}*

Kirkman MS, Weinberger M, Landsman PB, Samsa GP, Shortliffe EA, Simel DL, et al. A telephone-delivered intervention for patients with NIDDM. Effect on coronary risk factors. *Diabetes Care* 1994;**17**(8):840–6. [4491323; MEDLINE: 95044714]

Kjelsberg 1990 *{published data only}*

Kjelsberg MO. Mortality after 10 1/2 years for hypertensive participants in the multiple risk factor intervention trial. *Circulation* 1990;**82**(5):1616–28. [3224192]

Kulik 2013 *{published data only}*

Kulik A, Desai NR, Shrank WH, Antman EM, Glynn RJ, Levin R, et al. Full prescription coverage versus usual prescription coverage after coronary artery bypass graft surgery: analysis from the post-myocardial infarction free Rx event and economic evaluation (FREEE) randomized trial. *Circulation* 2013;**128**(Suppl 1):S219–S225. [4491324]

Kuznar 2002 *{published data only}*

Kuznar W. Protocol helps drug adherence. *Cardiology Review* 2002;**19**(3):6. [3224196]

Lee 2007 *{published data only}*

Lee JK. How should we measure medication adherence in clinical trials and practice?. *Therapeutics and Clinical Risk Management* 2007;**3**(4):2007. [4491325]

Lesaffre 2000 *{published data only}*

Lesaffre E, De Klerk E. Estimating the power of compliance - Improving methods. *Controlled Clinical Trials* 2000;**21** (6):540–51. [4491326]

Lin 2006 *{published data only}*

Lin EH, Katon W, Rutter C, Simon GE, Ludman EJ, Von Korff M, et al. Effects of enhanced depression treatment on diabetes self-care. *Annals of Family Medicine* 2006;**4**(1): 46–53. [4491327]

Lindholm 1996 *{published data only}*

Lindholm LH, Ekbom T, Dash C, Isacsson A, Schersten B. Changes in cardiovascular risk factors by combined pharmacological and nonpharmacological strategies: the main results of the CELL Study. *Journal of Internal Medicine* 1996;**240**(1):13–22. [3224206]

Merriam 1997 *{published data only}*

Merriam PA, Ockene IS, Hebert JR, Ma Y. A lipid trial tracking system. *Journal of Public Health Management and Practice* 1997;**3**(6):74–8. [3224208]

Moher 2001 *{published data only}*

Moher M, Yudkin P, Wright L, Turner R, Fuller A, Schofield T, et al. Cluster randomised controlled trial to compare three methods of promoting secondary prevention of coronary heart disease in primary care. *BMJ* 2001;**322** (7298):1338–42. [3224210]

Oi 1998 *{published data only}*

Oi K, Komori H. Escape phenomenon with pravastatin during long-term treatment of patients with hyperlipidemia associated with diabetes mellitus. *Current Therapeutic Research, Clinical and Experimental* 1998;**59**(2):130–8. [3224212]

Oosterhoff 2011 *{published data only}*

Oosterhof P, Van Boven JF, Visser ST, Hiddink EG, Stuurman-Bieze AG, Postma MJ, et al. Cost effectiveness of increasing statin adherence for secondary prevention in community pharmacies. Value in Health 2011; Vol. 14: A379. [4491329]

Polack 2008 *{published data only}*

Polack J, Jorgenson D, Robertson P. Evaluation of different methods of providing medication-related education to patients following myocardial infarction. *Canadian Pharmacists Journal / Revue des Pharmaciens du Canada* 2008;**141**:241. [4491330]

Rachmani 2002 *{published data only}*

Rachmani R, Levi Z, Slavachevski I, Avin M, Ravid M. Teaching patients to monitor their risk factors retards the progression of vascular complications in high-risk patients with Type 2 diabetes mellitus: a randomized prospective study. *Diabetic Medicine* 2002;**19**(5):385–92. [3224218]

Rastam 1996 *{published data only}*

Rastam L, Frick J-O. Nurses counseling for hypercholesterolemia: Efficient strategy in middle-aged men. *Cardiovascular Risk Factors* 1996;**6**(1):36–41. [3224220]

Rindone 1998 *{published data only}*

Rindone JP, Hiller D, Arriola G. A comparison of fluvastatin 40 mg every other day versus 20 mg every day in patients with hypercholesterolemia. *Pharmacotherapy* 1998;**18**(4): 836–9. [3224224; MEDLINE: 98355406]

Robin 2002 *{published data only}*

Robin DM, Giordani PJ, Lepper HS, Croghan TW. Patient adherence and medical treatment outcomes: a meta-analysis. *Medical Care* 2002;**40**(9):794–811. [3224226]

Rodgers 2000 *{published data only}*

Rodgers J. Pharmacological interventions in type 2 diabetes: the role of nurses. *British Journal of Nursing* 2000;**9**(13): 866–70. [3224228]

Rubenfire 2004 *{published data only}*

Rubenfire M, Impact of Medical Subspecialty on Patient Compliance to Treatment Study Group. Safety and compliance with once-daily niacin extended-release/lovastatin as initial therapy in the Impact of Medical Subspecialty on Patient Compliance to Treatment (IMPACT) study. *American Journal of Cardiology* 2004;**94** (3):306–11. [4491331]

Schectman 1996 *{published data only}*
Schectman G, Wolff N, Byrd JC, Hiatt JG, Hartz A. Physician extenders for cost-effective management of hypercholesterolemia. *Journal of General Internal Medicine* 1996;**11**(5):277–86. [3224232; MEDLINE: 96338658]

Scherwitz 1995 *{published data only}*
Scherwitz LW, Brusis OA, Kesten D, Safian PA, Hasper E, Berg A, et al. Life style changes in patients with myocardial infarct in the framework of intramural and ambulatory rehabilitation--results of a German pilot study [Lebensstilanderung bei Herzinfarktpatienten im Rahmen der stationaren und ambulanten Rehabilitation--Ergebnisse einer deutschen Pilotstudie]. *Zeitschrift fur Kardiologie* 1995;**84**(3):216–21. [3224234]

Shaffer 1995 *{published data only}*
Shaffer JW. Reducing low-density lipoprotein cholesterol levels in an ambulatory care system. Results of a multidisciplinary collaborative practice lipid clinic compared with traditional physician-based care. *Archives of Internal Medicine* 1995;**155**(21):2330–5. [4491332]

Simpson 2001 *{published data only}*
Simpson SH, Johnson JA, Tsuyuki RT. Economic impact of community pharmacist intervention in cholesterol risk management: an evaluation of the study of cardiovascular risk intervention by pharmacists. *Pharmacotherapy* 2001;**21** (5):627–35. [3224238]

Toobert 2000 *{published data only}*
Toobert DJ, Glasgow RE, Radcliffe JL. Physiologic and related behavioral outcomes from the women's lifestyle heart trial. Annals of Behavioural Medicine. 22 2000; Vol. 22, issue 1:1–16. [3224240]

Tsuyuki 1999 *{published data only}*
Tsuyuki RT, Johnson JA, Teo KK, Ackman ML, Biggs RS, Cave A, et al. Study of Cardiovascular Risk Intervention by Pharmacists (SCRIP): a randomized trial design of the effect of a community pharmacist intervention program on serum cholesterol risk. *Annals of Pharmacotherapy* 1999;**33** (9):910–9. [4491333]

Tully 2000 *{published data only}*
Tully MP, Seston EM. Impact of pharmacists providing a prescription review and monitoring service in ambulatory care or community practice. *Annals of Pharmacotherapy* 2000;**34**(11):1320–31. [3224244]

Vale 2002 *{published data only}*
Vale MJ, Jelinek MV, Best JD, Santamaria JD. Coaching patients with coronary heart disease to achieve the target cholesterol: a method to bridge the gap between evidence-based medicine and the "real world"--randomized controlled trial. *Journal of Clinical Epidemiology* 2002;**55**(3):245–52. [3224246]

Wahlstrom 1995 *{published data only}*
Wahlstrom R, Tomson G, Diwan VK, Beermann B, Sterky G. Hyperlipidaemia in primary care - a randomized controlled trial on treatment information in Sweden: Design and methodology. *Pharmacoepidemiology and Drug Safety* 1995;**4**(2):75–90. [4491334]

Weymiller 2007 *{published data only}*
Weymiller AJ. Helping patients with type 2 diabetes mellitus make treatment decisions: Statin choice randomized trial. *Archives of Internal Medicine* 2007;**167**(10):28. [4491335]

Wright 2002 *{published data only}*
Wright L. The specialist nurse in coronary heart disease prevention: Evidence for effectiveness. *British Journal of Cardiology* 2002;**9 Suppl 3**:S15–9. [3224252]

Wu 2006 *{published data only}*
Wu JY, Leung WY, Chang S, Lee B, Zee B, Tong PCY, et al. Effectiveness of telephone counselling by a pharmacist in reducing mortality in patients receiving polypharmacy: Randomised controlled trial. *BMJ* 2006;**333**(7567):522–7. [4491336]

Yigit 2004 *{published data only}*
Yigit F, Muderrisoglu H, Guz G, Bozbas H, Korkmaz ME, Ozin MB, et al. Comparison of intermittent with continuous simvastatin treatment in hypercholesterolemic patients with end stage renal failure. *Japanese Heart Journal* 2004;**45**(6):959–68. [3224256]

Yilmaz 2005 *{published data only}*
Yilmaz MB, Pinar M, Naharci I, Demirkan B, Baysan O, Yokusoglu M, et al. Being well-informed about statin is associated with continuous adherence and reaching targets. *Cardiovascular Drugs and Therapy* 2005;**19**(6):437–40. [3224258]

Zermansky 2002 *{published data only}*
Zermansky AG, Petty DR, Raynor DK, Lowe CJ, Freemantle N, Vail A. Clinical medication review by a pharmacist of patients on repeat prescriptions in general practice: A randomised controlled trial. *Health Technology Assessment* 2002;**6**(20):76. [3224260]

References to studies awaiting assessment

Harrison 2015 *{published data only}*
* Harrison TN, Green KR, Liu IA, Vansomphone SS, Handler J, Scott RD, et al. Automated outreach for cardiovascular-related medication refill reminders. *Journal of Clinical Hypertension* 2015;**18**(7):641–6. [4491338; DOI: 10.1111/jch.12723]
Reynolds K, Green KR, Vansomphone SS, Scott RD, Cheetham TC. Automated outreach for cholesterol-lowering medication refill reminders. *European Heart Journal* 2011;**32**(Abstract Suppl):230–1. [4491339]

Johnson 2006 *{published data only}*
Johnson SS, Driskell MM, Johnson JL, Dyment SJ, Prochaska JO, Prochaska JM, et al. Transtheoretical model intervention for adherence to lipid-lowering drugs. *Disease Management* 2006;**9**(2):102–14. [3224184]

Lee 2006 *{published data only}*

Lee JK. Effect of a pharmacy care program on medication adherence and persistence, blood pressure, and low-density lipoprotein cholesterol: a randomized controlled trial. *JAMA* 2006;**296**(21):2563–71. [4491340]

References to ongoing studies

ACTRN12616000233426 *{published data only}*

ACTRN12616000233426. INtegrated combination Therapy, Electronic General practice support tool, phaRmacy led intervention And combination Therapy Evaluation (INTEGRATE): A pragmatic cluster randomised controlled trial. www.anzctr.org.au/Trial/Registration/TrialReview.aspx?id=370068 19th February 2016. [4491342]

ACTRN12616000422426 *{published data only}*

ACTRN12616000422426. Text4Heart Partnership: a text messaging program to enhance self-management of cardiovascular disease. www.anzctr.org.au/Trial/Registration/TrialReview.aspx?id=370398 1st April 2016. [4491344]

Thom 2014 *{published data only}*

Thom S, Field J, Poulter N, Patel A, Prabhakaran D, Stanton A, et al. Use of a Multidrug Pill In Reducing cardiovascular Events (UMPIRE): rationale and design of a randomised controlled trial of a cardiovascular preventive polypill-based strategy in India and Europe. *European Journal of Preventive Cardiology* 2014;**21**:252–61. [3224262]

Additional references

4S 1994

Scandinavian Simvastatin Survival Study Group. Randomised trial of cholesterol lowering in 4444 patients with coronary heart disease: the Scandinavian Simvastatin Survival Study (4S). *Lancet* 1994;**344**(8934):1383–9.

ACC/AHA Guidelines 2013

Stone NJ, Robinson JG, Lichtenstein AH, Bairey Merz CN, Blum CB, et al. 2013 ACC/AHA Guideline on the Treatment of Blood Cholesterol to Reduce Atherosclerotic Cardiovascular Risk in AdultsA Report of the American College of Cardiology/American Heart Association Task Force on Practice Guidelines. *Circulation* 2014;**129**(25 Suppl 2):s1–45.

Armour 2007

Armour C, Bosnic-Anticevich S, Brilliant M, Burton D, Emmerton L, Krass I, et al. Pharmacy Asthma Care Program (PACP) improves outcomes for patients in the community. *Thorax* 2007;**62**:496–592.

Athyros 2002a

Athyros VG, Papageorgiou AA, Mercouris BR, Athyrou VV, Symeonidis AN, Basayannis EO, et al. Treatment with atorvastatin to the National Cholesterol Educational Program goal versus 'usual' care in secondary coronary heart disease prevention. The GREek Atorvastatin and Coronary-heart-disease Evaluation (GREACE) study. *Current Medical Research and Opinion* 2002;**18**(4):220–8.

Avorn 1998

Avorn J, Monette J, Lacour A, Bohn RL, Monane M, Mogun H, et al. Persistence of use of lipid-lowering medications. *JAMA* 1998;**279**(18):1458–62.

Baigent 2005

Baigent C, Keech A, Kearney PM, Blackwell L, Buck G, Pollicino C, et al. Cholesterol Treatment Trialists' (CTT) Collaborators. Efficacy and safety of cholesterol-lowering treatment: Prospective meta-analysis of data from 90 056 participants in 14 randomised trials of statins. *Lancet* 2005; **366**(9493):1267–78.

Benner 2002

Benner JS, Glynn RJ, Mogun H, Neumann PJ, Weinstein MC, Avorn J. Long-term persistence in use of statin therapy in elderly patients. *JAMA* 2002;**288**(4):455–61.

Blackburn 2005

Blackburn DF, Dobson RT, Blackburn JL, Wilson TW. Cardiovascular morbidity associated with nonadherence to statin therapy. *Pharmacotherapy* 2005;**25**(8):1035–43.

Brown 2011

Brown MT, Bussell JK. Medication adherence: WHO cares?. *Mayo Clinic Proceedings* 2011;**86**(4):304–14.

Cheng 2004

Cheng CW, Woo K-S, Chan JC, Tomlinson B, You JH. Association between adherence to statin therapy and lipid control in Hong Kong Chinese patients at high risk of coronary heart disease. *British Journal of Clinical Pharmacology* 2004;**58**(5):528–35.

Costa 2015

Costa E, Giardini A, Savin M, Menditto E, Lehane E, Laosa O, et al. Interventional tools to improve medication adherence: review of literature. *Patient Preference and Adherence* 2015;**9**:1303-14.

Dickersin 1994

Dickersin K, Scherer R, Lefebvre C. Identifying relevant studies for systematic reviews. *BMJ* 1994;**309**(6964): 1286–91.

Downs 1998

Downs JR, Clearfield M, Weis S, Whitney E, Shapiro DR, Beere PA, et al. Primary prevention of acute coronary events with lovastatin in men and women with average cholesterol levels: results of AFCAPS/TexCAPS. Air Force/Texas Coronary Atherosclerosis Prevention Study. *JAMA* 1998;**279**(20):1615–22.

Ebrahim 1998

Ebrahim S. Detection, adherence and control of hypertension for the prevention of stroke: a systematic review. *Health Technology Assessment* 1998;**2**(11):1–78. [www.hta.ac.uk/project.asp?PjtId=881]

Guyatt 2008

Guyatt GH, Oxman AD, Vist GE, Kunz R, Falck-Ytter Y, Alonso-Coello P, et al. GRADE: an emerging consensus on rating quality of evidence and strength of recommendations. *BMJ* 2008;**336**:924–6.

Higgins 2011

Higgins JPT, Green S, editor(s). Cochrane Handbook for Systematic Reviews of Interventions. Cochrane Handbook of Systemtic Reviess of Interventions Version 5.1.0 (updated March 2011). The Cochrane Collaboration, 2011. Available from handbook.cochrane.org.

Jackevicius 2002

Jackevicius CA, Mamdani M, Tu JV. Adherence with statin therapy in elderly patients with and without acute coronary syndromes. *JAMA* 2002;**288**(4):462–7.

Lefebvre 1996

Lefebvre C, McDonald S. Development of a sensitive search strategy for reports of randomized controlled trials in EMBASE. Paper presented at the Fourth International Cochrane Colloquium, 20-24 Oct 1996; Adelaide, Australia. 1996.

Lefebvre 2011

Lefebvre C, Manheimer E, Glanville J. Chapter 6: Searching for studies. In: Cochrane Handbook for Systematic Reviews of Interventions Version 5.1.0 (updated March 2011). The Cochrane Collaboration, 2011. Available from handbook.cochrane.org.

Lewis 2003

Lewis DK, Robinson J, Wilkinson E. Factors involved in deciding to start preventive treatment: qualitative study of clinicians' and lay people's attitudes. *BMJ* 2003;**327**(7419): 841–5.

LIPID 1998

Long-Term Intervention with Pravastatin in Ischaemic Disease (LIPID) study group. Prevention of cardiovascular events and death with pravastatin in patients with coronary heart disease and a broad range of initial cholesterol levels. The Long-Term Intervention with Pravastatin in Ischaemic Disease (LIPID) Study Group. *New England Journal of Medicine* 1998;**339**(19):1349–57.

Mahtani 2011

Mahtani KR, Heneghan CJ, Glasziou PP, Perera R. Reminder packaging for improving adherence to self-administered long-term medications. *Cochrane Database of Systematic Reviews* 2011, Issue 9. [DOI: 10.1002/14651858.CD005025.pub3]

Marinker 1997

Marinker M. *From Compliance to Concordance: Towards Shared Goals in Medicine taking*. London: Royal Pharmaceutical Society of Great Britain, 1997.

MRC/BHF 2002

Heart Protection Study Collaborative Group. MRC/BHF Protection Study of cholesterol lowering with simvastatin in 20536 high-risk individuals: a randomised placebo-controlled trial. *Lancet* 2002;**360**(9326):7–22.

Mullen 1997

Mullen PD. Compliance becomes concordance. *BMJ* 1997; **314**(7082):691–2.

Muller-Nordhorn 2005

Muller-Nordhorn J, Willich SN. Effectiveness of interventions to increase adherence to statin therapy. *Disease Management of Health Outcomes* 2005;**13**(2):72–82. [1173–8790/05/0002–0073/$34.95/0]

NICE 2014

National Institute for Health and Care Excellence (NICE). Cardiovascular Disease: risk assessment and reduction, including lipid modification. www.nice.org.uk/guidance/cg181 (accessed 18th December 2016).

Nieuwlaat 2014

Nieuwlaat R, Wilczynksi N, Navarro T, Hobson N, Jeffery R, Keepanasseril A, et al. Interventions for enhancing medication adherence. *Cochrane Database of Systematic Reviews* 2014, Issue 11. [DOI: 10.1002/14651858.CD000011.pub4]

Pasina 2014

Pasina L, Brucato AL, Falcone C, Cucchi E, Bresciani A, Sottocorno M, et al. Medication non-adherence among elderly patients newly discharged and receiving polypharmacy. *Drugs & Aging* 2014;**31**(4):283-9. [DOI: 10.1007/s40266-014-0163-7]

Primatesta 2000

Primatesta P, Poulter NR. Lipid concentrations and the use of lipid lowering drugs: evidence from a national cross sectional survey. *BMJ* 2000;**321**(7272):1322–5.

Rash 2016

Rash JA, Campbell DJ, Tonelli M, Campbell TS. A systematic review of interventions to improve adherence to statin medication: what do we know about what works? . *Preventive Medicine* 2016;**90**:155–69. [DOI: 10.1016/j.ypmed.2016.07.006]

Rosenson 2015

Rosenson R, Kent ST, Brown TM, Farkouh ME, Levitan EB, Yun H, et al. Underutilization of high-intensity statin therapy after hospitalization for coronary heart disease. *Journal of the American College of Cardiology* 2015;**65**(3): 270–7.

Rueda 2006

Rueda S, Park-Wyllie LY, Bayoumi A, Tynan A-M, Antoniou T, Rourke S, et al. Patient support and education for promoting adherence to highly active antiretroviral therapy for HIV/AIDS. *Cochrane Database of Systematic Reviews* 2006, Issue 3. [DOI: 10.1002/14651858.CD001442.pub2]

Sackett 1976

Sackett DL, Haynes RB. *Compliance with Therapeutic Regimens*. Baltimore: John Hopkins University Press, 1976.

Sacks 1996

Sacks FM, Pfeffer MA, Moye LA, Rouleau JL, Rutherford JD, Cole TG, et al. The effect of pravastatin on coronary events after myocardial infarction in patients with average cholesterol levels. Cholesterol and Recurrent Events Trial investigators. *New England Journal of Medicine* 1996;**335** (14):1001–9.

Schroeder 2004

Schroeder K, Fahey T, Ebrahim S. Interventions for improving adherence to treatment in patients with high blood pressure in ambulatory settings. *Cochrane Database of Systematic Reviews* 2004, Issue 3. [DOI: 10.1002/14651858.CD004804]

Shepherd 1995

Shepherd J, Cobbe SM, Ford I, Isles CG, Lorimer AR, MacFarlane PW, et al. Prevention of coronary heart disease with pravastatin in men with hypercholesterolemia. West of Scotland Coronary Prevention Study Group. *New England Journal of Medicine* 1995;**333**(20):1301–07.

SIGN 2007

Scottish Intercollegiate Guidelines Network (SIGN). Risk estimation and the prevention of cardiovascular disease. A national clinical guideline.. Available at www.sign.ac.uk/pdf/sign97.pdf. Edinburgh: Scottish Intercollegiate Guidelines Network, 2007 (accessed 11th January 2009).

Tsuyuki 2001

Tsuyuki RT, Bungard TJ. Poor adherence with hypolipidemic drugs: a lost opportunity. *Pharmacotherapy* 2001;**21**(5):576–82.

Vermeire 2001

Vermeire E, Hearnshaw H, Van Royen P, Denekens J. Patient adherence to treatment: three decades of research. A comprehensive review. *Journal of Clinical Pharmacy and Therapeutics* 2001;**26**(5):331–42.

Vermeire 2005

Vermeire EIJJ, Wens J, Van Royen P, Biot Y, Hearnshaw H, Lindenmeyer A. Interventions for improving adherence to treatment recommendations in people with type 2 diabetes mellitus. *Cochrane Database of Systematic Reviews* 2005, Issue 2. [DOI: 10.1002/14651858.CD003638.pub2]

Wei 2002

Wei L, Wang J, Thompson P, Wong S, Struthers AD, MacDonald TM. Adherence to statin treatment and readmission of patients after myocardial infarction: a six year follow up study. *Heart (British Cardiac Society)* 2002;**88**(3):229–33.

WHO Report 2002

World Health Organization. The World Health Report 2002 - Reducing risks, promoting healthy life. Available at www.who.int/whr/2002/en/whr02˙en.pdf?ua=1. Geneva: World Health Organization, 2002 (accessed 18th December 2016).

References to other published versions of this review

Schedlbauer 2003

Schedlbauer A, Schroeder K. Interventions to improve adherence to lipid lowering medication. *Cochrane Database of Systematic Reviews* 2003, Issue 2. [DOI: 10.1002/14651858.CD004371]

Schedlbauer 2004

Schedlbauer A, Schroeder K, Peters TJ, Fahey T. Interventions for improving adherence to lipid lowering medication. *Cochrane Database of Systematic Reviews* 2004, Issue 4. [DOI: 10.1002/14651858.CD004371.pub2]

Schedlbauer 2010

Schedlbauer A, Davies P, Fahey T. Interventions to improve adherence to lipid lowering medication. *Cochrane Database of Systematic Reviews* 2010, Issue 3. [DOI: 10.1002/14651858.CD004371.pub3]

* *Indicates the major publication for the study*

CHARACTERISTICS OF STUDIES

Characteristics of included studies *[ordered by study ID]*

Aslani 2010

Methods	Parallel cluster-randomised controlled clinical trial Randomisation ratio: 1:1 Equivalence design: 2-sided confidence interval Open-label
Participants	N recruited = 142 N randomised = 97 (49 control, 48 intervention) N reported outcomes = 97 Mean age 58 years (CI 55.2 to 60.8) for the intervention and 63.6 years (CI 60.1 to 67.1) for the control group INCLUSION CRITERIA "At least 18 years old, able to fluently speak and read English, taking a lipid-lowering medicine for at least 1 month prior to enrolment in the study." EXCLUSION CRITERIA Not reported COUNTRY/SETTING: Australia STUDY PERIOD: Not reported
Interventions	Number of study centres: 38 community pharmacies INTERVENTION GROUP In addition to routine care, participants received individualised adherence support service delivered at t = 1,2,3,4 (baseline and 3,6,9 months) to address issues identified from a questionnaire and come up with appropriate interventions recorded on data sheets. Interventions included counselling and advice about the disease, medicine, medicine use, adherence and lifestyle measures CONTROL GROUP Received routine care from pharmacist (blood lipid levels measured and reported to participant, participant completed the questionnaire)
Outcomes	TIME OF OUTCOME MEASUREMENTS "Repeated measures (baseline (t = 1), post-intervention at 3-monthly intervals (t = 2,3, 4))." PRIMARY OUTCOMES: lipid levels using Accutrend GC, participant adherence to therapy using MARS Medication Adherence Report Scale SECONDARY OUTCOME: lifestyle measures - potential factors affecting lipid levels
Notes	Commercial funding/non-commercial funding/other funding: "This project has been funded by the Australian Government Department of Health and Ageing as part of the Third Community Pharmacy Agreement, administered by the Pharmacy Guild of Australia." Participating pharmacists received reimbursement for every completed participant Stated aim for study: "This study aimed to evaluate the impact of a community pharmacist-delivered adherence support service on patients' adherence and total cholesterol levels."

Aslani 2010   *(Continued)*

Risk of bias

Bias	Authors' judgement	Support for judgement
Random sequence generation (selection bias)	Unclear risk	Not reported
Allocation concealment (selection bias)	Unclear risk	Not reported
Blinding (performance bias and detection bias) All outcomes	Unclear risk	Unblinded open-label study
Incomplete outcome data (attrition bias) All outcomes	Low risk	"A comparison of the demographics of patients who stayed in the study and those who dropped out, showed that they were mostly similar. Cross tabulation using Fishers Exact Test (two-sided) found that there were differences between the two groups on only one variable"
Selective reporting (reporting bias)	Low risk	All outcomes reported

Brown 1997

Methods	Cross-over randomised controlled clinical trial Randomisation ratio: 1:1 Equivalence design: 2-sided confidence interval Open-label
Participants	N recruited = 31 N randomised = 31 (cross-over - both groups received intervention) N reported outcomes = 29 Mean age 49 ± 7 yrs INCLUSION CRITERIA "All were men less than or equal to 65 years old at high risk for future cardiac events by virtue of: (1) an elevated apoprotein B greater than or equal to 125mg/dl, (2) at least 1 coronary lesion greater than or equal to 50% stenosis or 2 lesions greater than or equal to 30% stenosis, as documented in the baseline angiogram, and (3) a family history of premature cardiovascular events. All patients signed an approved written consent form." EXCLUSION CRITERIA Not reported COUNTRY/SETTING: USA STUDY PERIOD: Not reported
Interventions	Number of study centres: 1 "All patients received the 3-drug regimen listed above (niacin, lovastatin 20mg BD, colestipol 10g BD), using regular niacin, for 12 months, with dosage adjustment to a

Brown 1997   *(Continued)*

	target cholesterol of 150 to 175 mg/dl, and to minimize side effects." INTERVENTION (2) AND CONTROL (1) GROUP at 12 months: "At 12 months, patients were randomly assigned to: (1) continue with regular niacin at a dosage identical to that established in the 12 month dose-finding period, or (2) change to polygel controlled-release niacin at that daily dosage, but given twice rather than 4 times/day." INTERVENTION AND CONTROL GROUP at 20 months: "At 20 months, groups (1) and (2) were reversed (crossover)." "This regimen continued for 8 more months. Just before the clinic visit at 28 months, patients completed a mail-in questionnaire comparing the 2 niacin preparations in terms of a variety of possible side effects and specifying which of the 2 preparations they preferred. After 30 months, all these drugs were discontinued and a postdrug follow-up evaluation was performed 6 weeks later."
Outcomes	TIME OF OUTCOME MEASUREMENTS "Plasma very low-density lipoprotein (VLDL), LDL, and HDL cholesterol and triglycerides, apolipoprotein B, and aspartate aminotransferase were measured at baseline and every 4 months at the Northwest Lipid Research Laboratory. At entry (before treatment), at 6 months, 12 months, 20 months, 28 months, and 6 weeks after stopping the triple-drug regimen, the lipid and clinical laboratory determinations listed in Table II were obtained. HDL2 and HDL3 cholesterol were measured at baseline, at 1 and 2 years, and at 6 weeks after discontinuing therapy." PRIMARY OUTCOME: lipid levels SECONDARY OUTCOMES: compliance, side effects
Notes	Commercial funding/non-commercial funding/other funding: "The pharmaceutical supplies were provided by Merck Research Laboratories, Inc., West Point, Pennsylvania; Upjohn Co., Inc., and Upsher-Smith Inc., Minneapolis, Minnesota. This study was supported in part by grants from the National Heart, Lung, and Blood Institute and National Institutes of Health, Bethesda, Maryland; in part by the University of Washington Clinical Research Center (NIH #RR31), Seattle, Washington; and in part by a grant from the John L. Locke, Jr. Charitable Trust, Seattle, Washington." Stated aim for study: "To identify a regimen that is effective among such hyperlipidemic coronary disease patients (usually meets </-100 mg/dl target), is well tolerated, and is realistic, we have employed and evaluated a 3-drug combination with niacin, lovastatin, and colestipol, in moderate doses in such patients. Furthermore, we have objectively compared a polygel controlled-release niacin (Upsher-Smith, Minneapolis) with regular niacin used in this regimen in a randomized, crossover trial design."

Risk of bias

Bias	Authors' judgement	Support for judgement
Random sequence generation (selection bias)	Unclear risk	Not reported
Allocation concealment (selection bias)	Unclear risk	Not reported

Brown 1997 *(Continued)*

Blinding (performance bias and detection bias) All outcomes	Unclear risk	Unblinded open-label study
Incomplete outcome data (attrition bias) All outcomes	Unclear risk	"2 left the study during the 12-month run-in phase due to time conflict"
Selective reporting (reporting bias)	Low risk	All outcomes reported

Castellano 2014

Methods	Parallel randomised controlled clinical trial Randomisation ratio: 1:1 Equivalence design: 2-sided confidence interval Open-label
Participants	N recruited = 695 N randomized = 695 (345 control, 350 intervention) N reported outcomes = 695 included for intention-to-treat analysis, but only 458 completed all visits for per protocol analysis Mean age for Phase 1 is 64 ± 11 years (not reported for Phase 2) INCLUSION CRITERIA Participants previously included in Phase 1 (cross-sectional study of FOCUS) but not in Phase 2 (randomised controlled trial of FOCUS) EXCLUSION CRITERIA Secondary dyslipidaemia, contraindication to any of the components of the polypill, participation in another trial, previous percutaneous transluminal coronary angioplasty with a drug eluting stent within the previous year, severe congestive heart failure (New York Heart Association functional class III to IV), serum creatinine > 2 mg/dl, any condition limiting life expectancy < 2 years, and pregnancy or premenopause COUNTRY/SETTING: Argentina, Brazil, Italy, Paraguay, and Spain STUDY PERIOD: January 2011 to January 2014
Interventions	Number of study centres: 63 outpatient clinics in Argentina, Paraguay, Italy and Spain INTERVENTION GROUP FDC polypill containing aspirin 100 mg, simvastatin 40 mg, and rampiril at 3 different doses: 2.5,5, or 10 mg given once daily CONTROL GROUP Received aspirin, simvastatin, and ramipril as 3 separate drugs given once daily
Outcomes	TIME OF OUTCOME MEASUREMENTS Participants were followed at 1, 4, and 9 months PRIMARY OUTCOME: percentage of participants taking medication adequately at 9 months in each arm assessed by attendance at the final 9-month visit and the Morisky-Green questionnaire (MAQ) and pill count methods, simultaneously SECONDARY OUTCOMES: risk factor control in each study arm (BP and lipid LDL-cholesterol levels at months 1 and 9), incidence of adverse events (including death, reinfarction, and rehospitalisation for any CV cause), rate of treatment withdrawal,

Castellano 2014   *(Continued)*

	tolerability, and quality of life, economic end points (medical and nonmedical costs data not shown)
Notes	Commercial funding/non-commercial funding/other funding: Not reported; however, it is stated in the text that the FOCUS trial "provided both the polypill group and the control group with free medications." Stated aim for study: "This randomized trial aims to analyze the impact of a polypill strategy on adherence in post-MI patients."

Risk of bias

Bias	Authors' judgement	Support for judgement
Random sequence generation (selection bias)	Low risk	"a central electronic randomization service assigned participants to 1 of 2 arms"
Allocation concealment (selection bias)	Low risk	See above
Blinding (performance bias and detection bias) All outcomes	Unclear risk	Unblinded but "pill count enabled a more objective assessment of adherence during the trial"
Incomplete outcome data (attrition bias) All outcomes	Low risk	78 participants (43 intervention, 35 control) were lost to follow-up, 27 participants (14 intervention, 13 control) discontinued the medications due to an adverse effect
Selective reporting (reporting bias)	Low risk	All outcomes reported

Choudhry 2011

Methods	Parallel cluster-randomised controlled clinical trial Equivalence design: 2-sided confidence interval Open-label Randomisation occurred at the level of plan sponsor (i.e. the employer, union, government, or association that sponsors a particular benefits package) so that all eligible employees of a given plan sponsor received the same coverage after randomisation
Participants	N recruited = 6768 (13.5% excluded because plan sponsors declined to participate) N randomised = 5855 (2845 intervention, 3010 control) N reported outcomes = 5216 Mean age 53.6 years, 75% of participants were men INCLUSION CRITERIA: - patients discharged after myocardial infarction - patients receiving medical and prescription drug benefits through Aetna, a large commercial insurer in the United States EXCLUSION CRITERIA: Not stated

Choudhry 2011   *(Continued)*

COUNTRY/SETTING: USA
STUDY PERIOD: "We planned to recruit 7500 patients over a 1.5-year period and to follow them for a minimum of 1 year in order to achieve a power of 90% to detect a between-group difference of 20% in the relative risk of the primary outcome. Because of slower-than anticipated enrollment, the trial steering committee accepted a recommendation from the independent data and safety monitoring committee that equivalent power could be obtained if a total of 1000 primary outcome events were to occur. The steering committee then adapted the trial by extending enrollment by 15 months and reducing minimum follow-up to 3 months."
End of study was 30 November 2010.

Interventions	INTERVENTION GROUP: Pharmacy benefits for participants in the full-coverage group were changed so that they had no cost sharing for any brand-name or generic statin, betablocker, angiotensin-converting-enzyme (ACE) inhibitor, or angiotensin-receptor blocker (ARB) for every prescription after randomisation. All copayments and co-insurance were waived at the point of care (i.e. the pharmacy), as was any contribution to a participant's deductible CONTROL GROUP: Usual copayment arrangements
Outcomes	PRIMARY OUTCOME: first major vascular event or revascularisation SECONDARY OUTCOMES: rates of medication adherence: by calculating the mean medication possession ratio (number of days a participant had a supply of each medication class available) divided by the number of days of eligibility for that medication; ratios were multiplied by 100 to generate absolute adherence percentages. "We also calculated the proportion of patients who had full adherence (defined as a medication possession of ≥80%) to each and to all three study medication classes throughout follow-up.", total major vascular events or revascularisation, the first major vascular event, health expenditures The median duration of follow-up after randomisation was 394 days (interquartile range, 201 to 663)
Notes	All outcomes reported as ITT with GEE to adjust for clustering Funding: "Supported by unrestricted research grants from Aetna and the Commonwealth Fund to Brigham and Women's Hospital." COI: all authors report receiving funding from healthcare funds and pharmaceutical companies

Risk of bias

Bias	Authors' judgement	Support for judgement
Random sequence generation (selection bias)	Low risk	"use of a random-number generator"
Allocation concealment (selection bias)	Unclear risk	not reported

Choudhry 2011   *(Continued)*

Blinding (performance bias and detection bias) All outcomes	Unclear risk	not reported
Incomplete outcome data (attrition bias) All outcomes	Low risk	"A total of 133 patients (4.7%) in the full-coverage group and 151 (5.0%) in the usual-coverage group lost insurance eligibility between the time of hospital discharge and randomization, so data from these patients were not included in the follow-up analyses."
Selective reporting (reporting bias)	Low risk	all outcomes reported

Derose 2012

Methods	Parallel randomised controlled clinical trial Randomisation ratio: 1:1 Equivalence design: 2-sided confidence interval Open-label
Participants	N recruited = 28,750 (based on mean numbers for 10-week recruitment in weekly batches) N randomised = 5216 (2610 control, 2606 intervention) N reported outcomes = 5216 Mean age 56.1 years, 50.6% of participants were women INCLUSION CRITERIA "We identified a group of patients who were prescribed a statin as a new medication. A new medication was operationalized as a prescription for a statin or combination drug containing a statin and no record of such a drug dispensed within 365 days before the index prescription date. Participants were limited to those with 1 or more years of membership from the prescription date and no gap in enrolment more than 30 days during the past year. An age limit of 24 years and older at the time of the prescription was required because of infrequent statin prescriptions in younger individuals and controversial use of statins early in life. Members who had no record of the statin prescription being filled at a health plan pharmacy after 1 to 2 weeks were considered nonadherent and eligible for the study." EXCLUSION CRITERIA Not reported COUNTRY/SETTING: USA STUDY PERIOD: April to June 2010
Interventions	Number of study centres: Kaiser Permanente Southern California, an integrated healthcare system at 14 medical centres and 197 medical offices INTERVENTION GROUP "The intervention group received automated telephone calls followed 1 week later by letters for continued nonadherence." CONTROL GROUP

Derose 2012   *(Continued)*

	"The control group received no outreach."
Outcomes	TIME OF OUTCOME MEASUREMENTS The time frame for intervention was guided by prior work. In these analyses, 18.4% of new statin prescriptions remained unfilled after 12 weeks. Among those who filled their prescription, 82.2% to 90.1% did so by 1 to 2 weeks after the prescription date. With a plan to conduct the intervention in weekly batches, it was determined that contact 1 to 2 weeks after the prescription date was a practical time frame for initiating outreach PRIMARY OUTCOME: dispensation of a statin ("The primary outcome was dispensation of a statin between the first telephone call (day 0, the randomization day) and up to 2 weeks after delivery of the letter.") SECONDARY OUTCOME: refills at intervals up to 1 year
Notes	Commercial funding/non-commercial funding/other funding: This research was supported by grants from Merck Sharp & Dohme Corp, a subsidiary of Merck & Co Inc, Whitehouse Station, New Jersey Stated aim for the study: "We performed a randomized controlled trial to evaluate an automated system to decrease primary nonadherence to statins for lowering cholesterol. " Conflict of Interest Disclosures: Ms Marrett is an employee of Merck. Dr Tunceli is an employee of Merck and owns stock in the company

Risk of bias

Bias	Authors' judgement	Support for judgement
Random sequence generation (selection bias)	Low risk	"A study programmer used computer-generated random numbers to sort participants into the intervention and control groups in equal proportion (day 0)"
Allocation concealment (selection bias)	Low risk	See above
Blinding (performance bias and detection bias) All outcomes	Low risk	"Assignment was concealed from study investigators and analysts"
Incomplete outcome data (attrition bias) All outcomes	Unclear risk	Mean numbers were given for recruitment data in 10 weekly batches Attrition was not reported
Selective reporting (reporting bias)	Low risk	All outcomes reported

Eussen 2010

Methods	Parallel randomised controlled clinical trial Randomisation ratio: 1:1 Equivalence design: 2-sided confidence interval Open-label
Participants	N recruited = 1016 signed informed consent N randomised = 1016 (513 control group, 503 intervention group) N reported outcomes = 899 (460 control, 439 intervention) Mean age: 60.1 ± 11.3 (control) and 60.2 ± 10.9 (intervention) INCLUSION CRITERIA New users of statins age 18 and above "New users were defined as those who had not filled a prescription for statins in the preceding 6 months, verified by the pharmacist through a patient record check." EXCLUSION CRITERIA Not reported COUNTRY/SETTING: The Netherlands STUDY PERIOD: "Study enrollment started in September 2004 and was completed in March 2006."
Interventions	Number of study centres: 26 community pharmacies in the Netherlands CONTROL GROUP "Patients in the control group were provided usual care, consisting of verbal and written drug information according to the standard protocol in the pharmacies. Patients in the usual care group did not receive lipid measurements or counselling sessions." INTERVENTION GROUP "Patients in the intervention (pharmaceutical care) group were invited to visit the pharmacy for 5 individual counselling visits, each lasting 10-15 minutes. Counseling visits were scheduled at first prescription, at second prescription (after 15 days), and at subsequent refill dates at 3, 6, and 12 months after the start of statin therapy."
Outcomes	TIME OF OUTCOME MEASUREMENTS "At 3, 6, and 12 months, total cholesterol, high-density lipoprotein cholesterol, and triglyceride levels were measured from fasting fingerstick whole blood samples using Cholestech LDX Analyzers (Cholestech Corp., Hayward, CA) and low-density lipoprotein cholesterol (LDL-C) was estimated by the Friedewald formula.21 Measured lipid levels and treatment goals were recorded on a wallet card that was kept by all patients to monitor their progress in lowering lipid levels. In addition, medication adherence was assessed via unused pill counts, and the association between adherence and lipid levels was discussed to encourage patients to adhere to the prescribed dosing regimen." PRIMARY OUTCOMES: adherence in terms of time to discontinuation and medication possession ratio (MPR), lipid levels
Notes	Commercial funding/non-commercial funding/other funding: "This study was funded by a grant from the National Institute for Public Health and the Environment (RIVM). The Division of Pharmacoepidemiology and Clinical Pharmacology employing Mr. Eussen, Dr. Klungel, Dr. de Boer, and Dr. Bouvy has received unrestricted funding for pharmacoepidemiologic research from GlaxoSmithKline, Novo Nordisk, the private/public funded Top Institute Pharma (www.tipharma.nl, includes co-funding from universities, government, and industry), the Dutch Medicines Evaluation Board, and the Dutch Ministry of Health. The funding source had no role in the study design; in the

Eussen 2010   (*Continued*)

collection, management, analysis, or interpretation of the data; in the writing of the manuscript; or in the decision to submit the manuscript for publication."

Stated aim for study: "To implement and assess the effectiveness of a community pharmacy-based pharmaceutical care program developed to improve patients' adherence to statin therapy."

Risk of bias

Bias	Authors' judgement	Support for judgement
Random sequence generation (selection bias)	Low risk	"Once the informed consent form was received, each participant was randomly assigned to either the intervention or control group by a procedure that was built into the computer system and used a set of random numbers in a 1:1 ratio"
Allocation concealment (selection bias)	Low risk	See above
Blinding (performance bias and detection bias) All outcomes	Unclear risk	Unblinded "open-label study"
Incomplete outcome data (attrition bias) All outcomes	Low risk	"A total of 1016 subjects were enrolled in the trial, 513 (50%) of whom were randomized to the pharmaceutical care group and 503 (50%) to the usual care group (Figure 1). A total of 117 patients were excluded because no pharmacy dispensing data were available for these subjects, due to mismatch between data from the electronic records and the handwritten study entry forms. Thus, 899 patients (439 in the pharmaceutical care group and 460 in the usual care group) were eligible for analysis. Of the patients in the pharmaceutical care group, 62 (14%) did not attend any follow-up counselling session, whereas 29 (7%), 43 (10%), and 305 (69%) patients attended 3, 4, and all 5 counselling sessions, respectively."
Selective reporting (reporting bias)	Low risk	All outcomes reported

Fang 2015

Methods	Randomised controlled clinical trial (RCT) Randomisation ratio: 1:1:1 Equivalence design: (2-sided confidence interval) Open-label
Participants	N recruited = 596 N randomized = 280 (95 SMS, 92 SMS + ML, 93 phone) N reported outcomes = 271 Mean age not reported; 68% - 70% men INCLUSION CRITERIA "All study participants had CAD diagnoses of chronic stable angina consistent with the criteria of the Chinese Medical Association of Cardiovascular Disease guide (2007 edition). Their case histories included a history of angina, together with dual-source computed tomography or angiography examinations that revealed coronary artery stenosis of 75% or more. All patients were prescribed oral beta blockers, angiotensin-converting enzyme inhibitors (ACEIs), nitrates or lipid-lowering drugs to be taken at different times according to their doctors' suggestion. Statins were taken once daily in the evening because lipid metabolism by the human body is fastest at night. All patients functioned independently in their daily lives and were able to receive SMS and ML communications via mobile phone." EXCLUSION CRITERIA "The exclusion criteria were as follows: (1) nonconformance with the diagnostic standards for chronic stable angina established by the Chinese Medical Association of Cardiovascular Epidemiology, (2) history of mental illness, (3) infection, fever, operation, serious heart failure, respiratory failure or acute stroke in the prior month and (4) inability to use a mobile phone that accepts SMS." COUNTRY/SETTING: China STUDY PERIOD: March-December 2013
Interventions	Number of study centres: West China Hospital of Sichuan University CONTROL GROUP *Phone* "The phone group received a telephone call once a month to remind them of their medication schedule and upcoming appointments." INTERVENTION GROUPS *SMS* "The SMS group received medication reminders and educational materials via SMS." *SMS +ML* "The SMS + ML group received medication reminders via SMS and educational materials via a Micro Letter (ML). We built a public ML platform, from which we regularly released CAD-related information, including the hazards and methods of preventing hyperlipidaemia, the role, scope, usage, method of use, and side effects of lipid-lowering drugs and other related information. Patients in the SMS + ML group had open access to all information on the ML platform."
Outcomes	"We used the four-item dichotomous Morisky Medication Adherence Scale (MMAS) to assess drug compliance. Scaled scores were determined by digitally tabulating responses as yes (1) or no (0). Scores ranged from 0-4. A score of 0 indicated good compliance, scores of 1 and 2 indicated fair to medium compliance, and scores of 3 and 4 indicated poor compliance."

Fang 2015   *(Continued)*

	PRIMARY OUTCOME: medication adherence, phone (reference)
Notes	Commercial funding/non-commercial funding/other funding : Funding not reported Stated aim for study: "To compare drug adherence to lipid-lowering therapy among outpatients with coronary artery disease who received information via short message service, via short message service and Micro Letter, or via phone only."

Risk of bias

Bias	Authors' judgement	Support for judgement
Random sequence generation (selection bias)	Low risk	"Participants were randomised into three groups, SMS (n = 95), SMS + ML (n = 92), and phone (n = 93), by a computer-generated random number table."
Allocation concealment (selection bias)	Low risk	See above
Blinding (performance bias and detection bias) All outcomes	Unclear risk	Unblinded open-label study
Incomplete outcome data (attrition bias) All outcomes	Low risk	"During the study period, nine of the 280 enrolled subjects withdrew from the study, including four from the SMS group, two from the SMS + ML group, and three from the phone group. Reasons for withdrawal included unwillingness to complete the test (n = 6) and personal issues (n = 3). The overall response rate of the study was 96 78% (271/280)."
Selective reporting (reporting bias)	Low risk	All outcomes reported

Faulkner 2000

Methods	Parallel randomised controlled clinical trial Randomisation ratio: 1:1 Equivalence design: 2-sided confidence interval Open-label
Participants	N recruited = 30 N randomised = 30 (15 control group, 15 intervention group) N reported outcomes = 30 Mean age: 61 ± 12 (control group) and 64 ± 12 (intervention group) INCLUSION CRITERIA "Patients who had undergone coronary artery bypass graft (CABG) surgery or percutaneous transluminal coronary angioplasty (PTCA) in the previous 7-30 days were eligible.

Faulkner 2000 *(Continued)*

	Patients had to have a baseline fasting LDL above 130 mg/dl. They had to be able to read, understand, and speak English, and to have a telephone in their home. Written informed consent was obtained from each participant." EXCLUSION CRITERIA "Exclusion criteria were serum transaminase levels greater than 2 times the upper limit of normal; concomitant therapy with cyclosporine, warfarin, or erythromycin; and a history of significant gastrointestinal disease, including gastroesophageal reflux disease, peptic ulcer disease, Crohn's disease, and ulcerative colitis." COUNTRY/SETTING: university-affiliated tertiary care hospital in Omaha, Nebraska, USA STUDY PERIOD: Not reported
Interventions	Number of study centres: Coronary care unit at St.Joseph Hospital "While still hospitalized, all patients were prescribed lovastatin (Mevacor) 20 mg/day at bedtime and colestipol (Colestid) 5 g twice/day. All patients received dietary instruction before the start of drug therapy." CONTROL GROUP No telephone contact INTERVENTION GROUP "A pharmacist telephoned patients at their home every week for 12 weeks. To ensure consistency in the information requested of the patients, the same pharmacist was involved in each patient contact and a standard set of questions was asked. Emphasis was placed on the importance of therapy in reducing the risk of recurrent cardiac events. Patients were questioned about when and where prescriptions were filled, how they paid for their prescriptions, potential side effects, overall well-being, and specific reasons for noncompliance when applicable."
Outcomes	TIME OF OUTCOME MEASUREMENTS "Lipid profiles were measured at baseline, at 6 and 12 weeks after starting therapy, and at 1 and 2 years after enrolment. Compliance was determined by pill and packet counts (not performed within the patient's view) at the 6- and 12-week clinic visits. To assess long-term compliance, pharmacies at which patients filled their prescriptions were contacted at 1 and 2 years to document refill information." PRIMARY OUTCOMES: lipid levels, compliance - pill and packet counts and refill records
Notes	Commercial funding/non-commercial funding/other funding : Not reported Stated aim for study: "we assessed the impact of personalized telephone follow-up on the rate of compliance in high-risk, hypercholesterolemic patients receiving combination drug therapy."

Risk of bias

Bias	Authors' judgement	Support for judgement
Random sequence generation (selection bias)	Low risk	"Patients were randomized to telephone contact or no telephone contact using a computer-generated list of random numbers"

Faulkner 2000   *(Continued)*

Allocation concealment (selection bias)	Unclear risk	Not reported
Blinding (performance bias and detection bias) All outcomes	Unclear risk	Unblinded open-label study
Incomplete outcome data (attrition bias) All outcomes	Low risk	None of the 30 participants enrolled in the study were lost to follow-up
Selective reporting (reporting bias)	Low risk	All outcomes reported

Fischer 2014

Methods	Parallel randomised controlled clinical trial Randomisation ratio: 1:100 automated intervention; 1:40 live intervention Equivalence design: (2-sided confidence interval) Open-label
Participants	*Automated Intervention* N recruited = 861,894 N randomised = 861,894 (852,612 control, 9282 intervention) N reported outcomes = 861,894 *Live Intervention* N recruited = 124,131 N randomised = 124,131 (121,155 control, 2976 intervention) N reported outcomes = 124,131 INCLUSION CRITERIA All "Patients with newly prescribed cardiovascular medications received at CVS community pharmacies." EXCLUSION CRITERIA "A prescription was considered new if there were no claims in the same therapeutic class 6 months before the index date. Patients without at least 6 months of eligibility before the index date were excluded unless they had another prescription that satisfied the inclusion criteria." COUNTRY/SETTING: USA STUDY PERIOD: January 2008 to December 2010
Interventions	*Control group* "Control patients received usual care." *Automated Intervention* "Patients received automated phone calls on days 3 and 7 after the prescription was processed but remained unpurchased. The calls reminded patients that their prescription was ready and encouraged them to pick it up." *Live Intervention* "Identified patients who had not purchased a prescription 8 days after it was bottled, even after receiving automated calls on days 3 and 7. A pharmacist or technician called these patients to better understand barriers to medication adherence and provide counselling and solutions to encourage appropriate medication use. Messaging included education

Fischer 2014   *(Continued)*

	about the importance of treatment, suggestions about lower cost options when relevant, and efforts to engage and motivate patients to adhere to therapy."
Outcomes	PRIMARY OUTCOMES: proportion of abandoned prescriptions
Notes	**Publication details** Commercial funding/non-commercial funding/other funding: "The research was funded by the National Association of Chain Drug Stores Foundation. Study design, conduct, and reporting were determined independently by the research team." **Stated aim for study** "To determine whether 2 pharmacy-based interventions could decrease PMN." (Primary medication nonadherence)

Risk of bias

Bias	Authors' judgement	Support for judgement
Random sequence generation (selection bias)	Low risk	"Patients with randomly selected birthdays served as the control population"
Allocation concealment (selection bias)	Low risk	See above
Blinding (performance bias and detection bias) All outcomes	Unclear risk	Unblinded open-label study
Incomplete outcome data (attrition bias) All outcomes	Low risk	All randomised participants' outcome reported
Selective reporting (reporting bias)	Low risk	All outcomes reported

Goswami 2013

Methods	Parallel randomised controlled clinical trial Randomisation ratio: 1:1 Equivalence design: 2-sided confidence interval Open-label
Participants	N recruited = 500 N randomised = 500 (125 control group, 375 intervention group) N reported outcomes = 208 (53 control group, 155 intervention group) - eligible for analysis "Among the control group, the average age was 67.8 years, compared with 69.5 years for the intervention group. The sex distribution was predominantly male for both groups (67.9% of the controls and 58.7% of the intervention group)." INCLUSION CRITERIA "All subjects had to satisfy inclusion criteria to be considered eligible for participation by one of the ten participating physicians of the practice's study team: (1) be older

Goswami 2013   *(Continued)*

	than 21 years of age and, on the basis of clinical assessment by his or her physician, a candidate for statin therapy; (2) have received a first prescription for atorvastatin after study initiation at the practice, including patients who were new to the practice and returning practice patients (new versus continuing atorvastatin patients were deciphered by requiring claims activity 6 months before and after the index date); and (3) provide a personally signed and dated informed consent document indicating that the participant (or a legally acceptable representative) had been informed of all pertinent aspects of the study."
	EXCLUSION CRITERIA
	"Patients were excluded from the study if they were unwilling to participate in the adherence counseling or unwilling to give a written informed consent document."
	COUNTRY/SETTING: USA
	STUDY PERIOD: "The target sample was enrolled in the study from March 2010 through May 2011."
Interventions	Number of study centres: Prairie Heart Cardiovascular Consultants in Illinois
	INTERVENTION GROUP
	"All patients randomized to the intervention group were provided adherence counseling from a nurse (via a 5-10-minute discussion), and an adherence tip sheet. Patients in the intervention group were also given the opportunity to enroll in the My HeartWise™ Program,24 a 12-week guide to managing cholesterol (included monthly mailing of educational materials). The practice physicians also had the discretion to provide eligible patients in the intervention group with a copay relief card (usable with commercial payers, not Medicare)."
	CONTROL GROUP
	"The control group received usual care, with no additional adherence counseling or tip sheet."
Outcomes	TIME OF OUTCOME MEASUREMENTS
	t = 3, 6, 9, 12 months since index date
	PRIMARY OUTCOME: adherence to atorvastatin using PDC (proportion of days covered) and MPR (medication possession ratio)
	SECONDARY OUTCOME: persistence with the index therapy over the 6-month post-index period
Notes	Commercial funding/non-commercial funding/other funding :" This study was sponsored by Pfizer, Inc."
	Conflict of Interest: "NJG is a speaker for The Medicines Company, Medtronic, and Boston Scientific and is the medical director for SynvaCor. MDK and MRK are employees of IMS Health, which was a paid consultant to Pfizer in connection with the development of this article. AK, JM, LZL, and JV are employees of Pfizer, Inc, and own stock in Pfizer, Inc."
	Stated aim for study: "This trial evaluated the effectiveness of an integrated intervention program that included a 3-to-5-minute nurse counseling session, copay relief cards, and a monthly newsletter on adherence to atorvastatin treatment."
	Limitations:
	1) "As the control group's adherence was initially high, there was little room for improvement as a result of the intervention. The large number of continuing users at this particular cardiology practice group could explain the high adherence rate observed in

Goswami 2013   *(Continued)*

this study, which in turn could partially explain the lack of a significant impact due to the intervention. The literature confirms that new users often exhibit lower adherence rates as compared with continuing users."

2) "The frequency with which discount cards were given to control patients was not tracked. However, because many of the patients were older than 65 years of age, the impact of discount cards was likely limited, as Medicare patients did not qualify to receive them."

Risk of bias

Bias	Authors' judgement	Support for judgement
Random sequence generation (selection bias)	Low risk	"Eligible patients were randomized using a telephone randomization system to one of two groups: an intervention group and a control group (with a patient ratio of 3:1 intervention:control)"
Allocation concealment (selection bias)	Unclear risk	Not reported
Blinding (performance bias and detection bias) All outcomes	Unclear risk	Unblinded open-label study
Incomplete outcome data (attrition bias) All outcomes	Unclear risk	"The study initially included 500 patients (125 control patients and 375 patients who received the adherence intervention). After matching with the LRx database, 97 controls and 319 intervention patients remained eligible for analysis. However, only 93 controls and 300 intervention patients actually had any LRx claims available for analysis during the study window. Of this group, 57 controls and 180 intervention patients had an atorvastatin prescription after enrollment in the study, which served as the index date. After applying the study requirement of claims activity 6 months before and after the index date, only 53 controls (seven new users [first atorvastatin prescription after randomization] and 46 continuing users [evidence of atorvastatin prescription within 6 months prior to randomization]) and 155 intervention patients (14 new users and 141 continuing users) remained eligible for analysis (Figure 1)."
Selective reporting (reporting bias)	Low risk	All outcomes reported

Gujral 2014

Methods	Parallel randomised controlled clinical trial Randomisation ratio: 1:1 Equivalence design: 2-sided confidence interval Open-label
Participants	N recruited = 640 N randomised = 200 (100 control, 100 intervention) N reported outcomes = 137 (72 intervention group and 65 control group) at 12 months Mean age of participants in the intervention group was 58.4 (SD 11.3) and in the control group 60.4 (SD 11.0) years; respectively 77% and 80% men INCLUSION CRITERIA "The study population was a convenience sample of patients admitted to the coronary care unit, cardiology ward or general medical wards with a documented diagnosis of STelevated MI or Non-ST-elevated MI." "Participation in the study required patients to nominate and attend one community pharmacy for the study period." From protocol: 18 - 85 years old EXCLUSION CRITERIA Not reported in paper but from protocol: • People whose primary language is other than English (LOTE) • Children and/or young people (i.e. < 18 years) • People with an intellectual or mental impairment • Aboriginal and/or Torres Strait Islander peoples • Women who are pregnant COUNTRY/SETTING: Queensland, Australia STUDY PERIOD: Enrolment from October 2009 to August 2010
Interventions	INTERVENTION GROUP: "In the intervention group the community pharmacist reviewed the patient monthly when they collected their prescriptions, to assess if they were getting their MI medicines dispensed and whether they were experiencing any problems with their MI medicines. At 3 and 6 months, the pharmacist had a longer discussion with the patient tailored to their medication beliefs provided by the researcher from the repertory grid interview." CONTROL GROUP: " Patients in the control group did not have their medication beliefs communicated to their community pharmacist by the researcher. The community pharmacists for patients in the control group were asked to provide the patient with usual care when they collected their prescription medications."
Outcomes	PRIMARY OUTCOMES: medication non-adherence at 12 months SECONDARY OUTCOMES: medication non-adherence at 6 months and changes in adherence and medication beliefs between 6 to 12 months "Medication adherence was measured in two ways. A medication possession ratio (MPR) was determined from prescriptions filled by the patient over the study period for the lipid lowering agent and ACE-I/ARB or beta-blocker (if they were not prescribed an ACE-I/ARB)." "Patients were categorised as non-adherent based on the MPR of the lipid lowering drug." "Medication beliefs were elicited .... using the repertory grid technique and the BMQ Specific at the 6 and 12 month interviews."

Gujral 2014 *(Continued)*

	After discharge from hospital participants were followed for 12 months and participated in 3 interviews with the researcher (face-to-face at 5 - 6 weeks, by telephone at 6 and 12 months)
Notes	Funding: "This work was supported by the Pharmacy Board of Queensland Research Grants Program 2008, Brisbane, Queensland. The Pharmacy Board had no input in the research design, methodology or results. The ideas expressed in this manuscript are those of the authors and are not intended to represent the position of the Board or members of the Board."

Risk of bias

Bias	Authors' judgement	Support for judgement
Random sequence generation (selection bias)	Unclear risk	"Patients were randomly assigned into the pharmacy intervention or control group using block randomisation." From protocol: …"predetermined randomisation sequence.." "Will use an Excel data base to generate a permuted block randomisation sequence to ensure equal numbers of participants in both groups."
Allocation concealment (selection bias)	High risk	"Patients were randomly assigned into the pharmacy intervention or control group using block randomisation." From protocol: "Allocation was not concealed."
Blinding (performance bias and detection bias) All outcomes	Unclear risk	Not blinded
Incomplete outcome data (attrition bias) All outcomes	High risk	attrition 31.5% (137/200 analysed at primary endpoint)
Selective reporting (reporting bias)	Low risk	

Guthrie 2001

Methods	Parallel randomised controlled clinical trial Randomisation ratio: 1:1 Equivalence design: 2-sided confidence interval Open-label
Participants	N recruited = 13,100 N randomised = 13,100 (2765 control, 10335 intervention) N reported outcomes = 4548 (3635 in intervention group, 913 in control group) - returned 6-month patient survey forms

Guthrie 2001   *(Continued)*

	Mean age 57.9 years (intervention group), 58.3 years (control group) INCLUSION CRITERIA "Patients with risk scores ~4 on a scale of -1 to +16 for men and -1 to +17 for women on the First Heart Attack Risk Test were considered to be at increased risk for a first MI and suitable for enrollment in the registry program. An elevated total cholesterol level despite dietary interventions was an additional inclusion criterion." EXCLUSION CRITERIA "Previous MI, current therapy with a 3-hydroxy-3-methylglutaryl coenzyme A reductase inhibitor (i.e., statin), as well as membership in a federally funded health care program (except Medicare or plans for federal employees) constituted exclusion criteria. Medicaid patients were excluded in accordance with federal regulations prohibiting participation of such patients in programs involving prescription writing. Women of childbearing potential were similarly excluded from participation in the registry." COUNTRY/SETTING: USA STUDY PERIOD: December 1997 to December 1998
Interventions	Number of study centres: 2708 physicians INTERVENTION GROUP "Individuals randomized to the intervention group received telephone reminders at weeks 2 and 8, as well as reminder postcards at week 4, to reinforce these messages about coronary risk reduction. Each of these communications stressed the importance of following the physician's instructions and taking medications as prescribed. These reminders were issued by a national program-coordinating center. Reminder postcards were also mailed to both groups at 4 and 5 months after enrollment. Physicians completed follow-up evaluation forms after patient visits, which were scheduled according to their normal practices." CONTROL GROUP Usual care
Outcomes	TIME OF OUTCOME MEASUREMENTS "At 3 and 6 months or study discontinuation, registry participants completed patient-survey forms concerning compliance with care and mailed these to the program-coordinating center." PRIMARY OUTCOME: compliance SECONDARY OUTCOME: lifestyle modifications
Notes	Commercial funding/non-commercial funding/other funding: "This registry was funded by Bristol-Myers Squibb Co, Princeton, New Jersey." "For professional services and administrative activities conducted in association with the First MI Risk Reduction Program, each participating physician received an honorarium of $500 from the registry sponsor." Stated aim for study: "The purpose of the First Myocardial Infarction (MI) Risk Reduction Program, an open-label drug registry involving mainly primary-care patients at increased risk of a first MI, was to examine the effects of postal and telephone reminders, as well as demographic and other baseline characteristics, on patient self-reported compliance with pravastatin treatment."

Risk of bias

Guthrie 2001   *(Continued)*

Bias	Authors' judgement	Support for judgement
Random sequence generation (selection bias)	Unclear risk	Not reported
Allocation concealment (selection bias)	Unclear risk	Not reported
Blinding (performance bias and detection bias) All outcomes	Unclear risk	Unblinded "open-label" study
Incomplete outcome data (attrition bias) All outcomes	High risk	"-35% of the total number of patients enrolled who returned patient survey forms to the national program coordinating center at 6 months"
Selective reporting (reporting bias)	Low risk	All outcomes reported

Ho 2014

Methods	Parallel randomised controlled clinical trial Randomisation ratio: 1:1 Equivalence design: 2-sided confidence interval Open-label not reported
Participants	N recruited = 253 patients N randomised = 253 participants (124 control, 129 intervention) N reported outcomes = 241 participants) (119 control, 122 intervention) Mean age 64 yrs, 98% men INCLUSION CRITERIA "Patients admitted with ACS as the primary reason for hospital admission and used the VA for their usual care" EXCLUSION CRITERIA "1) patients admitted for primary non-cardiac diagnosis who developed ACS as a secondary condition 2) planned discharge to nursing home or skilled nursing facility 3) irreversible, noncardiac medical condition likely to affect 6-month survival or inability to execute study protocol 4) lack of telephone or cell phone 5) VA not a primary source of care in the future 6) fill medications at non-VA pharmacy 7) pregnancy" COUNTRY/SETTING: 4 Department of Veterans Affairs (VA) medical centers (Denver, Colorado; Little Rock, Arkansas; Seattle, Washington; and Durham, North Carolina), USA STUDY PERIOD: "Recruitment began July 1, 2010, in Denver and Seattle; September 1, 2010, in Little Rock; and July 1, 2011, in Durham."

Ho 2014   *(Continued)*

Interventions	Number of study centres: 4 "Department of Veterans Affairs medical centers located in Denver (CO), Seattle (WA), Durham (NC), and Little Rock (AK)" INTERVENTION GROUP "standard ACS hospital discharge instructions, a discharge medication list, and educational information about cardiac medications" and "1) pharmacist-led medication reconciliation and tailoring, 2) patient education, 3) collaborative care between pharmacist and a patient's primary care clinician and/or cardiologist, and 4) 2 types of voice messaging (educational and medication refill reminder calls)" CONTROL GROUP "standard ACS hospital discharge instructions, a discharge medication list, and educational information about cardiac medications"
Outcomes	TIME OF OUTCOME MEASUREMENTS: 12-month clinic visit PRIMARY OUTCOMES: "Proportion of patients adherent to medication regimens based on a mean proportion of days covered (PDC) greater than 0.80 in the year after hospital discharge using pharmacy refill data for 4 cardioprotective medications (clopidogrel, B-blockers, statins, and ACEI/ARB)" SECONDARY OUTCOMES: "Proportion of patients reaching blood pressure goals (<140/90mmHg) and LDL-C goals (<100mg/dL) at 12 months"
Notes	Commercial funding/non-commercial funding/other funding: "This study was funded by a Veterans Health Administration Health Service Research & Development Investigator Initiated Award. Dr. Bosworth was supported by a senior career scientist award." Stated aim for study: "To test a multifaceted intervention to improve adherence to cardiac medications"

Risk of bias

Bias	Authors' judgement	Support for judgement
Random sequence generation (selection bias)	Low risk	"Eligible patients with ACS were randomized using blocked randomization stratified by study site in a 1:1 ratio to INT or UC"
Allocation concealment (selection bias)	Low risk	"The allocation sequence was concealed until a patient consented to participate and was generated centrally using the graphical user interface implemented for the study"
Blinding (performance bias and detection bias) All outcomes	Unclear risk	Not reported
Incomplete outcome data (attrition bias) All outcomes	Low risk	"Of 253 patients, 241 (95.3%) completed the study (122 in INT and 119 in UC)"
Selective reporting (reporting bias)	Low risk	All outcomes reported

Kardas 2013

Methods	Parallel randomised controlled clinical trial Randomisation ratio: 1:1 Equivalence design: (2-sided confidence interval) Open-label
Participants	N recruited = 198 N randomised = 198 (89 control, 107 intervention) N reported = 196 Mean age 59.6 ± 9.1 years, 75.5% women INCLUSION CRITERIA Outpatients with untreated hyperlipidaemia (total cholesterol ≥ 250 mg/dL) aged 40 - 80 years (59.6 ± 9.1 years) were enrolled EXCLUSION CRITERIA Mental illness, dependence on other people's care, and/or medication taking, being at risk of not completing the study due to alcoholism, psychoactive substance abuse, homelessness etc., porphyria, unstable angina, NYHA class III or IV heart failure, acute infections, liver disease (cirrhosis), or significantly elevated transaminases (level ≥ 3 times above the normal values), allergy to simvastatin, or any other known contraindications to its use, pregnancy, and lactation COUNTRY/SETTING: primary care centers in Poland STUDY PERIOD: Not reported
Interventions	CONTROL GROUP All patients who were enrolled in the study were prescribed simvastatin at the initial dose of 20 mg to be taken once daily in the evening INTERVENTION GROUP Intervention group received counselling every 8 weeks and were instructed to adopt routine evening activity as a reminder
Outcomes	PRIMARY OUTCOME: adherence expressed as Medication Possession Ratio, calculated as the proportion of the number of days during which the participant was in possession of simvastatin, over the total number of days of the follow-up period
Notes	

Risk of bias

Bias	Authors' judgement	Support for judgement
Random sequence generation (selection bias)	Unclear risk	Not reported
Allocation concealment (selection bias)	Unclear risk	Not reported
Blinding (performance bias and detection bias) All outcomes	Unclear risk	Unblinded open-label study

Kardas 2013   *(Continued)*

Incomplete outcome data (attrition bias) All outcomes	Low risk	2 participants lost to attrition
Selective reporting (reporting bias)	Low risk	All outcomes reported

---

Kooy 2013

Methods	Parallel randomised controlled clinical trial Randomisation ratio: 1:1:1 Equivalence design: (2-sided confidence interval) Open-label
Participants	N recruited = 399 N randomised = 399 (134 control, 134 intervention-1, 131 intervention-2) N reported outcomes = 381 Mean age 76.5 (SD 6.3), 44.1% men INCLUSION CRITERIA ≤ 65 years old (Mean age 76.5) "We included patients who had started statins at least one year prior to inclusion and were non-adherent in the year prior to inclusion (refill rate between 50 and 80%)." EXCLUSION CRITERIA "We excluded patients who were not personally responsible for their medication intake or who received their medication in a dosing aid, patients with a life expectancy of less than 6 months and patients younger than 65 years. Life expectancy is difficult to assess but this assessment was based on personal knowledge about the patient and the prescription of drugs used in the palliative phase. Patients who had switched to a different statin in the 540 days before the inclusion date were also excluded." COUNTRY/SETTING: The Netherlands STUDY PERIOD: Patients recruited between January 2008 and March 2008
Interventions	Number of study centres: 24 community pharmacies *Counseling with ERD group (1)* "The pharmacist sent patients a written invitation and a follow up phone call was made 14 days after the written invitation. The intervention consisted of two elements: the first and most important element was the application of the stages of change model in non-adherence counseling. The second element was the Electronic Reminder Device (ERD)." "The 10-min counseling session by the pharmacist consisted of five phases. The patient received feedback on their previous drug dispensing data (1). Patients were asked if they were aware that they were non-adherent and reasons for non-adherence were discussed (2). Patients were informed about the benefits of statin use (3), received an ERD to help them with medication taking (4) and were informed that after one year they would be invited for a follow-up visit (5). The ERD is a medication reminder device that starts beeping every day at the same time until the patient switches it off. Patients can adjust the time." *ERD group (2)* "Patients received the ERD by mail with a written instruction about the use of the device."

Kooy 2013   *(Continued)*

Control group (3)
"Patients in the control group received usual care. In the Netherlands usual care entails: at the start of therapy, patients receive written and spoken information about the therapy and medication. After about 2 weeks, the patient should return for the first refill. The patient is then asked about his or her experience, concerns and need for information. Patients who use a statin for more than a year do not receive counselling on a regular basis."

Outcomes	"The pre-specified primary outcome was refill adherence to statins based on pharmacy dispensing records. Refill adherence was assessed by calculating the proportion of days covered of the 360 days following the index date by dividing the total days' supply by the number of days of study participation [PDC360 (Hess et al., 2006)]." PRIMARY OUTCOME: refill adherence SECONDARY OUTCOME: discontinuation
Notes	**Publication details** Commercial funding/non-commercial funding/other funding : "This trial was funded by Utrecht University." **Stated aim for study** "The aim of this study was to assess the effectiveness of an electronic reminder device (ERD) with or without counselling to improve refill adherence and persistence for statin treatment in non-adherent patients."

Risk of bias

Bias	Authors' judgement	Support for judgement
Random sequence generation (selection bias)	Low risk	"Patients were randomized into one of three groups: the Counseling with ERD group, the ERD group (with written instruction) or the control group (usual care) in a 1:1:1 ratio using a computer generated random number sequence. Patients were randomized in blocks based on baseline medication adherence (above or below 65%) and age [above or below 75 using the minimization method with equal weights assigned to both categories (Scott et al., 2002; Heritier et al., 2005)]."
Allocation concealment (selection bias)	Low risk	See above
Blinding (performance bias and detection bias) All outcomes	Unclear risk	Unblinded "open-label study"
Incomplete outcome data (attrition bias) All outcomes	Low risk	"A total of 399 patients considered eligible by the pharmacists were randomly assigned to one of the two intervention groups or the

Kooy 2013   *(Continued)*

		control group. Two patients were excluded because they did not fill any prescription after the selection date. A total of 16 patients were excluded because they started receiving medication weekly after the index date."
Selective reporting (reporting bias)	Low risk	All outcomes reported

Ma 2010

Methods	Parallel randomised controlled clinical trial Randomisation ratio: 1:1 Equivalence design: (2-sided confidence interval) Open-label
Participants	N recruited = 689 N randomised = 689 (338 control, 331 intervention) N reported outcomes = 559 Mean age 60 years, 60% men INCLUSION CRITERIA "A patient was eligible for the study if he/she was between the ages of 30 and 85 years and had CHD defined as the presence of at least one coronary lesion ≥50% at the time of coronary angiography. Patients could have a history of prior CHD, or this could have been their first such diagnosis." EXCLUSION CRITERIA "Patients were excluded if they were unable or unwilling to give informed consent in English, had a history of intolerance to two or more statin drugs, planned to move out of the area within one year of recruitment, had a poor prognosis such that life expectancy was estimated to be <5 years, had a major psychiatric illness, or had no telephone." COUNTRY/SETTING: tertiary care hospital in central Massachusetts, USA STUDY PERIOD: "The study was conducted between September 2000 and August 2005."
Interventions	Number of study centres: 1 INTERVENTION GROUP "In this two-condition randomized clinical trial, the intervention condition included: (1) a computer-based tracking system designed to facilitate follow-up of patients who were initially seen for a CHD clinical event at UMass Memorial Medical Center (UMMMC); (2) an initial inpatient contact and a series of coordinated patient-centered pharmacist-delivered telephone counseling contacts to improve adherence to prescribed medications." CONTROL GROUP "The UC condition consisted of normal clinical care as determined by the patient's provider."
Outcomes	*"The primary outcome* evaluated at one year included percentage of patients with a serum low-density lipoprotein cholesterol (LDL-C) level <100 mg/dl; *the secondary outcome* included the proportion of prescribed statin medication taken by patients as measured

Ma 2010   *(Continued)*

by a continuous multiple-interval (CMA) based on pharmacy records. The CMA is the ratio of days supply obtained to total days between refill records [22]. Other secondary outcomes evaluated at one year included the proportion of patients prescribed ACE inhibitor and beta-blocker medication. Adherence to these medications was also measured by CMA."

PRIMARY OUTCOME: LDL-C < 100 mg/dl

SECONDARY OUTCOMES: adherence with statin medication

Notes	**Publication details** Commercial funding/non-commercial funding/other funding : "The project described was supported by Award Number R01 HL66786-01 to Dr. Ira S. Ockene from the National Heart, Lung, and Blood Institute (NHLBI)." **Stated aim for study** "The overall goal of this study was to implement and evaluate the effects of a pharmacist-delivered intervention (PI) designed to improve LDL-C goal attainment according to the NCEP ATP-III Guidelines and prescribed lipid-lowering medi- cation adherence in patients with known CHD."

Risk of bias

Bias	Authors' judgement	Support for judgement
Random sequence generation (selection bias)	Low risk	"The patient was the unit of randomiza-tion and analysis. Randomization was con-ducted by a statistician who was not in-volved with the intervention. The study was conducted between September 2000 and August 2005. The Institutional Review Boards of the University of Massachusetts Medical School approved all subject re-cruitment, intervention, and data collec-tion procedures."
Allocation concealment (selection bias)	Low risk	See above
Blinding (performance bias and detection bias) All outcomes	Unclear risk	Unblinded "open-label study"
Incomplete outcome data (attrition bias) All outcomes	Low risk	"Of 689 patients recruited, 338 were ran-domized to the control condition and 351 to the intervention condition. A total of 559 (81%) had complete pharmacy records and were included in the final analysis."
Selective reporting (reporting bias)	Low risk	All outcomes reported

Márquez 1998

Methods	Parallel randomised controlled clinical trial Randomisation ratio: 1:1 Equivalence design: 2-sided confidence interval Open-label
Participants	N recruited = 110 N randomised = 110 (55 control, 55 intervention) N reported outcomes = 108 Mean age years 55.7 (intervention group), 56.1 years (control group) INCLUSION CRITERIA a) outpatients of both sexes from 18 - 75 years old b) diagnosed with new or uncontrolled hypercholesteraemia that can be treated according to the recommendation of the Spanish Society of Arteriosclerosis c) patients in whom pharmacological treatment of hypercholesteraemia is indicated by fluvastatin and can be initiated as new drug treatment d) agree to participate in the study by written and verbal consent EXCLUSION CRITERIA a) patients who want to join the study to control their lipid levels or get lipid-lowering drugs b) secondary hypercholesteraemia c) patient is known to have side effects from statins d) contraindicated for fluvastatin use or hypersensitive to fluvastatin e) pregnant or breastfeeding women f) patients in a pathological situation which could interfere with the study (i.e. disabled, alcoholic, drug user, chronic diseases) g) unwilling to grant informed consent or poor co-operation is expected h) patients who have participated in other studies from this investigation i) having a cohabitant who is taking the same lipid-lowering medication used in the study COUNTRY/SETTING: primary care centers in Spain STUDY PERIOD: Patients enrolled between January and March 1997
Interventions	Number of study centres: Primary Care setting INTERVENTION GROUP "HE (Health Education) was monitored by a) a group HE session and b) back-up letter sent to their homes." CONTROL GROUP "received HE from their family doctor"
Outcomes	TIME OF OUTCOME MEASUREMENTS: Pill counts over 4 months PRIMARY OUTCOME: compliance SECONDARY OUTCOMES: lipid levels, adverse effects
Notes	Commercial funding/non-commercial funding/other funding: Not reported Stated aim for study: "To analyse the efficacy of Health Education (HE) through group session with postal back-up in furthering compliance with therapy for Lipidemias."

Risk of bias

Márquez 1998   *(Continued)*

Bias	Authors' judgement	Support for judgement
Random sequence generation (selection bias)	Unclear risk	Not reported
Allocation concealment (selection bias)	Low risk	Randomisation performed blind
Blinding (performance bias and detection bias) All outcomes	Low risk	Generator and outcome assessor blinded to allocation
Incomplete outcome data (attrition bias) All outcomes	Unclear risk	2 were excluded for having no measurement count tablets
Selective reporting (reporting bias)	Low risk	All outcomes reported

Márquez 2004

Methods	Parallel randomised controlled clinical trial Radomisation ratio: 1:1 Equivalence design: (2-sided confidence interval)
Participants	N recruited = 126 N randomised = 126 (63 control, 63 intervention) N reported outcomes = 115 Mean age 57.7 (SD 8.7) years, 51.3% women INCLUSION CRITERIA Outpatients of both sexes, aged between 18 and 75 years Patients who, for the pharmacological treatment of hypercholesterolaemia this indicated the use of lipid-lowering pills, were recommended the use of simvastatin Patients gave their consent to participate in this study Patients requiring lipid-lowering medication treatment, as a function of the cardiovascular risk factors and presenting primary prevention, according to Spanish recommended by the Consensus guidelines for the control of blood cholesterol EXCLUSION CRITERIA Patients at baseline needed to control their lipid numbers with 2 or more lipid-lowering drugs Present known cardiovascular disease Secondary hypercholesterolaemia Side effects and contraindications to the use of statins Pregnant or lactating women COUNTRY/SETTING: Spain STUDY PERIOD: Recruitment between January and June 2001
Interventions	Number of study centres: 6 CONTROL GROUP "The control group ... received the doctor's normal treatment." INTERVENTION GROUP

Márquez 2004   *(Continued)*

	"The Intervention group ... received in addition a telephone call at 2 weeks, 2 months, and 4 months."
Outcomes	PRIMARY OUTCOMES: adherence, serum lipids SECONDARY OUTCOMES: number needed to intervene in order to avoid 1 non-complier
Notes	Aim: "To analyse the efficacy of the intervention through a telephone call about patients' compliance with lipaemia therapy." Funding: N/A Conflicts: None stated Language: Spanish

Risk of bias

Bias	Authors' judgement	Support for judgement
Random sequence generation (selection bias)	Low risk	Randomisation by providing numbers derived from tables by chance
Allocation concealment (selection bias)	Low risk	Randomisation performed blind
Blinding (performance bias and detection bias) All outcomes	Unclear risk	Unblinded open-label study
Incomplete outcome data (attrition bias) All outcomes	Low risk	11 out of 126 participants were excluded
Selective reporting (reporting bias)	Low risk	All outcomes reported

Márquez 2007

Methods	Parallel randomised controlled clinical trial Randomisation ratio: 1:1 Equivalence design: (2-sided confidence interval)
Participants	N recruited = 220 N randomised = 220 (110 control, 110 intervention) N reported outcomes = 186 Mean age 60.62 years (SD 11 yrs), 59.6% women INCLUSION CRITERIA Outpatients of both sexes, aged between 18 and 75 years Patients who, for the pharmacological treatment of hypercholesterolaemia this indicated the use of lipid-lowering pills, were recommended the use of simvastatin Patients gave their consent to participate in this study Patients requiring lipid-lowering medication treatment, as a function of the cardiovascular risk factors and presenting primary prevention, according to Spanish recommended

Márquez 2007   *(Continued)*

	by the Consensus guidelines for the control of blood cholesterol EXCLUSION CRITERIA Patients at baseline needed to control their lipid numbers with 2 or more lipid-lowering drugs Present known cardiovascular disease Secondary hypercholesterolaemia Side effects and contraindications to the use of statins Pregnant or lactating women COUNTRY/SETTING: Spain STUDY PERIOD: Recruitment between January and June 2006
Interventions	Number of study centres: 5 Intervention group received calendar reminder of medication taking received at the time of first prescription
Outcomes	PRIMARY OUTCOMES: adherence, serum lipids SECONDARY OUTCOMES: number needed to intervene in order to avoid 1 non-complier
Notes	Aim: To analyse the efficacy of the intervention with a calendar reminder of the medication taking in the treatment of hypercholesterolaemia Funding: N/A Conflicts: None reported Language: Spanish

Risk of bias

Bias	Authors' judgement	Support for judgement
Random sequence generation (selection bias)	Low risk	Randomisation by providing numbers derived from tables by chance
Allocation concealment (selection bias)	Low risk	Randomisation performed blind
Blinding (performance bias and detection bias) All outcomes	Unclear risk	Unblinded open-label study
Incomplete outcome data (attrition bias) All outcomes	Low risk	22 participants lost to follow-up
Selective reporting (reporting bias)	Low risk	All outcomes reported

Interventions to improve adherence to lipid-lowering medication (Review)   63

Nieuwkerk 2012

Methods	Parallel randomised controlled clinical trial Randomisation ratio: 1:1 Equivalence design: (2-sided confidence interval) Open-label
Participants	N recruited = 201 N randomised = 201 (100 control, 101 intervention) N reported outcomes = 181 Mean age 49.2 years (SD 1.3) in routine care (RC) group and 48.9 years (SD 1.2) in extended care (EC) group, 60% men in RC and 59% men in EC INCLUSION CRITERIA "Patients (aged > 18 years) with indications for statin use (primary or secondary prevention of cardiovascular events)." EXCLUSION CRITERIA "Patients with severe fasting dyslipidemia (total cholesterol >9.0 mmol/L or triglycerides >4.0 mmol/L) were excluded, as were those with fasting glucose >7.0 mmol/L. In addition, patients who had used statins for >3 months before inclusion, who had histories of drug and/or alcohol abuse, who were pregnant or breast-feeding, or who had life expectancies <2 years were excluded. In case patients had started statin therapy within 3 months, a washout period of 2 weeks was applied." COUNTRY/SETTING: The Netherlands STUDY PERIOD: Patients recruited from May 2002 to May 2004
Interventions	Number of study centres: outpatient clinics of 2 hospitals "All patients visited a study nurse practitioner at the Academic Medical Center in addition to their regular visits to their treating specialists. The baseline visit took place within 3 months after statin treatment had been indicated. Subsequent visits were scheduled after 3, 9, and 18 months." CONTROL GROUP *Routine Care (RC)* "RC consisted of measuring body weight and blood pressure and performing a capillary lipid profile at each visit (Cholestech; Alere Health BV, Tilburg, The Netherlands). Initially, all patients received atorvastatin 10 mg, unless baseline cholesterol levels were severe and more aggressive therapy was needed. Dose escalation during the study period was allowed if deemed appropriate by the treating physician." INTERVENTION GROUP *Extended Care (EC)* "In addition to RC, subjects in the EC group received multifactorial risk-factor counselling, during which the nurse practitioner explained the presence of unmodifiable risk factors, such as age, gender, and family history, and modifiable risk factors, such as lipid levels, diabetes mellitus, blood pressure, overweight, smoking habits, and physical activity. The study nurse was not blinded to the purpose of the study. The counselling focused on changing modifiable risk factors such as increasing medication adherence, reducing overweight, smoking cessation, and increasing physical activity. All obtained data were summarized in a personal risk-factor passport: a graphical presentation of the patient's calculated 10-year cardiovascular disease risk. It also showed the target risk that could be reached if all the patient's modifiable risk factors were optimally treated, as well as the standard age- and gender-related risk. Ten-year risk and target risk were calculated using the Framingham risk score. In addition, the risk-factor passport contained the

Nieuwkerk 2012   *(Continued)*

	most recent ultrasound image of the patient's carotid artery, as well as an example of a healthy and an unfavorable image of the carotid artery, which were both explained and discussed by the nurse practitioner. This risk-factor passport was updated during each follow-up visit."
Outcomes	"The objective of the present study was to investigate if nurse-led multifactorial cardio-vascular risk-factor counselling would improve adherence to lipid-lowering medication and lipid levels without increasing patients' anxiety compared to routine care (RC). We also investigated whether such an intervention would result in a lower body mass index; lower blood pressure; improved intima-media thickness (IMT) and flow-mediated di-latation (FMD); better quality of life (QoL), symptom scores, and beliefs about medi-cation; changed risk perception; and more smoking cessation compared with RC." PRIMARY OUTCOMES: Serum LDL, adherence to lipid-lowering medication SECONDARY OUTCOMES: BMI, BP, IMT, FMD, QoL, etc.
Notes	**Publication details** Commercial funding/non-commercial funding/other funding : "This study was funded in part by Pfizer (Capelle aan den IJssel, The Netherlands)." **Stated aim for study** "The aim of this study was to investigate whether nurse-led cardiovascular risk-factor counseling could improve statin adherence and lipid levels without increasing patients' anxiety."

Risk of bias

Bias	Authors' judgement	Support for judgement
Random sequence generation (selection bias)	Low risk	"After inclusion, patients were randomly assigned to RC or extended care (EC), us-ing a randomization computer program, to obtain an equal distribution of primary and secondary prevention patients, hospital ori-gin, and gender in the 2 groups"
Allocation concealment (selection bias)	Low risk	See above
Blinding (performance bias and detection bias) All outcomes	Unclear risk	Unblinded "open-label study"
Incomplete outcome data (attrition bias) All outcomes	Low risk	All randomised participants' outcomes re-ported
Selective reporting (reporting bias)	Low risk	All outcomes reported

Park 2013

Methods	Parallel randomised controlled clinical trial Randomisation ratio: 1:1:1 Superiority design: (2-sided confidence interval) Open-label
Participants	N recruited = 90 N randomised = 90 (30 control, 30 intervention-1, 30 intervention-2) N reported outcomes = 84 Mean age 59.2 years (SD 9.4, range 35 - 83), 24% women INCLUSION CRITERIA "Inclusion criteria were: (a) >/=21 years of age, (b) hospitalized for non-ST elevation MI, ST elevation MI, or PCI, (c) prescribed an antiplatelet medication [thienopyridine class of ADP receptor inhibitors and/or a cyclooxygenase inhibitor (i.e., aspirin)], (d) prescribed a statin medication (HMG-CoA reductase inhibitors), (e) owned a mobile phone with text messaging capability, and (f) were able to speak, read, and understand English." EXCLUSION CRITERIA "Exclusion criteria included: (a) cognitive impairment that limited ability to understand and complete questionnaires, and (b) inability to operate a mobile phone." COUNTRY/SETTING: USA STUDY PERIOD: "Recruitment took place between April 2012 and March 2013 until the final sample size was obtained."
Interventions	Number of study centres: 1 Text Message Reminders + Text Message Education*(1)* "Patients who received text messages (TM) for medication reminders and health education." TM Education Alone*(2)* "Patients who received TM for health education." *No TM (3)* "Patients who did not receive TM."
Outcomes	"First, data from the Medication Event Monitoring System (MEMS) provided four different indicators of adherence including: (1) total number of doses taken, (2) percentage of prescribed doses taken, (3) percentage of days correct number of doses were taken, and (4) percentage of doses taken on schedule. Second, the response rate to the TM medication reminders by the TM Reminders + TM Education group was to correspond to adherence. Third, medication adherence was assessed using the MMAS-8, a self-report measure completed at baseline and at follow-up. The MMAS-8 is a well-validated tool and correlates with other adherence measures such as medication refill rates and electronic monitoring devices (e.g., MEMS)." "For the secondary aim, feasibility and patient satisfaction were assessed by successful execution of the intervention, patient participation, and by the Mobile Phone Use Questionnaire. The latter questionnaire was developed for the purpose of the study and sought to obtain patients' experience with using mobile phones for medication reminders and/or education." PRIMARY OUTCOME: medication adherence SECONDARY OUTCOME: feasibility and patient satisfaction

Park 2013   *(Continued)*

Notes	**Publication details** Commercial funding/non-commercial funding/other funding : "Funding for research materials was provided by a grant from the Graduate Division of University of California, San Francisco and a scholarship from the UCSF/Hartford Center of Geriatric Nursing Excellence. CareSpeak Communications provided the use of the mobile Health manager platform, which is designed to improve medical therapy adherence using two-way text messaging." **Stated aim for study** "The primary aim was to compare medication adherence among three groups: (1) patients who received text messages (TM) for medication reminders and health education (TM Reminders + TM Education), (2) patients who received TM for health education (TM Education Alone), and (3) patients who did not receive TM (No TM). The secondary aim was to explore feasibility and patient satisfaction with mobile phone use to improve medication adherence among patients who received TM."

Risk of bias

Bias	Authors' judgement	Support for judgement
Random sequence generation (selection bias)	Low risk	"Group assignment was generated by random allocation sequence using blocks of six that was prepared by a biostatistician. The PI assigned patients to their groups by distributing envelopes in consecutive, numbered order."
Allocation concealment (selection bias)	Low risk	"Eligible patients opened sealed opaque envelopes that contained the assignment to one of three groups (TM Reminders + TM Education, TM Education Alone, or No TM)"
Blinding (performance bias and detection bias) All outcomes	Unclear risk	Unblinded "open-label study"
Incomplete outcome data (attrition bias) All outcomes	Low risk	"Ninety patients were recruited to participate and completed baseline questionnaires; however, six patients withdrew or were lost to follow-up"
Selective reporting (reporting bias)	Low risk	All outcomes reported

Interventions to improve adherence to lipid-lowering medication (Review)   67

Patel 2015

Methods	Parallel randomised controlled clinical trial Randomisation ratio: 1:1 Equivalence design: 2-sided confidence interval Open-label
Participants	N recruited = 731 N randomised = 623 (312 control, 311 intervention) N reported outcomes = 623 Median age: 63.4 years (intervention), 63.7 years (control) INCLUSION CRITERIA "Men and women aged 18 years at high CVD risk, defined as either established CVD (history of coronary, ischaemic cerebrovascular, or peripheral vascular disease) or an estimated five-year CVD risk of 15% (using the Framingham risk equation, including a 5% increment for Aboriginal or Torres Strait Islander identification) were eligible. Each participant had to have, in their doctor's view, indications for all and no contraindications to any component of at least one of two polypills - version 1 (containing aspirin 75 mg, simvastatin 40 mg, lisinopril 10 mg, atenolol 50mg) or version 2 (containing aspirin 75 mg, simvastatin 40 mg, lisinopril 10 mg, hydrochlorothiazide 12.5 mg)." EXCLUSION CRITERIA "Participants were excluded if it was felt clinically inappropriate to alter medications." COUNTRY/SETTING: Australia STUDY PERIOD: January 2010 - May 2012
Interventions	Number of study centres: 33 Australian centers (12 Aboriginal Medical Services) "Participants attended the primary healthcare centres for trial assessments at randomization and 12 month intervals thereafter. All participants were also reviewed one month post-randomization and at intervening six month intervals, but these could be conducted by telephone. BP and fasting lipids levels were obtained at baseline, 12 months, 24 months and the final visit (at 36 months)." INTERVENTION GROUP - "polypill-based strategy received a polypill containing aspirin 75 mg, simvastatin 40 mg, lisinopril 10 mg and either atenolol 50 mg or hydrochlorothiazide 12.5 mg" CONTROL GROUP - 'usual care' continued with separate medications and doses as prescribed by their doctor
Outcomes	PRIMARY OUTCOMES: self-reported combination treatment use, systolic blood pressure and total cholesterol SECONDARY OUTCOMES: "Secondary outcomes included self-reported combination treatment use at 12 months; combination treatment prescriptions at the study end; reasons for stopping cardiovascular medications; changes in lipid fractions; quality of life; serious adverse events; cardiovascular events (coronary heart disease, heart failure leading to death or hospitalization, cerebrovascular or peripheral arterial disease events); and renal events (new onset microalbuminuria (albumin:creatinine ratio 3.0-33.9mg/mmol), progression to macroalbuminuria (albumin:creatinine ratio >33.9mg/mmol) or at least a 50% decrease in estimated glomerular filtration rate from baseline to a level <60 ml/min per 1.73m2)."

Patel 2015   *(Continued)*

Notes	Commercial funding/non-commercial funding/other funding: "This work was supported by the National Health and Medical Research Council of Australia (grant numbers 457508, 571281 and 632810). The funder and Dr Reddy's Laboratories (who provided polypills free of charge for the trial) had no role in the study design, data collection and analysis, decision to publish, or preparation of the manuscript." Stated aim for study: "Most individuals at high cardiovascular disease (CVD) risk worldwide do not receive any or optimal preventive drugs. We aimed to determine whether fixed dose combinations of generic drugs ('polypills') would promote use of such medications."

Risk of bias

Bias	Authors' judgement	Support for judgement
Random sequence generation (selection bias)	Low risk	"Central, computer-based randomization to polypill based strategy or usual care"
Allocation concealment (selection bias)	Low risk	See above
Blinding (performance bias and detection bias) All outcomes	Unclear risk	Unblinded
Incomplete outcome data (attrition bias) All outcomes	Low risk	"The study failed to recruit the numbers of participants originally planned as a result of limited resources and was therefore underpowered to demonstrate significant differences in BP and cholesterol."
Selective reporting (reporting bias)	Low risk	All outcomes reported

PILL 2011

Methods	Parallel randomised controlled clinical trial Randomisation ratio: 1:1:1 Equivalence design: 2-sided confidence interval Double-blinded
Participants	N recruited = 859 N randomised = 378 (189 in each arm) N reported outcomes = 373 (at 12 weeks) Mean age 61.2 years (SD 7.2) in red heart pill (RHP) group and 61.6 years (SD 7.2) in placebo group 81% men in RHP group and 80% men in placebo group INCLUSION CRITERIA "..key eligibility criteria were raised cardiovascular risk together with no indication for or contraindication to treatment with component medicines in the polypill. Individuals were included if they were adults (18 years or older) with a cardiovascular disease (CVD)

PILL 2011   *(Continued)*

risk over 5 years of at least 7.5%, determined by the Framingham risk function using data on age, gender, blood pressure, total cholesterol, HDL cholesterol, diabetes status and cigarette smoking status..."

"To be included, the participants had to have no contraindication to treatment with low-dose aspirin, angiotensin-converting enzyme (ACE) inhibitor, low-dose diuretic or statin; nor any indication or recommendation under local guidance for treatment with any of these medicines."

EXCLUSION CRITERIA

"Participants taking other antiplatelet, blood pressure lowering or cholesterol lowering medicines were also excluded, as were patients with diabetes mellitus or GFR #30 ml/min/1.73 m2."

COUNTRY/SETTING: Trial was conducted in 7 countries - Australia (n = 21), Brazil (n = 8), India (n = 109), Netherlands (n = 102), New Zealand (n = 12), United Kingdom (n = 113) and United States (n = 13)

STUDY PERIOD: 17 October 2008 to 22 December 2009

Interventions	INTERVENTION: Red Heart Pill (RHP, a polypill comprising a bilayered tablet containing aspirin 75 mg, lisinopril 10 mg, hydrochlorothiazide 12.5 mg and simvastatin 20 mg) CONTROL: identical placebo. "The use of concomitant open-label therapy was allowed at the discretion of the responsible clinician. Without the need to unblind, additional treatment with open-label therapy was permitted -75 mg aspirin; any beta-blocker, calcium channel blocker, angiotensin receptor blocker or alpha-blocker; 10-20 mg lisinopril and/or 12.5 mg hydrochlorothiazide or 2.5 mg bendrofluazide; 10-20 mg simvastatin - if any of these treatments became indicated during the trial. If there was a need for higher doses of aspirin, ACE inhibitor, diuretic or simvastatin, these were provided as open label treatment and the trial treatment was stopped. Open-label fibrate (with the exception of gemfibrozil) could also be added, without the need to unblind or stop the trial treatment, provided that appropriate monitoring for rhabdomyolysis was instituted."
Outcomes	PRIMARY OUTCOMES: • change in systolic blood pressure (SBP), • change in LDL-cholesterol • tolerability (proportion who withdrew from trial treatment for any reason) SECONDARY OUTCOMES: • treatment adherence (% of prescribed treatment according to pill counts, with participants asked to return all used blisters and unused trial treatment to study visits) • diastolic blood pressure • total cholesterol • HDL cholesterol • total cholesterol: HDL cholesterol ratio • non-HDL cholesterol • triglycerides, • frequency of switching/adding open-label treatment • estimated effects on CVD risk Outcomes were assessed at 2, 6 and 12 weeks after randomisation A post-study follow-up appointment 4 weeks after the final 12-week visit

PILL 2011   *(Continued)*

Notes	"Participants were recruited from 17 October 2008 to 22 December 2009. Regulatory delays in importing trial treatment were prolonged and recruitment was 22 participants less than intended, since the study medication expiry date was reached." Commercial funding/non-commercial funding/other funding: "The trial was funded by The Wellcome Trust, the Health Research Council of New Zealand, the National Heart Foundation of New Zealand, the National Health and Medical Research Council of Australia, The Brazilian Ministry of Health (Projeto Hospitais de Excelencia) and the British Heart Foundation. The polypill and matching placebo were provided free of charge by Dr. Reddy's Laboratories, Hyderabad, India. None of these parties had any role in study design, data collection, data analysis, data interpretation, or writing of the report. The corresponding author had full access to all data in the study. The Steering Committee had final responsibility for the decision to submit for publication."

Risk of bias

Bias	Authors' judgement	Support for judgement
Random sequence generation (selection bias)	Low risk	"Study treatments were allocated using a central computer-based randomisation service at The Clinical Trials Research Unit, University of Auckland, accessible by Internet, using a minimisation algorithm including age, sex and centre."
Allocation concealment (selection bias)	Unclear risk	"Eligible participants were randomised to the Red Heart Pill..."
Blinding (performance bias and detection bias) All outcomes	Low risk	"Participants, research staff and and coordinating centre staff were all blinded to the allocation."
Incomplete outcome data (attrition bias) All outcomes	Low risk	Outcomes reported for 373 of 378 participants (98.7%)
Selective reporting (reporting bias)	Low risk	All outcomes reported

Pladevall 2014

Methods	Parallel randomised controlled clinical trial Randomisation ratio: 1:1:1 Equivalence design: 2-sided confidence interval Open-label
Participants	N recruited = 3799 N randomised = 1692 (567 usual care, 569 adherence information, 556 adherence information and motivational interviewing) N reported outcomes = 1692 Mean age 64.9 years (± 11.5) in UC group, 63.3 yrs (± 10.9) in AI group, 64.5 years (±

Pladevall 2014   *(Continued)*

	10.5) in AI+MI group 53% women in UC, 47% in AI and 48% in AI+MI group INCLUSION CRITERIA "age ≥ 18 years, a member of the health plan with prescription drug coverage in both 2007 and 2008, ≥ 1 A1C measurement with the last value ≥ 7%, ≥ 1 LDL-C measurement with the last value ≥ 100 mg/dL, and ≥ 1 prescription for both an oral diabetes medication and a lipid-lowering medication." EXCLUSION CRITERIA "Patients were not eligible to participate if they had been in hospice care or hospitalized ≥ 90 days, if they were participating in any other study involving diabetes management or medication adherence, or if their primary care provider did not consent to be part of the study." COUNTRY/SETTING: Michigan, USA STUDY PERIOD: Patients recruited between July 1, 2007, and January 1, 2008	
Interventions	Number of study centres: Henry Ford health system in southeast Michigan and metropolitan Detroit Arm 3 - 6 adherence sessions: initial face-to-face or phone and subsequent 5 sessions via phone every 3 months CONTROL GROUP - 'usual care' Medication adherence information (AI) provided to their physician to discuss with participants Medication AI and receive motivational interviewing (MI) provided directly to patients via an "adherence clinic" of nurses and pharmacists (AI + MI)	
Outcomes	PRIMARY OUTCOMES: A1C and LDL-C levels at 18 months post-randomisation SECONDARY OUTCOMES: medication adherence using total days' supply of medication in 3 month period divided by number of days of observation from pharmacy claims	
Notes	Commercial funding/non-commercial funding/other funding: "This project was made possible through funding from the National Institute of Diabetes and Digestive and Kidney (R01DK064695 to Drs Pladevall and Williams), the National Institute of Allergy and Infectious Diseases (R01AI079139 to Dr Williams), and the National Heart Lung and Blood Institute (R01HL079055 and R01HL118267 to Dr Williams), National Institutes of Health and the Fund for Henry Ford Hospital (to Drs Pladevall and Williams) ." Stated aim for study: "The purpose of this study was to assess whether providing medication adherence information with or without motivational interviewing improves diabetes and lipid control." Conflicts: None reported Language: English	

Risk of bias

Bias	Authors' judgement	Support for judgement

Pladevall 2014   *(Continued)*

Random sequence generation (selection bias)	Low risk	"2-step randomization process was used. A random number generator was first used to randomly sort each participating physician's list of enrolled patients. The order of treatment arm assignment was then randomly selected for each physician's patient list of participating patients."
Allocation concealment (selection bias)	Low risk	See above
Blinding (performance bias and detection bias) All outcomes	Unclear risk	Unblinded - "Because the study design involved interaction between the research team, adherence clinic staff, and patients, none of these groups were blinded to study arm assignment."
Incomplete outcome data (attrition bias) All outcomes	Unclear risk	"Patient participation in the AI + MI arm was low (49%) and limit the interpretation of the study results. For individuals who were lost to follow-up (57 patients UC, 69 patients AI, 54 patients AI + MI), the last available values were carried forward."
Selective reporting (reporting bias)	Low risk	All outcomes reported

Poston 1998

Methods	Parallel cluster-randomised controlled clinical trial (54 pharmacies (26 intervention group/28 control groups)) Randomisation ratio: 1:1
Participants	N recruited = 455 N randomised = 455 (224 control, 231 intervention) N reported outcomes = 455 Mean age 60.8 (SD 11) years, 43.8% women INCLUSION CRITERIA "Each pharmacist was asked to invite patients presenting new or refill Mevacor, Zocor, Prinvil, or Vasotec to participate in this study." EXCLUSION CRITERIA "Patients were excluded from this study if literacy was an issue, if they were visitors or indicated that they would be out of the region for several months during the study or if their medication was formally monitored on a daily basis." COUNTRY/SETTING: Ontario, Canada STUDY PERIOD: Not reported
Interventions	Number of study centres: 2 CONTROL GROUP Medication refill records were obtained and both groups received follow-up telephone

Poston 1998   *(Continued)*

	calls from pharmacy at 2, 5 and 8 months regarding medication behaviour and general demographics INTERVENTION GROUP "Pharmacists in London (test site) also provided each patient with a VI Program Kit, which included a videotape, information booklet, and newsletter. Later patients would receive two additional newsletters." Titration period: "Recruitment was initiated July 1996 and completed February 1997. Interviews were completed November 1997."
Outcomes	Results were only presented in subgroup analysis: adherence
Notes	Aim: This study examined the "effectiveness of the Vital Interests Program on patient adherence to prescribed medications for hypertension, congestive heart failure, and raised cholesterol." Funding: Merck Frosst Canada Incorporation Conflicts: None reported Language: English

Risk of bias

Bias	Authors' judgement	Support for judgement
Random sequence generation (selection bias)	Unclear risk	Cluster-0randomisation
Allocation concealment (selection bias)	Unclear risk	Not reported
Blinding (performance bias and detection bias) All outcomes	Unclear risk	Unblinded open-label study
Incomplete outcome data (attrition bias) All outcomes	Low risk	"Only 28 patients (2.8%) completely withdrew from this study, 38 could not be contacted, and 9 patients died"
Selective reporting (reporting bias)	Low risk	All outcomes reported

Powell 1995

Methods	Parallel randomised controlled clinical trial Randomisation ratio: 1:1 Equivalence Design: (2-sided confidence interval)
Participants	N recruited = 568 N randomised = 568 (297 control, 271 intervention) N reported outcomes = 568 Mean age 55 years (range 20 - 97) in control group and 54 years (range 20 - 94) in the intervention group

Powell 1995   *(Continued)*

	68% women in control group and 65% in intervention group INCLUSION CRITERIA "The subjects were drawn from a large (500,000) midwestern member Health Maintenance Organization; a member is a person receiving medical and prescription drug coverage through the plan." EXCLUSION CRITERIA Not reported COUNTRY/SETTING: USA STUDY PERIOD: Recruitment 1 July 1993 to 2 January 1994
Interventions	Number of study centres: 1 CONTROL GROUP Treatment before study: Standard care i.e. "Members with a pharmacy claim for benazepril, metoprolol, simvastatin, or transdermal estrogen" INTERVENTION GROUP "Subjects in the study group were mailed one of four videotape programs presenting information on the drugs prescribed and the inferred disease state. Refill data were collected over nine months." Titration period: "Enrollment occurred over a six-month period"
Outcomes	Time of outcome measurements: "total number of days' supply of a medication obtained by a member during the study divided by the number of days between the time the subject was enrolled and April 1, 1994 or the date the member was terminated from the plan, whichever came first" PRIMARY OUTCOME: Medication-Possession Ratio (> 80% equals compliance)
Notes	Aim: "The objective of this study was to assess the value of mailed educational videotapes as a means of enhancing medication compliance" Funding: Ciba-Geigy Corporation and Merck & Company Conflicts: None reported Language: English

Risk of bias

Bias	Authors' judgement	Support for judgement
Random sequence generation (selection bias)	Unclear risk	"Members ... randomly assigned to a study group or a control group"
Allocation concealment (selection bias)	Unclear risk	Not reported
Blinding (performance bias and detection bias) All outcomes	Low risk	"The study group was told that the videotapes were part of a patient education program but not that medication compliance was being assessed"
Incomplete outcome data (attrition bias) All outcomes	Low risk	Of 205 surveys mailed, 97 (47%) were returned

Powell 1995   *(Continued)*

Selective reporting (reporting bias)	Low risk	All outcomes reported

Schectman 1994

Methods	Parallel randomised controlled clinical trial
	Randomisation ratio: 1:1
	Equivalence design: (2-sided confidence interval)
Participants	N recruited = 164
	N randomised = 164 (81 control, 83 intervention)
	N reported outcomes = 162
	Mean age 61 years (SD 2) in telephone group and 59 (SD 2) in control group for the BAS subgroup;
	no sex distribution reported
	INCLUSION CRITERIA
	"Patients with hyperlipidemia requiring treatment with either niacin or BAS (bile acid sequestrants) were eligible to participate in the study if they had not been previously treated with, or were not currently taking, these agents. Access to a telephone was also a requirement for study entry. Patients taking other medications, including other lipid-lowering agents, were eligible for participation."
	EXCLUSION CRITERIA
	No additional exclusion criteria stated.
	COUNTRY/SETTING: USA
	STUDY PERIOD: September 1990 to September 1991
Interventions	Number of study centres: 1 active lipid clinic
	INTERVENTION GROUP
	"Patients randomized to the telephone contact group received five telephone calls within one month after drug therapy was started."
	CONTROL GROUP
	"The control group received no telephone calls."
Outcomes	"The drug discontinuance rate was defined as the percentage of patients unable to continue therapy because of noxious adverse effects. Tolerance was calculated as one minus the drug discontinuance rate, and was defined as the ability of the patient to continue the medication, regardless of whether any adverse effects were experienced."
	"Patient compliance was estimated by two different methods. First, patients were routinely asked at the clinical interview: "Patients often find it hard to take all of their medication without missing any doses. During the past week, how many doses of your medication have you missed?" The answer was recorded and then entered into the database. The second method employed a computerized check on the pharmacy prescription record. Because patients received all their medications on a monthly basis from the VAMC pharmacy, adherence was estimated by dividing the number of prescription refills by the duration of drug therapy."
	PRIMARY OUTCOMES: drug discontinuation, adherence, final dosage

Schectman 1994   *(Continued)*

Notes	**Publication details**
	Commercial funding/non-commercial funding/other funding : "This work was supported through HSR&D Grant 77-33-05P from the Veterans Administration, and through a grant from the Squibb-Bristol Company."
	Stated aim for study
	"We conducted a prospective, randomized, controlled study to determine whether telephone contact by an allied healthcare professional could improve patient acceptability and adherence to drug therapy with nicotinic acid and BAS."

Risk of bias

Bias	Authors' judgement	Support for judgement
Random sequence generation (selection bias)	Unclear risk	"Patients were randomized into two groups by the study coordinator: the telephone contact group and the control group"
Allocation concealment (selection bias)	Unclear risk	Not reported
Blinding (performance bias and detection bias) All outcomes	Low risk	"Lipid clinic staff were not made aware of the group assignment, and were instructed not to ask patients on subsequent visits whether they had been telephoned. Similarly, patients were instructed not to report that they had received telephone contact unless specific interventions were performed necessitating awareness of the staff."
Incomplete outcome data (attrition bias) All outcomes	Low risk	"Two subjects prescribed BAS and randomized to telephone contact moved shortly after randomization and did not attend subsequent clinic visits. These subjects were withdrawn from the study and are not included in the data analysis. Completing the study were 102 patients prescribed niacin and 60 patients prescribed BAS."
Selective reporting (reporting bias)	Low risk	All outcomes reported

Selak 2014

Methods	Parallel randomised controlled clinical trial Randomisation ratio: 1:1 Equivalence design: (2-sided confidence interval) Open-label
Participants	N recruited = 513 N randomised = 513 (257 control, 256 intervention) N reported outcomes = 513 Mean age 62 years (SD 8) in both groups, 39% women in FDC group and 34% in control group INCLUSION CRITERIA "Adults aged 18-79 years at high risk of cardiovascular disease (based on either established disease (coronary, cerebrovascular, or peripheral vascular) or $\geq 15\%$ five year risk of a cardiovascular event) were eligible for the trial." "Other inclusion criteria were that the patient's general practitioner considered all the drugs in at least one of the two versions of the fixed dose combination treatment available were recommended, and was uncertain if treatment was best provided as fixed dose combination based treatment or as usual care." "We included patients who had started statins at least one year prior to inclusion and were non-adherent in the year prior to inclusion (refill rate between 50 and 80%)." EXCLUSION CRITERIA "Exclusion criteria were contraindications to any of the components of the fixed dose combination, congestive heart failure, haemorrhagic stroke, active stomach or duodenal ulcer, receipt of an oral anticoagulant, concerns by the general practitioner about the risk to a patient of changing his or her cardiovascular disease drugs, impending alteration of a drug regimen for an important length of time (for example, planned coronary bypass graft operation), or the participant was unlikely to complete the trial or the trial procedures (for example, terminal illness)." COUNTRY/SETTING: New Zealand STUDY PERIOD: Randomisation between July 2010 and July 2012, follow-up concluded in August 2013
Interventions	Number of study centres: 54 general practices in the Auckland and Waikato regions of New Zealand CONTROL GROUP "After randomisation, the participant's cardiovascular drugs were reviewed by their usual general practitioner (who was encouraged to manage the participants irrespective of treatment allocation in accordance with New Zealand cardiovascular disease risk assessment and management guidelines). Changes or additions to a cardiovascular drug regimen were at the discretion of the general practitioner, who remained the principal ongoing healthcare provider, including overseeing the use of fixed dose combination treatment where appropriate." INTERVENTION GROUP "General practitioners had the choice of two fixed dose combinations. Both contained aspirin 75 mg, simvastatin 40 mg, and lisinopril 10 mg, with atenolol 50 mg additionally added to one combination and hydrochlorothiazide 12.5 mg to the other. General practitioners could select the combination to use, change combinations, or discontinue treatment at any stage during the trial. There were no limitations on the use of any concomitant (including cardiovascular) drugs the general practitioners considered ap-

Selak 2014   *(Continued)*

	propriate. Fixed dose combination treatment was prescribed according to the general practitioner's usual method."
Outcomes	PRIMARY OUTCOME: Adherence SECONDARY OUTCOME: mean change in LDL
Notes	**Publication details** Commercial funding/non-commercial funding/other funding: "The trial was funded by project grants from: New Zealand Health Research Council (06/582, 12/889), National Heart Foundation of New Zealand (1376), New Zealand Lotteries Grants Board (230904-310308), the Elsie Shrimpton Fund (University of Auckland), PHARMAC (New Zealand's Pharmaceutical Management Agency; A499735-QA24208), Te Kupenga Hauora Māori (University of Auckland), Auckland regional district health boards (Auckland, Counties Manukau, and Waitemata; 12/889), the Faculty Research Development Fund (University of Auckland), and the Auckland Medical Research Foundation." **Stated aim for study** "The IMPACT (IMProving Adherence using Combination Therapy) trial was designed to evaluate whether fixed dose risk factors in people with established cardiovascular disease or at similarly high risk treated in primary care, where the majority of care for patients with vascular disease occurs."

Risk of bias

Bias	Authors' judgement	Support for judgement
Random sequence generation (selection bias)	Low risk	A central randomisation service randomly assigned (1:1) participants to fixed dose combination based treatment or usual care. A minimisation algorithm included the stratification factors: primary health organisation (these provide business management and quality of care services to groups of general practices), history of cardiovascular disease (yes or no), self-reported adherence to recommended drugs (antiplatelet, statin, and ≥ 2 blood pressure-lowering drugs; yes or no), and ethnicity (indigenous Māori or non-Māori)
Allocation concealment (selection bias)	Low risk	See above
Blinding (performance bias and detection bias) All outcomes	Unclear risk	Unblinded open-label study
Incomplete outcome data (attrition bias) All outcomes	Low risk	"Between July 2010 and July 2012, we screened and randomised 513 (from 91 general practitioners) of 814 potentially el-

Selak 2014   *(Continued)*

igible patients invited by their doctors to participate in the trial and who had provided written informed consent. The median duration of follow-up was 23 months in both arms. Follow-up concluded in August 2013, 12 months after the last participant was randomised, as planned. Primary outcome data were available for 95-97% of participants."

Selective reporting (reporting bias)	Low risk	All outcomes reported

---

Sweeney 1991

Methods	Parallel randomised controlled clinical trial Randomisation ratio: ~1:1 Equivalence design: (2-sided confidence interval) Open-label
Participants	N recruited = 98 N randomised = 98 (39 control, 49 intervention) N reported outcomes = 83 Mean age 55.3 years (SD 1.9) in the Bar group and 55.5 years (SD 1.8) in the Powder group 49% men in the Bar group and 44% in the Powder group INCLUSION CRITERIA "Male and female subjects, 23 to 78 years of age, with hypercholesterolemia greater than the 90th percentile for LDL or total cholesterol were recruited." EXCLUSION CRITERIA "Subjects who had significant hypertriglyceridemia (more than 200 mg/dL), major gastrointestinal disorders, intolerance to bile acid-binding resins, or metabolic disorders were excluded." COUNTRY/SETTING: two sites: Emory Health Enhancement Program, Emory University in Atlanta, Georgia, and YMCA Cardiac Rehabilitation Center in Palo Alto, California, USA STUDY PERIOD: Not reported
Interventions	Number of study centres: 2 Treatment before study "After baseline medical history, physical examination, and comprehensive laboratory studies were obtained, all subjects were enrolled in a diet-only intervention phase utilizing the American Heart Association Step I diet for at least 6 weeks prior to randomization to medication. The diet composition was as follows: 15% protein, 55% carbohydrate, 30% fat, and 300 mg or less of dietary cholesterol per day. Subjects were instructed in the diet by experienced dietitians at the beginning of this period, and blood lipid levels were measured every 2 weeks. Serum cholesterol levels were maintained to within 10% of previous values for at least two visits prior to randomization." INTERVENTION AND CONTROL GROUPS

Sweeney 1991   *(Continued)*

"Subjects who qualified were randomly assigned to receive cholestyramine powder (two 4-g packets, twice daily) or confectionery bars (two 4-g bars, twice daily). Medication was taken in the morning and evening within ½ hour of a meal. Subjects had their choice of a mint- or maple-flavored bar, but were not permitted to switch flavors once the trial had begun. This comparative phase lasted for 8 weeks."

Outcomes	"Compliance to treatment was determined at each 2-week visit by counting the number of packets or bars not consumed and subtracting this from the amount of medication that had been dispensed. This number was divided by the amount that should have been consumed and multiplied by 100, yielding percent compliances." PRIMARY OUTCOMES: lipid changes, compliance SECONDARY OUTCOMES: changes in haemodynamic data and body weight
Notes	**Publication details** "This work was supported by a research grant from Bristol-Myers U.S. Pharmaceutical Group." **Stated aim for study** "The purpose of the study was to compare the powder and the bar forms of cholestyramine to determine efficacy and patient compliance."

Risk of bias

Bias	Authors' judgement	Support for judgement
Random sequence generation (selection bias)	Unclear risk	"Subjects who qualified were randomly assigned to receive cholestyramine powder (two 4-g packets, twice daily) or confectionery bars (two 4-g bars, twice daily)"
Allocation concealment (selection bias)	Unclear risk	Not reported
Blinding (performance bias and detection bias) All outcomes	Unclear risk	Unblinded open-label study
Incomplete outcome data (attrition bias) All outcomes	Low risk	"Overall, five of 39 subjects taking powder and six of 49 subjects taking bar prematurely discontinued the study. Of the five powder subjects, two were noncompliant, one had an intercurrent illness after 64 days, one had an allergic reaction after 14 days, and one experienced a syncopal episode of undetermined etiology after 14 days of therapy. Two of the six bar subjects were noncompliant, two experienced "heartburn" after approximately 14 days, one had epigastric pain after 13 days, and one disliked the bar and discontinued ther-

Sweeney 1991   *(Continued)*

		apy after 5 days. Eighty-three patients completed the study."
Selective reporting (reporting bias)	Low risk	All outcomes reported

Tamblyn 2009

Methods	Parallel cluster-randomised controlled trial Block design with randomly-selected block sizes of 6, 8, and 12 Equivalence design: (2-sided confidence interval)
Participants	N recruited = 2293 N randomised = 2293 (1127 control, 1166 intervention) N reported outcomes = 2293 Mean age 73.2 yrs (SD 8.6) in control group, 73.0 yrs (SD 8.6) in intervention group and 73.1 yrs (SD 8.6) combined 61.5% women INCLUSION CRITERIA "59 physicians and 15,486 patients in the MOXXI primary care research program (National EHR). 6372 patients had public drug insurance, and 2293 (36.0%) of these patients had active lipid-lowering or antihypertensive drugs at the index visit." "Patients were eligible for the study if they and their physicians had consented to participate in the MOXXI research program, they were insured with the provincial drug insurance program, and they had at least 1 active lipid-lowering or antihypertensive drug prescribed by the study physician in the 3 months prior to the index visit." EXCLUSION CRITERIA No specific exclusion criteria listed COUNTRY/SETTING: Quebec, Canada STUDY PERIOD: study started in April 2006
Interventions	INTERVENTION GROUP "In the intervention group, the primary care physician was provided with the drug profile: the patient's list of current prescribed and dispensed drugs, total costs of medications dispensed each month, the amount of out-of-pocket expenditures paid by the patient (deductibles and copayments), graphic representation of unfilled prescriptions, and days of drug supply for each medication, based on the start and end dates of dispensed medications. At each visit, patient adherence to lipid-lowering and antihypertensive drugs was calculated based on drugs dispensed in the past 3 months. If treatment adherence was less than 80%, the physician received an alert to check for potential adherence problems." CONTROL GROUP "In the control group, the primary care physician had access only to the current list of prescribed and dispensed drugs and did not receive alerts when patient adherence was less than 80%."
Outcomes	"Each patient was followed for 6 months after the index visit to assess the primary (drug profile review, change in therapy) and secondary study outcomes (medication adherence)"

Tamblyn 2009   *(Continued)*

Notes	Aim: "To determine if a cardiovascular medication tracking and nonadherence alert system, incorporated into a computerized health record system, would increase drug profile review by primary care physicians, increase the likelihood of therapy change, and improve adherence with antihypertensive and lipid-lowering drugs." Funding: N/A Conflicts: None reported Language: English

Risk of bias

Bias	Authors' judgement	Support for judgement
Random sequence generation (selection bias)	Low risk	"Patients within a primary care physician's practice were randomized to the intervention or control group." "The central database server conducted real-time assessment of patent eligibility at the first visit after the start of the study in April 2006, and eligible patients were randomized to intervention or control groups using a randomized block design with randomly selected block sizes of 6, 8, and 12."
Allocation concealment (selection bias)	Low risk	See above
Blinding (performance bias and detection bias) All outcomes	High risk	Single-blinded study design; "Physicians and patients were blind to the outcome assessed but not intervention status ... In particular, we suspect that physicians were more vigilant"
Incomplete outcome data (attrition bias) All outcomes	Unclear risk	Not reported
Selective reporting (reporting bias)	Low risk	All outcomes reported

Thom 2013

Methods	Parallel randomised controlled clinical trial Randomisation ratio: 1:1 Equivalence design: (2-sided confidence interval) Open-label
Participants	N = 2138 screened N = 2004 randomised (1002 control, 1002 intervention) N = 1921 reported outcomes for adherence Mean Age 62.1 yrs (SD 10.4) in the FDC group and 61.6 yrs (SD 10.8) in the control group

Thom 2013   *(Continued)*

	81.5% men in the FDC group and 82.3% in the control group INCLUSION CRITERIA "[Patients] aged 18 years or older with high cardiovascular risk, defined as either established CVD (history of coronary heart disease, ischemic cerebrovascular disease, or peripheral vascular disease) or an estimated 5-year CVD risk of 15%or greater; the risk score included age, sex, SBP, ratio of total to high-density lipoprotein cholesterol (HDL-C), diabetes, smoking, and a 5% adjustment for people from the Indian subcontinent" EXCLUSION CRITERIA N = 134 excluded (62 - cardiovascular risk too low, 38 - medication switch contraidicated, 18 - clinically unstable , 11 - patient changed plans, 5 - other) COUNTRY/SETTING: India; London, England; Dublin, Ireland; and Utrecht, the Netherlands STUDY PERIOD: Randomization between July 2010 and July 2011
Interventions	Random assignment to a FDC strategy (n = 1002) containing either (1) 75 mg aspirin, 40 mg simvastatin, 10 mg lisinopril, and 50 mg atenolol or (2) 75 mg aspirin, 40 mg simvastatin, 10 mg lisinopril, and 12.5 mg hydrochlorothiazide or to usual care (n = 1002) "Participants attended clinic visits for randomization, at 12 months, and at the end of the study. Telephone or clinic visits were conducted at 1 month, 6 months, and 18months. Self-reported adherence to all medications was recorded as the number of days medication was taken in the week prior to the visit (value between 0-7 days). During trial contacts, the research team asked about barriers to adherence, quality of life (measured using the self-administered EQ-5D questionnaire19), cardiovascular and other serious adverse events, and reasons for stopping cardiovascular medications."
Outcomes	PRIMARY OUTCOMES: "Primary outcomes included adherence to indicated medications (defined as taking the medication for at least 4 days during the week preceding the visit) at baseline and at the end of the trial and changes in SBP and LDL-C from baseline to the end of the trial." SECONDARY OUTCOMES: "Secondary outcomes: 12 month adherence, reasons for stopping medications, quality of life, serious adverse events, and changes in total cholesterol, HDL-C, triglycerides, and creatinine from baseline to 12 months and end of study and cardiovascular events (including coronary heart disease, heart failure leading to death or hospital admission, and cerebrovascular or peripheral arterial disease events)"
Notes	Aim: "To assess whether FDC delivery of aspirin, statin, and 2 blood pressure-lowering agents vs usual care improves long-term adherence to indicated therapy and 2 major CVD risk factors, systolic blood pressure (SBP) and low-density lipoprotein cholesterol (LDL-C)." Funding: "The project was funded by the European Commission Seventh Framework Programme (grant 241849). Dr. Reddy's Laboratories (Hyderabad, India) provided the FDCs and supported the trial start-up meetings in London and India." Conflicts: None reported Language: English

Risk of bias

Thom 2013 *(Continued)*

Bias	Authors' judgement	Support for judgement
Random sequence generation (selection bias)	Low risk	"Randomization to FDC or usual care was conducted in a 1:1 ratio and allocation was stratified by site and by the presence or absence of established CVD using a web-based clinical data management system (In-Form; PhaseForward Inc)"
Allocation concealment (selection bias)	Low risk	See above
Blinding (performance bias and detection bias) All outcomes	Unclear risk	Unblinded open-label study
Incomplete outcome data (attrition bias) All outcomes	Low risk	"The trial had 90% power overall to detect difference. Estimates all assumed ... up to 10% of patients having died or been lost to follow-up"
Selective reporting (reporting bias)	Low risk	All outcomes reported

Vollmer 2014

Methods	Randomised controlled clinical trial (RCT) Randomisation ratio: 1:1:1 Equivalence design: (2-sided confidence interval) Open label
Participants	N recruited = 45,051 N randomised = 21,752 (7255 control, 7247 IVR, 7250 IVR+) for all, 16,380 for statins, and 13,063 for ACEi/ARB N reported outcomes: Statin adherence = 16,366 and LDL levels = 13,776 Mean age 63.6 yrs (SD 12.2), 53% men INCLUSION CRITERIA ≥ 40 years old (Mean age 63.6) "Using each region's EMR, we identified participants 40 years and older with diabetes mellitus and/or cardiovascular disease (CVD), suboptimally (<90%) adherent to a statin or ACEI/ARB during the previous 12 months, and due or overdue for a refill" EXCLUSION CRITERIA "We excluded only individuals with medical conditions that might contraindicate the use of these medications, such as medication allergies, liver failure, cirrhosis, rhabdomyolysis, end-stage renal disease, chronic kidney disease and those on KP's "do not contact" list." COUNTRY/SETTING: 3 regions of the Kaiser Permanente (KP) health plan-Northwest (KPNW), Hawaii (KPH), and Georgia (KPG), USA STUDY PERIOD: "Study enrollment began in December 2011 and continued through May 2012. Intervention and outcome assessment continued through November 2012."

Vollmer 2014   *(Continued)*

Interventions	Number of study centres: 3 regions of the Kaiser Permanente (KP) health plan-Northwest (KPNW), Hawaii (KPH), and Georgia (KPG) CONTROL GROUP "UC participants had access to the full range of usual services, including each region's normal education and care management outreach efforts to encourage statin and ACEI/ARB use." INTERVENTION GROUPS *Interactive Voice Recognition (IVR) Calls* "VR participants received automated phone calls when they were due or overdue for a refill. The calls used speech-recognition technology to educate patients about their medications and help them refill prescriptions (we created separate "refill" and "tardy" calls). The flow of each call was determined by participants' responses; each call lasted 2 to 3 minutes. At randomization, IVR participants received a pamphlet explaining these calls Both call types offered a transfer to KP's automated pharmacy refill line. The tardy call also offered a transfer to a live pharmacist. With permission, obtained at the first successful call contact, the program left detailed messages on answering machines or with another household member." *Enhanced IVR (IVR+)* "In addition to IVR calls, participants in the IVR+ arm received a personalized re-minder letter if they were 60 to 89 days overdue and a live outreach call if they were $\geq$90 days overdue, as well as EMR-based feedback to their primary care provider. IVR+ participants received additional materials, including a personalized health report with their latest BP and cholesterol levels, a pill organizer, and bimonthly mailings."
Outcomes	"We used a modified version of the Proportion of Days Covered (PDC),16 defined from pharmacy dispensing records, for our primary measure. Because we were measuring adherence to chronic medications patients were known to be taking at randomization, we modified the PDC (mPDC) to include the whole follow- up period as the denominator time frame rather than time from first dispensing.17 We accounted for medication on hand at randomization and ignored any medication remaining at the end of follow-up. We computed mPDCs separately for statins and ACEI/ARBs." PRIMARY OUTCOMES: medication adherence SECONDARY OUTCOMES: lipid Levels, blood pressure
Notes	Commercial funding/non-commercial funding/other funding : "This project was sup-ported by grant number R01HS019341 from the Agency for Healthcare Research and Quality." Stated aim for study: "Evaluate the utility of 2 electronic medical record (EMR)-linked, automated phone reminder interventions for improving adherence to cardiovascular disease medications."

Risk of bias

Bias	Authors' judgement	Support for judgement
Random sequence generation (selection bias)	Low risk	"Computer-generated randomization as-signments were stratified by region and blocked to assure balance across treatment

Vollmer 2014 *(Continued)*

		arms"
Allocation concealment (selection bias)	Low risk	See above
Blinding (performance bias and detection bias) All outcomes	Unclear risk	Unblinded open-label study
Incomplete outcome data (attrition bias) All outcomes	Low risk	16,380 randomised for statins with adherence data for 16,366 at end of study
Selective reporting (reporting bias)	Low risk	All outcomes reported

Vrijens 2006

Methods	Parallel cluster-randomised controlled clinical trial Randomisation ratio: 1:1 Equivalence design: (2-sided confidence interval) Open-label
Participants	N recruited = 429 N randomised = 392 (198 control, 194 intervention) N reported outcomes = 392 Mean age 61.9 yrs (SD 9.9) in the intervention group and 60.4 yrs (SD 10.2) in the control group 55% men in the intervention group and 46% in the control group INCLUSION CRITERIA "All patients, aged 18 years or above, who had been taking atorvastatin for at least 3 months, and who had no contraindications to continuation of the treatment, could be included in the study provided they usually got their medication in one of the pharmacies participating in the study." EXCLUSION CRITERIA None reported COUNTRY/SETTING: Belgium STUDY PERIOD: Patients enrolled between 13 February 2000 and 26 June 2002
Interventions	Number of study centres: 35 pharmacies "In each linguistic region, one district was randomized to deliver care as usual (control group), while in the other district a patient intervention through a pharmaceutical care program was implemented (intervention group)." "The supportive intervention program consisted of review by the patients' pharmacist, jointly with the patient, of the electronically compiled dosing history, a 'beep-card' that reminds patient of the dosing time, and educational reminders. In the intervention group, the pharmacist delivered an educational message at each follow-up visit, updated the 'compliance passport' and analyzed, together with the patient, the electronically compiled dosing history of the past month/ 3 months."

Vrijens 2006   *(Continued)*

Outcomes	"The primary outcome parameter is 'post-baseline adherence' to prescribed therapy defined for each patient as the proportion of days during which the MEMS record showed that the patient had opened the pill container. The estimation of this variable started from the second pharmacy visit until an arbitrary cut-off point of 300 days after inclusion. 'Baseline adherence' is estimated between inclusion and the second visit to the pharmacy Adherence can vary in many different ways over time. Summarizing the history in just one measure may hide important features of adherence patterns, especially potential changes over time. We captured the temporal evolution of daily adherence to study this clinically relevant aspect of dosing history data Further we found it useful to define persistence as the length of time between onset and discontinuation of treatment execution." PRIMARY OUTCOMES: adherence, persistence
Notes	**Publication details** Commercial funding/non-commercial funding/other funding : "No conflict of interest was declared. Contract grant sponsor: Pfizer Belgium, Boulevard de la Plaine 17, BE 1050 Bruxelles-Ixelles, Belgium." **Stated aim for study** "The objective of this study was to estimate the effect of a pharmaceutical care program on the adherence of once-daily atorvastatin treatment in patients with elevated cholesterol levels."

Risk of bias

Bias	Authors' judgement	Support for judgement
Random sequence generation (selection bias)	Unclear risk	"In each linguistic region, one district was randomized to deliver care as usual (control group), while in the other district a patient intervention through a pharmaceutical care program was implemented (intervention group)" "While we realize that there might be bias in the selection of the participating patients resulting three of the nine baseline variables being statistically significantly different between the two groups, the intervention effect remained significant in a multiple Cox regression analysis controlling for the baseline variables"
Allocation concealment (selection bias)	Unclear risk	See above
Blinding (performance bias and detection bias) All outcomes	Unclear risk	Unblinded "open-label study"

Vrijens 2006   *(Continued)*

Incomplete outcome data (attrition bias) All outcomes	Low risk	"Between 13 February 2000 and 26 June 2002, 429 subjects were entered into the study, of whom 37 did not visit the pharmacy: hence, a total of 392 subjects are included in the ITT set, of whom 194 attended pharmacies that employed adherence enhancing interventions and 198 subjects had no intervention"
Selective reporting (reporting bias)	Low risk	All outcomes reported

Wald 2014

Methods	Parallel randomised controlled clinical trial Randomisation ratio: 1:1 Equivalence design: 2-sided confidence interval Open-label not reported
Participants	N recruited = 303 N randomized = 303 (152 control, 151 intervention) N reported outcomes = 301 (151 control, 150 intervention) Median age 60 yrs (range 54 - 68) in the intervention group and 61 yrs (49 - 69) in the control group 55% men in the intervention and 54% in the control group INCLUSION CRITERIA "patients who owned a mobile telephone with text message capability and who had been prescribed blood pressure and/or lipid-lowering medication" EXCLUSION CRITERIA None reported COUNTRY/SETTING: 7 primary care practices in London, UK STUDY PERIOD: Patients enrolled between February 2012 and August 2013, participant follow-up was completed in March 2014
Interventions	Number of study centres: 7 primary care practices in London INTERVENTION GROUP "Texts were sent daily for 2 weeks, alternate days for 2 weeks and weekly thereafter for 22 weeks (6 months overall), using an automated computer program." CONTROL GROUP No text reminders sent.
Outcomes	TIME OF OUTCOME MEASUREMENTS: "At 6 months, use of medication was assessed." Cholesterol and blood pressure was also measured PRIMARY OUTCOMES: "Medication use at 6 months, exceeding 80% of the prescribed regimen. Medication use was usually determined by personal enquiry at clinic visits, or failing that, using general practice electronic prescription records. Patients were asked whether they had stopped taking their medication and if not, the number of days in the previous 28 days that medication had been missed." SECONDARY OUTCOMES: "Secondary outcomes were i) the proportion of patients

Wald 2014   *(Continued)*

	continuing their medication regardless of the number of days missed and ii) among those continuing, the proportion taking >80% of their prescribed regimen." "Blood pressure measurements were taken at 6 months in patients on blood pressure lowering medication at randomization and similarly, serum cholesterol (total and LDL) in patients on cholesterol lowering medication at randomization."
Notes	Commercial funding/non-commercial funding/other funding: none reported Stated aim for study: "to assess the value of text messaging as a means of improving medication adherence in patients receiving blood pressure and/or lipid-lowering treatment for the prevention of cardiovascular disease"

Risk of bias

Bias	Authors' judgement	Support for judgement
Random sequence generation (selection bias)	Low risk	"The randomization schedule was computer generated in blocks of 4 and allocated centrally from the coordinating center by telephone"
Allocation concealment (selection bias)	Unclear risk	Not reported
Blinding (performance bias and detection bias) All outcomes	Unclear risk	Not reported
Incomplete outcome data (attrition bias) All outcomes	Low risk	"Two patients were lost to follow-up, providing data on 301 for analysis"
Selective reporting (reporting bias)	Low risk	All outcomes reported

Willich 2009

Methods	Parallel randomised controlled clinical trial Randomisation ratio: 1:1 Equivalence design: (2-sided confidence interval) Open-label
Participants	N recruited = 8108 N randomised= 8108 (4044 control, 4064 intervention) N reported outcomes = 6872 Mean age 60.8 yrs (SD 10.41), 56.1% men INCLUSION CRITERIA Low density lipoprotein cholesterol (LDL-C) > 115 mg/dl if statin-naïve or else > 125 mg/dl Participants were also required to have at least one of the following risk factors: history of CHD, other atherosclerotic disease, 10-year CHD risk Z20%, or diabetes EXCLUSION CRITERIA

Willich 2009 *(Continued)*

	Fasting triglycerides > 400 mg/dl (4.5 mmol/l); familial or secondary hypercholestero-laemia; active liver disease, defined as elevations of aspartate aminotransferase or alanine aminotransferase (ALT) Z1.5 upper limit of normal (ULN); creatine kinase greater than 3ULN; or unstable angina COUNTRY/SETTING: Germany STUDY PERIOD: Enrolment between April 2002 and February 2004
Interventions	INTERVENTION GROUP Participants in the intervention group received 10/20 mg rosuvastatin in addition to a starter pack containing a videotape, an educational leaflet, details of the free phone patient helpline and website, and labels with a reminder to take study medication. Participants also received regular personalised letters and phone calls throughout the study CONTROL GROUP The control group received 10/m20 rosuvastatin alone
Outcomes	PRIMARY OUTCOMES: Long-term cumulative direct and indirect disease related costs associated with rosuvastatin treatment either with or without additional compliance programme at 12 and 36 months SECONDARY OUTCOMES: Number (%) of participants achieving 1998 European LDL-C and total cholesterol goals after 3, 6, and 12 months of therapy; number (%) of participants increasing their dose of rosuvastatin at month 3; percentage change from baseline in lipids and lipoproteins; compliance with drug therapy (assessed by counting the number of pills returned by the patient at 6 and 12 months); and safety
Notes	Aim: "To determine whether a compliance-enhancing program could increase the level of lipid control patients treated with rosuvastatin" Funding: "This study was supported by a grant from AstraZeneca." Conflicts: None reported Language: English

Risk of bias

Bias	Authors' judgement	Support for judgement
Random sequence generation (selection bias)	Low risk	"For the 12-month intervention phase, consecutive patients were randomized 1 : 1, using a computer-generated randomization list, to receive rosuvastatin 10 mg daily (manufacturer AstraZeneca GmbH, D-22876 Wedel, Germany) either with or without a compliance program"
Allocation concealment (selection bias)	Low risk	See above
Blinding (performance bias and detection bias) All outcomes	Unclear risk	Unblinded open-label study

Willich 2009   *(Continued)*

Incomplete outcome data (attrition bias) All outcomes	Low risk	"Assuming a 20% dropout rate, at least 6608 patients were required to be recruited for 90% power"
Selective reporting (reporting bias)	Low risk	All outcomes reported

BAS bile acid sequestrants
BMI body mass index
BP blood pressure
CHD coronary heart disease
COI conflict of interest
FDC fixed-dose combination
FMD flow mediated dilatation
GEE generalised estimated equations
HDL-C high density lipoprotein cholesterol
IMT intima media thickness
ITT intention to treat
LDL-C low density lipoprotein cholesterol
MEMS Medication Event Monitoring System
MI myocardial infarction
RCT randomised controlled trial
SD standard deviation
SE standard error
TC total cholesterol
TRG triglycerides

DATA AND ANALYSES

Comparison 1. Intensified patient care vs usual care

Outcome or subgroup title	No. of studies	No. of participants	Statistical method	Effect size
1 Medication adherence at ≤ 6 months	7	11204	Odds Ratio (M-H, Random, 95% CI)	1.93 [1.29, 2.88]
2 Medication adherence at > 6 months	3	663	Odds Ratio (M-H, Random, 95% CI)	2.87 [1.91, 4.29]
3 Reduction in total serum cholesterol at ≤ 6 mos (mg/dL)	4	430	Mean Difference (IV, Random, 95% CI)	17.15 [1.17, 33.14]
4 Reduction in total serum cholesterol at > 6 mos (mg/dL)	2	127	Mean Difference (IV, Random, 95% CI)	17.57 [14.95, 20.19]
5 Reduction in LDL-C at ≤ 6 months (mg/dL)	3	333	Mean Difference (IV, Random, 95% CI)	19.51 [8.51, 30.51]
6 Reduction in LDL-C > 6 months (mg/dL)	1		Mean Difference (IV, Random, 95% CI)	Totals not selected
7 Attrition rate sensitivity analysis (medication adherence at ≤ 6 months)	6	6656	Odds Ratio (M-H, Random, 95% CI)	2.22 [1.41, 3.49]

Analysis 1.1.   Comparison 1 Intensified patient care vs usual care, Outcome 1 Medication adherence at ≤ 6 months.

Review: Interventions to improve adherence to lipid-lowering medication

Comparison: 1 Intensified patient care vs usual care

Outcome: 1 Medication adherence at ≤ 6 months

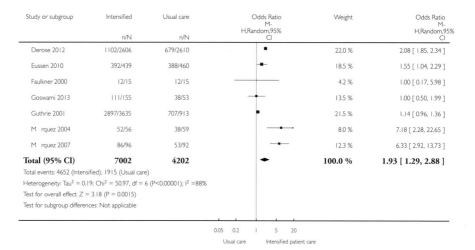

Study or subgroup	Intensified	Usual care	Odds Ratio M-H,Random,95% CI	Weight	Odds Ratio M-H,Random,95% CI
	n/N	n/N			
Derose 2012	1102/2606	679/2610		22.0 %	2.08 [1.85, 2.34]
Eussen 2010	392/439	388/460		18.5 %	1.55 [1.04, 2.29]
Faulkner 2000	12/15	12/15		4.2 %	1.00 [0.17, 5.98]
Goswami 2013	111/155	38/53		13.5 %	1.00 [0.50, 1.99]
Guthrie 2001	2897/3635	707/913		21.5 %	1.14 [0.96, 1.36]
M rquez 2004	52/56	38/59		8.0 %	7.18 [2.28, 22.65]
M rquez 2007	86/96	53/92		12.3 %	6.33 [2.92, 13.73]
Total (95% CI)	**7002**	**4202**		**100.0 %**	**1.93 [1.29, 2.88]**

Total events: 4652 (Intensified), 1915 (Usual care)

Heterogeneity: Tau^2 = 0.19; Chi^2 = 50.97, df = 6 (P<0.00001); I^2 =88%

Test for overall effect: Z = 3.18 (P = 0.0015)

Test for subgroup differences: Not applicable

```
         0.05   0.2    1    5    20
         Usual care    Intensified patient care
```

Analysis 1.2.   Comparison 1 Intensified patient care vs usual care, Outcome 2 Medication adherence at > 6 months.

Review: Interventions to improve adherence to lipid-lowering medication

Comparison: 1 Intensified patient care vs usual care

Outcome: 2 Medication adherence at > 6 months

Study or subgroup	Intensified n/N	Usual care n/N	Odds Ratio M-H,Random,95% CI	Weight	Odds Ratio M-H,Random,95% CI
Faulkner 2000	10/15	5/15		7.1 %	4.00 [0.88, 18.26]
Ho 2014	109/122	82/119		34.0 %	3.78 [1.89, 7.57]
Vrijens 2006	169/194	147/198		58.9 %	2.35 [1.38, 3.97]
Total (95% CI)	**331**	**332**		**100.0 %**	**2.87 [1.91, 4.29]**

Total events: 288 (Intensified), 234 (Usual care)

Heterogeneity: Tau^2 = 0.0; Chi^2 = 1.36, df = 2 (P = 0.51); I^2 =0.0%

Test for overall effect: Z = 5.10 (P < 0.00001)

Test for subgroup differences: Not applicable

```
        0.01    0.1     1     10    100
            Usual care    Intensified patient care
```

Analysis 1.3.   Comparison 1 Intensified patient care vs usual care, Outcome 3 Reduction in total serum cholesterol at ≤ 6 mos (mg/dL).

Review: Interventions to improve adherence to lipid-lowering medication

Comparison: 1 Intensified patient care vs usual care

Outcome: 3 Reduction in total serum cholesterol at ≤ 6 mos (mg/dL)

Study or subgroup	Intensified N	Mean(SD)	Usual care N	Mean(SD)	Mean Difference IV,Random,95% CI	Weight	Mean Difference IV,Random,95% CI
Aslani 2010	48	5.8 (6.5)	49	3.1 (6.8)		29.2 %	2.70 [0.05, 5.35]
Faulkner 2000	15	80 (21)	15	67 (29)		21.3 %	13.00 [-5.12, 31.12]
M rquez 2004	56	65 (35)	59	33 (37)		24.5 %	32.00 [18.84, 45.16]
M rquez 2007	96	72 (39)	92	49 (47)		25.0 %	23.00 [10.63, 35.37]
Total (95% CI)	**215**		**215**			**100.0 %**	**17.15 [1.17, 33.14]**

Heterogeneity: Tau^2 = 226.31; Chi^2 = 27.93, df = 3 (P<0.00001); I^2 =89%

Test for overall effect: Z = 2.10 (P = 0.035)

Test for subgroup differences: Not applicable

-100   -50   0   50   100

Usual care   Intensified patient care

Analysis 1.4.   Comparison 1 Intensified patient care vs usual care, Outcome 4 Reduction in total serum cholesterol at > 6 mos (mg/dL).

Review: Interventions to improve adherence to lipid-lowering medication

Comparison: 1 Intensified patient care vs usual care

Outcome: 4 Reduction in total serum cholesterol at > 6 mos (mg/dL)

Study or subgroup	Intensified		Usual care		Mean Difference	Weight	Mean Difference
	N	Mean(SD)	N	Mean(SD)	IV,Random,95% CI		IV,Random,95% CI
Aslani 2010	48	18 (6.5)	49	0.4 (6.8)		98.1 %	17.60 [14.95, 20.25]
Faulkner 2000	15	55 (22)	15	39 (30)		1.9 %	16.00 [-2.83, 34.83]
Total (95% CI)	**63**		**64**			**100.0 %**	**17.57 [14.95, 20.19]**

Heterogeneity: Tau² = 0.0; Chi² = 0.03, df = 1 (P = 0.87); I² =0.0%

Test for overall effect: Z = 13.14 (P < 0.00001)

Test for subgroup differences: Not applicable

```
        -100    -50     0      50     100
              Usual care       Intensified patient care
```

Analysis 1.5.   Comparison 1 Intensified patient care vs usual care, Outcome 5 Reduction in LDL-C at ≤ 6 months (mg/dL).

Review: Interventions to improve adherence to lipid-lowering medication

Comparison: 1 Intensified patient care vs usual care

Outcome: 5 Reduction in LDL-C at ≤ 6 months (mg/dL)

Study or subgroup	Intensified		Usual care		Mean Difference IV,Random,95% CI	Weight	Mean Difference IV,Random,95% CI
	N	Mean(SD)	N	Mean(SD)			
Faulkner 2000	15	62 (16)	15	53 (19)		34.6 %	9.00 [-3.57, 21.57]
M rquez 2004	56	63 (27)	59	36 (42)		34.0 %	27.00 [14.16, 39.84]
M rquez 2007	96	69 (41)	92	46 (55)		31.4 %	23.00 [9.09, 36.91]
Total (95% CI)	**167**		**166**			**100.0 %**	**19.51 [8.51, 30.51]**

Heterogeneity: Tau² = 49.82; Chi² = 4.23, df = 2 (P = 0.12); I² =53%
Test for overall effect: Z = 3.48 (P = 0.00051)
Test for subgroup differences: Not applicable

```
            -100   -50    0    50   100
                Usual care    Intensified patient care
```

Analysis 1.6.   Comparison 1 Intensified patient care vs usual care, Outcome 6 Reduction in LDL-C > 6 months (mg/dL).

Review: Interventions to improve adherence to lipid-lowering medication

Comparison: 1 Intensified patient care vs usual care

Outcome: 6 Reduction in LDL-C > 6 months (mg/dL)

Study or subgroup	Intensified		Usual care		Mean Difference IV,Random,95% CI	Mean Difference IV,Random,95% CI
	N	Mean(SD)	N	Mean(SD)		
Faulkner 2000	15	47 (18)	15	29 (18)		18.00 [5.12, 30.88]

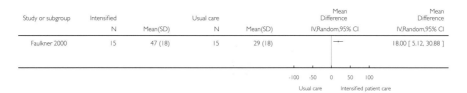

```
            -100   -50    0    50   100
                Usual care    Intensified patient care
```

Analysis 1.7.   Comparison 1 Intensified patient care vs usual care, Outcome 7 Attrition rate sensitivity analysis (medication adherence at ≤ 6 months).

Review: Interventions to improve adherence to lipid-lowering medication

Comparison: 1 Intensified patient care vs usual care

Outcome: 7 Attrition rate sensitivity analysis (medication adherence at ≤ 6 months)

Study or subgroup	Intensified n/N	Usual care n/N	Odds Ratio M-H,Random,95% CI	Weight	Odds Ratio M-H,Random,95% CI
Derose 2012	1102/2606	679/2610		28.2 %	2.08 [1.85, 2.34]
Eussen 2010	392/439	388/460		23.6 %	1.55 [1.04, 2.29]
Faulkner 2000	12/15	12/15		5.2 %	1.00 [0.17, 5.98]
Goswami 2013	111/155	38/53		17.2 %	1.00 [0.50, 1.99]
M rquez 2004	52/56	38/59		10.1 %	7.18 [2.28, 22.65]
M rquez 2007	86/96	53/92		15.6 %	6.33 [2.92, 13.73]
Total (95% CI)	**3367**	**3289**		**100.0 %**	**2.22 [1.41, 3.49]**

Total events: 1755 (Intensified), 1208 (Usual care)
Heterogeneity: Tau^2 = 0.19; Chi^2 = 19.56, df = 5 (P = 0.002); I^2 =74%
Test for overall effect: Z = 3.45 (P = 0.00056)
Test for subgroup differences: Not applicable

0.01   0.1   1   10   100
Usual care   Intensified patient care

ADDITIONAL TABLES

Table 1.   Matrix of comparisons in included studies

Comparator intervention	Intervention						
	1) simplification of drug regimen	2) patient education and information	3) intensified patient care[1]	4) complex behavioural approaches[2]	5) decision support systems[3]	6) administrative improvements[4]	7) pharmacy-led intervention
1) simplification of drug regimen	N/A						
2) patient educa-		N/A					

Table 1. Matrix of comparisons in included studies   *(Continued)*

tion and information							
3) intensified patient care[1]			N/A				
4) complex behavioural approaches[2]				N/A	Kooy 2013; Pladevall 2014		
5) decision support systems[3]					N/A		
6) administrative improvements[4]						N/A	
7) pharmacy-led intervention							N/A
8) usual care/ placebo	Brown 1997; Castellano 2014; Patel 2015; PILL 2011; Selak 2014; Sweeney 1991; Thom 2013	Gujral 2014; Park 2013; Poston 1998; Powell 1995; Willich 2009	Aslani 2010; Derose 2012; Eussen 2010; Fang 2015; Faulkner 2000; Goswami 2013; Guthrie 2001; Ho 2014; Kardas 2013; Ma 2010; Márquez 2004; Márquez 2007; Nieuwkerk 2012;	Márquez 1998			Choudhry 2011; Tamblyn 2009	Fischer 2014; Vollmer 2014

Table 1. Matrix of comparisons in included studies *(Continued)*

				Schectman 1994; Vrijens 2006; Wald 2014			

[1] Intensified patient care includes increased follow-up, sending out reminders, etc.

[2] Complex behavioural approaches include increasing motivation by arranging group sessions, giving out rewards, etc.

[3] Decision support systems include computer-based information systems aimed at support of decision-making.

[4] Administrative improvements include audit, documentation, computers.

N/A: not applicable

Table 2.   Intensified vs usual care: Medication adherence outcomes for pooled studies

Study	Intervention	Effective Y/N	Results
Faulkner 2000	Regular phone calls	Y	24% absolute difference (63% in intervention group vs 39% in control group; $P < 0.05$ reported; n = 30)
Márquez 2004	Regular phone calls	Y	29% absolute difference (93% in intervention group vs 64% in control group; $P < 0.001$ reported; n = 115)
Vrijens 2006	Regular review by the community pharmacist	Y	6.5% difference (95.9% in the intervention group vs 89.4% in the control group; $P < 0.001$ reported; n = 392)
Derose 2012	Automated telephone calls followed 1 week later by letters for continued nonadherence	Y	Statins were dispensed to 42.3% of intervention participants and 26.0% of control participants (absolute difference 16.3%; $P = 0001$; n = 5216)
Márquez 2007	Simple calendar reminder of medication taking given to patient at time of their first prescription	Y	32% difference (90% in intervention group vs 58% in control group; $P < 0.005$ reported; n = 186)
Guthrie 2001	Telephone and postal reminders	N	79.7% in intervention group vs 77.4% in control group; P value non-significant; n = 4548
Schectman 1994	Telephone and postal reminders	N	88% in intervention group vs 82% in control group; $P = 0.32$; n = 162
Aslani 2010	Individualised adherence support service delivered at baseline and 3, 6, 9 months to address issues identified from a questionnaire. Interventions included counselling and advice about the disease, medicine, medicine use, adherence and lifestyle measures	Y	Main effect $F_{2,178} = 4.3$; $P < 0.05$; contrast $F_{1,89} = 5.7$; $P < 0.05$; the intervention group reported that, compared with the control group, they were more liable to alter the dose of their medicine at the third reading compared to the second reading ($F_{1,89} = 4.97$; $P < 0.05$) (n = 142)

Table 2.   Intensified vs usual care: Medication adherence outcomes for pooled studies   *(Continued)*

Eussen 2010	Community pharmacy-based pharmaceutical care programme	Y	Lower rate of discontinuation within 6 months after initiating therapy versus usual care (HR 0.66; 95% CI 0.46 to 0.96; n = 899); no difference between groups at 12 months (HR 0.84; 95% CI 0.65 to 1.10)
Goswami 2013	Integrated intervention programme (nurse counselling, adherence tip sheet, copay relief card, opportunity to enrol in 12-week cholesterol management programme)	N	HR 0.66; 95% CI 0.46 to 0.96; No significant difference between groups in discontinuation at 12 months (HR 0.84; 95% CI 0.65 to 1.10) (n = 208)
Kardas 2013	Educational counselling at each visit (every 8 weeks) and asked to adopt a routine evening activity of choice for a reminder	Y	Mean ± SD MPR was 95.4 ± 53.7% and 81.7 ± 31.0%, for intervention and control group, respectively (P < 0.05; n = 196)
Ma 2010	Pharmacist-delivered telephone counselling calls post-hospital discharge	N	The continuous multiple interval (CMA) for statin medication use was 0.88 (SD = 0.3) in the PI condition (referring to the participant being 88% adherent to their statins medication), and 0.90 (SD = 0.3) in the usual care condition (P = 0.51) (n = 559)
Nieuwkerk 2012	Nurse-led cardiovascular risk-factor counselling	Y	Statin adherence was significantly higher (P < 0.01) and anxiety was significantly lower (P < 0.01) in the intervention group (n = 181)
Ho 2014	Pharmacist-led counselling, patient education, teamwork with participant's primary physician, and voice messaging	Y	89.3% in the intervention group were adherent vs 73.9% in the usual care group (P = 0.003) (n = 241)
Fang 2015	Short message service (SMS) and SMS plus Micro Letter (ML)	Y	SMS and SMS + ML groups had better cumulative adherence after 6 months than the phone group. The SMS + ML group had better cumulative adherence than the SMS group (n = 271)
Wald 2014	Texts sent daily for 2 weeks, alternate days for 2 weeks and weekly thereafter for 22 weeks using an automated computer programme	Y	improvement in adherence affecting 16 per 100 participants (95% CI 7 to 24), P = 0.001 (n = 301)

THE JOURNAL OF PEDIATRICS • www.jpeds.com

ORIGINAL ARTICLES

Impact of Erythropoiesis-Stimulating Agents on Behavioral Measures in Children Born Preterm

Jean R. Lowe, PhD[1], Rebecca E. Rieger, MS[2], Natalia C. Moss, MS[2], Ronald A. Yeo, PhD[2], Sarah Winter, MD[3], Shrena Patel, MD[3], John Phillips, MD[4], Richard Campbell, PhD[5], Shawna Baker, RN[3], Sean Gonzales, BS[1], and Robin K. Ohls, MD[1]

Objective To evaluate the impact of erythropoiesis-stimulating agents (ESAs) administered during initial hospitalization and family demographic factors on behavior at 3.5-4 years of age.

Study design Children were enrolled who had previously participated in a randomized study of ESAs (n = 35) or placebo (n = 14) in infants born preterm with birth weights of 500-1250 g. A term healthy control group (n = 22) also was recruited. Behavior was evaluated by parent report with the Behavioral Assessment System of Children-2. Principal component analyses identified 2 demographic factors, a Socioeconomic Composite (SEC) and a Family Stress Composite. A multivariate general linear model evaluated the impact of study group and sex on the 4 composite scales of the Behavioral Assessment System of Children-2. Demographic factors were treated as covariates and interactions with study group (ESA, placebo, and term) were examined.

Results The ESA group had significantly better scores than the placebo group on behavioral symptoms ($P = .04$) and externalizing scales ($P = .04$). An interaction was observed between study group and SEC ($P = .001$). A beneficial effect of ESAs was maximal in the children with lower SEC scores.

Conclusions The beneficial effects of ESAs on childhood behavior were maximal in children with lower SEC scores. ESAs seemed to ameliorate the adverse impact of lower SEC on behavioral domains seen in the placebo group. This effect was independent of the beneficial effect of ESAs on global cognition we reported previously. (*J Pediatr 2017;■■:■■-■■*).

Trial registration ClinicalTrials.gov: NCT01207778 and NCT00334737.

Infants born preterm are at risk for a variety of adverse outcomes, including motor, cognitive, and behavioral problems.[1] In a national cohort study from Finland, parents of 5-year-old children born with very low birth weight reported greater rates of behavioral difficulties including internalizing behavior (ie, anxiety, depression, withdrawal) and externalizing behavior (ie, conduct problems, aggression, hyperactivity) compared with children born term.[2] Behavioral problems in children with very low birth weight have been shown to persist through early childhood and adolescence and are not lessened by higher intelligence scores.[3] Several studies have shown that behavior problems in early childhood often are accompanied by cognitive, executive function, and motor difficulties, raising concerns about long-term outcomes.[4,5]

Erythropoiesis-stimulating agents (ESAs) such as erythropoietin (Epo) or darbepoetin (Darbe) have been used to increase red cell production and decrease transfusions in infants born preterm. Recent studies in animals and humans in which investigators evaluated the nonhematopoietic effects of ESAs suggest a neuroprotective potential through mechanisms of increased oligodendrogenesis, decreased inflammation, decreased oxidative injury, and decreased apoptosis.[6] Our group reported previously that the administration of ESAs (Epo or Darbe) shortly after birth significantly improved cognition and object permanence scores and decreased neurodevelopmental impairments at 2 years of age[7] in a randomized trial of children with birth weights of 500-1250 g.[8] These findings persisted at 3.5-4 years of age.[9]

The purpose of this study was to describe the effects of ESAs on behavioral and emotional functioning at 3.5-4 years of age. Because socioeconomic status has diverse and prominent effects on brain development,[10] the role of socioeconomic and family factors were investigated as possible modifiers of ESA effects.

Darbe	Darbepoetin alfa
Epo	Erythropoietin
ESA	Erythropoiesis-stimulating agents
BASC-2	Behavioral Assessment System of Children – Second Edition
SEC	Socioeconomic Composite

From the [1]Department of Pediatrics, University of New Mexico School of Medicine, Albuquerque, NM; [2]Department of Psychology, University of New Mexico, Albuquerque, NM; [3]Department of Pediatrics, University of Utah, Salt Lake City, UT; [4]Department of Neurology; and [5]Department of Psychiatry, University of New Mexico, Albuquerque, NM

Supported by the National Institutes of Health *Eunice Kennedy Shriver* National Institute of Child Health (R01 HD059856), the University of New Mexico Clinical Translational Science Center (UL1 TR000041), the University of Utah Center for Clinical and Translational Sciences (UL1TR001067), and the University of New Mexico Department of Pediatrics. The authors declare no conflicts of interest.

1

THE JOURNAL OF PEDIATRICS • www.jpeds.com   Volume ■■

Methods

Former infants born preterm (500-1250 g birth weight), enrolled at ≤48 hours of age in the original study[7] were eligible for the current BRITE study (Brain Imaging and Developmental Follow-up of Infants Treated with Erythropoietin; Clinicaltrials.gov: NCT01207778). Infants with genetic disorders, significant congenital anomalies (including known neurologic anomalies), hypertension, seizures, thrombosis, hemolytic disease, or who were already receiving Epo were ineligible for the original study. The number of children eligible for the study and evaluated at 3.5-4 years of age is shown in shown in **Figure 1** (available at www.jpeds.com).

A total of 49 former children born preterm from the original randomized controlled trial were recruited successfully. A group of children born at full term (n = 24) who had an uneventful newborn course also were recruited at age 3.5-4 years at the New Mexico site for the BRITE study. Questionnaires were missing from 2 of the term group and 4 of the preterm group; those subjects and were omitted from this analysis. The parents and examiners continued to be masked to the treatment assignment of the children. The study was approved by the institutional review boards at the University of Utah and the University of New Mexico, and informed consent was obtained from parents. Demographic and medical history data were obtained from the family.

Initial Study Procedures

Randomization of the participants born preterm to ESA vs placebo groups originally was performed during their initial hospitalization with the use of a computer-generated permuted block method, stratified by center. Twins were assigned to the same treatment group. Caregivers and investigators (except the research pharmacists and coordinators administering the study medicine) were masked to the treatment assignment. An investigational new drug application was approved by the Federal Drug Administration (IND #100138), and the study was registered at ClinicalTrials.gov (NCT00334737).

Dosing of Study Drug and Supplements

Infants were randomized to 1 of 3 groups: Epo, 400 units/kg, given subcutaneously 3 times a week; Darbe, 10 μg/kg, given subcutaneously once a week, with sham dosing 2 other times per week; or placebo, consisting of 3 sham doses per week. Dosing continued until 35 weeks of postmenstrual age, discharge, transfer to another hospital, or death. All infants received supplemental parenteral and enteral iron, folate, and vitamin E. All infants received study drug dosing through 35 weeks of postmenstrual age, for an average dosing length of 7.2 ± 1.8 weeks. After planned analyses showed no significant differences between Epo and Darbe recipients, they were combined as a single ESA group.

Present Study

The Behavioral Assessment of Children Scale–Second Edition (BASC-2) is a norm-referenced parent rating scale that assesses childhood behavioral and emotional issues.[11] The BASC-2 consists of 4 composite scales: adaptive skills (social skills, activities of daily living), behavioral symptoms (withdrawal or atypical behaviors), externalizing problems (hyperactivity, aggression, conduct problems), and internalizing problems (anxiety, depression, somatization). For the adaptive skills composite, greater scores are better; for other scales, greater scores are indicative of problems. Standardized t scores were used for analyses.

The Wechsler Preschool and Primary Scale of Intelligence – Third Edition, a widely used standardized scale of general cognitive abilities, was administered to each child.[12] Socioeconomic and demographic variables were obtained through maternal interviews, including maternal age and education, income level, the number of times the family moved since the index child's birth, the number of children in the household <6 years of age, and the primary language spoken in the home.

Data Analyses

The hypothesis of beneficial ESA treatment effects across all BASC-2 scales was tested with a multivariate general linear model with covariates (MANCOVA). With respect to the 4 dependent variables (BASC-2 scores) in the MANCOVA, preliminary analyses revealed that 3 of the 4 variables were not distributed normally, according to the Shapiro-Wilks test (all except the adaptive skills scale). A log transformation was performed for each BASC-2 scale; all transformed values correlated with the original t scores at r = 0.99.

Effect sizes from the MANCOVA are presented as partial eta-squared values with statistical significance of $P < .05$ for the Wilks' lambda multivariate tests. Fixed factors were study group and sex. Given the importance of demographic factors for BASC-2 scales,[13] these influences were considered systematically in the statistical model. Rather than including each of the 7 specific demographic variables in the model, which would reduce statistical power and complicate interpretation, these variables were reduced to 2 composites via the use of principal components analysis with direct oblimin rotation. Ethnicity was coded as either "Hispanic" or "non-Hispanic." Two factors emerged with eigenvalues >1, and these captured 37% and 23% of the shared variance (**Table I**, available at www.jpeds.com, provides details on factor loadings). For summary purposes, the first of these factors was termed "Socioeconomic Composite" (SEC) and the second "Family Stress Composite." Greater scores on the SEC indicated relatively greater income and education, and greater scores on the Family Stress Composite indicated more family moves, more children in the home, and younger maternal age. Preliminary analyses revealed that the second demographic factor was not related to any BASC-2 scale and did not interact with other factors, so this variable was dropped from further analysis.

In the MANCOVA, sex and study group (placebo, ESA, term) were fixed factors and SEC was a covariate. Interactions of sex with study group and SEC with study group were included because of concern that effects of ESA might be moderated by these factors. Planned comparisons contrasted the placebo and ESA groups (to reveal the effects of ESAs) and the ESA and term groups (to reveal whether ESA treatment improved scores

Table II. Demographic data

Factors	Placebo n = 14	ESA n = 35	Term n = 22	Placebo vs ESA	ESA vs term
Gestational age, wk	27.64 (1.52)	27.37 (1.74)	39.05 (1.35)	.40	<.001
Test age, mo	48.79 (3.26)	48.64 (3.69)	45.04 (2.10)	.72	<.001
Income*	4.00 (1.92)	4.59 (2.10)	5.09 (1.68)	.24	.74
Maternal education†	4.50 (1.09)	4.85 (1.20)	5.43 (1.38)	.24	.34
Maternal age, y	24.57 (4.11)	27.92 (6.87)	29.91 (7.62)	.02	.74
Number of family moves	2.29 (1.94)	1.31 (1.28)	1.22 (1.41)	.01	.69
Number of children < 6 y of age in home	2.07 (1.39)	1.59 (0.75)	1.65 (0.78)	.11	.19
Primary language				.10	.72
English	100%	83%	86%		
Spanish	0%	17%	14%		
Ethnicity				.92	.05
Hispanic	36%	37%	64%		
Non-Hispanic	64%	63%	36%		

Values shown are mean (SD) or percentiles.
*Income: <$10 000; $10 000-20 000; $20 000-30 000; $30 000-40 000; $40 000-50 000; $50 000-60 000; $60 000-70 000; $70 000.
†Maternal education: 0, less than high school; 1, completed high school; 2, completed 1 y of college, no degree; 3, associate's degree (2 y of college); 4, completed college; 5, some graduate school, no degree; 6, completed master's degree or greater.

on the set of dependent variables). For descriptive purposes independent-samples t tests and Pearson correlations and partial correlations also were conducted (significance level was $P < .05$).

Results

Infants were originally enrolled between July 2006 and May 2010. Demographic characteristics and statistical comparisons across study groups are shown in **Table II**. Maternal education level was not significantly different between the groups. For the full sample, 34% of the mothers had a high school education or less, and 39% had some college or a college degree. The characteristics of the children who returned for follow-up were similar to those who did not.[9] Tests of homogeneity (Levene test of equality of variances and Box test of equality of covariance matrices) indicated that statistical assumptions of MANCOVA were met.

The 3 study groups (ESA, placebo, and term controls) significantly differed on the 4 BASC-2 scales ($P = .001$; F[8, 112] = 3.546, partial eta-squared = 0.202). At the univariate level, the effect of study group was significant for all 4 BASC-2 scales (all P values < .001). SEC also had a significant effect ($P = .002$; F[4, 56] = 4.731, partial eta-squared = 0.253), and its interaction with study group also was significant ($P = .015$; F[8, 112] = 2.514, partial eta-squared = 0.152). There was no effect for sex ($P = .580$; F[4.56] = 0.724, $P = .580$, partial eta-squared = 0.049) or interaction of sex with study group ($P = .086$; F[8, 112] = 1.790, partial eta-squared = 0.113).

An additional multivariate generalized linear model was performed to compare the ESA and placebo groups. The effect of group fell just short of significance (F[4, 38] = 2.48, $P = .06$, partial eta-squared = 0.21). The effect of SEC was significant (F[4, 38] = 5.67, $P = .001$, partial eta-squared = 0.37), as was the interaction of SEC with group (F[4, 38] = 5.92, $P = .001$, partial eta-squared = 0.38). **Figure 2** shows the interaction of study group (ESA vs placebo) and the SEC factor on BASC-2 scales when SEC was split at the median to create high and low groups.

The ESA group had significantly better scores than the placebo group on behavioral symptoms ($P = .024$) and externalizing problems ($P = .018$), but the study groups did not differ on adaptive skills ($P = .221$) or internalizing problems ($P = .517$). The term group had better scores than the placebo and ESA groups on each of the BASC-2 scales (P values ranged from .009 to .002; **Table III**). There were differences in neurodevelopmental impairments between groups: 4 of 14 children (29%) in the placebo group had a Full-Scale IQ of <70, compared with 3 of 39 children (8%) in the ESA group ($P = .07$), and 3 children (21%) in the placebo group had mild cerebral palsy, compared with no children (0%) in the ESA group ($P = .016$).[9]

To evaluate the independence of these results on the BASC-2 from the ESA effects as we previously demonstrated for cognitive skills,[9] we conducted an additional multivariate general linear model analysis. Full-Scale IQ was added as a covariate, and significance levels were virtually unchanged in both analyses. Thus, the effects of ESAs on the BASC-2 were independent of the effects of ESAs on cognition.

We further analyzed the significant interaction of study group with SEC by examining correlations of SEC with the 4 BASC-2 scales, after co-varying for sex (**Table IV**). In the placebo group, these were all significant and negative (ranging from r = −0.807 for behavior problems to r = −0.671 for the reverse scored

Table III. BASC-2 composite scores across study groups

BASC-2 scales	Placebo n = 14	ESA n = 35	Term n = 22	P_1	P_2
Adaptive skills	50.86 (10.32)	53.40 (8.65)	60.45 (7.85)	.221	.003
Behavior symptoms	59.29 (16.23)	50.63 (11.77)	41.68 (7.23)	.024	.002
Externalizing problems	57.43 (13.32)	49.43 (11.41)	42.86 (6.83)	.018	.009
Internalizing problems	56.93 (10.51)	54.37 (11.48)	45.73 (8.60)	.517	.004

Values shown are standard score mean (SD). Significance levels were determined by independent samples t tests; P_1: placebo vs ESA; P_2: ESA vs term.

Impact of Erythropoiesis-Stimulating Agents on Behavioral Measures in Children Born Preterm   3

THE JOURNAL OF PEDIATRICS • www.jpeds.com   Volume ■■

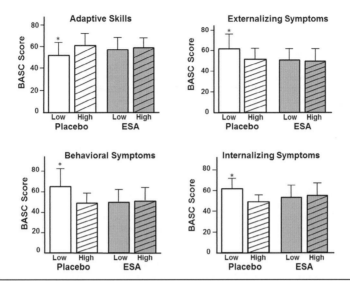

Figure 2. The interaction of study group (ESA vs placebo) and the SEC factor on BASC-2 scales. SEC was split at the median to create high and low groups. *Bars* represent SDs. Data from children in the placebo group are represented by *white columns* and from children in the ESA group by *gray columns*. *Hatched columns* represent high SEC data. *$P < .05$, low SEC placebo group vs the other 3 columns (high SEC placebo group, low SEC ESA group, and high SEC ESA group).

adaptive behavior scale; *P* values all < .02). In contrast, in the ESA group and the term group, none of these partial correlations with SEC approached significance. Thus, the placebo group seemed especially sensitive to the adverse effects of lower SEC for BASC-2 scales.

Discussion

In this study, we examined the effects of postnatal ESA administration on a parent rating scale tapping behavioral and emotional outcomes. Because it has been demonstrated that social and demographic variables affect behavioral functioning, we explored the impact of 2 important broad dimensions of social background, which included socioeconomic and stress variables. We also examined the possibility of interactions

Table IV. Correlations between the SEC factor and BASC-2 composite scores

BASC-2 scales	Placebo n = 14	P value	ESA n = 35	P value
Adaptive skills	0.67	.033	−0.01	NS
Behavior symptoms	−0.81	.003	−0.08	NS
Externalizing problems	−0.65	.01	−0.16	NS
Internalizing problems	−0.73	.003	−0.15	NS

NS, not significant.
Values shown are correlations with corresponding *P* value.

of ESAs and these 2 social factors. The overall effect of ESAs on the 4 BASC-2 composite scores, when we took into account the social factors and their interaction with ESA administration, fell just short of significance ($P = .06$), although the effect size fell in the medium-large range. The most significant effect was the interaction of ESA group with the SEC factor (**Figure 2**). This effect revealed that the beneficial aspects of ESAs were maximal in the low SEC group. ESAs apparently served to mitigate the adverse effects of low SEC in the ESA-treated children. Although we have described an effect of ESA on cognition in this same sample,[9] we found these cognitive effects were independent of the behavioral effects demonstrated here. Finally, despite these positive effects of ESAs, the ESA-treated children born preterm did not completely catch up to children born term on any BASC-2 scale.

In general, children born preterm had more behavioral symptoms, externalizing problems, and internalizing problems than did children born at term gestational age, similar to findings by Baron et al.[14] They observed that children born preterm had more problems than children born term on all 4 BASC-2 scales. Spittle et al[15] also found that toddlers born preterm (2 years' adjusted age) were rated by their parents on the Infant Toddler Social Emotional Assessment scale as having more internalizing and dysregulation problems. Another study that used the Strength and Difficulties Questionnaire noted that 5-year-old children born with very low birth weight had more internalizing, externalizing, and obsessive-compulsive behavior

4   Lowe et al

problems than a term control group.[2] The finding that the children born preterm treated with ESAs had less behavioral symptoms and externalizing problems on the BASC-2 than the children born preterm in the placebo group is unique to this study.

There is an expanding literature demonstrating that socioeconomic disadvantage can affect neurodevelopment adversely. In our sample, 34% of the mothers had a high school education or less, compared with 42% of the US population. We did find that 39% of the mothers had some college or a college degree, which is similar to the US population (38%).[16] A recent study demonstrated that children born to socioeconomically disadvantaged parents were more likely to exhibit neurologic abnormalities during the first 7 years of life.[17] A review article by Linsell et al[18] found that less parental education was related to lower cognitive development in children <5 years; this effect continued during school years. Compared with term-born children, 5-year-old children born preterm had significantly lower IQ scores (up to a 14-point difference) when their parents had less education. Moreover, higher parental education level was related to fewer parent-reported behavior problems in their children.[19] In the current study, we also found a significant SEC-by-study group interaction. Specifically, children with lower SEC benefited more from ESAs.

Consistent with this observation, significant correlations of SEC with BASC-2 composites were limited to the placebo group (**Table IV**). In a recent study, Noble et al[20] found that children from homes with lower family income and maternal education had differences in surface area in brain regions supporting language, executive function, and memory skills. A study in Switzerland by Leuchter et al[21] found that compared with infants born preterm treated with placebo, fewer infants born preterm treated with Epo during the neonatal period had abnormal term-equivalent age scores on magnetic resonance imaging for white matter injury, white matter signal intensity, periventricular white matter loss, and gray matter injury. O'Gorman et al[22] also reported improved white matter development as assessed by diffusion tensor imaging and tract-based spatial statistics in 24 of the infants treated with Epo compared with 34 infants treated with placebo. Our findings thus add to the evidence that ESAs may have beneficial effects in infants born preterm and, furthermore, suggest they have an enhanced beneficial effect related to behavior in infants from socially disadvantaged families.

Limitations of this study include the small number of children in each of our groups, which limits the generalizability of the findings. Also, there were differences in neurodevelopmental impairments between groups that may have impacted behavior: more children in the placebo group than the ESA group had a Full-Scale IQ < 70 ($P = .07$) or mild cerebral palsy ($P = .016$). Although our study had statistically significant results, confirmation in a larger study is needed. Although behavioral ratings are used widely, they have limitations and direct observation of the child's behaviors would be beneficial. We also did not have any measures of mother-child interactions, which have been found to impact a child's behavior and developmental outcome.[23,24]

Our findings may have implications for the medical treatment of children born preterm when considering the possible benefits of ESAs as one component in their comprehensive medical care during the neonatal period. Larger multicenter trials evaluating neuroprotective effects of high-dose Epo are under way (Preterm Epo Neuroprotection Trial, NCT01534481) and will provide additional evidence of the effect of ESAs on the neurodevelopment of infants born preterm. Our study suggests that it is important for early intervention programs to provide services to children from more disadvantaged environments that target strategies to improve externalizing behaviors such as hyperactivity and aggression, as well as behavioral problems such as withdrawal and mood abnormality. We found that children born preterm who were treated with ESAs in the neonatal period had cognitive improvement regardless of socioeconomic factors,[9] as well as behavioral improvements for those children from more impoverished backgrounds. It is possible that early treatment of infants born preterm with ESAs may mitigate the adverse effects of factors such as low maternal education and low income on behavior in early childhood. Although further investigation is needed, especially longitudinal studies through early school age,[25] these findings have important implications for improving outcomes of children born preterm. ■

The authors thank the research coordinators and bedside nurses involved in the original randomized study. We also thank Sarah Peceny for subject coordination, Kristi Watterberg for manuscript review, and Logan Radcliff for assistance in manuscript preparation. We are indebted to the parents for their willingness to allow their children to participate in this study. Finally, we acknowledge US taxpayers for providing the funding to support the National Institutes of Health and this study.

Submitted for publication May 9, 2016; last revision received Dec 9, 2016; accepted Jan 6, 2017

Reprint requests: Robin K. Ohls, MD, Department of Pediatrics, University of New Mexico Health Sciences Center, Albuquerque, NM 87131-0001. E-mail: rohls@salud.unm.edu

References

1. Aarnoudse-Moens CS, Oosterlaan J, Duivenvoorden HF, van Goudoever JB, Weisglas-Kuperus N. Development of preschool and academic skills in children born very preterm. Pediatrics 2011;158:51-6.
2. Rautava L, Hakkinen U, Korvenranta E, Gissler AM, Hallman M, Korvenranta H, et al. Health and the use of health care services in 5-year-old very-low-birth-weight infants. Acta Paediatr 2010;99:1073-9.
3. Conrad AL, Richman L, Lindgren S, Nopoulos P. Biological and environmental predictors of behavioral sequelae in children born preterm. Pediatrics 2010;125:e83-9.
4. Potharst ES, van Wassenaer-Leemhuis AG, Houtzager BA, Livesey D, Kok JH, Last BF, et al. Perinatal risk factors for neurocognitive impairments in preschool children born very preterm. Dev Med Child Neurol 2013;5:178-84.
5. Loe IM, Feldman HM, Huffman LC. Executive function mediates effects of gestational age on functional outcomes and behavior in preschoolers. J Dev Behav Pediatr 2014;35:323-33.
6. Messier AM, Ohls RK. Neuroprotective effects of erythropoiesis-stimulating agents in term and preterm neonates. Curr Opin Pediatr 2014;26:139-45.
7. Ohls RK, Kamath-Rayne BD, Christensen RD, Wiedmeier SE, Rosenberg A, Fuller J, et al. Cognitive outcomes of preterm infants randomized

THE JOURNAL OF PEDIATRICS • www.jpeds.com

Volume ■■

to darbepoetin, erythropoietin, or placebo. Pediatrics 2014;133:1023-30.

8. Nancy B. Bayley Scales of Infant and Toddler Development, Third Edition. San Antonio (TX): The Psychological Corporation; 2006.

9. Ohls RK, Cannon DC, Phillips J, Caprihan A, Patel S, Winter S, et al. Preschool assessment of preterm infants treated with darbepoetin and erythropoietin. Pediatrics 2016;137:1-9.

10. Hackman DA, Farah MJ, Meaney MJ. Socioeconomic status and the brain: mechanistic insights from human and animal research. Nat Rev Neurosci 2010;11:651-9.

11. Cecil RR. Behavior assessment system for children. 2nd ed. Minneapolis (MN): John Wiley & Sons, Inc.; 2004.

12. David W. The Wechsler Preschool and Primary Scale of Intelligence. 3rd ed. San Antonio (TX): The Psychological Corporation; 2002.

13. Arpi E, Ferrari F. Preterm birth and behaviour problems in infants and preschool-age children: a review of the recent literature. Dev Med Child Neurol 2013;55:788-96.

14. Baron IS, Erickson K, Ahronovich MD, Baker R, Litman FR. Neuropsychological and behavioral outcomes of extremely low birth weight at age three. Dev Neuropsychol 2011;36:5-21.

15. Spittle AJ, Treyvaud K, Doyle LW, Roberts G, Lee KJ, Inder TE, et al. Early emergence of behavior and social-emotional problems in very preterm infants. J Am Acad Child Adolesc Psychiatry 2009;48:909-18.

16. Ryan C, Bauman K. Educational attainment in the United States: 2015-2016. https://ask.census.gov/. Accessed 2015-2016.

17. Hung GCL, Hahn J, Alamiri B, Buka SL, Goldstein JM, Laird N, et al. Socioeconomic disadvantage and neural development from infancy through early childhood. Int J Epidemiol 2015;44:1889-99.

18. Linsell L, Malouf R, Morris J, Kurinczuk J, Marlow N. Prognostic factors for poor cognitive development in children born very preterm or with very low birth weight: a systematic review. JAMA Pediatr 2015;169:1162-72.

19. Potharst ES, van Wassenaer AG, Houtzager BA, van Hus JW, Last BF, Kok JH. High incidence of multi-domain disabilities in very preterm children at five years of age. Pediatrics 2011;159:79-85.

20. Noble KG, Houston SM, Brito NH, Bartsch H, Kan E, Kuperman JM, et al. Family income, parental education and brain structure in children and adolescents. Nat Neurosci 2015;18:773-8.

21. Leuchter RH, Gui L, Poncet A, Hagmann C, Lodygensky GA, Martin E, et al. Association between early administration of high-dose erythropoietin in preterm infants and brain MRI abnormality at term-equivalent age. JAMA 2014;312:817-24.

22. O'Gorman RL, Bucher HU, Held U, Koller BM, Hüppi PS, Hagmann CF, et al. Tract-based spatial statistics to assess the neuroprotective effect of early erythropoietin on white matter development in preterm infants. Brain 2015;138:388-97.

23. Treyvaud K, Doyle LW, Lee KJ, Roberts G, Cheong JL, Inder TE, et al. Family functioning, burden, and parenting stress 2 years after very preterm birth. Early Hum Dev 2011;87:427-31.

24. Lowe J, Erickson SJ, MacLean P, Duvall SW, Ohls RK, Duncan AF. Associations between maternal scaffolding and executive functioning in 3 and 4 year olds born very low birth weight and normal birth weight. Early Hum Dev 2014;90:587-93.

25. Delobel-Ayoub M, Arnaud C, White-Koning M, Casper C, Pierrat V, Garel M, et al. Behavioral problems and cognitive performance at 5 years of age after very preterm birth: the EPIPAGE Study. Pediatrics 2009;123:1485-92.

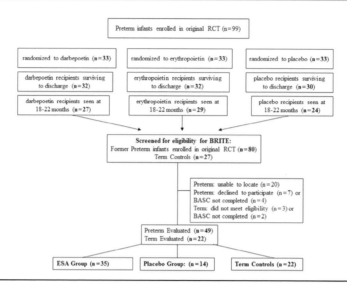

Figure 1. Numbers of infants that were screened for eligibility for the BRITE study, that were eligible for the study, and that were evaluated at 3.5-4 years with completed BASC-2 questionnaires. *RCT*, randomized controlled trial.

Table I. Loadings for the 2 sociodemographic factors used for principal component analysis

Factors	Socioeconomic Composite	Family Stress Composite
Income	0.70	−0.38
Maternal education	0.76	−0.37
Maternal age	0.21	−0.82
Number of family moves	−0.15	0.69
Number of children <6 y	−0.17	0.74
Ethnic background	0.72	−0.20
Primary language	−0.76	−0.30

Impact of Erythropoiesis-Stimulating Agents on Behavioral Measures in Children Born Preterm   6.e1

Applied Nursing Research 31 (2016) 52–59

Contents lists available at ScienceDirect

Applied Nursing Research

journal homepage: www.elsevier.com/locate/apnr

The effect of a translating research into practice intervention to promote use of evidence-based fall prevention interventions in hospitalized adults: A prospective pre–post implementation study in the U.S.

Marita G. Titler, PhD, FAAN [a,*], Paul Conlon, Pharm D, JD [b], Margaret A. Reynolds, PhD, FAAN [b], Robert Ripley, PharmD, BCPS [b], Alex Tsodikov, PhD [c], Deleise S. Wilson, PhD, RN [a], Mary Montie, PhD [a]

[a] School of Nursing, University of Michigan, USA
[b] Trinity Health, Novi, Michigan, USA
[c] Department of Biostatistics, School of Public Health, University of Michigan, USA

ARTICLE INFO

Article history:
Received 3 August 2015
Accepted 17 December 2015

Keywords:
Falls
Fall injuries
Fall prevention
Hospitals
Implementation
Translation

ABSTRACT

Background: Falls are a major public health problem internationally. Many hospitals have implemented fall risk assessment tools, but few have implemented interventions to mitigate patient-specific fall risks. Little research has been done to examine the effect of implementing evidence-based fall prevention interventions to mitigate patient-specific fall risk factors in hospitalized adults.
Objectives: To evaluate the impact of implementing, in 3 U.S. hospitals, evidence-based fall prevention interventions targeted to patient-specific fall risk factors (Targeted Risk Factor Fall Prevention Bundle). Fall rates, fall injury rates, types of fall injuries and adoption of the Targeted Risk Factor Fall Prevention Bundle were compared prior to and following implementation.
Design: A prospective pre–post implementation cohort design.
Setting: Thirteen adult medical-surgical units from three community hospitals in the Midwest region of the U.S.
Participants: Nurses who were employed at least 20 hours/week, provided direct patient care, and licensed as an RN (n = 157 pre; 140 post); and medical records of patients 21 years of age or older, who received care on the study unit for more than 24 hours during the designated data collection period (n = 390 pre and post).
Methods: A multi-faceted Translating Research Into Practice Intervention was used to implement the Targeted Risk Factor Fall Prevention Bundle composed of evidence-based fall prevention interventions designed to mitigate patient-specific fall risks. Dependent variables (fall rates, fall injury rates, fall injury type, use of Targeted Risk Factor Fall Prevention Bundle) were collected at baseline, and following completion of the 15 month implementation phase. Nurse questionnaires included the Stage of Adoption Scale, and the Use of Research Findings in Practice Scale to measure adoption of evidence-based fall prevention practices. A Medical Record Abstract Form was used to abstract data about use of targeted risk-specific fall prevention interventions. Number of falls, and number and types of fall injuries were collected for each study unit for 3 months pre- and post-implementation. Data were analyzed using multivariate analysis.
Results: Fall rates declined 22% (p = 0.09). Types of fall injuries changed from major and moderate to minor injuries. Fall injury rates did not decline. Use of fall prevention interventions improved significantly (p < 0.001) for mobility, toileting, cognition, and risk reduction for injury, but did not change for those targeting medications.
Conclusions: Using the Translating Research Into Practice intervention promoted use of many evidence-based fall prevention interventions to mitigate patient-specific fall risk factors in hospitalized adults.

© 2015 Published by Elsevier Inc.

1. Introduction

Falls are the most common reported patient safety incident in hospitals (Anonymous, 2011; Oliver, 2008a; Rubenstein, 2006), and are a major public health problem internationally (Caldevilla et al., 2013;

* Corresponding author. Tel.: +1 734 763 1188.
  E-mail address: mtitler@umich.edu (M.G. Titler).

http://dx.doi.org/10.1016/j.apnr.2015.12.004
0897-1897/© 2015 Published by Elsevier Inc.

Higaonna, 2015; Quigley & White, 2013; Shmueli et al., 2014). Up to 30% of falls result in injury including fractures, soft tissue trauma and death (Oliver, 2008a; Rubenstein, 2006). Additional consequences include prolonged hospital stay, discharge to long term care facilities, increased hospital costs, patient anxiety, and loss of confidence in mobility and activities of daily living (Boltz et al., 2014; Caldevilla et al., 2013; Oliver et al., 2004; Rubenstein, 2006; Tinetti & Kumar, 2010).

Hospitals have instituted fall risk assessment scales to identify patients at risk for falls followed by implementation of general fall

M.G. Titler et al. / Applied Nursing Research 31 (2016) 52–59   53

prevention interventions (e.g., putting signs on the door for those at risk) (Caldevilla et al., 2013; Oliver, 2008b). Although fall prevention interventions should be customized to the individual's identified risk factors (Anonymous, 2011; Cameron et al., 2012), hospitals have not yet promoted use of fall prevention interventions targeted to patient-specific risks (e.g., ambulation or refer to physical therapy for unsteady gait) (Coussement et al., 2008; Hempel et al., 2013; Oliver, Healey, & Haines, 2010). Because falls are complex and risks for falls are multifactorial, beneficial effects of fall reduction interventions may increase when interventions target patient-specific fall risk factors (Anonymous, 2011; Cameron et al., 2012; Coussement et al., 2008; Tinetti, 2003). Few studies however have examined the effect of implementing evidence-based fall prevention interventions to mitigate patient-specific fall risk factors in hospitalized adults (Dykes et al., 2010).

The purpose of this 18 month study was to implement evidence-based fall prevention interventions targeted to patient-specific fall risk factors (Targeted Risk Factor Fall Prevention Bundle) and evaluate the impact on reducing falls and fall related injuries. A multifaceted Translating Research Into Practice intervention was used to promote uptake and use of the Targeted Risk Factor Fall Prevention Bundle in 13 adult medical surgical units in three community hospitals in the U.S. Specific aims of the study were to (1) compare fall rates, fall injury rates, and types of fall injuries prior to and following implementation of the evidence-based Targeted Risk Factor Fall Prevention Bundle, and (2) evaluate adoption of the evidence-based Targeted Risk Factor Fall Prevention Bundle.

2. Fall Prevention Conceptual Framework

The conceptual framework used in this study was informed by a taxonomy that classifies types of fall prevention interventions (Cameron et al., 2012; Hook & Winchel, 2006; McCarter-Bayer, Bayer, & Hall, 2005). Interventions are conceptualized as Universal Fall Precautions (e.g., reducing environmental risks for falls such as patient room and hall free of clutter), General Fall Prevention Interventions (e.g., bedside table, call light and other personnel items within reach) and Targeted Individual Risk-Specific Interventions (interventions that target patient-specific fall risk factors).

Individual risk factors that consistently contribute to falls in hospitalized adults are gait instability and lower limb weakness; urinary incontinence, frequency or need for toileting assistance; previous fall history; agitation/confusion or impaired judgment; and polypharmacy and prescription of "culprit" drugs, in particular centrally acting sedatives and hypnotics (Oliver et al., 2004; Titler et al., 2011). Mitigating as many of these risk factors as possible is an effective way to reduce falling (Cameron et al., 2012; Oliver, 2008a).

The Targeted Risk Factor Fall Prevention Bundle, developed for this study, focused on interventions that reduce or modify patient-specific fall risk factors as outlined in Table 1. Fall prevention interventions were grouped by categories of risk to address (1) previous falls, (2) mobility limitations, (3) elimination, (4) medications, (5) factors that increase risk for serious injury from a fall (e.g., anticoagulants), and (6) cognitive and mental status. Some fall prevention interventions such as purposeful rounding are effective to address multiple risk factors (e.g., mobility impairments, elimination, comfort) (Fischer et al., 2005; Woodard, 2009). Others such as physical therapy referral, passive and active range of motions, and ambulation are important interventions targeted to mobility impairments, a risk factor for falls as well as functional decline (Markey & Brown, 2002; Ross & Morris, 2010; Tucker, Molsberger, & Clark, 2004). Medication management addresses vigilance and modification of types and number of medications that patients receive as well as the time of the day they are administered (e.g., diuretics) (Agostini, Concato, & Inouye, 2008; Agostini, Zhang, & Inouye, 2007). Medication reviews with pharmacist are helpful in decreasing falls (P.P.S. Advisory, 2008).

Table 1
Targeted risk factor fall prevention bundle.

Common risk factors[*]	Fall reduction interventions suggested for each risk factor type[**]
Mobility (gait instability, lower limb weakness or required assistance getting out of bed)	1. Ambulate 3 to 4 times per day with assistance as needed unless contraindicated. 2. Refer to Physical Therapy for assessment and gait and strength training as needed. 3. Active range of motion three times per day 4. Minimize use of immobilizing equipment (e.g., indwelling urinary catheters, restraints) 5. Assure proper assist equipment (e.g., walker, cane) is readily available and in proper working condition
Elimination: Fecal or urinary incontinence (urgency, need for toileting assistance, diuretics)	1. Schedule toileting and assistance to the bathroom (e.g., every two hours) 2. Bedside commode available for use 3. Administer diuretics before 5 p.m. to minimize nighttime toileting 4. Look for signs of urinary tract infection and notify physician 5. Stay within arm's reach during toileting
Medications (sedatives, anti-depressants, anticonvulsants, benzodiazepines and polypharmacy)	1. Pharmacy review of medications for recommendations 2. Review medications to minimize number. 3. Assist with toileting prior to administration of analgesics unless pain is too severe.
Cognition/mental status (agitation, confusion, disorientation, cognitive impairment,)	1. Delirium screen – use a delirium screening tool to assess 2. If possible avoid high risk drugs (e.g., opiates, sedatives, antidepressants) 3. Monitor electrolytes 4. Encourage nighttime sleep – use non-pharmacological mechanisms first 5. Encourage use of visual aids (e.g., glasses); use adaptive equipment such as large illuminated telephone key pads, and fluorescent tape on call button with reinforcement to use call button. 6. Assess pain control at regular intervals 7. Rounding every 1–2 hours
Risk for serious injury from a fall (osteoporosis or osteoporosis risk factors, medications/anticoagulants, postoperative.)	1. Indicate as high risk for injury from fall 2. Conduct hour toileting rounds 3. Use low bed (6 inches from the floor) 4. Consider placing a bedside mat on the floor when patient is in bed. 5. Assist with toileting prior to administration of analgesics.

[*] Factors repeatedly found as significant risk factors for falls in hospitalized older adults (Oliver et al., 2004; Tinetti & Kumar, 2010).
[**] Suggested interventions for each risk factor group (Cameron et al., 2012; Cumming, 2002; Dykes et al., 2010; Fischer et al., 2005; Healey et al., 2004; Hook & Winchel, 2006; Inouye, Brown, & Tinetti, 2009; Inouye et al., 2000; Oliver et al., 2004, 2007; Quigley et al., 2009; Ross & Morris, 2010; Shever et al., 2011; Tzeng, 2011).

3. Methods

A prospective, pre–post cohort implementation design using a participatory partnership research approach was used for this study. We chose a participatory partnership approach to foster engagement, ownership of the study, as well as use of findings to improve quality of care (Cornwall & Jewkes, 1995; Gold & Taylor, 2007; Green, Daniel, & Novick, 2001).

3.1. Setting

The study setting was three community hospitals in the Midwest region of the U.S. representing small (90 acute care beds), medium (243 acute care beds) and large (471 acute care beds) hospitals. Criteria for site inclusion were (1) acute care community hospital, (2) availability of at least one adult medical, surgical or medical-surgical unit, and (3) and interest in reducing falls.

Thirteen adult medical-surgical units from these 3 hospitals were invited to participate in the study. Exclusion criteria were critical care, obstetrics and pediatric units. Institutional review board (IRB) approval was obtained from the University of Michigan, as well as corresponding review boards at the participating hospitals.

3.2. Subjects

Nurses from the study units who met inclusion criteria were randomly selected from a list of eligible subjects to receive questionnaires prior to and following implementation of the Targeted Risk Factor Fall Prevention Bundle. Inclusion criteria for nurses were: (1) provided direct patient care on the study unit, (2) licensed as a registered nurse (RN), and (3) worked an average of 20 hours or more per week (.50 Full Time Equivalent).

Medical records of a randomly selected group of patients who met the following inclusion criteria were abstracted to determine what targeted, individual risk-specific fall prevention interventions were used for each patient: (1) age ≥ 21 years of age, (2) resided on the study unit >24 hours, and (3) care was received on the study unit during the designated data abstraction period. Medical records were abstracted for each day from admission to discharge from the study unit. Ten records/per unit/month reflecting 3 months of care delivered prior to implementation and 3 months at the end of implementation were abstracted (390 records at baseline; 390 records post-implementation).

3.3. Implementation Intervention

A Translating Research Into Practice (TRIP) multifaceted implementation intervention (see Fig. 1) was used to promote uptake and use of the fall prevention bundle, and was guided by the Translation Research Model (Titler, 2010; Titler & Everett, 2001; Titler et al., 2009) developed from Roger's Diffusion of Innovation Framework (Rogers, 2010). The Translation Research Model addresses four areas that effect adoption of evidence in practice: the *characteristics* of the evidence-based clinical topic (e.g., the fall prevention bundle), and how it is *communicated* to *users* in the *social system* (e.g., hospital, patient care unit) (Rogers, 2010; Titler et al., 2009).

The Translating Research Into Practice intervention, depicted in Fig. 1, consisted of multiple implementation strategies, organized by the Translation Research Model, and informed by prior research (Birken, Lee, & Weiner, 2012; Bradley et al., 2004; Dobbins et al., 2009a, 2009b; Dogherty et al., 2012; Dougherty & Conway, 2008; Farmer et al., 2008; Feldman & McDonald, 2004; Feldman et al., 2005; Flodgren et al., 2011; Forsetlund et al., 2009; Gifford et al., 2007, 2011; Greenhalgh et al., 2005; Grimshaw et al., 2006; Hysong, Best, & Pugh, 2006; Ivers et al., 2012; Jordan et al., 2009; Katz et al., 2009; Murtaugh et al., 2005; Ploeg et al., 2010; Rogers, 2010; Stetler et al., 2009; Titler, 2010; Titler et al., 2009). It was implemented over 15 months, as outlined in Table 2. To address the *social system*, a 60 minute meeting with the Chief Nursing Officer of each hospital was held at the beginning of implementation to overview the study, select the site opinion leader, and overview fall prevention interventions that mitigate patient-specific fall risk factors. All sites had an institution fall prevention quality improvement committee and the sites were encouraged to incorporate this project into the committee's work. A 60 minute education program was provided for the nurse managers of the study units to review the study, overview fall prevention interventions to mitigate patient-specific fall risks, and to explain the expectations of the site opinion leader and unit-based change champions. To address the *characteristics of the clinical topic*, (1) a set of six quick reference guides to assist clinicians with clinical decision-making were developed and organized by risk factor categories with suggested fall prevention interventions to address each; and (2) a set of 9 posters were developed about falls, patient-specific fall risk factors and fall prevention interventions to mitigate these risks. The posters were used in education of staff and posted in key areas on patient care units such as medication rooms and nurses' stations. To address *communication*, a nurse opinion leader for each hospital and nurse change champion for each of the 13 study units were selected in collaboration with the Chief Nursing Officer and Nurse Managers. A two-day train-the-trainer program for the opinion leaders and change champions was held with the overall purpose of increasing their knowledge and skills in fall prevention interventions to mitigate patient-specific fall risk factors, and to develop an implementation action plan for their respective practice sites. Staff education was done at each site by the opinion leader and change champions using inservices, point of care coaching with staff, and imparting knowledge through unit bulletin boards. Seven outreach visits to each of the hospitals were done by the first author in conjunction with the site opinion leader. These visits included rounding on each of the study units to address staff questions, reviewing progress in implementation of the fall prevention interventions, and discussion of strategies to promote use of the fall

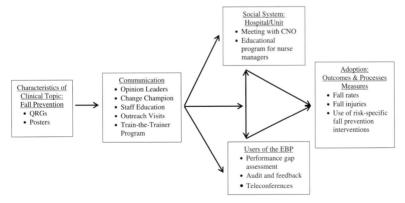

Fig. 1. Translation Research Model.

Table 2
TRIP intervention.

TRIP intervention implementation strategies	Translation research model component	Time during implementation phase of the study
Meeting with CNO and education of nurse managers of study units	Social system	Month 1
Selection of opinion leaders and unit-based change champions	Communication	Month 1
Train-the trainer program	Communication	Month 1
Performance Gap Assessment	Users of the EBP	Month 1
Quick reference guides	Characteristics of the clinical topic	Distributed in month 4
		Used months 4 through 15
Educational posters	Characteristics of the clinical topic	Distributed month 3
		Used months 3 through 11
Staff education	Communication	Month 3 to 4
Outreach/site visits every 6 weeks for a total of 7 visits per site	Communication	Month 4 through month 15
Audit and feedback — 6 reports	Users of the EBP	Month 5 through month 15
Monthly teleconferences total of 11	Users of the EBP	Month 3 through 14

prevention practices. To address the *users* component of the model, we used performance gap assessment, audit and feedback, and monthly teleconferences. Performance gap assessment informs practitioners, at the beginning of change, about a practice performance and opportunities for improvement (Titler et al., 2009). We provided unit fall rates, and types of fall injuries during the train-the-trainer program and used this as a focal point of discussion for improving fall prevention practices. Audit and feedback is ongoing auditing of performance indicators (e.g., use of fall prevention practices to mitigate patient-specific risks) and discussing the findings with practitioners during the practice change (Ivers et al., 2012). The change champions of each unit completed audits of five randomly selected medical records per month to ascertain if patient-specific fall risk factors were present and if so, were fall prevention interventions implemented to mitigate the specific risk factors. Completed audits were sent to the project office. Bar graphs were then developed regarding number of patient days with a specific fall risk (e.g., mobility issues) and the number of patient days with implementation of corresponding risk-specific fall prevention interventions (e.g., physical therapy referral; ambulation). These were discussed with staff during each of the outreach visits. Monthly 60 minute teleconferences among the opinion leaders and change champions from the study units were conducted to share implementation strategies and problem-solve issues that arose.

3.4. Dependent Variables and Instruments

The dependent variables for aim 1 were: (1) fall rates; (2) fall injury rates; and (3) types of fall injuries. A fall was defined as an unplanned descent to the floor, and was calculated, at the unit level, by the number of inpatient falls multiplied by 1000 and divided by the total number of inpatient days (Anonymous, 2004). Types of fall injuries were defined as minor (needs application of dressing, ice, cleaning of a wound, limb elevation, topical medication), moderate (results in suturing, steri-strips, fracture, or splinting), major (results in surgery, casting, or traction), and death (as a result of the fall) (Anonymous, 2004). A fall injury empirical rate was calculated by multiplying the number of inpatient falls with injuries by 1000 and dividing by total number of inpatient days (Anonymous, 2004).

The variables for aim 2 were: (1) number and type of risk-specific interventions (e.g., ambulation with assistance; physical therapy referral) delivered within and across each risk category (e.g., mobility); and (2) RNs level of adoption of the Targeted Risk Factor Fall Prevention Bundle. A Medical Record Abstract Form and detailed directions were designed to abstract data from medical records about use of fall prevention interventions that targeted patient-specific fall risk for each patient/medical record. Medical record abstraction is used by other investigators and the Center for Medicare and Medicaid Services to collect data on processes of care (Centers for Medicare & Medicaid Services: CMS.gov., 2014; Titler et al., 2009). The Medical Record Abstract Form was reviewed by 3 experts in fall prevention and then tested with 20 medical records for completeness and clarity. The Medical

Record Abstract Form and detailed instructions were then tested for inter-rater and intra-rater reliability using 30 medical records resulting in reliability of .92 and .95, respectively. Medical record data were used to calculate the number and type of risk-specific interventions (e.g., ambulation with assistance; physical therapy referral) delivered within and across each risk category (e.g., mobility; elimination) by number of patient days.

The RNs level of adoption of the targeted fall prevention interventions was measured by the *Stage of Adoption Instrument* and the *Use of Research Findings in Practice Scale*. The Stage of Adoption Instrument is based on Rogers' (Rogers, 2010) diffusion of innovation model, and measures stages of awareness, persuasion, and implementation for four evidence-based, fall prevention practices that target individual risk factors: ambulation; medication review; delirium screening; and post-fall huddle. It is scored on a 0 (low stage of adoption) to 4 (implementation) scale. Internal consistency is .95 to .76 with test–retest reliability (one week) of .83 (Rutledge & Donaldson, 1995; Rutledge et al., 1996; Titler et al., 2009). The Use of Research Findings in Practice Scale was used to measure nurses self-reported use of research findings for targeted risk factor fall prevention interventions (knowledge to implementation). Content validity and test–retest reliability (r = .87) have been demonstrated (Meyer & Goes, 1988; Titler et al., 2009). Nurses rate on a 9-point, Guttman type scale, the extent that they use evidence-based fall prevention interventions targeted to patient-specific risk factors to prevent or reduce falls. Each individual receives a score of 0–9 with lower scores reflecting knowledge awareness stage of adoption and higher scores reflecting implementation/use (Meyer & Goes, 1988; Titler et al., 2009).

3.5. Data Collection Procedures

The number of falls, number of injuries from falls, type of injuries from falls, and number of patient days per month were sent to the project director via secure electronic files for each of the study units for a 3 month period at baseline, midpoint and at the end of the implementation phase.

Medical record abstractions were conducted for care delivered 3 months prior to implementation (baseline) and at end of the implementation phase. The project director received a list of all eligible subjects/medical records from each study unit for each data collection period (baseline; post-implementation). Ten medical records per month were randomly selected for each study unit, using SPSS (SPSS, 1999) to generate a random sequence of medical records for each data collection period, and the list of eligible records were sent to the medical records department of each site. The trained research assistants were then provided access to the randomly selected medical records, and after confirming inclusion criteria of each record, data were abstracted using the Medical Record Abstract Form.

A list of nurses who met the inclusion criteria for each study unit was sent to the project director by the designated human resource person at each site. Thirty nurses per unit were randomly selected from this list.

M.G. Titler et al. / Applied Nursing Research 31 (2016) 52–59

For those units that did not have 30 eligible nurses, all that met inclusion were included in the sample (n = 336). Selected RNs were invited to complete a questionnaire consisting of the Stage of Adoption Instrument, the Use of Research Findings in Practice Scale, and demographic questions. At baseline (one month prior to implementation), a cover letter, the questionnaire, and a preaddressed, stamped, envelope were mailed to each selected nurse. The cover letter explained the study, invited the nurse to participate, and requested that the questionnaire be returned within 2 weeks. Return of the questionnaire signified consent to participate. Reminders were mailed to nurses who had not returned the questionnaire within 3 weeks. Post-implementation questionnaires were sent to RNs returning baseline questionnaires, with 1 reminder sent if questionnaires were not returned within 3 weeks of the first mailing. The return rate of questionnaires was 47% at baseline (n = 157) and 42% at follow-up (n = 140). Returned questionnaires were entered into a database and reviewed for accuracy by a trained research assistant.

Unit characteristics (e.g., bed capacity, average daily census, RN skill mix) were collected from nurse managers of the study unit. Patient characteristics (age, severity of illness) were acquired from the inpatient discharge abstract files (Balas et al., 2004; Titler et al., 2009; Vaughn et al., 2002). The All Patient Refined Diagnosis Related Groups (APR-DRG), the extent of physiological decompensation or organ system loss of function, was used to define severity of illness (1 = minor; 2 = moderate; 3 = major; 4 = severe) (All Patient DRG Definitions Manual, 2011).

3.6. Statistical Analyses

Data were first analyzed using descriptive statistics (e.g., mean, standard deviation, counts, percent) and examined for values out of range. A significance level (alpha) of <.05 was set a priori for all analyses.

For aim 1, multivariate analysis of fall rates was conducted using a Poisson regression model treating counts of falls and fall injuries as a response variable and the period of observation (baseline and post-implementation), as well as unit-level characteristics as explanatory variables. The model used an off-set term representing log-person-days of observation (e.g., patient days) contributing to the fall counts. Covariates included patient age, severity of illness (Minor, Moderate, Major, Severe, scored as 1–4, respectively), RN skill mix, and RN HPPD. Falls and fall injuries were used as dependent variables. Given the small numbers for type of injury, descriptive statistics were used to illustrate the number in each category (minor, moderate, major, death), from pre- to post-implementation.

To analyze data about risk-specific fall prevention interventions abstracted from medical records (aim 2), a set of appropriate interventions was identified for every type of fall risk. This resulted in the creation of risk-intervention pairs, where a specific risk profile corresponds to a specific fall prevention intervention to mitigate the fall risk. In addition, fall prevention interventions were analyzed by risk categories (e.g., mobility, elimination). For all patient days when a specific risk for falls was present, the presence of a fall prevention intervention targeted to a risk factor was treated as a correct response. Multivariate analyses of rates of correct interventions were conducted using a Poisson regression model using the count of correct interventions as the response variable and the period of observation (time before or after implementation), as well as unit-level characteristics (e.g., patient age, severity of illness, RN skill mix) as explanatory variables.

To analyze nurses' self-reported level of adoption (aim 2), multivariate analysis was conducted using a linear mixed model with a random intercept modeling the effect of the unit. The model takes into account the fact that nurses from the same unit may have unmeasured characteristics that make their responses to the questionnaire within the unit more alike than across different units. Multivariate linear mixed model analyses were run separately for each response variable

(e.g., ambulation, medication review, Use of Research Findings in Practice) to evaluate the effect of time (before versus after implementation). Covariates included years of work experience as an RN, education, and age. Gender and race were excluded, because the overwhelming majority was white and female.

4. Results

Demographics of the nurses and study units did not differ significantly between pre- and post-implementation. Patients on the study units were 65 years of age or older ($\bar{X}$ = 65.6; SD = 2.8), and the majority (68%) were in the moderate or major severity of illness category. The average RN skill mix was 75% and the mean RN hours per patient days was 6.8 (SD = 0.81). The majority of nurses were white (>90%), female (>90%), between 30 and 40 years of age, and with an average of over eight years work experience as an RN. Fifty-five percent of the nurses had an education of a baccalaureate degree or higher.

4.1. Impact on Falls (Aim 1)

As shown in Table 3, the decline in fall rates from pre- ($\bar{X}$ = 3.69; SD = 1.43) to post- implementation ($\bar{X}$ = 2.7; SD = 1.34) was not statistically significant (−0.251 on the log scale; SE = 0.15), but demonstrated a trend toward significance (p = 0.09) with a 22% decline in fall rates. Severity of illness and RN skill mix were significant. For example, a 1% increase in RN skill mix was associated with a 2.3% decrease in fall rates. Since injuries from falls are a rare event, their analysis carries less power compared to the overall analysis of fall rates. The decline in fall injury rates was not significant (pre: $\bar{X}$ = .70 SD = .71; post: $\bar{X}$ = .59 SD = .5; p = 0.73). Age was positively associated with fall injury rates (p = 0.046). A one year increase in age was associated with a 12% increase in injury from a fall. Although fall injury rates did not decline significantly, there were reductions in the severity of fall injury for major and moderate categories from 26% pre-implementation to 11% post-implementation (see Fig. 2 supplemental).

4.2. Adoption of the Targeted Risk Factor Fall Prevention Bundle (Aim 2)

Analysis of medical record data indicating adoption of fall prevention interventions targeting patient-specific fall risk factors showed significant improvements (p < 0.001) from pre- to post-implementation indicating that fall prevention interventions were implemented to address patient-specific fall risk factors for all risk categories except medications (see Table 4). For example, prior to implementation, there were 1285 patient days when patients had some mobility fall risk factor; fall prevention interventions to mitigate mobility risk were implemented 31 times per 100 patient days. In contrast, post-implementation, there were 1333 patient days when patients had some mobility fall risk factor

Table 3
Multivariate analysis of fall and fall injury rates.

Variables/category	Estimates of coefficient in the model	Std. Error	p Value
Fall rates			
Intercept	−4.14619	1.49725	0.005
Time period (after)	−0.251	0.15115	0.09
Patient age	−0.01369	0.02187	0.53
Severity of illness	**0.41152**	**0.20609**	**0.045**
RN skill mix	**−2.29978**	**0.85774**	**0.007**
RN HPPDs	0.01780	0.04811	0.711
Fall injury rates			
Intercept	−15.0001	3.7964	<0.001
Time period (after)	0.1118	0.3207	0.727
Patient age	**0.1144**	**0.0574**	**0.046**
Severity of illness	0.3323	0.5335	0.533
RN skill mix	−0.3864	1.7102	0.821
RN HPPDs	−0.0624	0.1100	0.571

M.G. Titler et al. / Applied Nursing Research 31 (2016) 52–59

57

Table 4
Fall prevention interventions by risk categories.

Risk-specific interventions [†]	Before implementation (n = 1638 patient days)		CI	After implementation (n = 1606 patient days)		CI	p Value
	Patient days [+]	Rate per 100 patient days [¥]		Patient days	Rate per 100 patient days		
History of previous fall	133	0.6	0–1.8	209.7	82	77–87	<0.001
Mobility	1285	31	29–33	1333	88	87–90	<0.001
Toileting/elimination	853.7	50	47–53	917.7	66	63–69	<0.001
Cognition/mental status	769	2.3	1.3–3.2	531	77	74–80	<0.001
Medication	1525	0.11	0–0.25	1562	0.1	0–0.25	0.981
Risk for injury	1142	66	64–69	1285	88	86–89	<0.001

CI — confidence interval.
N = 1638 total patient days before intervention; N = 1606 total patient days after intervention.
[+] Patient days are the number of days of labeled risk (denominator).
[¥] Number of times intervention(s) was received per 100 patient days (example: received a mobility intervention 88 times per 100 patient days).
[†] Received fall prevention interventions targeted to patient-specific risk (e.g., based on risk profile).

with a fall prevention intervention implemented 88 times per 100 patient days.

Specific types of fall prevention interventions implemented within each risk category as well as the sum of correct interventions by category are reported in Table 5 (supplemental materials). Specific types of interventions with counts greater than 5 were used in this analysis. For example, use of fall prevention interventions targeted to mobility risk increased for physical therapy, use of assistive equipment, and periodic rounding, as well as the overall sum of fall prevention interventions in the mobility risk category. Overall, the rate of correct interventions across risk categories increased by .27 per 100 patient days (SE = 0.4, $p < 0.001$) (see Table 5 supplemental).

Nurses' mean adoption scores increased significantly for: *ambulation* from 2.03 (1.2) pre-implementation to 2.54 (1.0) post-implementation (SE = .1405; $p = 0.002$); *post-fall huddles* from 2.81 (1.2) pre-implementation to 3.1 (1.0) post-implementation (SE = 0.1375; $p = 0.03$); and *Use of Research Findings in Practice* scores from 6.4 (2.9) pre-implementation to 7.4 (2.3) post-implementation (SE = .3345; $p = 0.04$). No covariates were significant, and adoption scores did not change significantly for medication review and delirium screening.

5. Discussion

The Translating Research Into Practice intervention used in this study was effective in promoting use of fall prevention interventions that target patient-specific fall risk factors. Increased use included fall prevention interventions for history of previous falls, mobility, elimination, cognition/mental status, and risk for injury from a fall. Targeted risk factor fall prevention interventions were designed to mitigate patient-specific risks factors for falls, which goes beyond general fall prevention interventions typically implemented for those designated at risk (Coussement et al., 2008; Hempel et al., 2013; Oliver, 2008a). Although investigators have demonstrated the effectiveness of translation interventions to improve use of evidence-based practices for a variety of other clinical topics (Birken et al., 2012; Dobbins et al., 2009a, 2009b; Dogherty et al., 2012; Farmer et al., 2008; Flodgren et al., 2011; Forsetlund et al., 2009; Gifford et al., 2007, 2011; Ivers et al., 2012; Jordan et al., 2009; Katz et al., 2009; Ploeg et al., 2010; Stetler et al., 2009), few studies have demonstrated improved uptake and use of fall prevention interventions that target patient-specific fall risk factors through a translation research approach (Dykes et al., 2010).

This study demonstrated a 22% reduction in fall rates from pre- to post-implementation with changes in types of injuries from major and moderate to minor injuries. Although the reduction in fall rates and change in types of fall injuries were not statistically significant, these changes are clinically meaningful (Coussement et al., 2008; Cumming et al., 2008; Dykes et al., 2010; Koh et al., 2009). These findings support those of Dykes and colleagues (Dykes et al., 2010) that demonstrated the effectiveness of targeted interventions for reducing falls.

Fall rates were associated with severity of illness and patient age. These findings are congruent with those of other investigators that suggest that falls and injuries from falls are influenced by patient age as well as the number and severity of other conditions (Hanlon et al., 2002; Lee, Cigolle, & Blaum, 2009).

Our study did not demonstrate statistically significant improvements in use of some fall prevention interventions, particularly those targeted to medications such as pharmacy review of medications, avoiding use of medications that increase fall risk (e.g., benzodiazepines), and toileting prior to administration of analgesics. Based upon nurses' self-report and medical record data, findings did not demonstrate increased use of specific fall prevention interventions related to mental status risk such as physician consultation for mental status changes, and scheduled rounding. The explanations for failing to see an increased use of these interventions may be due to complexity and the interdisciplinary nature of these fall prevention interventions (Quigley & White, 2013). Medication review requires multidisciplinary practices (e.g., pharmacy and physicians) and implementation by nurses alone may be difficult. Even though our study included pharmacy representatives to facilitate communication, it might not have been enough to support medication review. Although cognitive status is a fall risk factor that has been emphasized (Inouye et al., 1999), implementing interventions to screen and address cognitive status of hospitalized patients is complex and remains a challenge noted by others (Bradley et al., 2006; Carroll, Dykes, & Hurley, 2012).

Ambulation is an intervention that is recommended to prevent falls related to mobility limitations (Boltz et al., 2014; Oliver et al., 2004; Tinetti & Kumar, 2010). Nurses' self-reported use of ambulation increased from "persuaded" to "used sometimes" stage of adoption. Data from medical records also demonstrated an improvement in use of ambulation, although this change was not statistically significant ($p = 0.08$). These findings are similar to those of other investigators who have demonstrated that ambulation is one of several missed nursing care interventions (Kalisch, 2006; Kalisch, Landstrom, & Hinshaw, 2009). Boltz and colleagues (Boltz et al., 2014) demonstrated several factors that patients report as limiting mobility and physical activity during hospitalization, including elevated bed height, lack of assistive devices, and lack of available staff. Hospital leaders and staff must prioritize and value ambulation and physical activity interventions to prevent falls and functional decline.

6. Limitations

The study findings are not generalizable to other types of healthcare settings, such as ambulatory and long-term care agencies. Given the pre–post design of the study, it is difficult to rule out effects from other factors in the environment occurring simultaneously with this study. Lastly, although medical records are used by regulatory agencies

M.G. Titler et al. / Applied Nursing Research 31 (2016) 52–59

to measure care delivery, some of the fall prevention interventions may have been implemented, but not documented.

7. Conclusions

The Translating Research Into Practice intervention improved use of fall prevention interventions targeted to patient-specific fall risk factors. The study also demonstrated improvement in reduction of fall rates and types of fall injuries. To make significant gains in reducing falls in hospitals, clinicians must do more than arriving at a fall risk score with subsequent implementation of general fall reduction interventions; they need to know each patient's risk factors for falls and implement fall prevention interventions to mitigate those risks.

Appendix A. Supplementary data

Supplementary data to this article can be found online at http://dx.doi.org/10.1016/j.apnr.2015.12.004.

References

Agostini, J. V., Concato, J., & Inouye, S. K. (2008). Improving sedative-hypnotic prescribing in older hospitalized patients: provider-perceived benefits and barriers of a computer-based reminder. *Journal of General Internal Medicine*, 23(Suppl. 1), 32–36.

Agostini, J. V., Zhang, Y., & Inouye, S. K. (2007). Use of a computer-based reminder to improve sedative-hypnotic prescribing in older hospitalized patients. *Journal of American Geriatrics Society*, 55(1), 43–48.

All Patient DRG Definitions Manual (2011). *Version 29.0*. Available from: 3 M Health Information Systems (http://www.3m.com/us/healthcare/his/).

National voluntary consensus standards for nursing-sensitive care: an initial performance measure set: a consensus report. (2004).National Quality Forum.

Summary of the Updated American Geriatrics Society/British Geriatrics Society clinical practice guideline for prevention of falls in older persons. *Journal of the American Geriatrics Society*. (pp. 148–157)(2011).American Geriatrics Society & British Geriatrics, Society; Panel on Prevention of Falls in Older Persons.

Balas, E. A., et al. (2004). Computerized knowledge management in diabetes care. *Medical Care*, 42(6), 610–621.

Birken, S. A., Lee, S. Y., & Weiner, B. J. (2012). Uncovering middle managers' role in healthcare innovation implementation. *Implementation Science*, 7, 28.

Boltz, M., et al. (2014). Activity restriction vs. self-direction: hospitalised older adults' response to fear of falling. *International Journal of Older People Nursing*, 9(1), 44–53.

Bradley, E. H., et al. (2004). Translating research into clinical practice: making change happen. *Journal of American Geriatrics Society*, 52(11), 1875–1882.

Bradley, E. H., et al. (2006). Patterns of diffusion of evidence-based clinical programmes: a case study of the Hospital Elder Life Program. *Quality & Safety in Health Care*, 15(5), 334–338.

Caldevilla, M. N., et al. (2013). Evaluation and cross-cultural adaptation of the Hendrich II Fall Risk Model to Portuguese. *Scandinavian Journal of Caring Sciences*, 27(2), 468–474.

Cameron, I. D., et al. (2012). Interventions for preventing falls in older people in care facilities and hospitals. *Cochrane Database of Systematic Reviews*, 12, CD005465.

Carroll, D. L., Dykes, P. C., & Hurley, A. C. (2012). An electronic fall prevention toolkit: effect on documentation quality. *Nursing Research*, 61(4), 309–313.

Centers for Medicare & Medicaid Services: CMS.gov. (2014). Available from: http://www.cms.hhs.gov/

Cornwall, A., & Jewkes, R. (1995). What is participatory research? *Social Science and Medicine*, 41(12), 1667–1676.

Coussement, J., et al. (2008). Interventions for preventing falls in acute-and chronic-care hospitals: a systematic review and meta-analysis. *Journal of the American Geriatrics Society*, 56(1), 29–36.

Cumming, R. G. (2002). Intervention strategies and risk-factor modification for falls prevention. A review of recent intervention studies. *Clinics in Geriatric Medicine*, 18(2), 175–189.

Cumming, R. G., et al. (2008). Cluster randomised trial of a targeted multifactorial intervention to prevent falls among older people in hospital. *BMJ*, 336(7647), 758–760.

Dobbins, M., et al. (2009a). A description of a knowledge broker role implemented as part of a randomized controlled trial evaluating three knowledge translation strategies. *Implementation Science*, 4, 23.

Dobbins, M., et al. (2009b). A randomized controlled trial evaluating the impact of knowledge translation and exchange strategies. *Implementation Science*, 4, 61.

Dogherty, E. J., et al. (2012). Following a natural experiment of guideline adaptation and early implementation: a mixed-methods study of facilitation. *Implementation Science*, 7, 9.

Dougherty, D., & Conway, P. H. (2008). The "3 T's" road map to transform US health care: the "how" of high-quality care. *JAMA*, 299(19), 2319–2321.

Dykes, P. C., et al. (2010). Fall prevention in acute care hospitals: a randomized trial. *JAMA*, 304(17), 1912–1918.

Farmer, A. P., et al. (2008). Printed educational materials: effects on professional practice and health care outcomes. *Cochrane Database of Systematic Reviews*, 3, CD004398.

Feldman, P. H., & McDonald, M. V. (2004). Conducting translation research in the home care setting: lessons from a just-in-time reminder study. *Worldviews on Evidence-Based Nursing*, 1(1), 49–59.

Feldman, P. H., et al. (2005). Just-in-time evidence-based e-mail "reminders" in home health care: impact on patient outcomes. *Health Services Research*, 40(3), 865–885.

Fischer, I. D., et al. (2005). Patterns and predictors of inpatient falls and fall-related injuries in a large academic hospital. *Infection Control and Hospital Epidemiology*, 26(10), 822–827.

Flodgren, G., et al. (2011). Local opinion leaders: effects on professional practice and health care outcomes. *Cochrane Database of Systematic Reviews*, 8, CD000125.

Forsetlund, L., et al. (2009). Continuing education meetings and workshops: effects on professional practice and health care outcomes. *Cochrane Database of Systematic Reviews*, 2, CD003030.

Gifford, W., et al. (2007). Managerial leadership for nurses' use of research evidence: an integrative review of the literature. *Worldviews on Evidence-Based Nursing*, 4(3), 126–145.

Gifford, W., et al. (2011). Developing team leadership to facilitate guideline utilization: planning and evaluating a 3-month intervention strategy. *Journal of Nursing Management*, 19(1), 121–132.

Gold, M., & Taylor, E. F. (2007). Moving research into practice: lessons from the US Agency for Healthcare Research and Quality's IDSRN program. *Implementation Science*, 2, 9.

Green, L., Daniel, M., & Novick, L. (2001). Partnerships and coalitions for community-based research. *Public Health Reports*, 116(Suppl. 1), 20–31.

Greenhalgh, T., et al. (2005). Storylines of research in diffusion of innovation: a meta-narrative approach to systematic review. *Social Science and Medicine*, 61(2), 417–430.

Grimshaw, J., et al. (2006). Toward evidence-based quality improvement. Evidence (and its limitations) of the effectiveness of guideline dissemination and implementation strategies 1966-1998. *Journal of General Internal Medicine*, 21(Suppl. 2), S14–S20.

Hanlon, J. T., et al. (2002). Falls in African American and white community-dwelling elderly residents. *Journals of Gerontology. Series A, Biological Sciences and Medical Sciences*, 57(7), M473–M478.

Healey, F., et al. (2004). Using targeted risk factor reduction to prevent falls in older inpatients: a randomised controlled trial. *Age and Ageing*, 33(4), 390–395.

Hempel, S., et al. (2013). Hospital fall prevention: a systematic review of implementation, components, adherence, and effectiveness. *Journal of American Geriatrics Society*, 61(4), 483–494.

Higaonna, M. (2015). The predictive validity of a modified Japanese Nursing Association fall risk assessment tool: a retrospective cohort study. *International Journal of Nursing Studies*, 52(9), 1484–1494.

Hook, M. L., & Winchel, S. (2006). Fall-related injuries in acute care: reducing the risk of harm. *Medsurg Nursing*, 15(6), 370–377.

Hysong, S. J., Best, R. G., & Pugh, J. A. (2006). Audit and feedback and clinical practice guideline adherence: making feedback actionable. *Implementation Science*, 1, 9.

Inouye, S. K., Brown, C. J., & Tinetti, M. E. (2009). Medicare nonpayment, hospital falls, and unintended consequences. *New England Journal of Medicine*, 360(23), 2390–2393.

Inouye, S. K., et al. (1999). A multicomponent intervention to prevent delirium in hospitalized older patients. *New England Journal of Medicine*, 340(9), 669–676.

Inouye, S. K., et al. (2000). The Hospital Elder Life Program: a model of care to prevent cognitive and functional decline in older hospitalized patients. Hospital Elder Life Program. *Journal of American Geriatrics Society*, 48(12), 1697–1706.

Ivers, N., et al. (2012). Audit and feedback: effects on professional practice and healthcare outcomes. *Cochrane Database of Systematic Reviews*, 6, CD000259.

Jordan, M. E., et al. (2009). The role of conversation in health care interventions: enabling sensemaking and learning. *Implementation Science*, 4, 15.

Kalisch, B. J. (2006). Missed nursing care: a qualitative study. *Journal of Nursing Care Quality*, 21(4), 306–313.

Kalisch, B. J., Landstrom, G. L., & Hinshaw, A. S. (2009). Missed nursing care: a concept analysis. *Journal of Advanced Nursing*, 65(7), 1509–1517.

Katz, D., et al. (2009). A before-after implementation trial of smoking cessation guidelines in hospitalized veterans. *Implementation Science*, 4, 58.

Koh, S. L., et al. (2009). Impact of a fall prevention programme in acute hospital settings in Singapore. *Singapore Medical Journal*, 50(4), 425–432.

Lee, P. G., Cigolle, C., & Blaum, C. (2009). The co-occurrence of chronic diseases and geriatric syndromes: the health and retirement study. *Journal of American Geriatrics Society*, 57(3), 511–516.

Markey, D. W., & Brown, R. J. (2002). An interdisciplinary approach to addressing patient activity and mobility in the medical-surgical patient. *Journal of Nursing Care Quality*, 16(4), 1–12.

McCarter-Bayer, A., Bayer, F., & Hall, K. (2005). Preventing falls in acute care: an innovative approach. *Journal of Gerontological Nursing*, 31(3), 25–33.

Meyer, A. D., & Goes, J. B. (1988). Organizational assimilation of innovations: a multilevel contextual analysis. *Academy of Management Journal*, 31(4), 897–923.

Murtaugh, C. M., et al. (2005). Just-in-time evidence-based e-mail "reminders" in home health care: impact on nurse practices. *Health Services Research*, 40(3), 849–864.

Oliver, D. (2008a). Falls risk-prediction tools for hospital inpatients. Time to put them to bed? *Age and Ageing*, 37(3), 248–250.

Oliver, D. (2008b). Evidence for fall prevention in hospitals. *Journal of the American Geriatrics Society*, 56(9), 1774–1775.

Oliver, D., Healey, F., & Haines, T. P. (2010). Preventing falls and fall-related injuries in hospitals. *Clinics in Geriatric Medicine*, 26(4), 645–692.

Oliver, D., et al. (2004). Risk factors and risk assessment tools for falls in hospital inpatients: a systematic review. *Age and Ageing*, 33(2), 122–130.

Oliver, D., et al. (2007). Strategies to prevent falls and fractures in hospitals and care homes and effect of cognitive impairment: systematic review and meta-analyses. *BMJ*, 334(7584), 82.

Medication assessment: one determinant of falls risk. P.P.S. Advisory (Ed.). (2008). Pennsylvania Patient Safety Authority.

Ploeg, J., et al. (2010). The role of nursing best practice champions in diffusing practice guidelines: a mixed methods study. *Worldviews on Evidence-Based Nursing, 7*(4), 238–251.

Quigley, P. A., & White, S. V. (2013). Hospital-based fall program measurement and improvement in high reliability organizations. *Online Journal of Issues in Nursing, 18*(2), 5.

Quigley, P. A., et al. (2009). Reducing serious injury from falls in two veterans' hospital medical-surgical units. *Journal of Nursing Care Quality, 24*(1), 33–41.

Rogers, E. M. (2010). *Diffusion of innovations.* Simon and Schuster.

Ross, A. G., & Morris, P. E. (2010). Safety and barriers to care. *Critical Care Nurse, 30*(2), S11–S13.

Rubenstein, L. Z. (2006). Falls in older people: epidemiology, risk factors and strategies for prevention. *Age and Ageing, 35*(Suppl. 2), ii37–ii41.

Rutledge, D. N., & Donaldson, N. E. (1995). Building organizational capacity to engage in research utilization. *Journal of Nursing Administration, 25*(10), 12–16.

Rutledge, D. N., et al. (1996). Use of research-based practices by oncology staff nurses. *Oncology Nursing Forum, 23*(8), 1235–1244.

Shever, L. L., et al. (2011). Fall prevention practices in adult medical-surgical nursing units described by nurse managers. *Western Journal of Nursing Research, 33*(3), 385–397.

Shmueli, T., et al. (2014). Reporting adverse events at geriatric facilities: categorization by type of adverse event and function of reporting personnel. *International Journal of Health Care Quality Assurance, 27*(2), 91–98.

SPSS (1999). *SPSS Base 10.0 for Windows User's Guide.* Chicago, IL: SPSS, Inc.

Stetler, C. B., et al. (2009). Institutionalizing evidence-based practice: an organizational case study using a model of strategic change. *Implementation Science, 4,* 78.

Tinetti, M. E. (2003). Preventing falls in elderly persons. *New England Journal of Medicine, 348*(1), 42–49.

Tinetti, M. E., & Kumar, C. (2010). The patient who falls: "it's always a trade-off". *JAMA, 303*(3), 258–266.

Titler, M. G. (2010). Translation science and context. *Research and Theory for Nursing Practice, 24*(1), 35–55.

Titler, M. G., & Everett, L. Q. (2001). Translating research into practice. Considerations for critical care investigators. *Critical Care Nursing Clinics of North America, 13*(4), 587–604.

Titler, M. G., et al. (2009). Translating research into practice intervention improves management of acute pain in older hip fracture patients. *Health Services Research, 44*(1), 264–287.

Titler, M. G., et al. (2011). Factors associated with falls during hospitalization in an older adult population. *Research and Theory for Nursing Practice, 25*(2), 127–148.

Tucker, D., Molsberger, S. C., & Clark, A. (2004). Walking for wellness: a collaborative program to maintain mobility in hospitalized older adults. *Geriatric Nursing, 25*(4), 242–245.

Tzeng, H. M. (2011). A feasibility study of providing folding commode chairs in patient bathrooms to reduce toileting-related falls in an adult acute medical-surgical unit. *Journal of Nursing Care Quality, 26*(1), 61–68.

Vaughn, T. E., et al. (2002). Organizational predictors of adherence to ambulatory care screening guidelines. *Medical Care, 40*(12), 1172–1185.

Woodard, J. L. (2009). Effects of rounding on patient satisfaction and patient safety on a medical-surgical unit. *Clinical nurse specialist, 23*(4), 200–206.

BRIEF REPORT

Improving Exercise Prescribing in a Rural New England Free Clinic

Patricia Thompson Leavitt, DNP, FNP

ABSTRACT

This quality improvement project was undertaken to improve exercise prescribing frequency and quality in a rural New England free clinic. Prescribing guidelines from the American College of Sports Medicine and the American Academy of Family Physicians were used. Following a provider education program and workgroup-implemented documentation changes, overall exercise prescription frequency increased significantly from 34.6% in the pre-intervention group to 65.0% in the post-intervention group ($P < .05$). The use of some prescription elements (frequency, intensity, and timing) improved significantly ($P < .05$). Further study from the patient perspective is warranted.

Keywords: exercise prescription, FITT-PRO mnemonic, free clinic, inactivity, quality improvement, rural
© 2016 Elsevier Inc. All rights reserved.

INTRODUCTION

Background Knowledge

The World Health Organization (WHO) identifies inactivity as the fourth leading cause of mortality, accounting for 6% of deaths worldwide.[1] This places inactivity behind only high blood pressure (13%) and tobacco use (9%) as causative factors for mortality and is equal to high blood glucose (6%). Although obesity logically follows from a sedentary lifestyle, inactivity is a risk factor for abdominal adiposity and coronary heart disease independent of body mass index (BMI).[2]

Multiple factors and antecedents contribute to inactivity, including lack of time or motivation, increasing use of technology for work and recreation, and lack of knowledge.[3] For lower income persons, barriers to daily exercise exist in terms of money, time, and access to exercise equipment, yet most intervention studies have not accessed disadvantaged populations.[4,5] Barriers to exercise notwithstanding, research findings suggest that advice from respected health care professionals can have a positive impact on exercise rates.[6,7]

Despite evidence supporting the benefits of exercise, providers use exercise prescribing on a limited basis. In 2010, only 9.2% of provider office visits in the United States included counseling patients to participate in regular physical activity.[8] One reason for providers' failure to prescribe is lack of time,

even when structured programs are in place to assure consistency and follow-up.[9-12] Provider knowledge deficits about the specifics of exercise prescribing and confidence in prescribing abilities also play a role.[13]

Providers are most adept at utilizing the first 2 elements of the "Ask-Advise-Agree-Assist-Arrange" model used for change coaching[12]; they are not as comfortable at assessing readiness to change ("Agree") or providing follow-up ("Assist" and "Arrange"). Ackermann et al[14] found that providers were more likely to prescribe exercise for patients who were in the contemplation stage of change. In addition, providers are generally more inclined to target activity prescribing for obese individuals or those suffering from chronic disease.[8,15]

The American College of Sports Medicine (ACSM) has published recommendations for exercise prescribing in all populations.[6] The prescribing mnemonic "FITT-PRO" (Frequency, Intensity, Type, Time, and PROgression), as described by the American Academy of Family Physicians guideline, instructs the provider to consider each type of exercise (aerobic or endurance, flexibility, strengthening, and balance) and develop a prescription.[16] For example, a provider may create a prescription that reads: "Aerobic activity such as walking (Type), daily (Frequency) for 30 minutes per day (Timing). Exercise hard enough so that you cannot sing but are still able to talk (Intensity). Start

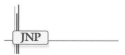

with 10 minutes per day as tolerated; increase by 5 minutes every 3 days until you reach 30 minutes daily" (Progression).

Local Problem

As part of ongoing quality improvement (QI) efforts before this project, gaps were identified in addressing leisure time physical activity with each patient. The Leavitt's Mill Free Health Center (LMFHC) patient baseline activity rates (36%) and documentation of provider exercise prescribing (32%) were comparable to national statistics for similar populations (N = 50).[8,17]

Intended Improvement

The aim of this QI project was to improve exercise prescribing frequency and improve exercise prescribing quality at LMFHC by implementing the ACSM exercise prescribing guidelines and the prescribing mnemonic FITT-PRO from the American Academy of Family Physicians.[6,16] The target for improvement was to double exercise prescribing rates from baseline.

METHODS

Ethical Issues

Approval for this project was granted by the institutional review board of Simmons College and the board of directors of the LMFHC. Potential bias by the project investigator, who also served as the health center's director, was safeguarded by the use of graduate assistants who managed all primary data and de-identified data before analysis.

Setting

The setting for this project, LMFHC, is a nurse-managed, rural free clinic located in southern Maine. With an active patient roster of 250, LMFHC has served over 1,700 patients in its 12-year history. The majority of patients are working adults living at or below 250% of the federal poverty level. Six part-time volunteer primary care providers and 3 part-time nursing support staff form the patient care team. Patient care documentation is paper-based, with selected patient statistics and visit data maintained in an encrypted database.

Planning the Intervention

Needs assessment interviews and educational session. After receiving informed consent, clinic staff (n = 9) were interviewed to ascertain their comfort and knowledge about exercise prescribing and advising. The data from these interviews formed the basis of the 90-minute educational intervention. The educational session was provided, which included a brief overview of current evidence regarding exercise benefits and the principles of exercise prescribing using the ACSM exercise prescribing guidelines, and the FITT-PRO mnemonic.[6,16] Specific information was offered regarding the particular absolute and relative contraindications to an exercise prescription. Strategies for incorporating the FITT-PRO elements of a complete exercise prescription were presented with an emphasis on timing and progression, components unfamiliar to this group of providers.

QI workgroup. Monthly staff meeting/QI workgroups began in the first month of the project and continued throughout the 7 months of the project. The focus of the staff QI workgroups involved systems improvements such as documentation tools, patient resources, and workflow changes. Standardized exercise prescription forms (basic and advanced) were adopted from the Veterans Administration's MOVE! website.[18] The forms were paper-based using a check-box format for "Frequency, Intensity, and Timing" and requiring free text entry for "Type and Progression." Initially, the forms were made available for use in a central cabinet, but the QI group soon recommended they be placed on the chart to cue providers at the annual wellness visit.

Data Collection and Analysis

Patient records were audited using a convenience sampling method. Records of the most recently occurring history and physical were audited pre-intervention (n = 52) and post-intervention (n = 42). Chart audit data elements included: patient age and gender; body mass index (BMI); chronic illnesses/comorbidities; baseline leisure time physical activity; and documentation of exercise prescribing and inclusion of the FITT-PRO elements. Data from chart audits were analyzed using chi-square testing to detect differences.

OUTCOMES

Overall, there were no significant differences ($P < .05$) in the demographic profiles of the pre- and post-intervention audited charts. Achievement of practice improvement goals was variable. Overall, the frequency of provider exercise prescribing closely approached the target improvement goal, with the overall frequency of prescribing improved from the previous level of 34.6% to 65.0% ($\chi^2 = 8.365$, $P = .004$).

Documentation of all 5 of the FITT-PRO elements as targeted in the project goals did not improve as dramatically. Statistically significant ($P < .05$) improvements were gained in frequency, intensity, and time. However, the inclusion of specific exercise and progression remained at low levels. Documentation of specific exercise type deteriorated and there was no improvement in the use of progression in exercise prescription from pre-intervention to post-intervention.

No significant differences in exercise prescribing frequency in the post-intervention group were noted when correlated with age, BMI, or chronic illness burden. An increase in prescriptions for female patients was noted, but this could be correlated with providers who only have women in their panel.

DISCUSSION

The relative success of this quality improvement project adds some practice-based evidence to knowledge about improving exercise prescribing in a primary care environment.

Clinic system changes in this project included the revision of the discharge form to emphasize healthy lifestyles and the implementation of the exercise prescription forms. Overall, the use of the forms improved adherence with guideline recommendations for documentation of recommended exercise frequency, intensity, and time (duration), but fell short in capturing discussions about exercise types and progression of the exercise plan. One factor that likely contributed to this discrepancy was the open-ended nature of the Type and PROgression sections of the form, as compared with the forced-choice check-boxes supplied for the FIT section of the form.

Since the conclusion of this project, the exercise prescription forms have been revised to simplify the process. The basic and advanced forms were collapsed to one "Physical Activity Prescription" form (see Figure). Checkboxes were inserted to clarify the prescription elements of type and progression. This QI change has not yet been studied formally but has met with informal approval from provider and staff members.

The QI workgroup successfully provided oversight for the project. For example, the workgroup recognized early in the improvement process that cueing the prescribers by placing the prescription form on the chart for completion increased the likelihood of exercise prescriptions being written as part of the encounter. The use of physical and visual cues to change human behavior, whether directly for patients or in terms of provider behavior, has been supported in a number of studies.[19-21]

The deep commitment of the staff, their caring, and immersion in the needs of the population may

Figure. Physical Activity Prescription form.

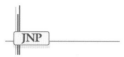

contribute to the discrepancy of the results of this project in comparison to other studies. These providers did not appear to selectively prescribe exercise to those with higher BMI, lower or higher chronic disease burden, or lower or higher pre-prescription activity levels, in contrast to earlier research.[15]

Limitations

This project had a number of limitations. Due to time constraints and low clinic volume, the chart audit was small. The project design included only 1 formal measurement of change. Ideally, several Plan-Do-Study-Act (PDSA) cycles should be included to provide incremental measurement of organizational change.[22]

As this was a provider-based project, patients were only indirectly involved. Ideally, patients would participate in the design of the intervention. Further, the project design did not include gathering data to ascertain patients' adherence to the exercise prescription.

Implications

The results of this project form a practical framework for the implementation of basic clinic support items, which can improve exercise prescribing practices. Although many primary care practices do not rely on paper-and-pencil forms, the revised exercise prescription template is well suited to the electronic environment by the use of check-boxes. Few nurse practitioners report that they utilize clinical guidelines in practice,[23] but implementation of easy-to-follow templated guidelines that could be embedded into an electronic medical record system could encourage adoption of the exercise prescribing guideline.

This project reinforces the value of time spent working with patients on encouraging lifestyle changes that are low cost and effective. By providing evidence of the success of such a project, and its minimal impact on the cost of care, policymakers can be further encouraged to support and incentivize primary care providers' inclusion of health promotion activities.

The increase in exercise prescribing at LMFHC was an encouraging finding. However, patient-centered research is needed to assess the impact exercise prescription and dispensing of the printed materials had upon patient readiness to exercise or actual activity levels. An area of future research should include measurement of patient change in all FITT-PRO elements via chart audits, focus group interviews, or surveys.

Most studies have concluded that primary care interventions involving intensive follow-up, personal attention, and social interaction are important factors in promoting positive changes in physical activity levels among community-dwelling adults.[24] Some studies have shown that the use of technology, such as text messaging, has potential as an adjunct in improving exercise rates.[25,26] It would be useful to know patients' perceptions regarding healthy lifestyle adoption and what additional interventions are warranted to improve physical activity levels in this population.

CONCLUSION

This small-scale, reproducible QI project resulted in a positive practice change through implementation of national guidelines for exercise prescribing in a primary care environment. Engaging patients to improve physical activity levels offers numerous patient health benefits and aligns philosophically with nurse practitioner practice. The FITT-PRO exercise prescription model provides a practical approach to brief intervention in a primary care environment. JNP

References

1. World Health Organization. Facts on physical activity. http://www.who.int/features/factfiles/physical_activity/facts/en/. Accessed September 2016.
2. Chomistek AK, Henschel B, Eliassen AH, Mukamal KJ, Rimm EB. frequency, type, and volume of leisure-time physical activity and risk of coronary heart disease in young women. *Circulation.* 2016;134:290-299.
3. Knight JA. Physical inactivity: associated diseases and disorders. *Ann Clin Lab Sci.* 2012;42(3):320-337.
4. Cleland V, Grenados A, Crawford D, Winzenberg T, Ball K. Effectiveness of interventions to promote physical activity among socioeconomically disadvantaged women: a systematic review and meta-analysis. *Obes Rev.* 2013;14:197-212. http://dx.doi.org/10.1111/j.1467-789X.2012.01058.x.
5. Orzeck KM, Vivian J, Torres CH, Armin J, Shaw SJ. Diet and exercise adherence and practices among medically underserved patients with chronic disease: variation across four ethnic groups. *Health Educ Behav.* 2012;40(1):56-66. http://dx.doi.org/10.1177/1090198112436970.
6. Garber CE, Blissmer B, Deschenes MR, et al. American College of Sports Medicine position stand. Quantity and quality of exercise for developing and maintaining cardiorespiratory, musculoskeletal, and neuromotor fitness in apparently healthy adults: guidance for prescribing exercise. *Med Sci Sports Exerc.* 2011;43(7):1334-1359. http://dx.doi.org/10.1249/MSS.0b013e318213fefb.
7. Orrow G, Kinmonth AL, Sanderson S, Sutton S. Effectiveness of physical activity promotion based in primary care: systematic review and meta-analysis of randomised controlled trials. *BMJ.* 2012;344:e1389. http://dx.doi.org/10.1136/bmj.e13892012.
8. Office of Disease Prevention and Health Promotion. Healthy People 2020. https://www.healthypeople.gov/2020/data-search/Search-the-Data#objid=5056/. Accessed September 2016.
9. Lobelo F, Stoutenberg M, Hutber A. The exercise is medicine global health initiative: a 2014 update. *Br J Sports Med.* 2014;48:1627-1633. http://dx.doi.org/10.1136/bjsports-2013-093080.

10. Carroll JK, Winters PC, Sanders MR, Decker F, Ngo T, Sciamanna CN. Clinician-targeted intervention and patient-reported counseling on physical activity. *Prev Chron Dis.* 2014;11:130302. doi, http://dx.doi.org/10.5888/pcd11.130302.

11. Goodman C, Davies SL, Dinan S, Tai SS, Iliffe S. Activity promotion for community-dwelling older people: a survey of the contribution of primary care nurses. *Br J Commun Nurs.* 2011;16(1):12-17.

12. Carroll JK. Evaluation of physical activity counseling in primary care using direct observation of the 5As. *Ann Fam Med.* 2011;9:416-422. http://dx.doi.org/10.1370/afm.1299.

13. Dacey M, Arnstein F, Kennedy MA, Wolfe J, Phillips E. The impact of lifestyle medicine continuing education on provider knowledge, attitudes, and counseling behaviors. *Med Teacher.* 2013;35(5):e1149-e1156. http://dx.doi.org/10.3109/0142159X.2012.733459.

14. Ackermann RT, Deyo RA, LoGerfo JP. Prompting primary providers to increase community exercise referrals for older adults: a randomized trial. *J Am Geriatr Soc.* 2005;53(2):283-289. http://dx.doi.org/10.1111/j.1532-5415.2005.53115.x.

15. Patel A, Schofield GM, Kolt GS, Keogh JWL. General practitioners' views and experiences of counselling for physical activity through the New Zealand Green Prescription program. *BMC Fam Pract.* 2011;12:119-119. http://dx.doi.org/10.1186/1471-2296-12-119.

16. McDermott AY, Mernitz H. Exercise and older patients: prescribing guidelines. *Am Fam Phys.* 2006;74(3):437-444.

17. National Center for Health Statistics. Lack of leisure-time physical activity: adults. Health Indicators Warehouse. http://www.healthindicators.gov/Indicators/Leisure-time-physical-activity-none-percent_1313/Profile/Data. Accessed November 18, 2012.

18. Veterans Administration MOVE! Reference tools. http://www.move.va.gov/ReferenceTools.asp#MOVE!23. Accessed September 2016.

19. Bellicha A, Kieusseian A, Fontvieille AM, et al. A multistage controlled intervention to increase stair climbing at work: effectiveness and process evaluation. *Int J Behav Nutr Phys Activ.* 2016;13:47. http://dx.doi.org/10.1186/s12966-016-0371-0.

20. Marteau TM, Hollands GJ, Fletcher PC. Changing human behavior to prevent disease: the importance of targeting automatic processes. *Science.* 2012;337(6101):1492-1495. http://dx.doi.org/10.1126/science.1226918.

21. Rozin P, Scott S, Dingley M, Urbanek JK, Jiang H, Kaltenbach M. Nudge to nobesity I: Minor changes in accessibility decrease food intake. *Judgm Decis Mak.* 2011;6(4):323-332.

22. Langley G, Moen R, Nolan K, Nolan T, Norman C, Provost L. *The Improvement Guide: A Practical Approach to Enhancing Organizational Performance. 2nd ed.* San Francisco: Jossey-Bass; 2009.

23. Facchiano L, Snyder CH. Evidence-based practice for the busy nurse practitioner: Part one: Relevance to clinical practice and clinical inquiry process. *J Am Acad Nurse Pract.* 2012;24:579-586. http://dx.doi.org/10.1111/j.1745-7599.2012.00748.x.

24. Neidrick TJ, Fick DM, Loeb SJ. Physical activity promotion in primary care targeting the older adult. *J Am Acad Nurse Pract.* 2012;24(7):405-416. http://dx.doi.org/10.1111/j.1745-7599.2012.00703.x.

25. Fjeldsoe BS, Miller YD, Graves N, Barnett A, Marshall AL. Randomized controlled trial of an improved version of MobileMums, an intervention for increasing physical activity in women with young children. *Ann Behav Med.* 2015;49:487-499. http://dx.doi.org/10.1007/s12160-014-9675-y.

26. Buchholz SW, Wilbur J, Ingram D, Fogg L. Physical activity text messaging interventions in adults: a systematic review. *Worldviews Evidence-Based Nurs.* 2013;10(3):163-173.

Patricia Thompson Leavitt, DNP, FNP, is executive director of the Leavitt's Mill Free Health Center in Bar Mills, ME, and an assistant professor at the University of Southern Maine School of Nursing in Portland. She can be reached at patricia.thompsonleavitt@maine.edu. *The author gratefully acknowledges the contribution of the University of Southern Maine's Graduate Assistant Program for providing funds to support 2 graduate assistants for the duration of this project. In compliance with national ethical guidelines, the author reports no relationships with business or industry that would pose a conflict of interest.*

1555-4155/16/$ see front matter
© 2016 Elsevier Inc. All rights reserved.
http://dx.doi.org/10.1016/j.nurpra.2016.09.014

ARTICLE IN PRESS

YJPDN-01532; No of Pages 4

Journal of Pediatric Nursing xxx (2017) xxx–xxx

Contents lists available at ScienceDirect

Journal of Pediatric Nursing

SPN Department

Application of the EBP Process: Maximizing Lactation Support with Minimal Education☆,☆☆

Frances M. Ullman, Ullman BSN, RN, IBCLC, RLC [b], MaryDee Fisher, DNP, RN, CPN [a,*]

[a] Chatham University, Pittsburgh, PA
[b] Children's Hospital of Pittsburgh of UPMC, United States

Background

The many advantages to providing breast milk instead of engineered infant formula for both the medically fragile and healthy term infant are well documented (Lawrence & Lawrence, 2016; Mcguire, 2011). Historically, educational efforts within neonatal intensive care units (NICUs) focused on critical diseases and conditions, as well as the highly technological management of fragile neonates. The International push to promote both the value and superiority of breast milk for infant feeding began over 3 decades ago (WHO, 1981). Early in the 21st century, the Joint Commission's Perinatal Care core measure set was adopted. It requires every birth hospital to track and then improve exclusive breastfeeding rates of the mother/baby couplet, thereby promoting population health (JCAHO, 2013). The 2011 U.S. Surgeon General's Call to Action emphasized the need for all healthcare professionals to have meaningful, influential interactions with the breastfeeding family. In addition, the health care communities' fundamental responsibilities to increase breastfeeding initiation and duration rates among all couplets were detailed (Mcguire, 2011). The directive was to be accomplished through education provided for all health care personnel that have contact with pregnant and post-partum women.

Among the educational topics assigned were breastfeeding practices and related short-term and long-term benefits (American Academy of Pediatrics, 2012). To accomplish this goal required changes in the academic curriculum, as well as clinical expectations and experiences for students and continuing education programs for active health care providers. The push to promote breastfeeding and staff education continues as core requirements as evidenced by the multiple federal and state sponsored programs (American Academy of Pediatrics, 2012). These widespread efforts are targeted to impact present clinical practices and enrich overall population health levels throughout society.

Identified benefits of human breast milk feeding include decreased rates of infections, gastrointestinal illness, childhood obesity, and juvenile diabetes (American Academy of Pediatrics, 2012). Positive effects have also been found to reach well into middle age for both mother and baby, including decreased incidences of multiple sclerosis, insulin and non-insulin-dependent diabetes, as well as several types of cancer (American Academy of Pediatrics, 2012). In addition, fragile infants in the NICU have the most to gain from the numerous health benefits that have been attributed to human breast milk feedings including enhanced resistance to infections.

The Question

The fundamental yet all-encompassing question for nurse educators in the NICU is: What is the most appropriate way to provide the education and clinical skills to equip nurses to best teach and promote breastfeeding to all mother-infant couplets?

Evidence-Based Practice Project

It was determined that an evidence-based practice (EBP) project would provide the most helpful information to guide nurse educators in constructing a focused program. The goal of this approach was to maximize the research findings that outline the positive effects of enhanced breastfeeding and support acquisition of clinical skills and practices to support the breastfeeding couplet, while minimizing the clinicians' time away from the bedside.

Literature Review

The first step of any EBP project is to gather and appraise available literature and relevant data from other practice sites. A literature search in late 2011 was completed using CINAHL and PubMed

---

☆ The mission of the Society of Pediatric Nurses is to support its members in their practice. One means of accomplishing this mission is to keep membership informed of innovative initiatives involving the board, committees, and members that promote research, clinical practice, education, and advocacy within the larger pediatric healthcare community. This department serves that purpose.

☆☆ Editor's Note: The following manuscript is another in our series of novice manuscripts. The authors worked with Dr. Sandy Mott and Dr. Nancy Blake over the past 9 months to craft the initial submission into one that demonstrates quality, rigor and logic in presentation. Among the lessons learned in writing is that writing takes time, multiple editing, and numerous iterations. Each rewrite makes the final manuscript better. SPN is thrilled with the response to this initiative, as there are always multiple manuscripts in process. Our purpose is to provide feedback that is instructive and supportive and encourages the membership to share their clinical inquiry experiences. The nurses that are responsible for patient care ask the most important questions. Sharing your questions and search for information benefits others and advance the science of nursing. Asking questions promotes learning and benefits patients, their families, and the nurses that provide care. The SPN Department pages in the journal are a mechanism for staying informed, sharing insights, and interacting with peers.

* Corresponding author: MaryDee Fisher, DNP, RN, CPN.
E-mail address: mfisher@Chatham.edu (M. Fisher).

http://dx.doi.org/10.1016/j.pedn.2017.01.003
0882-5963/© 2017 Elsevier Inc. All rights reserved.

ARTICLE IN PRESS

2   F.M. Ullman, M. Fisher Journal of Pediatric Nursing xxx (2017) xxx–xxx

databases. Key words included breastfeeding, lactation, education, and NICU nurses. Twenty-five articles were located, and 16 were subsequently deemed potentially related to this project and were reviewed. In preparation for this manuscript submission, an updated literature search was completed in 2016, so that no key articles and/or evidence were overlooked.

NICU nurses entrusted to care for the most vulnerable infants traditionally receive little education beyond their pre-licensure academic programs (Cricco-Lizza, 2009; Hellings & Howe, 2004). Subsequently, NICU nurses often lack sufficient updated information, experience and commitment to properly assist the breastfeeding couplet. As reported by Spatz, two of the three children's hospitals examined offered only basic annual competency demonstrations as the sole means for nursing staff education about breast feeding (2005). Additionally, clinical inquiry has noted that NICU nurses tend to have less supportive attitudes toward breastfeeding (BF), when compared to their pediatric and obstetric nurse counterparts (Sigman-Grant & Kim, 2016; Spear, 2004). This lack of on-going education and prior experience can readily contribute to NICU nurses conveying misinformation to parents or being nominally supportive about the breastfeeding process.

Overall, the healthcare industry aims to maximize resources while at the same time minimize costs; therefore, systems are hesitant to add new programs. All too often this challenge results in staff and parents having limited or no access to qualified lactation professionals despite the Surgeon General's directive. The concern in an urban tertiary level 3+ NICU, which is one not associated with an obstetrical unit was that insufficient lactation support personnel may compromise the ability to meet patient care demands for quality.

Standardized formal lactation education and support programs have been developed and are available for use by request. The programs include a broad and extensive education focus and vary in length from 8 to 40 hours. Most of them include a basic didactic component and demonstration that require numerous nursing hours away from bedside patient care. Some of these programs offer continuing nursing education credits or award certificates of completion (Spatz, 2005).

There were two potential consequences of enhanced breastfeeding education of NICU nurses evident in the literature. First, the likelihood that with an increased knowledge base, the NICU bedside nurse would approach breastfeeding with a more informed and supportive attitude was recognized as a benefit (Spear, 2004). Second, once the nurse had the appropriate knowledge and tools to embrace the documented benefits of breastfeeding practice, the behaviors become enmeshed into routine standards of care. The nurses' efforts become directly focused on assisting and properly supporting the breastfeeding couplet. The increase in support from bedside nurses led to increased success for overall breastfeeding practices, as nurses were able to properly demonstrate positioning techniques after acquiring the knowledge and learned skill associated with the breastfeeding process (Benner, 1984). With this increased support, parents had a more overall satisfying experience in the NICU (Spatz, 2005).

The responsibility to provide staff education tends to rest with hospitals that are already faced with the challenge of providing adequate staffing in tertiary level 3+ NICUs. These are the same NICUs that are experiencing dwindling staffing resources as noted above. The new graduate nurse traditionally has received limited lactation education as evidenced by the NCLEX–RN test plan for examination (National Council of State Board of Nursing, 2016). Nevertheless, the one common denominator, routinely available for a new mother requiring lactation support, remains the bedside nurse. The bedside nurse therefore needs to be knowledgeable and understand the benefits, mechanisms, and immediate and long-term effects of breastfeeding practices. In addition to providing knowledge that a mother may need for lactation success, the nurses' support or lack thereof, can impact a mother's ultimate determination to succeed at breastfeeding. In the primary author's experience as a Certified Lactation Consultant, it is not uncommon for mothers to identify the attitude of healthcare workers toward their breastfeeding efforts as a reason they quit or continue to breastfeed.

Implementation

After the review of literature, the International Board Certified Lactation Consultant, in conjunction with a fellowship team, evaluated the appropriateness and effectiveness of various education curriculums available. The group determined the two most important factors affecting the implementation and success of a breastfeeding program were the education content and support for staff to have time off of the unit. To minimize the effect on bedside unit staffing, the education sessions were limited to 2 hours. This focused the content of education to the information most beneficial at the bedside, clinician to breastfeeding couplet. Due to staffing constraints, bedside nurses needed to use non-scheduled hours to attend these valuable educational offerings. Thus, the decision was made to offer the breastfeeding education as a voluntary program. To partially compensate the nurses for time in attendance, Continuing Nursing Education (CNE) contact hours were awarded for the successful completion of the breastfeeding program. Each participant also received a recognition pin to wear with the hospital ID badge. The unit directors were informed who participated and completed the program so these clinicians would receive credit at the time of their yearly personal evaluation.

This project for staff education was submitted and approved by the internal Quality Review Committee. The initial implementation of the program yielded a total of 22 nurses who completed two 1-hour sessions. This number represents 17% of the total NICU bedside nursing staff. The lecture and demonstration content during the first education hour included the medical benefits of breastfeeding, anatomy and physiology, proper nipple shield application, breast pump usage, and breast milk storage. Participants were afforded the opportunity of return demonstration for assembly and cleaning of the breast pump units. The second hour addressed frequently encountered breastfeeding issues such as sore nipples, low milk supply, and the demonstration of basic latch support holding practices. Multiple opportunities to attend each of the 1-hour sessions were offered, including before and after a variety of shifts. This approach provided nurses the flexibility to choose the best educational option to support their lifestyle. These multiple educational sessions continue to be offered routinely at our tertiary NICU 3+ level hospital.

Program Evaluation

In order to measure the impact of the EBP project, evaluation tools were necessary. The primary author initially crafted two evaluation tools. They were then reviewed and further revised by the fellowship group. The group included eight other nurses whose specialty areas of practice included the care of the neonate, infant, and child populations. An advanced practice nurse, qualified to conduct the fellowship program, oversaw the process of tool development as well as reviewed the tools for content reliability. A statistician reviewed the proposed measurement tools and provided guidance for the design structure of the two tools.

The multiple-choice knowledge evaluation tool consisted of five questions, each with six options of which only three of the options were correct. The directions stated to choose all the correct responses for each of the questions. The second evaluation tool was a seven-point Likert scale self-evaluation of the nurse's comfort level in the following five areas: likely to help a mother with breastfeeding issues, confident to provide accurate information to breastfeeding mothers, initiate conversation about breastfeeding with the mother of a hospitalized baby, confident to provide breast pump use directions, and likely to help fellow staff with a breastfeeding issue that patient's mother is experiencing.

Please cite this article as: Ullman, F.M., & Fisher, M., Application of the EBP Process: Maximizing Lactation Support with Minimal Education, Journal of Pediatric Nursing (2017), http://dx.doi.org/10.1016/j.pedn.2017.01.003

ARTICLE IN PRESS

F.M. Ullman, M. Fisher Journal of Pediatric Nursing xxx (2017) xxx–xxx   3

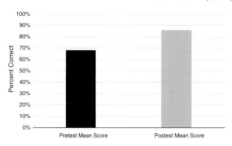

Figure 1. Mean RN Knowledge: Pre and Post Test Percent Scores.

there was an increased frequency in initiation of appropriate interventions by the bedside nurse, prior to an official consult for the lactation professional. Second, the staff sought lactation resources and information more readily than previously. Third, parents shared more positive comments regarding lactation support in follow-up phone calls. Although there was no significant change in the Press Ganey results, the leadership and staff observed a clinically significant change in attitude and behavior. And finally, the staff asked for more education sessions to be provided to further enhance their knowledge base and support practice changes.

Dissemination and Follow-Up

The limited focus and education provided in this program does not replace qualified lactation professionals, nor is it meant to undermine the value of comprehensive educational programs. It is unrealistic and not acceptable to expect under educated bedside professionals to provide the critically ill neonate and family with supportive education for breastfeeding practices. The value of this EBP focused program, which can be replicated in other centers, demonstrated that an investment of time, along with focused resources and receptivity, has the potential to improve the quality, access, and effectiveness of breastfeeding practices for in-patient care. Providing lactation information and skills to the nurse at the bedside has the potential to multiply and strengthen the resources available to the breastfeeding family, increase the incidence of breastfeeding practices and positively affect long-term outcomes.

The results of this program have been presented both locally and nationally in poster as well as podium formats. Clearly, supporting breastfeeding practices has far reaching implications for mothers and infants alike. The breastfeeding program continues to be offered as a voluntary education opportunity for NICU staff. Staff members in the NICU continue to have opportunities to earn CNE credit and be awarded recognition pins. The program is being incorporated into a three-tiered lactation support program, and is the initial step in lactation support for all mothers in this level 3+ NICU. The program demonstrated how a clinical question could indeed inform and change practice. This EBP project incorporated sound research evidence and family's preferences

Staff scores on both posttest measures increased overall. Participating staff completed pre (N = 24) and post (N = 22) knowledge tests. Their scores revealed an increase of 17.7 percent on overall paired *t* test scores (Figure 1). Results for the self-evaluation of perceptions of their level of comfort also revealed statistical significance from a paired t test analysis, with differences in means significant in all five questions with p values <0.05 (Figure 2).

Finally, families' perceived experience was quantified by tracking the aggregated results of a parental satisfaction survey. Press Ganey© Inpatient Pediatric Survey scores were collected and compared for the 3 months before as well as the 3 months after the breastfeeding educational sessions. The question "Nursing Support: Breastfeeding" showed no significant score differences between pre and post program implementation. Pre-implementation Press Ganey scores of 73 parents revealed a 93% average score. Post-implementation Press Ganey scores of 60 parents revealed a 92.5% average score on this same question. It is possible that the Press Ganey question identified to measure outcomes is more global in nature and is not specific enough to measure the actual educational impact of this EBP project, as was initially anticipated.

Empirically, there were several clinically significant changes noted by both the lactation consultant and the NICU clinical leaders. First,

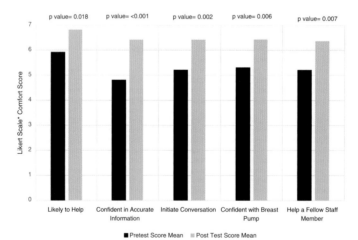

*Seven point Likert scale values ranged from 1-not at all likely to 4-neutral to 7-extremely likely

Figure 2. Mean RN Perceptions of Comfort Levels: Pre and Post Likert Scores.

Please cite this article as: Ullman, F.M., & Fisher, M., Application of the EBP Process: Maximizing Lactation Support with Minimal Education, *Journal of Pediatric Nursing* (2017), http://dx.doi.org/10.1016/j.pedn.2017.01.003

ARTICLE IN PRESS

4 F.M. Ullman, M. Fisher Journal of Pediatric Nursing xxx (2017) xxx–xxx

which are intrinsic within the definition of EBP, as well as clinicians' commitment to improved patient care. EBP provides the data that supports change and evidence to sustainable outcomes. The results of this project have the potential to positively impact the health of current and future generations.

References

American Academy of Pediatrics (2012). Policy statement breastfeeding and the use of human milk. *Pediatrics, 129*(3), 827–841. http://dx.doi.org/10.1542/peds.2011-3552.

Benner, P. (1984). *From novice to expert: excellence and power in clinical nursing practice.* Menlo Park, CA: Addison-Wesley.

Cricco-Lizza, R. (2009). Formative infant feeding experiences and education of NICU nurses. *The American Journal of Maternal/Child Nursing, 34*(4), 236–242. http://dx.doi.org/10.1097/01.nmc.0000357916.33476.a3.

Hellings, P., & Howe, C. (2004). Breastfeeding knowledge and practice of pediatric nurse practitioners. *Journal of Pediatric Health Care, 18*(1), 8–14. http://dx.doi.org/10.1016/s0891-5245(03)00108-1.

Joint Commission on Accreditation of Hospitals [JCAHO] (2013). Perinatal care: exclusive breast milk feeding. Retrieved 7/9/16 from https://manual.jointcommission.org/releases/TJC2015B2/DataElem0273.html

Lawrence, R., & Lawrence, R. (2016). *The revolution of infant feeding – in breastfeeding: a guide for the medical profession* (8th ed.). Philadelphia, PA: Mosby.

Mcguire, S. (2011). U.S. Dept. of health and human services. The surgeon General's call to action to support breastfeeding. *Advances in Nutrition: An International Review Journal, 2*(6), 523–524. http://dx.doi.org/10.3945/an.111.000968.

National Council of State Board of Nursing (2016). NCLEX-RN® examination test plan for the National Council Licensure Examination for registered nurses. Retrieved from https://www.ncsbn.org/RN_Test_Plan_2016_Final.pdf

Sigman-Grant, M., & Kim, Y. (2016). Breastfeeding knowledge and attitudes of Nevada health care professionals remain virtually unchanged over 10 Years. *Journal of Human Lactation, 32*(2), 350–354. http://dx.doi.org/10.1177/0890334415609916.

Spatz, D. L. (2005). Report of a staff program to promote and support breastfeeding in the Care of Vulnerable Infants at a Children's hospital. *Journal of Perinatal Education, 14*(1), 30–38. http://dx.doi.org/10.1624/105812405x23630.

Spear, H. J. (2004). Nurses' attitudes, knowledge, and beliefs related to the promotion of breastfeeding among women who bear children during adolescence. *Journal of Pediatric Nursing, 19*(3), 176–183. http://dx.doi.org/10.1016/j.pedn.2004.01.006.

World Health Organization (1981). *International code of Marketing of Breast-Milk Substitutes.* Geneva: World Health Organization.

Normothermia for NeuroProtection
It's Hot to Be Cool

Juliet G. Beniga, BSN, RN, CNRN, CCRN[a,*],
Katherine G. Johnson, MS, RN, APRN, CCRN, CNRN, CNS-BC[b],
Debra D. Mark, PhD, RN[c]

KEYWORDS

- Normothermia • NeuroProtection • Evidence • Brain injury

KEY POINTS

- Nurses are essential in the care of individuals with neurologic injury. Severe traumatic brain injury and stroke are major health problems in the United States and a common cause of disability and death.
- Fever is a significant contributor to secondary brain insult and management is a challenge for the neurocritical care team.
- The absence of standardized guidelines likely contributes to poor surveillance and under-treatment of increased temperature.

INTRODUCTION

Nurses are essential in the care of individuals with neurologic injury. Severe traumatic brain injury (TBI) and stroke are major health problems in the United States and a common cause of disability and death. In 2003, the US Centers for Disease Control and Prevention estimated that 1.5 million people sustain a TBI each year, and approximately 50,000 people die, accounting for a mortality of about 30%. At least 5.3 million Americans, have long-term needs for assistance to perform activities of daily living because of TBI-related cognitive, physical, and psychological disabilities. The direct cost of acute care, the loss of potential income, the ongoing costs of rehabilitation, and the indirect costs to the caregivers are substantial and at times not measurable.[1]

Funding Source: The Queen's Medical Center and University of Hawaii School of Nursing & Dental Hygiene Cooperative Research Partnership Grant (439381).
The authors have no additional disclosures.
[a] Neuroscience Institute, Neuroscience Intensive Care Unit, The Queen's Medical Center, 1301 Punchbowl Street, Honolulu, HI 96813, USA; [b] Neuroscience Institute, The Queen's Medical Center, 1301 Punchbowl Street, Honolulu, HI 96813, USA; [c] University of Hawaii at Manoa, School of Nursing & Dental Hygiene, 2528 McCarthy Mall, Webster Hall 402, Honolulu, HI 96822, USA
* Corresponding author.
E-mail addresses: julietsmail51@gmail.com; jbeniga@queens.org

Nurs Clin N Am 49 (2014) 399–413
http://dx.doi.org/10.1016/j.cnur.2014.05.013
0029-6465/14/$ – see front matter © 2014 Elsevier Inc. All rights reserved.

nursing.theclinics.com

Each year, about 795,000 people have a stroke, the leading cause of serious, long-term disability in the United States.[2] Stroke costs the United States an estimated $38.6 billion each year, which includes the cost of health care services, medications, and missed days of work.[3] In Hawaii, major cardiovascular disease, which includes coronary heart disease and stroke is the leading cause of death, with a statewide mortality of 45 per 100,000 deaths in 2005.[4]

Fever is a normal immunologic response to an infectious or inflammatory process; however, increased body temperature in the presence of neurologic injury can lead to secondary brain injury.[5] Hyperthermia contributes to a state of increased cerebral metabolism that, at the cellular level, may lead to ischemia, excitotoxicity, energy failure, cerebral swelling, inflammation, and neuronal death.[6] Regardless of the cause, fever can be harmful and is associated with poor outcomes, neurologic impairment, and prolonged intensive care unit (ICU) and hospital lengths of stay.[7,8] Thus, temperature management in neurologically vulnerable patients is both a prevalent challenge and a priority.

The primary treatment goal for the care of critically ill neurocritical patients is to prevent or minimize progression of brain insult for which fever is a cause. Therefore, the purpose of this project was to develop and institutionalize a standardized evidence-based practice (EBP) protocol to reduce temperature and to maintain normothermia in the neurocritical care patient population.

EVIDENCE FOR PRACTICE IMPROVEMENT

The Iowa Model of Evidence Based Practice was used as a framework to guide the process of developing a normothermia EBP guideline. The process begins with the recognition of a problem or trigger, which may be an identified practice issue or a knowledge deficit. The organizational mission and goals are explored to determine whether the problem is a priority for the organization. If addressing the practice issue is deemed a priority, a team of stakeholders, clinicians, educators, and other advocates of EBP are assembled. The next significant step is to compile, synthesize, and critique levels of the evidence relating to the practice issue. A pilot of the practice change occurs if there is sufficient evidence to support the change. Outcomes from the implementation of a practice change are monitored, evaluated, and reported for dissemination. The Iowa model provides an algorithm that highlights key decision points helpful to facilitate progression to the next step.[9]

Knowledge and Problem Triggers

Every year nearly all patients with severe TBI and a large number of patients with a stroke diagnosis are admitted to the 500-bed tertiary medical center located in the heart of downtown Honolulu, Hawaii. It is the state's designated level II trauma center, and approximately 40 patients with severe TBI are admitted to the 8-bed neuroscience ICU (NSICU) per year (2006–2009). The NSICU mean length of stay for patients with severe TBI is 18 days with a mortality of 28%, average age of 36 years (ranging from 14–69 years), and 95% of patients are male.[10] National statistics differ from these figures, reporting an incidence of TBI of 66% men and 23% women.[1]

As a primary stroke facility and Joint Commission–certified stroke center, an average of 500 patients with stroke diagnosis are admitted per year, with the NSICU admitting an average of 100 patients per year. About 75% of these patients have ischemic disease and 25% of patients have hemorrhagic stroke.[11]

Knowledge and problem triggers underscored the need for an evidence-based treatment protocol to manage fever in the NSICU. While establishing a TBI database for the NSICU, a high incidence and prolonged temperature increase was noted. The database and electronic medical record audits also revealed trends of fever under treatment and inadequate documentation. In the absence of a temperature management protocol, the current practice in the NSICU provided the nurse with a standing order for Tylenol to treat temperature greater than 38.6°C (101.5°F). Adjusting the room thermostat, ice packs, and the use of a circulating fan were noted interventions used by nurses. The use of cooling blankets was infrequent. Current literature confirmed that the issues experienced related to temperature management are not unique to this NSICU.

Forming a Team

A team consisting of 7 neurocritical nurses, a neuroscience clinical nurse specialist (CNS), 2 neuroscience research nurses, and a PhD nurse research mentor met for a total of 12 2-hour meetings during a period of 8 months. The team reviewed and synthesized relevant articles, decided on recommendations for best practices, and developed a written EBP guideline.

Assemble, Critique, and Synthesize Literature

A medical librarian was consulted to assist with assembling the literature. Key words used for the literature search were traumatic brain injury, nursing management, hyperthermia, fever, temperature management, normothermia, and shivering using CINAHL, Medline, PubMed, and the Cochrane databases, with a focus on the past 10 years.

A total of 42 relevant studies were assembled and critiqued using Mosby levels of evidence (Table 1).[12] To facilitate literature synthesis, information was organized into a matrix that proved valuable as a quick reference during development of the EBP guideline. Articles were categorized and assigned to a team member to read, critique, and summarize. Categories included scope of the problem, fever definitions, environmental cooling, pharmacologic treatment of fever, ice saline, surface cooling, intravascular cooling, shivering, outcomes, and timing of fever treatment. Each study was critiqued by 2 team members and then discussed as a group to ensure accuracy of grading the evidence. The recurring theme encountered in the literature review validated the need to promote normothermia and nursing management of increased temperature in the neurocritical care patient.

High incidence of fever

The high incidence of fever and secondary injury that results from fever in the neurocritical care patient population is well documented in the literature. Albrecht and

Table 1 Level of evidence	
Number of Articles	**Level of Evidence**
1	Level I: meta-analysis
9	Level II: randomized controlled trial
5	Level III: controlled trial, no randomization
7	Level IV: case control or cohort study, longitudinal studies
5	Level V: correlation study
11	Level VI: descriptive studies
0	Level VII: authority opinion or expert committee reports
4	Reviews: other

From Melnyk B. A focus on adult acute and critical care. Worldviews Evid Based Nurs 2004;1(3):194–7; with permission.

colleagues[13] (1998) reported that fever occurred in 68% of patients with TBI within 72 hours of hospitalization. In a retrospective study of 846 patients with TBI, Jiang and colleagues[14] (2002) reported a 67.5% incidence of fever (>37°C) in the first 48 hours of hospitalization, with a fever greater than 39°C occurring in 25% of the patients. In a retrospective analysis of 110 patients admitted within 24 hours of stroke, fever, and sub-febrility (temperatures 37.5–38°C) were associated with more severe symptoms.[15,16]

Nursing management

Nursing interventions to manage fever are often delayed, and consensus definitions of normothermia, fever, and the temperature at which to initiate protocols varied between institutions, regions, and personal clinical decision making.[17] In a retrospective chart review of 108 neurocritical care patients, only 31% of patients with fever received any documented intervention and delay in implementing a treatment protocol occurred in 58% of patients.[18] A questionnaire mailed to nurses working in neurocritical care units showed that fewer than 20% have a fever management protocol in place for neurologic patients, variations in temperature ranges to start treatment were 37 to 40°C, and choice of pharmacologic therapy was inconsistent. Common findings for treatment across studies are the use of acetaminophen every 4 hours, ice packs, water cooling blankets, and tepid bathing.[19]

Normothermia recommended

Current strategies to improve neurologic outcomes following TBI are multidisciplinary and include the application of the Guidelines for the Management of Severe Traumatic Brain Injury.[20] TBI guidelines cite maintenance of normothermia as the minimum standard of care and recommend mild to moderate hypothermia for neuroprotection and improved patient outcomes.[20] In addition, ischemic stroke guidelines by the American Heart Association state that fever should be treated pharmacologically and with cooling measures such as cooling blankets and cooling devices.[21]

Sufficient evidence

The literature clearly supported the necessity to treat fever and maintain normothermia. However, there is no definitive research for the steps to achieve normothermia in this population. Findings across studies supported the clinical relevance and need for the development of temperature management guidelines for the neurocritical care patient population.[14–21] A retrospective chart audit of 81 patients with severe TBI in the NSICU at our facility revealed an average daily maximum temperature of 37.6°C, and only 3% of temperature greater than 37.0°C (n = 4247) were noted to have a documented fever reduction intervention (Table 2).

IMPLEMENTATION STRATEGIES
Development of the EBP Guideline

There is no clear definition for fever in the literature so defining normothermia and fever was a challenge. A literature summary for fever control and its outcome by Aiyagari and Diringer[5] (2007) provided a range for fever definition between 37°C and 38.5°C. Hoedemaekers and colleagues[22] (2007) defined normothermia at 37.0°C in their temperature management study. Diringer[23] (2004) defined fever at greater than 38.0°C when conducting a studying to determine effectiveness of a catheter-based system in reducing increased temperature. After much discussion, the team defined the normothermia threshold at 37.0°C and concluded that it was a valid starting point for a preventive phase of fever management.

Before this project, temperature readings were measured every 4 hours with a tympanic thermometer or sporadically with a continuous brain temperature/intracranial

Table 2
Preguideline and postguideline data

	Before Guideline (2006–2009) n = 4247[a]	After Guideline (2011) n = 4590[a]	After Guideline (2013) n = 300[b]
Age (y)	44 ± 18	55 ± 17	47
Male gender (%)	79	43	66
Diagnosis	100% TBI	10% TBI 10% ischemic stroke 22% ICH 55% SAH	16% TBI 25% ischemic stroke 25% ICH 33% SAH
Admission temperature (°C)	36.3 ± 1	36.4 ± 1	36.5
Admission GCS	6 ± 2	11 ± 6	10
Discharge GCS	14 ± 2	14 ± 2	—
ICU LOS (d)	18 ± 11	13 ± 7	—
Mortality (%)	25	24	—
Average daily maximum temperature (°C)	37.6	37.8	37.9
T ≥37.0°C (%)	40	69	—
T ≥37.0°C (% treated[c])	3	9.4	—
T ≥37.5°C (% treated[d])	10	15.5	30
Guideline compliance (%)	—	9.4	30
Average temperature nursing treated (°C)	37.8	37.8	38.3
Average temperature nursing did not treat (°C)	37.5	37.6	38.0

Abbreviations: GCS, Glasgow Coma Score; ICH, intracranial hemorrhage; LOS, length of stay; SAH, subarachnoid hemorrhage; T, temperature.
  [a] n = temperature episode ≥37.0°C.
  [b] n = temperature episode ≥37.5°C.
  [c] Initial normothermia definition and threshold T ≥37.0°C.
  [d] Revised normothermia definition and threshold T ≥37.5°C.

pressure monitor. Foley catheters with continuous temperature sensors were made available to our facility as this project evolved. This equipment allowed continuous temperature measurement, which is most suitable for monitoring trends.

The efficacy of pharmacologic interventions alone for fever management is inconclusive,[5] but a retrospective review of temperature interventions in the NSICU suggested that acetaminophen (Tylenol) in combination with external measures, such as surface cooling, cool cloth bath, and reducing the room temperature, may be more effective than acetaminophen (Tylenol) alone (Fig. 1). This finding is consistent with an experimental study conducted by Price and colleagues[24] (2003) examining cooling methods for critically ill patients with cerebral insults. Despite the small sample size of 67 patients, the study suggests that acetaminophen in combination with evaporative cooling reduces body core temperature in adult, ventilated patients. The same study discounted the effectiveness of circulating fans.

The use of the Blanketrol III cooling blanket was supported by a prospective, randomized controlled trial, evaluating efficacy and safety of 5 different cooling methods for induction and maintenance of hypothermia and normothermia in critically ill patients.[22] The study results showed that temperature decreased faster in patients

404   Beniga et al

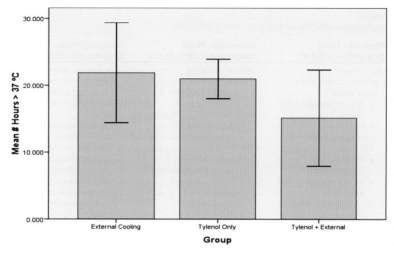

Fig. 1. Temperature interventions in the NSICU. SE, standard error.

cooled with water-circulating blankets, gel-coated cooling pads, and intravascular cooling devices compared with air-circulating cooling devices and conventional methods. Conventional cooling consisted of rapid infusion of cooled intravenous (IV) solution followed by surface cooling using icepacks.

The resulting EBP guideline, entitled *Normothermia for NeuroProtection*, outlines 3 phases of increased temperature with recommended interventions consisting of environmental and evaporative therapies, pharmacologic interventions, surface cooling, and intravascular cooling. The preventive phase (temperature [T] >37°C) primarily consists of environmental, evaporative, and pharmacologic interventions. The therapeutic phase (T>38°C–38.6°C) adds surface cooling with the Blanketrol III cooling vest and blanket. The refractory phase (T>38.6°C) expands the cooling blanket arsenal and includes a cooling head wrap and considerations for intravascular cooling (Table 3).

Impact of Shivering

Shivering can occur at normothermic or even hyperthermic stages of temperature because of increases in the hypothalamic thermoregulator set point (fever) and leads to an increasing threshold zone and rewarming.[25] Shivering dramatically increases the amount of heat transfer required to maintain normothermia, and may be associated with adverse effects on level of consciousness, defeat the cooling process, eliminate the potential benefits of therapeutic normothermia, and in extreme cases may be more detrimental than the fever.[26]

In addition to the normothermia guideline, a practice standard to address shivering was also constructed from existing literature recommendations (Table 4).[27–33] The Bedside Shivering Assessment Scale (BSAS), a clinical tool that measures severity of shivering, is the basis for the EBP shivering guideline.[28] Evidence-based recommendations for treatment of shivering include pharmacologic and therapeutic interventions, such as counterwarming. Efforts should be focused on avoiding shivering and halting it as soon as it starts; therefore, early recognition, prevention, and treatment are imperative to maximize normothermia interventions.

Table 3
Normothermia for NeuroProtection: NSICU guideline

Preventive Phase Temperature >37.0°C	Therapeutic Phase Temperature >38°C–38.6°C	Refractory Phase Temperature >38.6°C

Environment +
  pharmacologic therapies
1. Cool room
  • Adjust thermostat dial
    to cool
  • Fan not recommended
2. Administer Tylenol per
  MD order
  • 650 mg q 4 h
    (recommended)
  • Do not exceed
    3900 mg/d
3. Cool cloth bath (evapo-
  rative cooling)
  • Remove clothing
  • Use cool tap water to
    wash all skin surfaces
  • Pad dry to prevent
    shivering
  • Place cool cloth on
    forehead; replace
    when it becomes
    warm
Combination therapies
  may be more effective
  (eg, cool cloth bath
  and Tylenol)
Points to remember:
• Baseline CBC with
  differential
• Institute shivering
  management
  guidelines
	Surface therapies
	Institute interventions 1,
	  2, and 3 listed for the
	  preventive phase
	4. Surface cooling: Blanke-
	  trol III blanket and vest
	  • Apply blanket on top
	    of patient, set target
	    temperature to 37°C
	  • Apply vest to patient
	  • Set temperature
	    gradient to 20°C with
	    smart mode
	  • Assess skin q 4
	Points to remember:
	• Monitor for S/S of
	  infection
	• Monitor skin integrity
	• Institute shivering
	  management
	  guidelines
		Core focused therapies
		Institute interventions 1,
		  2, 3, and 4 then:
		5. Add Blanketrol III head
		  wrap
		6. Consider cooled NG
		  instilled fluids
		7. Consider cooled IV fluids
		8. Suggest Coolgard intra-
		  vascular cooling for
		  normothermia
		Target temperature = 37°C
		Points to remember:
		• Monitor for S/S of
		  infection
		• Monitor skin integrity
		• Institute shivering
		  management
		  guidelines

Abbreviations: CBC, complete blood count; MD, Doctor of Medicine; NG, nasogastric; Q, every; S/S, signs & symptoms.

Educational Strategies and Marketing

A month-long campaign, launched in January 2010, introduced the *Normothermia for NeuroProtection* and *Shivering Management* guidelines to the NSICU nursing staff. The campaign was evident on entrance into the NSICU because nurses were greeted with icicles, snowflakes, and large blue campaign buttons hanging from the ceiling. Inscribed on the button is the campaign theme, "It's Hot to be COOL 37°C" (**Fig. 2**). The event was highlighted with hospital-wide presentations at monthly nursing grand rounds, unit based registered nurse (RN) and advanced practice RN (APRN) in-services, and inclusion of content into the annual competency fair. Laminated copies of the guidelines were placed in each patient room, providing easy access.

A contest with incentives was established to encourage staff to adhere to the guide-line and draw attention to the campaign. Staff nurses received a point each time a tem-perature reduction intervention was initiated as per the guideline. The neuro-CNS kept a cumulative point tally for a period of 4 weeks, which culminated with 2 nurses with

406   Beniga et al

Table 4
Shivering management: NSICU guideline

	0 = Absent	1 = Mild	2 = Moderate	3 = Severe
	Absence of shivering on neck or pectoral muscles	Localized to the neck and/or thorax. May be present only on palpation	Involvement of the UE ± neck or pectoralis muscles	Generalized whole-body involvement
	Goal = BSAS ≤1 Every hour: palpate masseter, pectoralis, deltoids, and quadriceps muscles for shivering. Watch for fine quivering in electrocardiogram, or BIS tracing			
Interventions[a]	Optimize sedation and analgesia	Acetaminophen Buspar + meperidine Magnesium IV gtt	Buspar + meperidine Magnesium IV continuous Dexmedetomidine Fentanyl	Must be on ventilator: Propofol Paralytics
Counterwarming	—	Place warm socks or blanket on hands and feet	Place warm socks or blanket on hands and feet	Consider Bair Hugger at 40–43°C

Buspirone (Buspar; pharmacologically reduces the shiver threshold; best if given with Demerol). Suggested dosing:
- Initial dose of 30 mg feeding tube then, 15–20 mg q 8
- Usual dose required is 20–30 mg/d in 2–3 divided doses; maximum dose 60 mg/d

Meperidine (Demerol; pharmacologically reduces the shiver threshold; synergistic with Buspar). Suggested dosing:
- 12.5–50 mg intravenously 3–4 times a day or as a continuous infusion up to 24 h
- if CR <2 and UOP >30 mL/h, reduce dose

Magnesium IV (vasodilation; improves efficacy of cooling and increases patient comfort; maintain high normal levels). Suggested dosing:
- 12 g in 250 mL NS; continuous infusion at 0.5–1.0 g/h (10 mL/h); titrate to maintain a serum magnesium level of 3–4 mg/dL
- Monitor levels

Dexmedetomidine (Precedex; reduces both the vasoconstriction and shivering thresholds). Suggested dosing:
- 0.2–1.5 μg/kg/h IV. Hold for HR <50 bpm or SBP <90 mm Hg

Propofol (Diprivan; to provide shiver suppression and continuous sedation). Suggested dosing:
- 20 μg/kg/min IV, titrate by 5 μg/kg/min as needed (not to exceed 50 μg/kg/min)

Vecuronium (Nocuron; only after adequate sedation is achieved; BIS ≤60). Suggested dosing:
- 0.1 mg/kg (up to 10 mg) IVP intermittent boluses prn shivering

Abbreviations: BIS, bispectral index; bpm, beats per minute; BSAS, Bedside Shivering Assessment Scale; CR, creatinine; gtt, drip; HR, heart rate; IVP, IV push; NS, normal saline; prn, as needed; SBP, systolic blood pressure; UE, upper extremities; UOP, urine output.
[a] Requires MD order.
Data from Refs.[27–33]

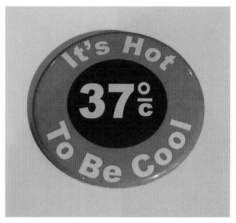

Fig. 2. Normothermia for NeuroProtection and Shivering Management campaign button.

the most points receiving a first prize Apple Store gift card and second prize with a spa gift certificate. The contest produced a tie with 2 first-place winners who were very engaged and set the tone for healthy competition. All the contest winners proved to be enthusiastic supporters of the new practice change. Feedback on the guideline was solicited at this time.

A hallmark of the normothermia guideline is the use of the Blanketrol III, a surface cooling device. Ongoing in-services about the use of the machine were provided on the unit and one-on-one training occurred at the bedside in the rooms of patients requiring cooling measures. Collaboration with the central supply department to ensure availability of supplies was essential to success. The increased use of the Blanketrol III required purchasing of additional machines and upgrades for older models. Introduction of expanded uses of surface cooling included use of a cooling vest and head wrap to supplement the traditional body blanket.

EVALUATION

The new practice changes created initial excitement but maintaining the momentum proved challenging. Many applauded the 3-phase intervention model, which places emphasis on prevention and early intervention when the patient's temperature begins to trend up. The staff recognized the impact of early treatment and acknowledged that it was less laborious to prevent a fever spike than to bring down a high fever. The following are examples of the initial feedback received from staff: "Guidelines are great…the emphasis to treat temperatures greater than 37°C is smart, then we avoid having to chase high fevers such as 38–40°C." "I love the whole concept of the preventive phase…when I treat temps as soon as they're greater than 37°C, the treatments are effective (Tylenol, cool wash cloths under armpits or on head) and I don't even have to do anything more physical such as (place a Blanketrol III)." "It great!!! Sometimes we work harder than we really need to… why wait to have to turn a heavy patient and place the Blanketrol III when we can give Tylenol or a cool bath as soon as we see the temp rising? Thanks again!"

Monitoring Practice Change

An anonymous survey to identify facilitators and barriers to guideline adherence was administered to 28 eligible NSICU nurses. To be eligible, RNs must have worked in the

NSICU as a staff nurse during the entire implementation period of the EBP guidelines (normothermia and shivering), must consent to participate, and be willing to speak up regarding their perceptions on use of the EBP guidelines. Twenty-seven surveys were returned for analysis. Box 1 list the 5 questions included in the staff nurse survey, which produced responses with common themes. The facilitators and barriers to guideline implementation are summarized in Box 2.

Nursing Compliance

To determine the impact of the practice change, it was important to measure nursing compliance with the temperature management guideline. A retrospective chart audit 10 months after guideline implementation identified temperature points greater than 37.0°C. Of the 4590 temperatures taken, there was a daily average maximum temperature of 37.8°C. Compared with 3% compliance with 4247 temperatures taken at the preintervention data collection point, 9.4% of temperature increases greater than or equal to 37.0°C were treated with fever reduction interventions (see Table 2). Continued monitoring 18 months after guideline implementation revealed an average daily maximum temperature of 37.9°C and 30% compliance with the guideline for temperatures greater than or equal to 37.5°C. This is an improvement from the 10% before the guideline, and the 15.5% after the guideline in 2011 when evaluating compliance with treating temperature greater than or equal to 37.5°C. The difference in the patient sampling was attributed to the literature supporting temperature management for all patients with neurologic injury and especially patients with a stroke diagnosis.

LESSONS LEARNED
What Worked?

Introduction of a new practice and sustaining the change is challenging and ongoing. Numerous factors contribute to the success of the implementation of normothermia and shivering guidelines in the NSICU. Credit is given to the team involved in the project, especially the staff nurses engaged at the bedside and recognizing the importance of being proactive in the management of increased temperature.

The It's Hot to be Cool campaign was a successful vehicle to launch the new practice recommendations. It created attention, excitement, and a source of discussion during the first few weeks. The campaign buttons that were distributed left a lasting impression, because name tags and back packs were decorated with them weeks thereafter. The campaign was primarily targeted for the NSICU, but presenting the project at monthly nursing grand rounds provided hospital-wide exposure and produced interest from other departments.

Box 1
Staff RN survey

Thoughts on implementing the temperature management EBP guideline

Your initial date of hire at the NSICU, Queen's Medical Center: (month, year)

1. When you hear the words, temperature management, what comes to mind?
2. When you hear the words, evidence-based practice guideline, what comes to mind?
3. Tell me about those processes that have facilitated the implementation of the temperature management guideline.
4. Tell me about those processes that have created barriers to guideline implementation.
5. When implementing an EBP guideline, what do you think is most important?

Box 2
Summary of barriers and facilitators to guidelines

What created barriers to guideline implementation?

- Old habits are hard to break
- Some staff with negative opinion of guidelines
- Increased nurse workload
- Increased patient acuity
- Equipment malfunction and unavailable
- Inadequate supplies
- Lack of order sets
- MD (Doctor of Medicine) orders not consistent with guideline
- Lack of support and reinforcement from MD

What facilitated implementation of guideline?

- Printed accessible guideline algorithm
- Functional equipment
- Continuous bladder temperature monitor
- MD support
- Education, competency inclusion
- Nurse manager and education council support
- Accessible guideline algorithm
- Motivating staff
- Physician support

A hospital-wide team was concurrently in the process of developing hypothermia after cardiac arrest (HACA) guidelines that included cooling and shivering management. Although the focus of HACA is hypothermia, the aggressive cooling outlined in the refractory phase of the NSICU normothermia guideline outlines use of the Coolgard intravascular device and was used in the HACA protocol as a primary intervention. A modified version of NSCIU's shivering guideline was adopted by the team.

Designing simple 1-page algorithms accessible in all patient rooms proved helpful in facilitating implementation of the guidelines. The tiered phases of temperature intervention received positive feedback from the nursing staff. The nurse is given a starting point that supports autonomy in selecting interventions appropriate for the temperature range. It encourages nurses to consider combinations of interventions focused on prevention, which is less tedious than having to reduce a highly increased temperature.

The introduction of temperature-sensing urinary catheters in the critical care units also proved timely and advantageous to our guideline launching. The availability of continuous temperature readings facilitated surveillance of escalating trends and helped trigger early intervention. In addition, the newly purchased Blanketrol III hypothermia machines provided a compatible connection to the urinary catheter.

What Were the Challenges?

The process of implementing new practice change presented new challenges for the NSICU staff. One challenge identified by staff as being evident early after implementation was the increase in workload attributed to early intervention, but necessary for the maintenance of normothermia and the required escalating treatments. Supported by the NSICU nurse manager and a patient acuity system, adjustment to staffing assignments were made to accommodate the additional workload.

Controlling shivering contributes significantly to patient acuity and created frustration among staff who verbalized shivering as a significant barrier to guideline implementation. In addition, varying physician approaches for shivering prevention and treatment were often viewed by nurses as inconsistent and contrary to the shivering guideline, which may have discouraged nurses from aggressive temperature intervention. There are several nurse-driven interventions in the guideline that combat shivering; however, many are pharmacologic and require a physician order.

The creation of order sets to initiate normothermia and shivering management were requested by staff. However, varying patient conditions and differences in practice preferences among the neurointensivists in the NSICU hindered the use of standard order sets. Staff feedback included, "Different doctors have different treatment modalities and don't follow guidelines/protocols" and "(There are) inconsistent orders because we have three different MDs."

Operational concerns with the use of the Blanketrol III hypothermia machine were initial contributors to workflow challenges. To accommodate workflow, some thought and planning was required for placement of the machine and the hose attachments in an already crowded room. The use of the vest and head wrap was considered cumbersome by the staff and the different modes of operation complex and difficult to set up, which became problematic when nurses, in an effort to speed up cooling, would attempt to manually adjust the blanket temperature, causing a drastic reduction and often triggering early shivering. To address these issues, company representatives were consulted and provided additional in-services for the staff. These issues are now mostly resolved.

Recommendations

The guideline does not fit all patients, especially those who are awake and not sedated. The use of the hypothermia blanket recommended in the therapeutic phase may be particularly counterproductive in this patient group because of shivering. The nurse must consider the distress and discomfort this would cause the patient. Interventions listed in the preventive phase may be more appropriate and are less likely to cause shivering.

Note the amendment of the normothermia threshold from 37.0°C to 37.5°C. The expectation to begin temperature reduction interventions at 37.0°C was not practical and premature treatment may mask initial signs of infections. Reexamination of the existing literature revealed that a large number of studies used 37.5°C as the fever threshold. Thus, we have now revised our normothermia guideline.

Although cost is not readily recognized at the bedside, the impact on patient hospitalization must be acknowledged. Once initiated, normothermia management is likely to continue for several days or more. There is an additional nursing resource requirement caused by increased patient acuity. There is also a need for additional equipment and supplies for pharmacologic use for both normothermia management and shivering prevention. However, these additional costs may be offset by earlier discharge from the NSICU and/or hospital, less loss of disability, and improved long-term function. It would be beneficial to include a cost-benefit analysis in future projects.

SUMMARY

Fever is a significant contributor to secondary brain insult and management is a challenge for the neurocritical care team. The absence of standardized guidelines likely contributes to poor surveillance and undertreatment of increased temperature. A need for practice change was identified and this EBP project was initiated to compile sufficient evidence to develop, implement, and evaluate a treatment guideline to manage fever and maintain normothermia in the neurocritical care population. Sustaining and monitoring the use of the normothermia and shivering management guidelines are ongoing processes. The improvement in guideline compliance is encouraging and the goal is to continue to monitor performance through quality improvement audits. Ongoing education, inclusion in NSICU staff annual competency, and staff update on compliance performance is essential to maintain and sustain the practice change achieved through this project.

ACKNOWLEDGMENTS

The authors would like to acknowledge the following individuals for their support of this project. EBP team: Susan Asai, RN; Dan Choe, RN; Jodie Kaalekahi, RN; Kim Nguyen, RN; Lyle Oshita, RN; Sandra Talavera, RN; Cherylee Chang, MD, Director, Neuroscience Institute; Johnna DeCastillo; Cindy Kamikawa, RN, CNO, The Queen's Medical Center; Kawehi Kauhola, RN, Manager, Neuroscience ICU; Matthew Koenig, MD; Renee Latimer, RN, Director, Queen Emma Nursing Institute; Dongmei Li, MS, PhD; Joseph Mobley Jr, PhD; Kazuma Nakagawa, MD; Dalnam Park; Neuroscience ICU staff.

REFERENCES

1. Langlois JA, Rutland-Brown W, Thomas KE. Traumatic brain injury in the United States: emergency department visits, hospitalizations, and deaths. Atlanta (GA): Centers for Disease Control and Prevention, National Center for Injury Prevention and Control; 2006.
2. Roger VL, Go AS, Lloyd-Jones DM, et al. Heart disease and stroke statistics—2012 update: a report from the American Heart Association. Circulation 2012; 125:e2–220.
3. Heidenreich PA, Trogdon JG, Khavjou OA, et al. Forecasting the future of cardiovascular disease in the United States: a policy statement from the American Heart Association. Circulation 2011;123:933–44.
4. Balabis J, Pubotsky A, Baker KK, et al. The burden of cardiovascular disease in Hawaii 2007. Honolulu (HI): Hawaii State Department of Health; 2007.
5. Aiyagari V, Diringer MN. Fever control and its impact on outcomes: what is the evidence? J Neurol Sci 2007;261:39–46.
6. Fritz HG, Bauer R. Secondary injuries in brain trauma: effects of hypothermia. J Neurosurg Anesthesiol 2004;16:43–52.
7. Greer DM, Funk SE, Reaven NL, et al. Impact of fever on outcome in patients with stroke and neurologic injury: a comprehensive meta-analysis. Stroke 2008;39: 3029–35.
8. Diringer MN, Reaven MA, Funk SE, et al. Elevated body temperature independently contributes to increased length of stay in neurologic intensive care unit patients. Crit Care Med 2004;32:1489–95.
9. Titler MG, Kleiber C, Rakel B, et al. The Iowa Model of evidence-based practice to promote quality care. Crit Care Nurs Clin North Am 2001;13:497–509.

412 Beniga et al

10. The Queen's Medical Center, Trauma Database. Traumatic Brain Injury Quality Improvement Program: TBI-trac™, 2006–2009.

11. The Queen's Medical Center, Neuroscience Institute, Stroke Database, 2009.

12. Melnyk BM. A focus on adult acute and critical care. Worldviews Evid Based Nurs 2004;1(3):194–7 Modified from Guyatt & Rennie (2002), Harris et al. (2001).

13. Albrecht RF 2nd, Wass CT, Lanier WL. Occurrence of potentially detrimental temperature alterations in hospitalized patients at risk for brain injury. Mayo Clin Proc 1998;73:629–35.

14. Jiang JY, Gao GY, Li WP, et al. Early indicators of prognosis in 846 cases of severe traumatic brain injury. J Neurotrauma 2002;19:869–74.

15. Hindfelt B. The prognostic significance of subfebrility and fever in ischemic cerebral infarction. Acta Neurol Scand 1976;53:72–9.

16. Ginsberg MD, Busto R. Combating hyperthermia in acute stroke: a significant clinical concern. Stroke 1998;29:529–34.

17. Thompson HJ, Kirkness CJ, Mitchell PH. Intensive care unit management of fever following traumatic brain injury. Intensive Crit Care Nurs 2007;23:91–6.

18. Thompson HJ, Kirkness CJ, Mitchell PH, et al. Fever management practices of neuroscience nurses: national and regional perspectives. J Neurosci Nurs 2007;39:151–62.

19. Thompson HJ, Kirkness CJ, Mitchell PH, et al. Fever management practices of neuroscience nurses, part II: nurse, patients, and barriers. J Neurosci Nurs 2007;39:196–201.

20. Brain Trauma Foundation, American Association of Neurological Surgeons, Congress of Neurological Surgeons, et al. Guidelines for the management of severe traumatic brain injury. XV. Steroids. J Neurotrauma 2007;24(Suppl 1):S91–5.

21. Adams HP Jr, del Zoppo G, Alberts MJ, et al. Guidelines for the early management of adults with ischemic stroke: a guideline from the American Heart Association/American Stroke Association Stroke Council, Clinical Cardiology Council, Cardiovascular Radiology and Intervention Council, and the Atherosclerotic Peripheral Vascular Disease and Quality of Care Outcomes in Research Interdisciplinary Working Groups: the American Academy of Neurology affirms the value of this guideline as an educational tool for neurologists. Stroke 2007;38: 1655–711.

22. Hoedemaekers CW, Ezzahti M, Gerritsen A, et al. Comparison of cooling methods to induce and maintain normo- and hypothermia in intensive care patients: a prospective intervention study. Crit Care 2007;1:R91.

23. Diringer MN. Treatment of fever in the neurologic intensive care unit with a catheter-based heat exchange system. Crit Care Med 2004;32:559–64.

24. Price T, McGloin S, Izzard J, et al. Cooling strategies for patients with severe cerebral insult in ICU (Part 2). Nurs Crit Care 2003;8:37–45.

25. Holtzclaw BJ. Shivering in acutely ill vulnerable populations. AACN Clin Issues 2004;15:267–79.

26. Badjatia NJ, Kowalski RG, Schimidt JM, et al. Predictors and clinical implications of shivering during therapeutic normothermia. Neurocrit Care 2007;6:186–91.

27. Badjatia N, Strongilis E, Prescutti M, et al. Metabolic benefits of surface counter warming during therapeutic temperature modulation. Crit Care Med 2009;37:1–5.

28. Badjatia NJ, Strongilis E, Gordon E, et al. Metabolic impact of shivering during therapeutic temperature modulation. Stroke 2008;39:3242–7.

29. Choi H, Ko S, Presciutti M, et al. Prevention of shivering during therapeutic temperature modulation: the Columbia Anti-Shivering Protocol. Neurocrit Care 2011; 14:389–94.

30. Doufas A, Wadhwa A, Lin C, et al. Neither arm nor face warming reduces the shivering threshold in unanesthetized humans. Stroke 2003;34:1736–40.
31. Kizilirmak S, Karakas S, Akca O, et al. Magnesium sulfate stops post anesthetic shivering. Ann N Y Acad Sci 1997;813:799–806.
32. Mokhtarani M, Mahgoub A, Morioka N, et al. Buspirone and meperidine synergistically reduce the shivering threshold. Anesth Analg 2001;93:1233–9.
33. Talke P, Tayefeh S, Sessler D, et al. Dexmedetomidine does not alter the sweating threshold, but comparably and linearly decreases the vasoconstriction and shivering thresholds. Anesthesiology 1997;87:835–41.

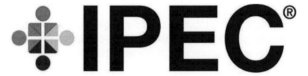

Interprofessional Education Collaborative

Connecting health professions for better care

Core Competencies for
Interprofessional Collaborative Practice:

2016 Update

This document may be reproduced, distributed, publicly displayed and modified provided that attribution is clearly stated on any resulting work and it is used for non-commercial, scientific or educational—including professional development—purposes. If the work has been modified in any way all logos must be removed.

Contact ip@aamc.org for permission for any other use.

Suggested Citation:
Interprofessional Education Collaborative. (2016).
Core competencies for interprofessional collaborative practice: 2016 update. Washington, DC: Interprofessional Education Collaborative.

Contents

Executive Summary

In 2009, six national associations of schools of health professions formed a collaborative to promote and encourage constituent efforts that would advance substantive interprofessional learning experiences. The goal was, and remains, to help prepare future health professionals for enhanced team-based care of patients and improved population health outcomes. The collaborative, representing dentistry, nursing, medicine, osteopathic medicine, pharmacy, and public health, convened an expert panel of representatives from each of the six IPEC sponsor professions to create core competencies for interprofessional collaborative practice, to guide curriculum development across health professions schools. The competencies and implementation recommendations subsequently published in the 2011 *Core Competencies for Interprofessional Collaborative Practice* have been broadly disseminated.

In this 2016 release, the IPEC Board updates the document with a three-fold purpose, to:

- Reaffirm the value and impact of the core competencies and sub-competencies as promulgated under the auspices of IPEC.

- Organize the competencies within a singular domain of **Interprofessional Collaboration**, encompassing the topics of values and ethics, roles and responsibilities, interprofessional communication, and teams and teamwork. These four topical areas were initially proposed as domains within interprofessional education (IPE). However, in the time since publication, it has become clear that interprofessional collaboration stands as a domain unto itself. Furthermore, creating shared taxonomy among the health professions serves to streamline and synergize educational activities and related assessment and evaluation efforts.

- Broaden the interprofessional competencies to better achieve the Triple Aim (improve the patient experience of care, improve the health of populations, and reduce the per capita cost of health care), with particular reference to population health.

Since the 2011 report was issued, IPEC has made substantive headway in interprofessional education and the crucial partnerships that will further its progress:

- There have been over 550 citations of the report in the peer-reviewed and related literature between May 2011 and December 2015. It has also been translated into several languages and used in professional development by the health insurance industry.

- Meaningful interprofessional learning experiences in the required curriculum has increased, as reported in *JAMA* and the *Journal of Dental Education*.

- The IPEC Faculty Development Institutes have hosted 339 multi-professional teams with 1,457 participants to design institutionally-based projects that advance IPE at their local institutions.

- With funding from the Josiah Macy Jr. Foundation, the IPE PORTAL collection of peer-reviewed educational resources and materials supporting IPE instruction, which are mapped to the IPEC Competencies, was launched in December 2012.

- In February 2016, IPEC welcomed 9 new institutional members, expanding the professional representation from 6 to 15:

  o American Association of Colleges of Podiatric Medicine (AACPM)
  o American Council of Academic Physical Therapy (ACAPT)
  o American Occupational Therapy Association (AOTA)
  o American Psychological Association (APA)
  o Association of American Veterinary Medical Colleges (AAVMC)
  o Association of Schools and Colleges of Optometry (ASCO)
  o Association of Schools of Allied Health Professions (ASAHP)
  o Council on Social Work Education (CSWE)
  o Physician Assistant Education Association (PAEA)

Introduction

The intent of the Interprofessional Education Collaborative (IPEC) that came together in 2009 to develop core competencies for interprofessional collaborative practice was to build on each profession's expected disciplinary competencies. The development of interprofessional collaborative competencies necessarily required moving beyond profession-specific educational efforts to engage students of different professions in interactive learning with each other.

In 2016 the IPEC Board aims to: reaffirm the original competencies, ground the competency model firmly under the singular domain of Interprofessional Collaboration, and broaden the competencies to better integrate population health approaches across the health and partner professions so as to enhance collaboration for improving both individual care and population health outcomes.

The original 2011 IPEC report grew out of the commitment of six founding professional educational organizations to define interprofessional competencies for their professions: dentistry, nursing, medicine, osteopathic medicine, pharmacy, and public health. The hope then, which is still apt today, was that other professional education organizations and a broader group of stakeholders in the quality of health professions education would see the value of these competencies and adopt the recommendations in their own work. The competencies were intentionally general enough in nature to allow flexibility within the professions and at the institutional level. This would allow faculty and administrators to develop a program of study for their profession or institution that is aligned with the general interprofessional competency statements but in a context appropriate to particular professional, clinical, practitioner, or institutional circumstances. This would broaden the scope and increase the momentum of the transformation of interprofessional education of health professionals.

In the five years since the original report's release, significant developments—from broad citation of the report and dissemination of the competencies to endorsement from accreditation bodies and robust attendance at team-based faculty development institutes—stand as demonstrations of just the kind of transformation and increased momentum IPEC initially envisioned. Specifically, additional organizations have signed on as IPEC supporting organizations, and most of those subsequently joined IPEC in 2016 as institutional members. The 2011 report has been widely cited throughout the health professions literature, translated into multiple languages, and reprinted in part and in whole in over a dozen educational textbooks. And, most importantly, initial findings from dentistry and medicine indicate that increased attention is being given to IPE within the required curriculum.

CORE COMPETENCIES FOR INTERPROFESSIONAL COLLABORATIVE PRACTICE: 2016 UPDATE

Because of these developments, the IPEC Board carried out an update in 2016. This 2016 update, like the initial 2011 IPEC report, is inspired by the vision that interprofessional collaborative practice is key to the safe, high-quality, accessible, patient-centered care desired by all. It also reflects the changes that have occurred in the health system since the release of the original report, two of the most significant of which are the increased focus on the Triple Aim (improving the experience of care, improving the health of populations, and reducing the per capita cost of health care) and implementation of the Patient Protection and Affordable Care Act in 2010. In reviewing the competencies in light of the new environment, the IPEC Board recognized that population health approaches need to be strengthened in the model. This updated version integrates explicit population health outcomes alongside individual care competencies into an expanded competency model that is needed to achieve today's health system goals of improved health and health equity across the life span.

Achieving that vision requires the continuous development of interprofessional competency by health professions students and students in other professional fields as part of the learning process, so that they enter the workforce ready for collaborative practice that helps to ensure health. The new population health content is grounded in the Framing the Future's Population Health across All Professions' Expert Panel, which included representation from each IPEC Board member. That panel's 2015 report aims to prepare professionals in health and other fields (e.g., law, business, architecture, urban planning, teaching, and engineering, including dual-degree students) for professional activities that impact population health, and to work together across disciplines, organizations, and sectors on innovative strategies to improve population health.

Perhaps the most important outcome of this updated orientation in IPEC's expanded competency model towards population health is providing an enabling framework for clinical care providers, public health practitioners, and professionals from other fields to collaborate more effectively and creatively across disciplines to optimize health care and advance population health.

This update retains most of the original wording of the general competency statements and related sub-competencies, revised to integrate population health concepts, recognizing that these statements have been used in mapping curricula or as an organizing framework for efforts such as the IPE PORTAL resource collection, IPEC Faculty Development Institutes, and the American Association of Colleges of Pharmacy's (AACP's) Professions Quest.

And this treatment differs in that Interprofessional Collaboration is pushed forward as the *central domain* under which the original four core general competencies and related sub-competencies are arrayed. This approach is consistent with what Englander et al. found in their 2013 exhaustive review of health professions' competency frameworks. They explored the degree of existing overlap in domains of competence and specific competency expectations between the health professions and within medicine's specialties and subspecialties. Through mapping 153 different competency lists that covered nine health professions and medicine specialties, subspecialties, and related initiatives, **Interprofessional Collaboration** emerged as a viable general domain.

Integration of the IPEC Core Competencies

Dissemination and Impact

From the outset, the report has been well received and broadly cited. In addition to having been translated into Japanese and Spanish, it has also been used by the medical and dental health insurance industries for professional development. Notably, the report has been cited in the peer-reviewed literature and other key publications well over 550 times. While many of these citations come from health science professions, it has also been picked up in the social sciences.

Increasingly, IPE learning experiences, once largely elective if offered at all, have begun to make substantive inroads into the required curriculum. A 2012 survey of dental education programs revealed that 34 percent of IPE offerings for dental students were required. In 2014, that profile dramatically shifted to 69 percent (Palatta et al 2015). In a similar vein, Barzansky and Etzel (2015) found the percentage of reporting medical schools with required IPE experiences rose from 76 percent to 92 percent between 2011 and 2014.

Support from the Health Professions' Education Community

Immediately after the 2011 report release, 12 organizations signed on as supporting organizations, and, significantly, in February 2016, IPEC officially expanded to include 9 institutional members:
- American Association of Colleges of Podiatric Medicine (AACPM)
- American Council of Academic Physical Therapy (ACAPT)
- American Occupational Therapy Association (AOTA)
- American Psychological Association (APA)
- Association of American Veterinary Medical Colleges (AAVMC)
- Association of Schools and Colleges of Optometry (ASCO)
- Association of Schools of Allied Health Professions (ASAHP)
- Council on Social Work Education (CSWE)
- Physician Assistant Education Association (PAEA)

The 2011 supporting organizations follow:
- Academic Consortium for Complementary & Alternative Health Care (ACCAHC)
- American Association of Colleges of Podiatric Medicine (AACPM)
- American Council of Academic Physical Therapy (ACAPT)
- American Physical Therapy Association (APTA)
- American Podiatric Medical Association (APMA)
- American Psychological Association (APA)
- American Speech-Language-Hearing Association (ASHA)
- Association of Schools and Colleges of Optometry (ASCO)
- Association of Schools of Allied Health Professions (ASAHP)
- Council on Social Work Education (CSWE)
- Physician Assistant Education Association (PAEA)
- Society of Simulation in Healthcare (SSH)

Interprofessional Education Reflected in Accreditation

"After reviewing each participating agency's accreditation standards regarding IPE, HPAC members agreed that the definition of IPE and competencies for health profession students identified in the 2011 Interprofessional Education Collaborative (IPEC) report are fundamental to educational programs in the health professions accredited by the HPAC members."

HPAC Press Release, December 2014

In late 2014, the independent accreditation bodies from the six IPEC-sponsoring associations formed the Health Professions Accreditors Collaborative (HPAC) to establish a standing relationship that enables stakeholders to readily communicate and engage activities in support of interprofessional education, with the shared goal of preparing graduates for meaningful collaborative practice. Though the initial composition of HPAC includes the founding IPEC professions' accreditors, HPAC anticipates the need for expanding to other professions' accreditation entities in order to develop meaningful collective activities.

Current members of the Health Professions Accreditors Collaborative (HPAC) include:

- Accreditation Council for Pharmacy Education (ACPE) www.acpe-accredit.org
- Commission on Collegiate Nursing Education (CCNE) www.aacn.nche.edu/ccne-accreditation
- Commission on Dental Accreditation (CODA) www.ada.org/en/coda
- Commission on Osteopathic College Accreditation (COCA) www.osteopathic.org
- Council on Education for Public Health (CEPH) www.ceph.org
- Liaison Committee for Medical Education (LCME) www.lcme.org

IPEC Faculty Development Institutes

The IPEC core competencies framework has served as a cornerstone for 10 IPEC Faculty Development Institutes hosted since May 2012. The Faculty Development Institutes are designed to bring together multi-profession teams for the express purpose of creating an institutionally based project to advance IPE. Since May 2012, the Institutes have hosted 339 teams and 1,457 participants coming from 185 cities in 48 states, Washington, DC, and Puerto Rico. (New Hampshire and Montana are the only states without representation in an Institute cohort.) The Institutes have also hosted international teams from Lebanon, Canada, and South Africa.

While the majority of the Institutes have focused on IPE 101, three have been dedicated to quality improvement and patient safety in IPE and one on population health IPE.

In addition to the initial 6 IPEC professions, more than 60 other professions have participated on Institute teams, including:

- Allied Health
- Architecture
- Athletic Training, Sports Studies, and Exercise Science
- Basic Science, Genetics, Microbiology
- Behavioral and Community Health
- Chiropractic Care
- Communication Science and Disorders
- Curriculum Evaluation and Education Research
- Dental Hygiene
- Education Administration and Leadership
- Global Health
- Health and Environmental Sciences
- Health Services Administration and Research
- Law
- Library Science

- Nurse Anesthesia
- Nursing and Law
- Nutrition and Dietetics
- Occupational Therapy
- Optometry
- Palliative Care
- Physical Therapy
- Physician Assistant
- Psychology
- Radiologic Sciences
- Rehabilitation Services
- Respiratory Therapy
- Social Work
- Speech-Language Pathology
- Veterinary Medicine

IPEC PORTAL Collection

To create a readily available source of free, high-quality teaching materials, the Josiah Macy Jr., Foundation awarded development funding for IPE modules that had been implemented by at least three health professions and could be used as stand-alone instructional sources or integrated into broader IPE activities. Hosted on the AAMC's MedEdPORTAL® platform, the IPE PORTAL collection launched in December 2012 with 28 fully developed modules directly linked to the Interprofessional Collaboration Competencies promulgated by the 2011 IPEC report.

The IPE PORTAL collection is based on MedEdPORTAL's peer-review model. By design it facilitates efforts to coordinate authentic educational experiences across disciplinary boundaries in supplying credible educational resources that are validated by content experts for use with learners from multiple health professions. Access to these educational materials can be especially useful for regional campuses that may not have other disciplines on the same campus.

Modules range from case-based resources, evaluation tools, and multimedia resources to presentations, lab guides, references, and tutorials. Primary topic listings include communication skills, curriculum development or evaluation, health education, and evaluation of clinical performance. Additional topics cover ambulatory education, assessment; cognition, human learning, and problem solving, counseling, evidence-based medicine, health care quality improvement, health care systems, patient safety and medical errors, physician-patient relationship, professionalism, teaching skills, and veterans' health and wellness.

Competency-Based Interprofessional Education: Definitional Framework

Operational Definitions

Interprofessional education:
"When students from two or more professions learn about, from and with each other to enable effective collaboration and improve health outcomes." (WHO 2010)

Interprofessional collaborative practice:
"When multiple health workers from different professional backgrounds work together with patients, families, [careers], and communities to deliver the highest quality of care." (WHO 2010)

Interprofessional teamwork:
The levels of cooperation, coordination and collaboration characterizing the relationships between professions in delivering patient-centered care.

Interprofessional team-based care:
Care delivered by intentionally created, usually relatively small work groups in health care who are recognized by others as well as by themselves as having a collective identity and shared responsibility for a patient or group of patients (e.g., rapid response team, palliative care team, primary care team, and operating room team).

Professional competencies in health care:
Integrated enactment of knowledge, skills, values, and attitudes that define the areas of work of a particular health profession applied in specific care contexts.

Interprofessional competencies in health care:
Integrated enactment of knowledge, skills, values, and attitudes that define working together across the professions, with other health care workers, and with patients, along with families and communities, as appropriate to improve health outcomes in specific care contexts.

The 2011 charge to the expert panel was to identify individual-level interprofessional competencies for future health professionals in training that are specifically relevant to the pre-licensure/pre-credentialed student. The expert panel also identified eight reasons why it is important to agree on a set of core competencies across the professions, which still hold true today. They are needed to:

1. Create a coordinated effort across the health professions to embed essential content in all health professions education curricula.

2. Guide professional and institutional curricular development of learning approaches and assessment strategies to achieve productive outcomes.

3. Provide the foundation for a learning continuum in interprofessional competency development across the professions and the lifelong learning trajectory.

4. Acknowledge that evaluation and research work will strengthen the scholarship in this area.

5. Prompt dialogue to evaluate the "fit" between educationally identified core competencies for interprofessional collaborative practice and practice needs/demands.

6. Find opportunities to integrate essential interprofessional education content consistent with current accreditation expectations for each health professions education program.

7. Offer information to accreditors of educational programs across the health professions that they can use to set common accreditation standards for interprofessional education and to know where to look in institutional settings for examples of implementation of those standards.

8. Inform professional licensing and credentialing bodies in defining potential testing content for interprofessional collaborative practice.

Interprofessional Collaboration Domain

Recognizing that educators and IPE development teams have used the 2011 competencies extensively for curriculum design and mapping, the original structure is retained in this 2016 update. The two changes are to present **Interprofessional Collaboration** as a domain in and of itself and to better integrate population health competencies. The first change flows from the work of Englander et al (2013). Instead of depicting four domains within interprofessional collaborative practice (values/ethics, roles/responsibilities, interprofessional communication, teams and teamwork), the four topical areas fall under the single domain of interprofessional collaboration in which four core competencies and related sub-competencies now reside. The second change responds to shifts in the health system since the 2011 report was released, most prominently the increased focus on the Triple Aim and implementation of the Patient Protection and Affordable Care Act in 2010.

Interprofessional Collaboration Competency Domain

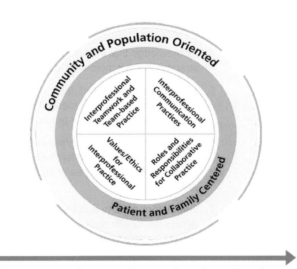

The Learning Continuum pre-licensure through practice trajectory

Four Core Competencies

The core competencies and sub-competencies feature the following desired principles: patient and family centered (hereafter termed "patient centered"); community and population oriented; relationship focused; process oriented; linked to learning activities, educational strategies, and behavioral assessments that are developmentally appropriate for the learner; able to be integrated across the learning continuum; sensitive to the systems context and applicable across practice settings; applicable across professions; stated in language common and meaningful across the professions; and outcome driven.

NOTE: The 2016 updates to the competencies and sub-competencies appear in **bold.**

Competency 1

Work with individuals of other professions to maintain a climate of mutual respect and shared values. (Values/Ethics for Interprofessional Practice)

Competency 2

Use the knowledge of one's own role and those of other professions to appropriately assess and address the health care needs **of patients** and **to promote and advance the health of populations.** (Roles/Responsibilities)

Competency 3

Communicate with patients, families, communities, **and professionals in health and other fields** in a responsive and responsible manner that supports a team approach to the **promotion and** maintenance of health and the **prevention and** treatment of disease. (Interprofessional Communication)

Competency 4

Apply relationship-building values and the principles of team dynamics to perform effectively in different team roles to **plan, deliver, and evaluate** patient/population-centered care **and population health programs and policies** that **are** safe, timely, efficient, effective, and equitable. (Teams and Teamwork)

IPEC Core Competencies for Interprofessional Collaborative Practice

Work with individuals of other professions to maintain a climate of mutual respect and shared values. (Values/Ethics for Interprofessional Practice)

Values/Ethics Sub-competencies:

VE1.	Place interests of patients and populations at center of interprofessional health care delivery **and population health programs and policies, with the goal of promoting health and health equity across the life span.**
VE2.	Respect the dignity and privacy of patients while maintaining confidentiality in the delivery of team-based care.
VE3.	Embrace the cultural diversity and individual differences that characterize patients, populations, and the **health team**.
VE4	Respect the unique cultures, values, roles/responsibilities, and expertise of other health professions **and the impact these factors can have on health outcomes**.
VE5	Work in cooperation with those who receive care, those who provide care, and others who contribute to or support the delivery of prevention and health services **and programs**.
VE6	Develop a trusting relationship with patients, families, and other team members (CIHC, 2010).
VE7.	Demonstrate high standards of ethical conduct and quality of care in contributions to team-based care.
VE8	Manage ethical dilemmas specific to interprofessional patient/ population centered care situations.
VE9.	Act with honesty and integrity in relationships with patients, families, **communities**, and other team members.
VE10.	Maintain competence in one's own profession appropriate to scope of practice.

Use the knowledge of one's own role and those of other professions to appropriately assess and address the health care needs **of patients** and **to promote and advance the health of populations.** (Roles/Responsibilities)

Roles/Responsibilities Sub-competencies:

RR1.	Communicate one's roles and responsibilities clearly to patients, families, **community members**, and other professionals.
RR2.	Recognize one's limitations in skills, knowledge, and abilities.
RR3.	Engage **diverse professionals** who complement one's own professional expertise, as well as associated resources, to develop strategies to meet specific **health and healthcare** needs **of patients and populations**.
RR4.	Explain the roles and responsibilities of other providers and how the team works together to provide care, **promote health, and prevent disease**.
RR5.	Use the full scope of knowledge, skills, and abilities of **professionals from health and other fields** to provide care that is safe, timely, efficient, effective, and equitable.
RR6.	Communicate with team members to clarify each member's responsibility in executing components of a treatment plan or public health intervention.
RR7.	Forge interdependent relationships with other professions **within and outside of the health system** to improve care and advance learning.
RR8.	Engage in continuous professional and interprofessional development to enhance team performance **and collaboration**.
RR9.	Use unique and complementary abilities of all members of the team to optimize **health and** patient care.
RR10.	**Describe how professionals in health and other fields can collaborate and integrate clinical care and public health interventions to optimize population health.**

Communicate with patients, families, communities, **and professionals in health and other fields** in a responsive and responsible manner that supports a team approach to the **promotion and** maintenance of health and the **prevention and** treatment of disease. (Interprofessional Communication)

Interprofessional Communication Sub-competencies:

CC1.	Choose effective communication tools and techniques, including information systems and communication technologies, to facilitate discussions and interactions that enhance team function.
CC2.	**Communicate** information with patients, families, **community members,** and **health team** members in a form that is understandable, avoiding discipline-specific terminology when possible.
CC3.	Express one's knowledge and opinions to team members involved in patient care **and population health improvement** with confidence, clarity, **and** respect, working to ensure common understanding of information, treatment, care decisions, **and population health programs and policies.**
CC4.	Listen actively, and encourage ideas and opinions of other team members.
CC5.	Give timely, sensitive, instructive feedback to others about their performance on the team, responding respectfully as a team member to feedback from others.
CC6.	Use respectful language appropriate for a given difficult situation, crucial conversation, or conflict.
CC7.	Recognize how one's uniqueness (experience level, expertise, culture, power, and hierarchy within the **health** team) contributes to effective communication, conflict resolution, and positive interprofessional working relationships (University of Toronto, 2008).
CC8.	Communicate the importance of teamwork in patient-centered **care and population health programs and policies.**

Apply relationship-building values and the principles of team dynamics to perform effectively in different team roles to **plan, deliver, and evaluate** patient/population-centered care **and population health programs and policies** that **are** safe, timely, efficient, effective, and equitable. (Teams and Teamwork)

Team and Teamwork Sub-competencies:

TT1.	Describe the process of team development and the roles and practices of effective teams.
TT2.	Develop consensus on the ethical principles to guide all aspects of **team work**.
TT3.	**Engage health and other professionals** in shared patient-centered **and population-focused** problem-solving.
TT4.	Integrate the knowledge and experience of **health and** other professions to inform **health and** care decisions, while respecting patient and community values and priorities/preferences for care.
TT5.	Apply leadership practices that support collaborative practice and team effectiveness.
TT6.	Engage self and others to constructively manage disagreements about values, roles, goals, and actions that arise among **health and other** professionals and with patients, **families, and community members.**
TT7.	Share accountability with other professions, patients, and communities for outcomes relevant to prevention and health care.
TT8.	Reflect on individual and team performance for individual, as well as team, performance improvement.
TT9.	Use process improvement to increase effectiveness of interprofessional teamwork and team-based **services, programs, and policies.**
TT10.	Use available evidence to inform effective teamwork and team-based practices.
TT11.	Perform effectively on teams and in different team roles in a variety of settings.

Resources

Association of Schools and Programs of Public Health (ASPPH). 2015. *Population Health across All Professions Expert Panel Report.* Washington, DC: ASPPH. http://www.aspph.org/app/uploads/2015/02/PHaAP.pdf

Barzansky,B. and Etzel, S. Medical Schools in the United States, 2014-2015. JAMA. 2015; 314(22): 2426-2435.

Canadian Interprofessional Health Collaborative. 2010. A national interprofessional competency framework. www.cihc.ca/resources/publications

Englander R, Cameron T, Ballard AJ, Dodge J, Bull J, Aschenbrener CA. Toward a common taxonomy of competency domains for the health professions and competencies for physicians. Academic Medicine. 2013; 88: 1088–1094.

Interprofessional Education Collaborative Expert Panel. 2011. *Core Competencies for Interprofessional Collaborative Practice: Report of an Expert Panel.* Washington, DC: IPEC.

Interprofessional Professionalism Collaborators. 2016. *Interprofessional Professionalism Behaviors.* Alexandria, VA: Interprofessional Professionalism Collaborative. http://www.interprofessionalprofessionalism.org/

Institute of Medicine (IOM). 2013. *Interprofessional Education for Collaboration: Learning How to Improve Health from Interprofessional Models Across the Continuum of Education to Practice: Workshop Summary.* Washington, DC: The National Academies Press.

Institute of Medicine (IOM). 2014. *Establishing Transdisciplinary Professionalism for Improving Health Outcomes: Workshop Summary.* Washington, DC: The National Academies Press.

Institute of Medicine (IOM). 2015. *Measuring the Impact of Interprofessional Education on Collaborative Practice and Patient Outcomes.* Washington, DC: The National Academies Press.

Palatta A, Cook B, Anderson E, Valachovic R. 20 years beyond the crossroads: the path to interprofessional education at U.S. Dental schools. Journal of Dental Education. 2015; 79(8):982-996.

University of Toronto. 2008. *Advancing the interprofessional education curriculum.* Toronto, Canada: University of Toronto.

World Health Organization (WHO). 2010. Framework for action on interprofessional education & collaborative practice. Geneva, Switzerland: WHO.

Appendix

FOR IMMEDIATE RELEASE
Contact: Dr. Sherin Tooks
CODA
tookss@ada.org
December 15, 2014

Press Release: Formation of the Health Professions Accreditors Collaborative (HPAC), 2014

New Health Professions Accreditors Collaborative Forms to Stimulate Interprofessional Engagement

Chicago, IL, Washington, DC and Silver Spring, MD – In an effort to strengthen ties across the health professions and better serve the public good, several of the nation's leading accrediting agencies are pleased to announce the formation of Health Professions Accreditors Collaborative (HPAC). Members of HPAC include the:

- Accreditation Council for Pharmacy Education (ACPE)
- Commission on Collegiate Nursing Education (CCNE)
- Commission on Dental Accreditation (CODA)
- Commission on Osteopathic College Accreditation (COCA)
- Council on Education for Public Health (CEPH)
- Liaison Committee for Medical Education (LCME)

HPAC members are committed to discussing important developments in interprofessional education (IPE) and exploring opportunities to engage in collaborative projects. It is anticipated that as HPAC evolves and develops activities, additional members from other health care accreditation organizations would join. HPAC will communicate with stakeholders around issues in IPE with the common goal to better prepare students to engage in interprofessional collaborative practice. After reviewing each participating agency's accreditation standards regarding IPE, HPAC members agreed that the definition of IPE and competency domains for health profession students identified in the Interprofessional Education Collaborative (IPEC) report (https://ipecollaborative.org/uploads/IPEC-Core-Competencies.pdf) are fundamental to educational programs in the health professions accredited by the HPAC members.

The participating agencies will meet regularly and host meetings on a rotating schedule. HPAC will respect the independence of accreditation standards, procedures, and decision-making of each participating accrediting agency.

About Members of the Health Professions Accreditors Collaborative (HPAC)

The **Accreditation Council for Pharmacy Education (ACPE)** is the national agency for the accreditation of professional degree programs in pharmacy and providers of continuing pharmacy education. ACPE is an autonomous and independent agency whose Board of Directors is derived through the American Association of Colleges of Pharmacy (AACP), the American Pharmacists

16

Association (APhA), the National Association of Boards of Pharmacy (NABP), and the American Council on Education (ACE). To learn more about ACPE, visit www.acpe-accredit.org.

The **American Osteopathic Association (AOA) Commission on Osteopathic College Accreditation (COCA)** serves as the accrediting agency for colleges of osteopathic medicine. The COCA reviews, evaluates, and takes final action on accreditation status, and communicates such action to appropriate state and federal education regulatory bodies. In addition, the COCA approves the standards, policies and procedures for college accreditation. The COCA reviews policy directions on predoctoral osteopathic medical education, and monitors and maintains high-quality osteopathic predoctoral education through the college accreditation process. Learn more at www.osteopathic.org.

The **Commission on Collegiate Nursing Education (CCNE)** is an autonomous accrediting agency that ensures the quality and integrity of baccalaureate, graduate, and residency programs in nursing. CCNE serves the public interest by assessing and identifying programs that engage in effective educational practices. CCNE accreditation supports and encourages continuing self-assessment by nursing programs and supports continuing growth and improvement of collegiate nursing education and post-baccalaureate nurse residency programs. Visit http://www.aacn.nche.edu/ccne-accreditation to learn more about CCNE.

The **Commission on Dental Accreditation (CODA)** is recognized by the United States Department of Education as the national accreditor for dental education programs, including predoctoral dental education programs, advanced dental education programs and allied dental education programs. The Commission functions independently and autonomously in matters of developing and approving accreditation standards, making accreditation decisions on educational programs and developing and approving procedures that are used in the accreditation process. It is structured to include an appropriate representation of the communities of interest. Learn more at www.ada.org/en/coda.

The **Council on Education for Public Health (CEPH)** is an independent agency recognized by the US Department of Education to accredit schools of public health and public health programs offered in settings other than schools of public health. These schools and programs prepare students for entry into careers in public health. The primary professional degree is the Master of Public Health (MPH) but other baccalaureate, masters and doctoral degrees are offered as well. Visit www.ceph.org for more information.

The **Liaison Committee on Medical Education (LCME)** accredits medical education programs leading to the MD degree in the United States and Canada. The LCME provides continuous quality improvement through its accreditation activities for medical education programs leading to the MD whose students are geographically located in the United States or Canada. Learn about LCME by visiting www.lcme.org.

###

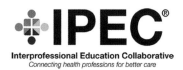
IPEC®
Interprofessional Education Collaborative
Connecting health professions for better care

FOR IMMEDIATE RELEASE
Contact: Shelley McKearney
February 22, 2016
smckearney@aacn.nche.edu
(202) 463-6930 ext. 269

Press Release: Institutional Members Join Interprofessional Education Collaborative (IPEC)

Interprofessional Education Collaborative Announces Expansion
Nine new members join organization dedicated to improving patient care

The Interprofessional Education Collaborative (IPEC) has approved nine additional members through a new institutional membership category, expanding its representation of associations of schools of the health professions to 15. Established in 2009 by six organizations committed to advancing interprofessional learning experiences and promoting team-based care, IPEC now includes the following national associations:

Founding members:
- American Association of Colleges of Nursing (AACN)
- American Association of Colleges of Osteopathic Medicine (AACOM)
- American Association of Colleges of Pharmacy (AACP)
- American Dental Education Association (ADEA)
- Association of American Medical Colleges (AAMC)
- Association of Schools and Programs of Public Health (ASPPH)

New institutional members:
- American Association of Colleges of Podiatric Medicine (AACPM)
- American Council of Academic Physical Therapy (ACAPT)
- American Occupational Therapy Association (AOTA)
- American Psychological Association (APA)
- Association of American Veterinary Medical Colleges (AAVMC)
- Association of Schools and Colleges of Optometry (ASCO)
- Association of Schools of Allied Health Professions (ASAHP)
- Council on Social Work Education (CSWE)
- Physician Assistant Education Association (PAEA)

"To actually deliver on the promise of interprofessional education and practice to improve health of individuals and populations as well as reduce health disparities, we have to ensure that this framework is central in the education of all health professionals," said Harrison C. Spencer, MD, MPH, DTM&H, CPH, IPEC Board Chair and President and CEO, Association of Schools and Programs of Public Health. "Changing and making all health professional education more consistent can help set the stage for the health system of the future we want to create together."

IPEC's mission is to ensure that new and current health professionals are proficient in the competencies essential for patient-centered, community and population oriented, interprofessional, collaborative practice. Eligible institutional members must be associations that represent and serve academic units at institutions of higher education that provide an educational program leading to the award of one or more academic degrees to students in one or more of the health professions that provide direct care to patients.

"Today marks a significant and growing commitment across the health professions in the United States to make collaborative, patient-centered care a reality," added Richard W. Valachovic, DMD, MPH, President of IPEC and President and CEO of the American Dental Education Association. "Including such a diverse and comprehensive group of new associations in IPEC's work brings us that much closer to success."

Health Professions Networks
Nursing & Midwifery
Human Resources for Health

Framework for Action on Interprofessional Education & Collaborative Practice

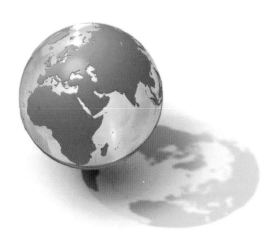

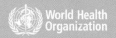
World Health
Organization

Framework for Action on Interprofessional Education & Collaborative Practice (WHO/HRH/HPN/10.3)

This publication is produced by the Health Professions Network Nursing and Midwifery Office within the Department of Human Resources for Health.

This publication is available on the Internet at: http://www.who.int/hrh/nursing_midwifery/en/

Copies may be requested from:
World Health Organization, Department of Human Resources for Health, CH-1211 Geneva 27, Switzerland

Edited by: Diana Hopkins, Freelance Editor, Geneva Switzerland

Layout: Monkeytree Creative Inc.
Cover design: S&B Graphic Design, Switzerland, www.sbgraphic.ch (illustration © Eric Scheurer)

Health Professions Networks
Nursing & Midwifery
Human Resources for Health

Framework for Action on Interprofessional Education & Collaborative Practice

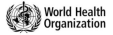 World Health Organization

4

Contents

5

Framework
for Action on
Interprofessional
Education and
Collaborative
Practice

6

Acknowledgements

The *Framework for Action on Interprofessional Education and Collaborative Practice* is the product of the WHO Study Group on Interprofessional Education and Collaborative Practice (see Annex 1 for a complete list of members). The Framework was prepared under the leadership of John HV Gilbert and Jean Yan, with support from a secretariat led by Steven J Hoffman.

Preparation of background papers and project reports was led by: Marilyn Hammick (lead author, Glossary and IPE Working Group Report), Steven J Hoffman (co-author, IPE International Scan), Lesley Hughes (co-author, IPE Staff Development Paper), Debra Humphris (lead author, SLSS Working Group Report), Sharon Mickan (co-author, CP Case Studies), Monica Moran (co-author, IPE Learning Outcomes Paper), Louise Nasmith (lead author, CP Working Group Report and CP Case Studies), Sylvia Rodger (lead author, IPE International Scan), Madeline Schmitt (co-author, IPE Staff Development Paper) and Jill Thistlethwaite (co-author, IPE Learning Outcomes Paper).

Significant contributions were also made by Peter Baker, Hugh Barr, David Dickson, Wendy Horne, Yuichi Ishikawa, Susanne Lindqvist, Ester Mogensen, Ratie Mpofu, Bev Ann Murray and Joleen Tirendi. Considerable support was provided by the Canadian Interprofessional Health Collaborative.

Administrative and technical support was provided by Virgie Largado-Ferri and Alexandra Harris. Layout and graphics were designed by Susanna Gilbert.

The main writers were Andrea Burton, Marilyn Hammick and Steven J Hoffman.

Interprofessional education... is an opportunity to not only change the way that we think about educating future health workers, but is an opportunity to step back and reconsider the traditional means of health-care delivery. I think that what we're talking about is not just a change in educational practices, but a change in the culture of medicine and health-care.

—Student Leader

7

Key messages

* The World Health Organization (WHO) and its partners recognize interprofessional collaboration in education and practice as an innovative strategy that will play an important role in mitigating the global health workforce crisis.

* Interprofessional education occurs when students from two or more professions learn about, from and with each other to enable effective collaboration and improve health outcomes.

* Interprofessional education is a necessary step in preparing a "collaborative practice-ready" health workforce that is better prepared to respond to local health needs.

* A collaborative practice-ready health worker is someone who has learned how to work in an interprofessional team and is competent to do so.

* Collaborative practice happens when multiple health workers from different professional backgrounds work together with patients, families, carers and communities to deliver the highest quality of care. It allows health workers to engage any individual whose skills can help achieve local health goals.

* After almost 50 years of enquiry, the World Health Organization and its partners acknowledge that there is sufficient evidence to indicate that effective interprofessional education enables effective collaborative practice.

* Collaborative practice strengthens health systems and improves health outcomes.

* Integrated health and education policies can promote effective interprofessional education and collaborative practice.

* A range of mechanisms shape effective interprofessional education and collaborative practice. These include:
  - supportive management practices
  - identifying and supporting champions
  - the resolve to change the culture and attitudes of health workers
  - a willingness to update, renew and revise existing curricula
  - appropriate legislation that eliminates barriers to collaborative practice

* Mechanisms that shape interprofessional education and collaborative practice are not the same in all health systems. Health policy-makers should utilize the mechanisms that are most applicable and appropriate to their own local or regional context.

* Health leaders who choose to contextualize, commit and champion interprofessional education and collaborative practice position their health system to facilitate achievement of the health-related Millennium Development Goals (MDGs).

* The *Framework for Action on Interprofessional Education and Collaborative Practice* provides policy-makers with ideas on how to implement interprofessional education and collaborative practice within their current context.

Framework for Action on Interprofessional Education and Collaborative Practice

9

Executive summary

At a time when the world is facing a shortage of health workers, policy-makers are looking for innovative strategies that can help them develop policy and programmes to bolster the global health workforce. The *Framework for Action on Interprofessional Education and Collaborative Practice* highlights the current status of interprofessional collaboration around the world, identifies the mechanisms that shape successful collaborative teamwork and outlines a series of action items that policy-makers can apply within their local health system (Figure 1). The goal of the Framework is to provide strategies and ideas that will help health policy-makers implement the elements of interprofessional education and collaborative practice that will be most beneficial in their own jurisdiction.

Figure 1.   Health and education systems

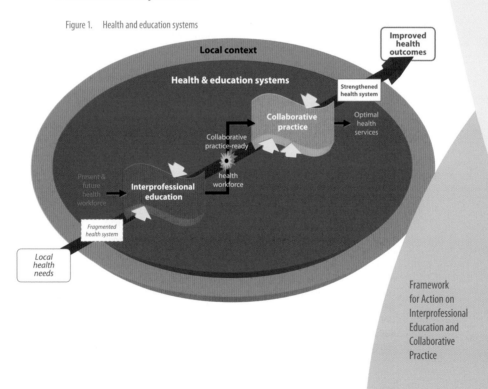

Framework
for Action on
Interprofessional
Education and
Collaborative
Practice

10

The case for interprofessional education and collaborative practice for global health

The *Framework for Action on Interprofessional Education and Collaborative Practice* recognizes that many health systems throughout the world are fragmented and struggling to manage unmet health needs. Present and future health workforce are tasked with providing health-services in the face of increasingly complex health issues. Evidence shows that as these health workers move through the system, opportunities for them to gain interprofessional experience help them learn the skills needed to become part of the collaborative practice-ready health workforce.

A collaborative practice-ready workforce is a specific way of describing health workers who have received effective training in interprofessional education. Interprofessional education occurs when students from two or more professions learn about, from and with each other to enable effective collaboration and improve health outcomes. Once students understand how to work interprofessionally, they are ready to enter the workplace as a member of the collaborative practice team. This is a key

step in moving health systems from fragmentation to a position of strength. Interprofessional health-care teams understand how to optimize the skills of their members, share case management and provide better health-services to patients and the community. The resulting strengthened health system leads to improved health outcomes.

Moving forward with integrated health and education policies

The health and education systems must work together to coordinate health workforce strategies. If health workforce planning and policymaking are integrated, interprofessional education and collaborative practice can be fully supported.

A number of mechanisms shape how interprofessional education is developed and delivered. In this Framework, examples of some of these mechanisms have been divided into two themes: educator mechanisms (i.e. academic staff training, champions, institutional support, managerial commitment, learning outcomes) and curricular mechanisms (i.e. logistics and scheduling, programme content, compulsory attendance, shared objectives, adult learning principles, contextual learning,

*T*he faculty development interprofessional education program was an expanding (mind and soul) experience for me to interact with other health workers in various health professions…an opportunity to share with like-minded people in other professions who value interprofessional education and are committed to bringing it about.

– Educator

11

assessment). By considering these mechanisms in the local context, policy-makers can determine which of the accompanying actions would lead to stronger interprofessional education in their jurisdiction.

Likewise, there are mechanisms that shape how collaborative practice is introduced and executed. Examples of these mechanisms have been divided into three themes: institutional support mechanisms (i.e. governance models, structured protocols, shared operating resources, personnel policies, supportive management practices); working culture mechanisms (i.e. communications strategies, conflict resolution policies, shared decision-making processes); and environmental mechanisms (i.e. built environment, facilities, space design). Once a collaborative practice-ready health workforce is in place, these mechanisms will help them determine the actions they might take to support collaborative practice.

The health and education systems also have mechanisms through which health-services are delivered and patients are protected. This Framework identifies examples of health-services delivery mechanisms (i.e. capital planning, remuneration models, financing, commissioning, funding streams) and patient safety mechanisms (i.e. risk management, accreditation, regulation, professional registration).

A call to action

It is important that policy-makers review this Framework through a global lens. Every health system is different and new policies and strategies that fit with and address their local challenges and needs must be introduced. This Framework is not intended to be prescriptive nor provide a list of recommendations or required actions. Rather it is intended to provide policy-makers with ideas on how to *contextualize* their existing health system, *commit* to implementing principles of interprofessional education and collaborative practice, and *champion* the benefits of interprofessional collaboration with their regional partners, educators and health workers.

Interprofessional education and collaborative practice can play a significant role in mitigating many of the challenges faced by health systems around the world. The action items identified in this Framework can help jurisdictions and regions move forward towards strengthened health systems, and ultimately, improved health outcomes. This Framework is a call for action to policy-makers, decision-makers, educators, health workers, community leaders and global health advocates to take action and move towards embedding interprofessional education and collaborative practice in all of the services they deliver.

Framework
for Action on
Interprofessional
Education and
Collaborative
Practice

12

Learning together to work together for better health

The need to strengthen health systems based on the principles of primary health-care has become one of the most urgent challenges for policy-makers, health workers, managers and community members around the world. Human resources for health are in crisis. The worldwide shortage of 4.3 million health workers has unanimously been recognized as a critical barrier to achieving the health-related Millennium Development Goals (1,2). In 2006, the 59th World Health Assembly responded to the human resources for health crisis by adopting resolution WHA59.23 which called for a rapid scaling-up of health workforce production through various strategies including the use of "innovative approaches to teaching in industrialized and developing countries" (3).

Governments around the world are looking for innovative, system-transforming solutions that will ensure the appropriate supply, mix and distribution of the health workforce. One of the most promising solutions can be found in interprofessional collaboration.

Figure 2.   Interprofessional education

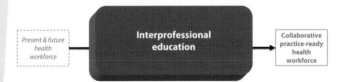

Figure 3.   Collaborative practice

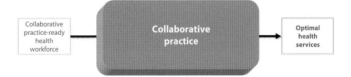

13

Key concepts

Health worker is a wholly inclusive term which refers to all people engaged in actions whose primary intent is to enhance health. Included in this definition are those who promote and preserve health, those who diagnose and treat disease, health management and support workers, professionals with discrete/unique areas of competence, whether regulated or non-regulated, conventional or complementary (1).

Interprofessional education occurs when two or more professions learn about, from and with each other to enable effective collaboration and improve health outcomes.

  * Professional is an all-encompassing term that includes individuals with the knowledge and/or skills to contribute to the physical, mental and social well-being of a community.

Collaborative practice in health-care occurs when multiple health workers from different professional backgrounds provide comprehensive services by working with patients, their families, carers and communities to deliver the highest quality of care across settings.

  * Practice includes both clinical and non-clinical health-related work, such as diagnosis, treatment, surveillance, health communications, management and sanitation engineering.

Health and education systems consist of all the organizations, people and actions whose primary intent is to promote, restore or maintain health and facilitate learning, respectively. They include efforts to influence the determinants of health, direct health-improving activities, and learning opportunities at any stage of a health worker's career (47–48).

  * Health is a state of complete physical, mental and social well-being and not merely the absence of disease or infirmity (World Health Organization, 1948) (49).
  * Education is any formal or informal process that promotes learning which is any improvement in behaviour, information, knowledge, understanding, attitude, values or skills (United Nations Educational, Scientific and Cultural Organization, 1997) (50).

A greater understanding of how this strategy can be implemented will help WHO Member States build more flexible health workforces that enable local health needs to be met while maximizing limited resources.

For health workers to collaborate effectively and improve health outcomes, two or more from different professional backgrounds must first be provided with opportunities to learn about, from and with each other. This *interprofessional education* is essential to the development of a "collaborative practice-ready" health workforce, one in which staff work together to provide comprehensive services in a wide range of health-care settings. It is within these settings where the greatest strides towards strengthened health systems can be made.

Policy-makers and those who support this innovative approach to human resources for health planning can use this Framework to move towards optimal health-services and better health outcomes by:

  * examining their local context to determine their needs and capabilities
  * committing to building interprofessional collaboration into new and existing programmes
  * championing successful initiatives and teams.

Framework
for Action on
Interprofessional
Education and
Collaborative
Practice

14

The *Framework for Action on Inter-professional Education and Collaborative Practice* provides a unique opportunity for all levels in the health and education systems to reflect on how they might better utilize interprofessional education and collaborative practice strategies to strengthen health system performance and improve health outcomes (Figures 2,3).

The need for interprofessional collaboration

Health policy-makers have shifted their focus from traditional delivery methods to innovative strategies that will strengthen the health workforce for future generations (4–7).

Although there is a great deal of interest in moving interprofessional collaboration forward, the desire to engage in this type of long-term planning is often sidelined by urgent crises such as epidemics of HIV/AIDS and/or tuberculosis, spiralling health-care costs, natural disasters, ageing populations, and other global health issues. Fortunately, many policy-makers are recognizing that a strong, flexible and collaborative health workforce is one of the best ways to confront these highly complex health challenges. In recent years, a number of local, national and regional associations

*B*uilding a regional network to support interprofessional collaboration not only ensured there was no competition for funding between projects, it also made it possible for all interprofessional projects to share best practices, challenges and opportunities.

–Regional Health Leader

and academic centres of excellence have been launched, demonstrating the growing momentum for interprofessional collaboration.

Interprofessional education and collaborative practice can positively contribute to some of the world's most urgent health challenges. For example:

Family and community health

Maternal and child health are essential to the overall well-being of a country. Every day 1500 women worldwide die from complications in pregnancy or childbirth. Health workers who are able to jointly identify the key strengths of each member of the health-care team and use those strengths to manage the complex health issues of the entire birthing family, will play a key role in reducing these alarming and preventable statistics.

HIV/AIDS, tuberculosis and malaria

The detection, treatment and prevention of global diseases, such as HIV/AIDS, tuberculosis and malaria, requires the collaboration of every type of worker within the health system. Interprofessional teams that have the expertise and resources to tailor their response to the local environment will be critical to the success of disease management programmes, education and awareness.

15

Health action in crisis

In situations of humanitarian crisis and conflict, a well-planned emergency response is essential. To overcome water, food and medical supply gaps, health workers must have the knowledge and skills to mobilize whatever resources and expertise are available within the health system and the broader community. Interprofessional education provides health workers with the kind of skills needed to coordinate the delivery of care when emergency situations arise.

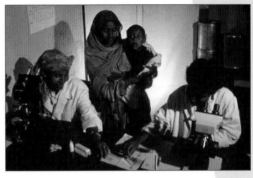

© WHO/DRT/Martel

Health security

Epidemics and pandemics place sudden and intense demands on the health system. Individuals who regularly work on a collaborative practice team can enhance a region's capacity to respond to health security issues such as outbreaks of avian influenza. In the event of a global epidemic or natural disaster, collaboration among health workers is the only way to manage the crisis.

Non-communicable diseases and mental health

Interprofessional teams are often able to provide a more comprehensive approach to preventing and managing chronic conditions such as dementia, malnutrition and asthma. These conditions are complex and often require a collaborative response.

Health systems and services

Interprofessional education and collaborative practice maximize the strengths and skills of health workers, enabling them to function at the highest capacity. With a current shortage of 4.3 million health workers, innovations of this nature will become more and more necessary to manage the strain placed on health systems.

The *Framework for Action on Interprofessional Education and Collaborative Practice* lists a range of practice- and system-level mechanisms that can help policy-makers implement and sustain progress in interprofessional collaboration. Recognizing that health and education systems should reflect local needs and aspirations, this Framework has been designed to help decision-makers worldwide apply key mechanisms and actions according to the needs of their unique jurisdictions. This Framework provides internationally relevant ideas for health policy-makers to consider and adapt as appropriate.

Team-based learning at Jimma University, Ethiopia

Since 1990, Jimma University has placed 20 to 30 final year students in medicine, nursing, pharmacy, laboratory science and environmental health in district health centres. Students deliver services ranging from nutrition promotion to primary care and basic laboratory services while becoming familiar with regional health centres and other students from a wide range of disciplines (51).

Framework for Action on Interprofessional Education and Collaborative Practice

16

International environmental scan of interprofessional education practices

To capture current interprofessional activities at a global level, the WHO Study Group on Interprofessional Education and Collaborative Practice conducted an international environmental scan between February and May 2008. The aim of this scan was to:

* Determine the current status of interprofessional education globally
* Identify best practices
* Illuminate examples of successes, barriers and enabling factors in interprofessional education.

A total of 396 respondents, representing 42 countries from each of the six WHO regions, provided insight about their respective interprofessional education programmes. These individuals represent various fields including practice (14.1 per cent), administration (10.6 per cent), education (50.4 per cent) and research (11.6 per cent).

Results indicate that interprofessional education takes place in many different countries and health-care settings across a range of income categories.* It involves students from a broad range of disciplines including allied health, medicine, midwifery, nursing and social work.

For most respondents, interprofessional education was compulsory. Student engagement occurs mainly at the undergraduate level, with a relatively even distribution among undergraduate years. Students are typically assessed in group situations (46.9 per cent in developed and 36.8 per cent in developing countries), followed by individual assignments, written tests and other methods. Although interprofessional education is normally delivered face-to-face, information technology is emerging as another valuable option.

Figure 4.   Types of learners who received interprofessional education at the respondents' insitutions

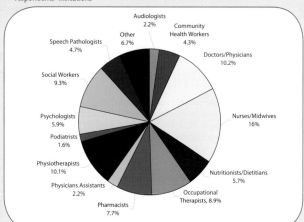

---

* The countries of the respondents were categorized according to the World Bank's Income Classification Scheme.

17

Figure 5.   Providers of staff training on interprofessional education

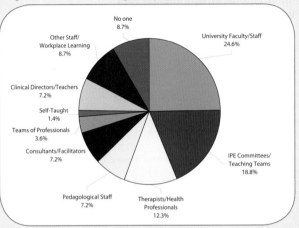

Internationally, preparing staff to deliver interprofessional education is uncommon. Courses are usually short and variable in nature and interprofessional education activities are not yet systematically delivered. In addition, routine evaluation of interprofessional education's impact on health outcomes and service delivery are rare.

Despite this, respondents reported that they had experienced many educational and health policy benefits from implementing interprofessional education. For example:

Educational benefits

* Students have real world experience and insight
* Staff from a range of professions provide input into programme development
* Students learn about the work of other practitioners

Health policy benefits

* Improved workplace practices and productivity
* Improved patient outcomes
* Raised staff morale
* Improved patient safety
* Better access to health-care

Significant effort is still required to ensure interprofessional initiatives are developed, delivered and evaluated in keeping with internationally recognized best practice.

The 42 countries represented by the respondents

Armenia, Australia, Bahamas, Belgium, Canada, Cape Verde, Central African Republic, China, Croatia, Denmark, Djibouti, Egypt, Germany, Ghana, Greece, Guinea, India, Iran (Islamic Republic of), Iraq, Ireland, Japan, Jordan, Malaysia, Malta, Mexico, Nepal, New Zealand, Norway, Pakistan, Papua New Guinea, Poland, Portugal, Republic of Moldova, Saudi Arabia, Singapore, South Africa, Sweden, Thailand, United Arab Emirates, United Kingdom, United States of America, Uruguay.

Framework
for Action on
Interprofessional
Education and
Collaborative
Practice

18

Interprofessional education and collaborative practice for improved health outcomes

After almost 50 years of inquiry, there is now sufficient evidence to indicate that interprofessional education enables effective collaborative practice which in turn optimizes health-services, strengthens health systems and improves health outcomes (Figure 6) (6–21). In both acute and primary care settings, patients report higher levels of satisfaction, better acceptance of care and improved health outcomes following treatment by a collaborative team (22).

Research evidence has shown a number of results:

* Collaborative practice can improve:
  - access to and coordination of health-services
  - appropriate use of specialist clinical resources
  - health outcomes for people with chronic diseases

- patient care and safety (23–25).
* Collaborative practice can decrease:
  - total patient complications
  - length of hospital stay
  - tension and conflict among caregivers
  - staff turnover
  - hospital admissions
  - clinical error rates
  - mortality rates (18–20, 22,23, 26–29).
* In community mental health settings collaborative practice can:
  - increase patient and carer satisfaction
  - promote greater acceptance of treatment
  - reduce duration of treatment
  - reduce cost of care
  - reduce incidence of suicide (17,21)
  - increase treatment for psychiatric disorders (30)
  - reduce outpatient visits (30).

Figure 6.   Health and education systems

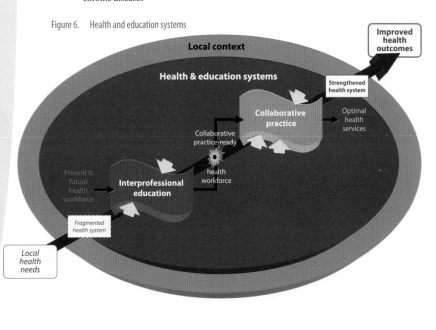

19

Cross-sectoral interprofessional collaboration during health crises

In 2005, northern Pakistan experienced a severe earthquake resulting in thousands of injuries. Relief efforts were particularly challenging in isolated mountain communities. A wound clinic was eventually opened within a partially constructed hotel, but had no source of water, making infection control extremely difficult. One of the volunteer health workers took the initiative to locate a trained plumber who was able to provide the clinic with a constant source of clean water within 48 hours. In this situation, seeking expertise outside of the conventional health-care team ensured earthquake victims were able to receive quality health-services in spite of the difficult circumstances (52). This is a common occurrence in emergency situations where collaboration across sectors can be essential to improving health outcomes (48).

* Terminally and chronically ill patients who receive team-based care in their homes:
  - are more satisfied with their care
  - report fewer clinic visits
  - present with fewer symptoms
  - report improved overall health (24,31).

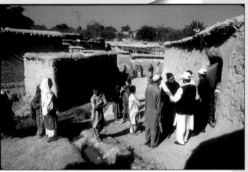

© Jean-Marc Giboux

* Health systems can benefit from the introduction of collaborative practice which has reduced the cost of:
  - setting up and implementing primary health-care teams for elderly patients with chronic illnesses (31)
  - redundant medical testing and the associated costs (32)
  - implementing multidisciplinary strategies for the management of heart failure patients (19)
  - implementing total parenteral nutrition teams within the hospital setting (18).*

This evidence clearly demonstrates the need for a collaborative practice-ready health workforce, which may include health workers from regulated and non-regulated professions such as community health workers, economists, health informaticians, nurses, managers,

*A*ny project that encompasses different specialties or jurisdictions needs to coordinate activities to achieve the greatest effectiveness. This is particularly the case with emergency situations. It is in that capacity that interprofessional teams may have the greatest impact on a public health emergency. The increased coordination and smoother functioning will facilitate a more efficient and effective response, as well as delivering assistance more quickly to those in need.

– National Chief Public Health Officer

---

* Summary charts of research evidence from systematic reviews related to interprofessional education and collaborative practice can be found in Annexes 6 and 7 respectively. The Canadian Interprofessional Health Collaborative has also recently prepared an evidence synthesis for policy-makers on the effects of interprofessional education, including 181 studies from 1974–2005, that can be accessed at http://www.cihc.ca/resources-files/the_evidence_for_ipe_july2008.pdf

Framework for Action on Interprofessional Education and Collaborative Practice

20

social workers and veterinarians. Cross-sectoral interprofessional collaboration between health and related sectors is also important because it helps achieve the broader determinants of health such as better housing, clean water, food security, education and a violence-free society.

Interprofessional education can occur during pre- and post-qualifying education in a variety of clinical settings (e.g. basic training programmes, post-graduate programmes, continuing professional development and learning for quality service improvement). Interprofessional education is generally well-received by participants who develop communication skills, further their abilities to critically reflect, and learn to appreciate the challenges and benefits of working in teams. Effective interprofessional education fosters respect among the health professions, eliminates harmful stereotypes, and evokes a patient-centred ethic in practice (8).

Many health workers already practice in teams and actively communicate with colleagues. While coordination and cooperation lay the foundation for collaboration, they are not the same as collaborative practice, which takes cooperation one step further by engaging a collaborative practice-ready health workforce, poised to take on complex or emergent problems and solve them

> Having a personal relationship with the team members helped to build trust among us, and colleagues that trust each other are much more inclined to seek collaboration.
> – Rural health worker

together. These health workers know how to collaborate with colleagues from other professions, have the skills to put their interprofessional knowledge into action and do so with respect for the values and beliefs of their colleagues. They can interact, negotiate and jointly work with health workers from any background.

Interprofessional education and collaborative practice are not panaceas for every challenge the health system may face. However, when appropriately applied, they can equip health workers with the skills and knowledge they need to meet the challenges of the increasingly complex global health system.

The role of health and education systems

Regional issues, unmet health needs and local background influence how health and education systems are organized around the world. No two contexts are exactly the same, yet all share six common building blocks. Collaborative practice can be seen in each of the six building blocks of the health systems:

1. health workforce
2. service delivery
3. medical products, vaccines and technologies
4. health systems financing
5. health information system
6. leadership and governance (32)

Critical reflection on collaborative practice

Several primary health-care clinics in Denmark maintain records on the services that each of its health workers provide to facilitate reflection, open discussion and improvement among its staff in how they work collaboratively. This process facilitates the sharing of best practices and fosters a team spirit (53).

21

Because of the unique nature of each health region, collaborative practice strategies must be considered according to local needs and challenges. In some regions, this may mean that collaborative, team-based approaches to care are driven by efforts to promote patient safety (34,35), maximize limited health resources, move care from acute to primary care settings or encourage greater integrated working (36,37). In others, the focus may be on human resource benefits such as increased health worker job satisfaction or greater role clarity for health workers when working in teams (22).

Regardless of the context in which policy-makers choose to introduce collaborative practice, research evidence and experience have demonstrated that a team-based approach to health-care delivery maximizes the strengths and skills of each contributing health worker. This enhances the efficiency of teams through reduced service duplication, more frequent and appropriate referral patterns, greater continuity and coordination of care and collaborative decision-making with patients (22). It can also assist in recruitment and retention of health workers (29) and possibly help mitigate health workforce migration.

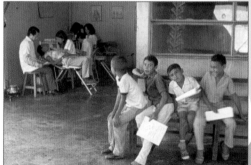

© WHO/photo by ALMASY P.

Framework
for Action on
Interprofessional
Education and
Collaborative
Practice

22

A culture shift in health-care delivery

One of the benefits of implementing interprofessional education and collaborative practice is that these strategies change the way health workers interact with one another to deliver care. Both strategies are about people: the health leaders and policy-makers who strive to ensure there are no barriers to implementing collaborative practice within institutions; the health workers who provide services; the educators who provide the necessary training to health workers; and most importantly, the individuals and communities who rely on the service. By shifting the way health workers think about and interact with one another,

the culture of the working environment and attitudes of the workforce will change, improving the working experience of staff and benefiting the community as a whole.

Internationally, interprofessional education and collaborative practice are now considered credible strategies that can help mitigate the global health workforce crisis. The growing evidence and research base continues to identify interprofessional collaboration as beneficial to health workers, systems and communities. In order to move interprofessional education and collaborative practice forward, this Framework outlines the mechanisms that policy-makers and civil society leaders can use to begin making the shift to system-wide interprofessional collaboration.

It made me more aware of how important the process of change is. Teams can benefit patients if they are working well. If the team is not working well it can also affect the patient. It also makes me more aware of how I will want to practice in the future.

- Pharmacy Student

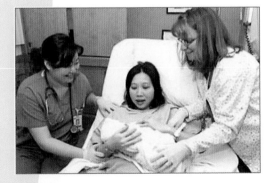

Moving forward

23

Achieving interprofessional education and collaborative practice requires a review and assessment of the mechanisms that shape both. For this Framework, a number of key mechanisms were identified from a review of the research literature, results of an international environmental scan of interprofessional education practices, country case studies and the expertise of key informants. These mechanisms have been organized into broad themes and grouped into three sections: 1) interprofessional education, 2) collaborative practice, and 3) health and education systems. For each

section, possible action items have been identified that health policy-makers can implement in their local context. However, while the mechanisms and actions have been assigned under the broad categories of interprofessional education and collaborative practice, there is a great degree of overlap, and many of the mechanisms influence both sections (Figure 7). As these strategies are introduced and expanded, interprofessional education and collaborative practice will become more embedded, strengthening health systems and improving health outcomes.

Figure 7.   Examples of mechanisms that shape interprofessional education at the practice level

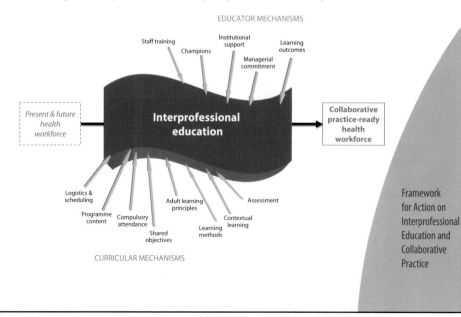

Framework
for Action on
Interprofessional
Education and
Collaborative
Practice

24

Staff training for interprofessional education

An interprofessional preceptor development course for East Carolina University's Rural Health Training Program in the United States of America consisted of four three-hour sessions over four months. Educators learned how to increase student comfort with the interprofessional curriculum and one another. Content included regular meetings to discuss shared cases and provide feedback (59).

Interprofessional education: achieving a collaborative practice-ready health workforce

Interprofessional education is shaped by mechanisms that can be broadly classified into those driven by:

* staff responsible for developing, delivering, funding and managing interprofessional education
* the interprofessional curricula.

Educator[†] mechanisms. Developing interprofessional education curricula is a complex process, and may involve staff from different faculties, work settings and locations. Sustaining interprofessional education can be equally complex and requires:

* supportive institutional policies and managerial commitment (38)
* good communication among participants
* enthusiasm for the work being done
* a shared vision and understanding of the benefits of introducing a new curriculum
* a champion who is responsible for coordinating education activities and identifying barriers to progress (39).

Careful preparation of instructors for their roles in developing, delivering and evaluating interprofessional education is

also important (10,14,40,41). For most educators, teaching students how to learn about, from and with each other is a new and challenging experience. For interprofessional education to be successfully embedded in curricula and training packages, the early experiences of staff must be positive. This will ensure continued involvement and a willingness to further develop the curriculum based on student feedback.

Curricular mechanisms. Health-care and education around the world are provided by different types of educators and health workers who offer a range of services at different times and locations. This adds a significant layer of coordination for interprofessional educators and curriculum developers. Evidence has shown that making attendance compulsory and developing flexible scheduling can prevent logistical challenges from becoming a barrier to effective interprofessional collaboration.

Research indicates that interprofessional education is more effective when:

* principles of adult learning are used (e.g. problem-based learning and action learning sets)
* learning methods reflect the real world practice experiences of students (39)
* interaction occurs between students.

Effective interprofessional education relies on curricula that link learning activities, expected outcomes and an

---

† The term "educator" includes all instructors, trainers, faculty, preceptors, lecturers and facilitators who work within any education or health-care institution, as well as the individuals who support them.

25

assessment of what has been learned (42). It is important to remember that expected outcomes will be influenced by the student's physical and social environment as well as their level of education. Well-constructed learning outcomes assume students need to know: what to do (i.e. knowledge); how to apply their knowledge (i.e. skills); and when to apply their skills within an appropriate ethical framework using that knowledge (i.e. attitudes and behaviour).

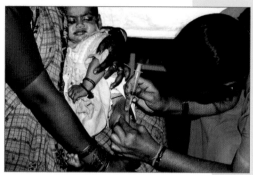

© WHO/P. Virot

Interprofessional education offers students real-world experience

In 1996, Linköping University in Sweden implemented an extensive commitment to interprofessional education for all health science students. Up to 12 weeks of the curriculum for all students is devoted to interprofessional education (60). A part of this commitment was the launch of the first interprofessional student training ward at the Faculty of Health Sciences at Linköping University (61).

A similar training program has been offered at the nearby Karolinska Institutet since 1998, where a two week mandatory interprofessional course for medical, nursing, physiotherapy and occupational therapy students is delivered on a training ward. Five to seven students work in teams to plan and organize patient care while their supervisors act as coaches. At the end of every shift the student teams reflect on their learning experience with their supervisors (62).

Interprofessional curriculum development and delivery

At Tribhuvan University's Maharajgunj Nursing Campus in Nepal, the curricula on newborn care was updated at a workshop that included nursing and medical faculty. Participants worked together to identify essential components of a new curriculum. They found that the nursing faculty were more knowledgeable and skilled in areas like essential newborn care while the medical faculty were more knowledgeable and skilled in advanced care (63).

At Christian Medical College in Vellore, India, nursing students are taught about interprofessional teamwork and the role of interpersonal relationships when communicating with patients and colleagues. They learn about different ways to improve collaboration, including strengthening referral services. (64).

The New Generation Project at the University of Southampton is at the forefront of making common learning across the health-care practices a reality. The project comprises a team of educationalists and researchers who have created and are developing a new syllabus that brings the distinct health-care professions closer together through common understanding, mutual respect and communication (65).

Mandatory interprofessional education

In Sweden, the Centres for Clinical Education Project conducted evaluations of a two week interprofessional course for medical, nursing, physiotherapy and occupational therapy students. Evaluators noted that in making the interprofessional clinical course mandatory, there was greater contact among faculty, staff and students – who expressed an interest in having these interactions continue (66).

Framework
for Action on
Interprofessional
Education and
Collaborative
Practice

26

These outcomes may be seen in the following examples grouped under the interprofessional learning domains.

1. Teamwork:
   - being able to be both team leader and team member
   - knowing the barriers to teamwork
2. Roles and responsibilities:
   - understanding one's own roles, responsibilities and expertise, and those of other types of health workers
3. Communication:
   - expressing one's opinions competently to colleagues
   - listening to team members
4. Learning and critical reflection:
   - reflecting critically on one's own relationship within a team
   - transferring interprofessional learning to the work setting
5. Relationship with, and recognizing the needs of, the patient:
   - working collaboratively in the best interests of the patient
   - engaging with patients, their families, carers and communities as partners in care management
6. Ethical practice:
   - understanding the stereotypical views of other health workers held by self and others
   - acknowledging that each health workers views are equally valid and important

We welcome white brothers and sisters who are working together to improve the health of our people. We will go out with you – we will guide and support you – we will introduce you to the community. You will find that each of our communities share a sense of humor – we hang on to it – we are a resilient people and we welcome working together on this journey towards interprofessional collaboration."

– Aboriginal Community Leader

Interprofessional education provides learners with the training they need to become part of the collaborative practice-ready health workforce. Once health workers are ready to practice collaboratively, additional mechanisms and actions can help shape their experience (Table 1). In developing collaborative practice, health system planners and health educators must engage in discussions about how they can help learners transition from education to the workplace.

27

Table 1.   Actions to advance interprofessional education for improved health outcomes

ACTION	PARTICIPANTS	LEVEL OF ENGAGEMENT EXAMPLES	POTENTIAL OUTCOMES
1. Agree to a common vision and purpose for interprofessional education with key stakeholders across all faculties and organizations	• Decision-makers • Policy-makers • Health facility directors and managers • Education leaders • Educators • Health workers	CONTEXTUALIZE • Vision: "Whether students are in the classroom or participating in practice education, interprofessional education will be encouraged and collaborative practice principles upheld"	• All health-worker education is directed by an interprofessional vision and purpose
2. Develop interprofessional education curricula according to principles of good educational practice	• Curriculum developers • Educators • Education leaders • Researchers	CONTEXTUALIZE • Link with local researchers to understand how best practices in interprofessional education can be applied to their local context • Develop curricula based on existing resources and local needs	• An interprofessional education framework that is specific to the local region and takes into account culture, geography, history, challenges, etc. • Engagement of numerous community layers, such as health workers, researchers and facilities
3. Provide organizational support and adequate financial and time allocations for: • the development and delivery of interprofessional education • staff training in interprofessional education	• Health facility directors and managers • Education leaders	COMMIT • Set aside a regular time for interprofessional champions, staff and others to meet • Provide incentives for staff to participate in interprofessional education	• A collaborative practice-ready health workforce • Improved workplace health and satisfaction for health workers
4. Introduce interprofessional education into health worker training programmes: • all pre-qualifying programmes • appropriate post-graduate and continuing professional development programmes • learning for quality service improvement	• Government leaders • Policy-makers • Education leaders • Educators • Curricula developers • Health facility directors and managers	COMMIT • Introduce new system-wide curricula • Manage senior health worker resistance to 're-education'	• A collaborative practice-ready health workforce • Interprofessional education and collaborative practice embedded into health-system delivery
5. Ensure staff responsible for developing, delivering and evaluating interprofessional education are competent in this task, have expertise consistent with the nature of the planned interprofessional education and have the support of an interprofessional education champion	• Educators • Education leaders	COMMIT • Provide educators and training staff with opportunities to discuss shared challenges and successes • Provide resources for educators and staff • Focus on continuous improvement using appropriate evaluation tools	• Strengthened education with a focus on interprofessional education and collaborative practice
6. Ensure the commitment to interprofessional education by leaders in education institutions and all associated practice and work settings	• Education leaders • Health facility directors and managers	CHAMPION • Allow educators, clinical supervisors and staff to share positive interprofessional experiences with their supervisors and leaders	• Improved attitudes toward other health professions • Improved communication among health workers

Framework
for Action on
Interprofessional
Education and
Collaborative
Practice

28

Collaborative practice: achieving optimal health-services

Collaborative practice works best when it is organized around the needs of the population being served and takes into account the way in which local health-care is delivered. A population-based or needs-based approach is necessary when determining the best way to introduce new interprofessional concepts. While a collaborative practice-ready health workforce is an essential mechanism towards shaping the effectiveness of collaborative practice, by itself it will not guarantee the provision of optimal health-services (Figure 8).

Other practice-level mechanisms, such as institutional supports, working culture and environment can enable the effectiveness of collaborative practice (Table 2).

Institutional supports. Institutional mechanisms can shape the way a team of people work collaboratively, creating synergy instead of fragmentation (43). Staff participating in collaborative practice need clear governance models, structured protocols and shared operating procedures. They need to know that management supports teamwork and believes in sharing the responsibility for health-care service delivery among team members. Adequate time and space is needed for interprofessional

Delivery of interprofessional education using information communication technologies

In the virtual learning environment, students from different health professional groups gain an understanding of the roles and responsibilities of each member of the health-care team. Experiences from the Universitas 21 global consortium of universities show that information communication technology can be used to help break down established stereotypes and promote equal partnership in patient care (67).

Effective communication strategies

At a psychiatry hospital in Tamilnadu, India, a mental health team works interprofessionally to deliver patient care. In this setting clinical rounds are done together, allowing all professions to be engaged in the decision-making process. Individuals from this team have emphasized that their success is largely due to a clear understanding of responsibilities, trust between professions, open and honest communication, and inclusion of the family in patient care (68).

Students' views of interprofessional education

At the University of Queensland in Australia, students reported gaining a better understanding of the need for 'communication and listening' following an interprofessional workshop about children who have developmental coordination disorders (69).

Structures for shared decision-making

In an urban community health clinic in India, care is managed by a team of health workers. Each practitioner has a caseload of over 3,000 patients, and physicians provide weekly support during clinic hours (64).

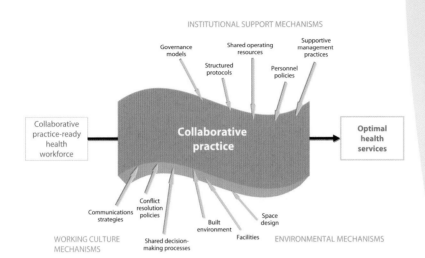

Figure 8.   Examples of mechanisms that shape collaboration at the practice level

collaboration and delivery of care. At the same time, personnel policies need to recognize and support collaborative practice and offer fair and equitable remuneration.

Working culture. Collaborative practice is effective when there are opportunities for shared decision-making and routine team meetings. This enables health workers to decide on common goals and patient management plans, balance their individual and shared tasks, and negotiate shared resources. Structured information systems and processes, effective communication strategies, strong conflict resolution policies and regular dialogue among team and community members play an

important role in establishing a good working culture.

Environment. Space design, facilities and the built environment can significantly enhance or detract from collaborative practice in an interprofessional clinic. In some cases, effective space design has included input and recommendations from the community and patients, as well as members of the health-care team. Most notably, physical space should not reflect a hierarchy of positions. Additional considerations could include developing a shared space to better facilitate communication or organizing spaces and rooms in ways that eliminate barriers to effective collaboration (44).

*T*he course was very helpful in gaining an understanding of the roles and perspectives of other health professions, working as a team, and developing efficient relationships in the workplace.

– Physiotherapy Student

Framework for Action on Interprofessional Education and Collaborative Practice

30

Table 2.   Actions to advance collaborative practice for improved health outcomes

ACTION	PARTICIPANTS	LEVEL OF ENGAGEMENT EXAMPLES	POTENTIAL OUTCOMES
1. Structure processes that promote shared decision-making, regular communication and community involvement	• Health facility managers and directors • Health workers	CONTEXTUALIZE • Discuss and share ideas for improved communication processes • Develop a sense of community through interaction and staff support	• A model of collaborative practice that recognizes the principles of shared decision-making and best practice in communication across professional boundaries
2. Design a built environment that promotes, fosters and extends interprofessional collaborative practice both within and across service agencies	• Policy-makers • Health facility managers and directors • Health workers • Capital planners • Architects/space planners	CONTEXTUALIZE • Relocate and rearrange equipment to better facilitate communication flow	• Improved communication channels • Improved satisfaction among health workers
3. Develop personnel policies that recognize and support collaborative practice and offer fair and equitable remuneration models	• Government • Health facility managers and directors • Policy-makers • Regulatory/labour bodies	COMMIT • Review personnel policies and consider innovative remuneration and incentive plans	• Improved workplace health and well-being for workers • Improved working environment
4. Develop a delivery model that allows adequate time and space for staff to focus on interprofessional collaboration and delivery of care	• Health facility managers and directors • Policy-makers • Health workers	COMMIT • Set aside time for staff to meet together to discuss cases, challenges and successes • Provide opportunity for staff to be involved in development of new processes and strategic planning	• Improved interaction between management and staff • Greater cohesion and communications between health workers
5. Develop governance models that establish teamwork and shared responsibility for health-care service delivery between team members as the normative practice	• Health facility managers and directors • Policy-makers • Government leaders	CHAMPION • Review and update the existing governance model • Develop a strategic plan for an interprofessional education and collaborative practice model of care	• A sustained commitment to embedding interprofessional collaboration in the workplace • Updated governance model, job descriptions, vision, mission and purpose

Vision and programme aims

In Nepal, a national strategy called Saving Newborn Lives was implemented to address high rates of newborn mortality. Bringing together nursing and medical faculty, this common goal became the catalyst for the development of an integrated curriculum and strengthened relationships between the two professions (56).

Collaborative practice and the built environment

The physical setting for collaborative practice plays an important role in the quality of care provided by interprofessional teams. For health workers providing services to patients and family dealing with sensitive health issues such as mental illness or chronic disease, a private, quiet area is essential in order to provide quality, compassionate, patient-centred care (47).

31

Legislation to support collaborative practice

In 2008, the Government of British Columbia in Canada passed legislation that included a provision on interprofessional collaboration. Each of the province's health professional regulatory colleges are now asked, "(k) in the course of performing its duties and exercising its powers under this Act or other enactments, to promote and enhance the following: (ii) interprofessional collaborative practice between its registrants and persons practising another health profession" (45).

Government mechanisms shaping interprofessional education in norway

In 1972, the Norwegian Government stated that to prepare students to work across boundaries and to further interprofessional collaboration, health professional students should be educated together. In 1995 they recommended that all undergraduate allied health, nursing and social work programmes include a common core curricula that covered: scientific theory; ethics; communication and collaboration; and scientific methods and knowledge about the welfare state. All university colleges adopted the common core. Government encouraged shared studies, but provided a great degree of flexibility for university colleges that had too few professions or were located far from potential partner institutions (70).

Health and education systems: achieving improved health outcomes

The health and education systems must coordinate their efforts in order to ensure the future health workforce consists of appropriately qualified staff, positioned in the right place at the right time. Institutions and individuals working within the health and education systems can help foster a supportive climate for interprofessional collaboration. In developing collaborative practice, health workers and health educators must discuss how to make the transition from education to the work environment. Key principles that can guide the movement towards interprofessional education and collaborative practice include context relevance, policy integration, multi-level system change and collaborative leadership. It is also important to note that service users, patients and carers

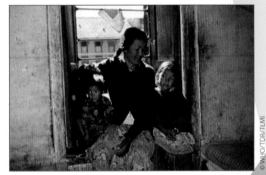

© WHO/TDR/TLMI

and families are all engaged in the collaborative practice process.

Legislation is a key mechanism through which health and education systems are organized, monitored and managed. Because legislative changes can influence how health workers are educated, accredited, regulated and remunerated, legislation has a significant impact on the development, implementation and sustainability of interprofessional education and

Framework for Action on Interprofessional Education and Collaborative Practice

32

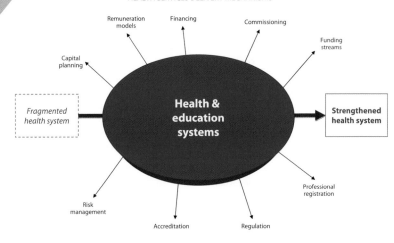

Figure 9.   Examples of influences that affect interprofessional education and collaborative practice at the system level

collaborative practice (Figure 9). It can also play an important role in championing interprofessional collaboration when government agrees to develop legislation that removes barriers to collaborative practice. Regulation is often an important part of the legislative agenda. As the health workforce diversifies, policy-makers must address the role that regulation could or should play in recognizing and supporting new and emerging professions, particularly those that include a unique mix of skills.

Health-services delivery. The way in which health and education services are financed, funded and commissioned[‡] can influence the success of interprofessional education and collaborative practice. For example, how health workers are remunerated can affect the amount of time they spend collaborating with one another and demonstrating "teamwork in practice" to students. Reviewing how different workforce remuneration models, funding streams and risk management processes may impact patient care and student learning is

‡   Financing is how money is raised, funding is how money is spent, and commissioning is the process of choosing service providers.

33

essential to moving interprofessional education and collaborative practice forward. At the same time, coordinating policies for health-services that support the development and delivery of integrated team-based services would:

* engage other areas of public policy such as social care, education, housing and justice
* systematize interprofessional collaboration in education and health as a national strategic direction
* facilitate the commissioning of health and education services that support the principles of collaborative practice.

*I*t was an encouraging feeling to have the support, camaraderie and cooperation of the other students and preceptors in the community, and it gave us the opportunity to experience both learning and teaching roles with each other. It helped make me aware of some of the misconceptions existing between professions and the limitations of our own profession.

– Medical Student

Patient safety. Governance mechanisms that establish system-wide standards and support patient safety can be used to embed interprofessional education and collaborative practice within the health-care system. Many of the governance mechanisms that are enacted throughout the world exist to protect patients and the community. If regulation is too rigid, processes may become fragmented and result in an escalation of costs and additional strain on the health system. Alternately, if regulation is reasonably flexible, opportunities to embed interprofessional education into practice increase.

Sustained political commitment

In Japan, the Kobe Municipal Government committed to a collaborative practice model for maternal and child health to help reduce infant mortality rates. This programme, called The Supporting Room, provides comprehensive services (prenatal, postpartum and during early childhood) delivered by staff from different professions in a collaborative setting (71).

Integrated health and education policies as supportive mechanisms

An explicit change in health policy in England required all universities who train health professionals to develop and integrate interprofessional education in the classroom and in practice (6). In Canada, one of the outcomes of the Romanow Commission (72) which reviewed and advised on a future model for the Canadian health-care system, was the recommendation that interprofessional education be taken forward with the explicit intention to promote team-based working (73–74).

In Thailand, Khon Kaen University is responding to the worldwide shortage of health workers by coordinating meetings between community hospitals, administrative organizations and faculty to develop programmes to support local practitioners and educators (75).

Framework for Action on Interprofessional Education and Collaborative Practice

34

Interprofessional education and patient safety

In the United States of America, the Institute of Medicine issued a landmark report in 2003 titled, *Health Professions Education: A Bridge to Quality* (76), which emphasized the need for interprofessional education and collaborative practice. This publication was a follow-up to two earlier reports on patient safety, *To Err is Human* (77) and *Crossing the Quality Chasm* (78), released in 1999 and 2001 respectively.

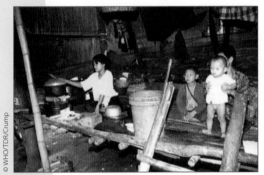

© WHO/TDR/Crump

Before this [interprofessional education] project, people didn't really see each other as people. They saw each other as a "doctor" or a "nurse" and forgot about the human side. Now, they go beyond the job title and communicate with each other with more respect. Because of this project, they see each other as people now and that's a big change.

– Education Leader

In almost every country there are legal and regulatory structures that can be both barriers to and enablers of interprofessional education and collaborative practice. Accreditation requirements for health centres and registration criteria for students can also transform education and practice (42). One government, for example, has included a clause in their health legislation that requires regulatory bodies to include interprofessional education as part of their bylaws (45). Another includes a requirement that community members be part of the selection panel for student admission into health professional education programmes and, alongside the professional bodies that oversee health professional education, strongly indicates that students should experience interprofessional education as part of their initial professional education (46–48). By embedding interprofessional education and collaborative practice in legislation, accreditation requirements and/or registration criteria, policy-makers and government leaders can be champions of interprofessional collaboration. In response to issues raised around patient safety in *To err is human*, in 2003 the United States Institute of Medicine issued a landmark report *Health professions education: a bridge to quality* which emphasized the need for interprofessional education and collaborative practice (Table 3).

35

Table 3.   Actions to support interprofessional education and collaborative practice at the system-level

ACTION	PARTNERSHIPS	LEVEL OF ENGAGEMENT EXAMPLES	POTENTIAL OUTCOMES
1. Build workforce capacity at national and local levels	• Government leaders • Health facility managers and directors • Education leaders • Policy-makers	CONTEXTUALIZE • engage in focused discussions with partners and health-care leaders • develop short and long term planning strategies for recruitment, retention and education	• Short-, medium- and long-term planning for an interprofessional workforce • Clear and defined direction for human resources for health planning
2. Create accreditation standards for health worker education programmes that include clear evidence of interprofessional education	• Education leaders • Regulatory bodies • Legislators • Government leaders • Researchers	CONTEXTUALIZE • Review current accreditation standards and ensure future standards include interprofessional education and collaborative practice components • Ensure accreditation standards of all professions include similar language on interprofessional education and collaborative practice	• Updated accreditation standards for all professions with a shared theme of interprofessional education and collaborative practice
3. Create policy and regulatory frameworks that support educators and health workers to promote and practice collaboratively, including new and emerging roles and models of care	• Government leaders • Professional associations • Regulatory authorities • Education leaders • Legislators	COMMIT • Encourage legislators to develop appropriate legislative models to support collaborative practice • Engage partners and health workers in discussions around roles and responsibilities of new and emerging professions	• Legislative and regulatory frameworks that support interprofessional education and collaborative practice
4. Create frameworks and allocate funding for clear interprofessional outcomes as part of life long learning for the health workforce	• Professional associations • Regulatory bodies • Government leaders • Government agencies • Education leaders • Legislators	COMMIT • Develop programmes and courses that suit pre- and post-qualifying education	• Lifelong learning for health workers to enable them to become and remain collaborative-practice ready throughout their career
5. Create an environment in which to share best practices from workforce planning, financing, funding and remuneration which are supportive of interprofessional education and collaborative practice	• Government leaders • Researchers • Education leaders • Health facility managers and directors	CHAMPION • Host meetings that bring together regional champions to share successes and challenges	• A coherent funding model for interprofessional collaboration • Improved communication between all levels of the health system • Development of a database of best practices/evidence

Framework
for Action on
Interprofessional
Education and
Collaborative
Practice

36

Conclusion

The World Health Organization recognizes interprofessional collaboration in education and practice as an innovative strategy that will play an important role in mitigating the global health crisis. The purpose of the *Framework for Action on Interprofessional Education and Collaborative Practice* is to provide policy-makers with a broad understanding of how interprofessional education and collaborative practice work in a global context. This Framework uses research evidence and a range of examples from existing projects around the world to provide readers with new ideas on how to implement and integrate these strategies in their region.

Interprofessional education and collaborative practice can be difficult concepts to explain, understand and implement. Many health workers believe themselves to be practicing collaboratively, simply because they work together with other health workers. In reality, they may simply be working within a group where each individual has agreed to use their own skills to achieve a common goal. Collaboration, however, is not only about agreement and communication, but about creation and synergy. Collaboration occurs when two or more individuals from different backgrounds with complementary skills interact to create a shared understanding that none had previously possessed or could have come to on their own. When health workers collaborate together, something is there that was not there before. The only way health workers can achieve an understanding of how collaboration applies to health-care, is to participate in interprofessional education which will enable them to be collaborative-practice ready.

This Framework focuses on the importance of introducing interprofessional education and collaborative practice as strategies that can transform the health system. It is no longer enough for health workers to be professional. In the current global climate, health workers also need to be interprofessional. By working collaboratively, health workers can

> We know that inter-professional collaboration is key to providing the best in patient care. That means we need to ensure our health and human services students gain the knowledge and skills they need through interprofessional education that begins at the earliest stages of their schooling.
> – Assistant Deputy Minister for Health and Education

37

A role for global health organizations

Health policy is increasingly influenced by international health organizations. Global health institutions, non-governmental organizations and donor agencies can play an important role in supporting and championing interprofessional education and collaborative practice.

Examples of how global health organizations might consider taking a leading role in interprofessional collaboration include:

* Support national health policy-makers in their efforts to introduce, enable and sustain interprofessional education and collaborative practice.
* Ensure projects and programmes are developed that include interprofessional education and collaborative practice and link education and practice initiatives.
* Provide funding streams that facilitate regional, national and local level collaborative practice efforts.
* Support coordination between health and education systems.
* Advocate for interprofessional education and collaborative practice and ensure it remains a priority on the global health agenda.
* Work across organizations to identify possibilities and harness opportunities where interprofessional education and collaborative practice could strengthen existing and new programmes.
* Take a global leadership role by committing and championing interprofessional education and collaborative practice internationally.

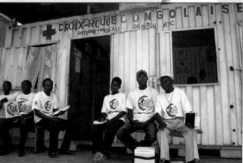

© WHO

positively address current health challenges, strengthening the health system and improving health outcomes.

Ultimately, interprofessional education and collaborative practice are about people: the health workers who provide services and work together to ensure patients and the community receive the best treatment as efficiently as possible; the educators who understand the importance of bringing together students from a range of disciplines to learn about, from and with one another; the health leaders and policy-makers who strive to ensure there are no barriers to implementing collaborative practice within institutions; and most importantly, the individuals who require and use health-services, trusting that their health workers are working together to provide them with the best service possible (Table 4).

Rather than providing a set of instructions or recommendations for the introduction and implementation of interprofessional education and collaborative practice, this Framework instead seeks agreement from policy-makers around the world to act now. Policy-makers will move towards optimal health-services and better health outcomes by examining their local context to determine their needs and capabilities; committing to building interprofessional collaboration into new and existing programmes; and championing successful initiatives and teams.

Framework
for Action on
Interprofessional
Education and
Collaborative
Practice

38

Table 4.   Summary of identified mechanisms that shape interprofessional education and collaborative practice

INTERPROFESSIONAL EDUCATION	COLLABORATIVE PRACTICE	HEALTH AND EDUCATION SYSTEMS
Educator mechanisms	**Institutional supports**	**Health-services delivery**
• Champions	• Governance models	• Capital planning
• Institutional support	• Personnel policies	• Commissioning
• Managerial commitment	• Shared operating procedures	• Financing
• Shared objectives	• Structured protocols	• Funding streams
• Staff training	• Supportive management practices	• Remuneration models
Curricular mechanisms	**Working culture**	**Patient safety**
• Adult learning principles	• Communication strategies	• Accreditation
• Assessment	• Conflict resolution policies	• Professional registration
• Compulsory attendance	• Shared decision-making processes	• Regulation
• Contextual learning	**Environment**	• Risk management
• Learning outcomes	• Built environment	
• Logistics and scheduling	• Facilities	
• Programme content	• Space design	

Contextualize

No two health systems in the world are exactly alike. Structure, processes, key health issues, types of health workers and the cultural context are just some of the factors which may influence how health-care is delivered. Countries seeking to move towards more collaborative types of practice are all at different starting points, with different challenges to overcome.

For this reason, the Framework suggests that those who wish to develop and engage a collaborative practice-ready health workforce begin by assessing what is readily and currently available, and building on what they have. Moving to implement interprofessional education and collaborative practice will only work if there is a realistic possibility of achieving success and an authenticity around how and what needs to be achieved. Developing, maintaining and nurturing strong partnerships within

the community is key to health system transformation.

Examples of actions that policy-makers might take to contextualize interprofessional education and collaborative practice in their local jurisdiction could include:

* agreeing on why interprofessional education and collaborative practice could benefit the local community and how key stakeholders in local regional facilities and organizations can work together to achieve this

* considering how to structure processes in a way that promotes shared decision-making, regular communication and community involvement

* introducing integrated workforce capacity and capability planning across the health and education systems at regional, national and local levels.

39

Commit

Once policy-makers feel they have contextualized their own health system and have identified areas where they can move forward, a commitment can be made to pursue interprofessional collaboration as an innovative strategy for health system transformation (Figure 10).

This type of commitment may come in a variety of forms. In some regions, there is a demonstrated need for evidence (especially research and evaluation) that supports interprofessional education and collaborative practice. While we know a lot about the positive impact of effective interprofessional education and collaborative practice, particularly from those who have personally benefitted from this type of practice, there is still much we do not know. Health workers and policy-makers could benefit from a strong global commitment to support this research.

The commitment by leaders in health and education to work together to implement innovative ways of

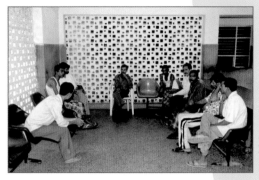

© WHO/P. Virot

delivering interprofessional education and collaborative practice is often one of the most important steps toward a strengthened health system. Together, leadership can ensure that traditional barriers to collaborative practice, such as legislation and regulation, are reconsidered. Without coordination between the two systems, which are linked at the core, it can be challenging for health workers to follow the necessary steps to achieve collaborative practice readiness.

Examples of actions that policy-makers might take to demonstrate their

Figure 10.   Implementation of integrated health workforce strategies

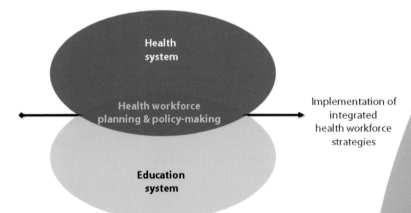

Health system

Health workforce planning & policy-making

Implementation of integrated health workforce strategies

Education system

Framework for Action on Interprofessional Education and Collaborative Practice

40

Student leaders as partners for change

Thousands of health professional students from across Canada came together in 2005 to form the National Health Sciences Students' Association as a grassroots movement to champion interprofessional education. Drawing on a network of 22 university/college-based chapters and over 20 health professions, student leaders design and deliver local academic, social and community service programmes that promote collaborative practice. The Association's University of Toronto chapter, for example, hosted a series of social events coinciding with the university's interprofessional 'Pain Week' curriculum. The Dalhousie University chapter recruited hundreds of health professional students to participate in a breast cancer charity run while learning about, from and with one another. The local chapter at the University of British Columbia partnered with its provincial Ministry of Health to coordinate innovative health programming for elementary and high school students (79).

commitment to interprofessional education and collaborative practice in their local jurisdiction could include:

* introducing interprofessional education into all health-related education and training programmes
* updating personnel policies to recognize and support collaborative practice and offer fair and equitable remuneration models
* harmonizing the way in which health programmes are funded, financed and commissioned to ensure there are no barriers to collaborative practice.

Champion

Like most innovative ideas, interprofessional education and collaborative practice require advocates who recognize that the health system is not ideal or sustainable in its current form, and that the move to build a collaborative health workforce is one of the ways to strengthen and transform the system. Over time, the goal is for collaborative practice to become an integral part of every health worker's education and practice, so that it is embedded in the training of every health worker and the delivery of every appropriate health-service. Collaborative practice should be the norm, but to achieve this goal, changes are needed in attitudes, in systems and in operations.

Politics and policy can play a huge role in advocating for change. Identifying and supporting interprofessional education and collaborative practice champions, ensuring appropriate collaborative practice-friendly policies are in place, and sharing the positive outcomes of successful collaborative programmes are small but significant steps towards broadening the use of interprofessional collaboration around the world.

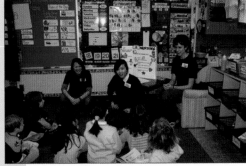

© NaHSSA

41

Examples of actions policy-makers might take to champion interprofessional education and collaborative practice in their local jurisdiction could include:

* encouraging leaders in education institutions, governments and practice settings to share their commitment to interprofessional education, and actively seek to embed it in related programmes and discussion;

* sharing the lessons learned from models of health workforce planning, financing, funding, commissioning and remuneration that are supportive of interprofessional education and collaborative practice;

* encouraging management to support teamwork and the sharing of responsibility for health-care service delivery among team members.

Interprofessional education and collaborative practice can play a significant role in mitigating many of the challenges faced by health systems around the world. Now is the time to act,

to implement these strategies which have the potential to transform health-care delivery, strengthen health systems and ultimately improve health outcomes. While every jurisdiction, region and country has unique challenges and needs, the goal of this Framework is to provide suggestions and ideas that will build on the work currently underway and open dialogue and discussion around key interprofessional education and collaborative practice initiatives that could be implemented in the future. It is the hope of the WHO Study Group on Interprofessional Education and Collaborative Practice that this Framework will be the impetus for policy-makers throughout the world to embrace interprofessional education and collaborative practice. By implementing strategies that promote interprofessional collaboration, the system will begin to move from a fragmented state to one where health systems are strengthened and health outcomes are improved.

> **W**atching the excitement of these future health-care leaders learning from and about each other, it is exciting to think what the next few years will bring in terms of changes and renewal in our health-care system. Which at the end of the day, is what it is all about!
>
> – Chief Nursing Officer

Championing interprofessional collaboration

In the Muscat Region of Oman, several clinics identified strong support for collaborative practice among high-level policy-makers as an enabling factor for achieving effective teamwork among their health workers. The availability and willingness of health managers and health system planners to meet with front-line staff was also recognized as being important (80).

Framework
for Action on
Interprofessional
Education and
Collaborative
Practice

42

References

1   World Health Organization. *World health report 2006 – working together for health.* Geneva, 2006.

2   Global Health Workforce Alliance. *GHWA welcomes G8 commitment for action on chronic health worker shortages.* Geneva, World Health Organization, 2008 (http://www.who.int/workforcealliance/news/g82008/en/index.html, accessed 12 August 2008).

3   Resolution WHA59.23. Rapid scaling up of health workforce production. In: *Fifty-ninth World Health Assembly, Geneva, 22–27 May 2006. Resolutions and decisions, annexes.* Geneva, World Health Organization, 2006 (WHA59/2006/REC/1).

4   Matthews Z, Channon A, Van Lerberghe W. *Will there be enough people to care? Notes on workforce implications of demographic change 2005–2050.* Geneva, World Health Organization, 2006 (http://www.who.int/hrh/resources/workforce_implications.pdf, accessed on 11 August 2008).

5   *Strategic principles for workforce development in New Zealand.* Wellington, Health Workforce Advisory Committee, 2005.

6   *Working together, learning together: a framework for lifelong learning for the NHS.* London, Department of Health, 2001 (http://www.dh.gov.uk/en/Publicationsandstatistics/Publications/PublicationsPolicyAndGuidance/DH_4009558, accessed 27 July 2008).

7   *The primary health care package for South Africa – a set of norms and standards.* Pretoria, South Africa, Department of Health, 2000 (http://www.doh.gov.za/docs/policy/norms/full-norms.html, accessed on 31 July 2008).

8   Reeves S et al. Interprofessional education: effects on professional practice and health care outcomes. *Cochrane Database of Systematic Reviews,* 2008, Issue 1.

9   Barr H et al. *Evaluations of interprofessional education: a United Kingdom review for health and social care.* London, BERA/CAIPE, 2000.

10 Reeves S. Community-based interprofessional education for medical, nursing and dental students. *Health and Social Care in the Community,* 2001, 8:269–276.

11 Reeves S. A systematic review of the effects of interprofessional education on staff involved in the care of adults with mental health problems. *Journal of Psychiatric Mental Health Nursing,* 2001, 8:533–542.

12 Cooper H et al. Developing an evidence base for interdisciplinary learning: a systematic review. *Journal of Advanced Nursing,* 2001, 35:228–237.

13 Barr H et al. *Effective interprofessional education: assumption, argument and evidence.* Oxford, Blackwell Publishing, 2005.

14 Hammick M et al. A best evidence systematic review of interprofessional education. *Medical Teacher,* 2007, 29:735–751.

15 Reeves S et al. *Knowledge transfer and exchange in interprofessional education: synthesizing the evidence to foster evidence-based decision-making.* Vancouver, Canadian Interprofessional Health Collaborative, 2008.

16 Zwarenstein M, Bryant W. Interventions to promote collaboration between nurses and doctors. *Cochrane Database of Systematic Reviews,* 2000, Issue 1.

17 Simmonds S et al. Community mental health team management in severe mental illness: a systematic review. *The British Journal of Psychiatry,* 2001, 178:497–502.

18 Naylor CJ, Griffiths RD, Fernandez RS. Does a multidisciplinary total parenteral nutrition team improve outcomes? A systematic review. *Journal of Parenteral and Enteral Nutrition,* 2004, 28:251–258.

19 McAlister FA et al. Multidisciplinary strategies for the management of heart failure patients at high risk for admission. *Journal of the American College of Cardiology,* 2004, 44:810–819.

20 Holland R et al. Systematic review of multidisciplinary interventions in heart failure. *Heart,* 2005, 91:899–906.

21 Malone D et al. Community mental health teams (CMHTs) for people with severe mental illnesses and disordered personality.

43

Cochrane Database of Systematic Reviews, 2007, Issue 2. (Art. No.: CD000270. DOI: 10.1002/14651858.CD000270.pub2)

22 Mickan SM. Evaluating the effectiveness of health care teams. *Australian Health Review,* 2005, 29(2):211-217.

23 Lemieux-Charles L et al. What do we know about health care team effectiveness? A review of the literature. *Medical Care Research and Review,* 2006, 63:263–300.

24 Hughes SL et al. A randomized trial of the cost-effectiveness of VA hospital-based home care for the terminally ill. *Health Services Research,* 1992, 26:801–817.

25 Jansson A, Isacsson A, Lindholm LH. Organisation of health care teams and the population's contacts with primary care. *Scandinavian Journal of Health Care,* 1992, 10:257–265.

26 *Teamwork in healthcare: Promoting effective teamwork in healthcare in Canada.* Ottawa, Canadian Health Services Research Foundation, 2006 (http://www.chsrf.ca/research_themes/pdf/teamwork-synthesis-report_e.pdf, accessed 30 July 2009).

27 Morey JC et al. Error reduction and performance improvements in the emergency department through formal teamwork training: Evaluation results of the MedTeams project. *Health Services Research,* 2002, 37:1553–1581.

28 West MA et al. Reducing patient mortality in hospitals: the role of human resource management. *Journal of Organisational Behaviour,* 2006, 27:983–1002.

29 Yeatts D, Seward R. Reducing turnover and improving health care in nursing homes: The potential effects of self-managed work teams. *The Gerontologist,* 2000, 40:358–363.

30 Jackson G et al. A new community mental health team based in primary care: a description of the service and its effect on service use in the first year. *British Journal of Psychiatry,* 1993, 162:375–384.

31 Sommers LS et al. Physician, nurse, and social worker collaboration in primary care for chronically ill seniors. *Archives of Internal Medicine,* 2000, 160:1825–1833.

32 Loxley A. *Collaboration in health and welfare.* London, Jessica Kingsley Publishers, 1997.

33 *Everybody's business – strengthening health systems to improve health outcomes: WHO's framework for action.* Geneva, World Health Organization, 2007 (http://www.who.int/healthsystems/strategy/everybodys_business.pdf, accessed 12 August 2008).

34 *Learning from Bristol: the report of the public inquiry into children's heart surgery at the Bristol Royal Infirmary 1984-1995 [Command Paper: CM 5207].* London, Department of Health, 2001 (http://www.bristol-inquiry.org.uk/, accessed 27 July 2008).

35 Borrill C, West M. *Team working and effectiveness in health care: findings from the Healthcare Team Effectiveness Project.* Birmingham, Aston Centre for Health Service Organisation Research, 2002.

36 Ham C. *Clinically integrated systems: The next step in English health reform?* London, The Nuffield Trust, 2005 (http://www.nuffieldtrust.org.uk/ecomm/files/Clinically_Integrated_Systems.pdf, accessed 31 July 2008).

37 Fabbricotti I, Helderman J. Integrated care for elderly. *Health Policy Monitor,* October 2003 (http://www.hpm.org/survey/nl/b1/3, accessed 30 July 2008).

38 Stone M. Coming in from the interprofessional cold in Australia. *Australian Health Review,* 2007, 31:332–340.

39 Freeth D et al. *Effective interprofessional education: development, delivery and evaluation.* Oxford, Blackwell Publishing, 2005.

40 Davidson M et al. Interprofessional pre-qualification clinical education: a systematic review. *Australian Health Review,* 2008, 32:111–120.

W ith my student and I, it sparked a good discussion about peoples' roles in the workplace, and how to manage that communication back and forth better. We spent quite a while talking about that and the fact that when things go wrong, it's often because there's a lack of understanding of the other guy's job and if you had some idea of what they were going through to try and streamline things together, how all the pieces fit, you'd have a more cohesive workplace."

–Nurse Preceptor

Framework for Action on Interprofessional Education and Collaborative Practice

44

41 Steinert Y. Learning together to teach together: interprofessional education and faculty development. *Journal of Interprofessional Care*, 2005, 19(Suppl. 1): 60–75.

42 Gilbert JHV. Interprofessional learning and higher education structural barriers. *Journal of Interprofessional Care*, 2005, 19(Suppl. 1):87–106.

43 D'Amour D, Oandasan I. Interprofessionality as the field of interprofessional practice and interprofessional education: an emerging concept. *Journal of Interprofessional Care*, 2005, 19(Suppl. 1):8–20.

44 Newton C, Bainbridge L. *Space design can enhance interprofessional health education and collaborative practice.* (In preparation.)

45 *Health Professions Act*, R.S.B.C. 2008, c. 183, s. 16(2)(k). Victoria, Government of British Columbia, 2008.

46 Wenman H. *Working towards full participation.* London, General Social Care Council, 2005/*Tomorrow's doctors.* London, General Medical Council, 2003/ *Statement of common purpose for subject benchmark statements for the health and social care professions.* Gloucester UK, Quality Assurance Agency for Higher Education, 2006.

47 *World health report 2000 – health systems: improving performance.* Geneva, World Health Organization, 2000.

48 *World health report 2007 – a safer future: global public health security in the 21st century.* Geneva, World Health Organization, 2007.

49 Preamble to the Constitution of the World Health Organization as adopted by the International Health Conference, New York, 19 June - 22 July 1946. Signed on 22 July 1946 by the representatives of 61 States and entered into force on 7 April 1948. *Official Records of the World Health Organization*, 1946, No. 2, p. 100.

50 *International standard classification of education.* Paris, United Nations Educational, Scientific and Cultural Organization, 1997 (http://www.unesco.org/education/information/nfsunesco/doc/isced_1997.htm, accessed 13 August 2008).

51 Global Health Workforce Alliance. *Scaling up, saving lives: Task Force for Scaling Up Education and Training for Health Workers.* Geneva, World Health Organization, 2008 (http://www.who.int/workforcealliance/documents/Global_Health%20FINAL%20REPORT.pdf, accessed 9 August 2008).

52 Redwood-Campbell L. [unpublished data: personal communication], 8 August 2008.

53 Ledderer L et al. *Collaborative practice in general practice in Denmark.* Odense, University of Southern Denmark, 2008.

54 Borril C et al. Team working and effectiveness in health care. *British Journal of Health Care Management*, 2000, 6:34–37.

55 Haward R et al. Breast cancer teams: the impact of constitution, new cancer work-load, and methods of operation on their effectiveness. *British Journal of Cancer*, 2003, 89:15–22.

56 Taylor J, Blue I, Misan G. Approach to sustainable primary health care service delivery for rural and remote South Australia. *Australian Journal of Rural Health*, 2001, 9:304–310.

57 Lobato L, Burlandy L. The context and process of health care reform in Brazil. In: Fleury S, Belmartino S, Baris E, eds. *Reshaping health care in Latin America: a comparative analysis of health care reform in Argentina, Brazil, and Mexico.* Ottawa, International Development Research Centre, 2000 (http://www.idrc.ca/fr/ev-35305-201-1-DO_TOPIC.html, accessed 11 August 2008).

58 Lehmann U, Saunders D. *Community health workers: what do we know about them? The state of evidence on programmes, activities, costs and impact on health outcomes of using community health workers.* Geneva, World Health Organization, 2007 (http://www.who.int/hrh/documents/community_health_workers.pdf, accessed 11 August 2008).

59 Clay MC et al. Applying adult education principles to the design of a preceptor development program. *Journal of Interprofessional Care*, 1999, 13:405–415.

60 Areskog NH. Multiprofessional education at the undergraduate level – the Linköping model, *Journal of Interprofessional Care*, 1994, 8:279–282.

61 Wahlström O, Sandén I, Hammar M. Multiprofessional education in the medical curriculum. *Medical Education* 1997, 31:425–429.

62 Ponzer, S et al. Interprofessional training in the context of clinical practice: goals and student's perception on clinical education wards. *Medical Education*, 2004, 38:727–736.

63 Shrestha S. *A case study of collaborative practice from Nepal.* Kathmandu, Tribhuvan University, 2008.

45

64   Jacob B, Vijayakumar C, Jayakaran R. *A collaborative practice case study describing the College of Nursing Community Health Programme in India*. Vellore, Christian Medical College, 2008.

65   O'Halloran C, Hean S, Humphris D, Macleod-Clark J. Developing common learning: the New Generation Project undergraduate curriculum model. *Journal of Interprofessional Care*, 2006, 20:12–28.

66   Mogensen E et al. Centre for Clinical Education: developing the health care education of tomorrow. *Education for Health*, 2002, 15:19–26.

67   Ho K et al. Opportunities for global academic contribution to interprofessional education in e-health: case study of Universitas 21. *Journal of Interprofessional Care*. (In press.)

68   Chandy S, Jacob B. *A collaborative practice case study from a mental health centre in India*. Vellore, Christian Medical College, 2008.

69   Rodger S et al. Enhancing teamwork among allied health students: evaluation of an interprofessional workshop. *Journal of Allied Health*, 2005, 34:230–235.

70   Almås S, Barr H. Differential implementation and differential outcomes in undergraduate health and social care education. *Journal of Interprofessional Care*. (In press.)

71   Ishikawa Y. [unpublished data: personal communication], 9 July 2008.

72   *Commission on the Future of Health Care in Canada: The Romanow Commission*. Ottawa, Health Canada, 2002 (http://www.hc-sc.gc.ca/hcs-sss/hhr-rhs/strateg/romanow-eng.php, accessed 27 July 2008).

73   Ontario Interprofessional Care Steering Committee. *Interprofessional care: a blueprint for action in Ontario*. Toronto, HealthForceOntario, 2007 (http://www.healthforceontario.ca/upload/en/whatishfo/ipc%20blueprint%20final.pdf, accessed 11 August 2008).

74   Mable AL, Marriott J. *Steady state – finding a sustainable balance point: international review of health workforce planning*. Ottawa, Health Canada, 2001 (http://www.hc-sc.gc.ca/hcs-sss/alt_formats/hpb-dgps/pdf/pubs/2002-steadystate-etatstable/2002-steadystate-etatstable-eng.pdf, accessed 11 August 2008).

75   Khanitta N. *A collaborative practice case study from Thailand*. Khon Kaen, Khon Kaen University, 2008.

76   Institute of Medicine. *Health professions education: a bridge to quality*. Washington DC, National Academy Press, 2003.

77   Institute of Medicine. *To err is human: building a safer health system*. Washington DC, National Academy Press, 1999.

78   Institute of Medicine. *Crossing the quality chasm: a new health system for the 21st century*. Washington DC, National Academy Press, 2001.

79   Hoffman SJ et al. Student leadership in interprofessional education: benefits, challenges and implications for educators, researchers and policymakers. *Medical Education*, 2008, 42:654–661.

80   Tawilah J. [unpublished data: personal communication], 13 September 2008.

Framework
for Action on
Interprofessional
Education and
Collaborative
Practice

46

Annexes

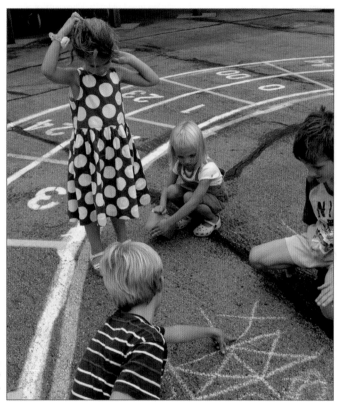

47

ANNEX 1 Membership of the WHO Study Group on Interprofessional Education and Collaborative Practice

Central Leadership Team

* John HV Gilbert, University of British Columbia, Canada (Co-Chair)
* Jean Yan, Human Resources for Health, World Health Organization (Co-Chair)
* Steven J Hoffman, Human Resources for Health, World Health Organization (Project Manager)

Interprofessional Education Working Group

* Peter G Baker, University of Queensland, Australia (Theme Leader)
* Marilyn Hammick, Centre for the Advancement of Interprofessional Education, the United Kingdom
* Wendy Horne, Auckland University of Technology, New Zealand
* Lesley Hughes, University of Hull, the United Kingdom
* Monica Moran, University of Queensland, Australia
* Sylvia Rodger, University of Queensland, Australia
* Madeline Schmitt, University of Rochester, the United States
* Jill Thistlethwaite, University of Sydney, Australia

Collaborative Practice Working Group

* Yuichi Ishikawa, Kobe University, Japan (Theme Leader)
* Susanne Lindqvist, University of East Anglia, the United Kingdom
* Sharon Mickan, Oxford Brookes University, the United Kingdom
* Ester Mogensen, Karolinska Institutet, Sweden
* Ratie Mpofu, University of the Western Cape, South Africa
* Louise Nasmith, University of British Columbia, Canada

System-level Supportive Structures Working Group

* Debra Humphris, University of Southampton, the United Kingdom (Co-Theme Leader)
* Jill Macleod Clark, University of Southampton, the United Kingdom (Co-Theme Leader)
* Hugh Barr, *Journal of Interprofessional Care*, the United Kingdom
* Vernon Curran, Memorial University of Newfoundland, Canada
* Denise Holmes, Association of Academic Health Centers, the United States
* Lisa Hughes, Department of Health (England), the United Kingdom
* Sandra MacDonald-Rencz, Health Canada, Canada
* Bev Ann Murray, Health Canada, Canada

Framework
for Action on
Interprofessional
Education and
Collaborative
Practice

48

ANNEX 2   Partnering organizations

Australasian Interprofessional Practice and Education Network (AIPPEN)

AIPPEN is a network of individuals, groups, institutions and organizations committed to researching, delivering, promoting and supporting interprofessional learning, education and practice. The primary aim of the network is to promote better health-care outcomes and to enhance interprofessional practice through interprofessional learning in Australia and New Zealand by developing a network to promote communication and collaboration among members.

AIPPEN aims to:

* promote the development of a network that can link health professional education and care sectors, universities, vocational education and training sector, government, practitioners and service users (patients);
* organize a series of seminars and conferences to share information and experiences;
* influence workforce policy and practice change in Australia and New Zealand;
* encourage research, evaluation and collaboration between different teams that can demonstrate the health-care and economic advantages of interprofessional learning;
* disseminate information on interprofessional learning.

Canadian Interprofessional Health Collaborative (CIHC)

CIHC is a pan-Canadian collaborative of partners advancing the evidence base related to Interprofessional Education for Collaborative Patient-Centred Practice (IECPCP) towards improved health education, improved health services, and improved health for Canadians.

CIHC's focus is on building a representative Collaborative, identifying and sharing best practices in interprofessional education and collaborative practice, and translating this knowledge to people who can use it to transform health-care.

CIHC aims to:

* facilitate knowledge production, exchange and application in interprofessional education and collaborative practice;
* foster strategic and innovative partnerships that enable interprofessional collaboration in education, research and practice;
* promote a coordinated approach to curriculum development and reform;
* articulate, advance, and advocate a research and evaluation agenda for interprofessional education and collaborative practice;
* develop support for leadership in interprofessional education and collaborative practice;
* build the Canadian Interprofessional Health Collaborative and model interprofessional collaborative approaches within and among organizations and sectors.

49

European Interprofessional Education Network (EIPEN)

EIPEN aims to establish a sustainable inclusive network of people and organizations in partner countries to share and develop effective interprofessional learning and teaching for improving collaborative practice and multi agency working in health-care. EIPEN has two interlinked aims to:

* develop a transnational network of universities and employers in the participating countries;
* promote good practices in interprofessional learning and teaching in health-care.

Higher education and employer partners come from Belgium, Finland, Greece, Hungary, Ireland, Poland, Slovenia, Sweden and the United Kingdom.

Journal of Interprofessional Care

The *Journal of Interprofessional Care* is the vehicle for worldwide dissemination of experience, policy, research evidence and theoretical and value perspectives. The journal informs collaboration in education, practice and research between medicine, nursing, veterinary science, allied health, public health, social care and related professions to improve health status and quality of care for individuals, families and communities.

The Journal's scope continues to widen in response to calls for closer collaboration by a growing number of national governments in ever more fields of practice, e.g. care for children and for older people, criminal justice, education for special needs, HIV/AIDS, juvenile justice, mental health, palliative care, physical and learning disabilities among others. This is reflected in the range of contributors and readers from different fields, professions and countries.

Framework
for Action on
Interprofessional
Education and
Collaborative
Practice

50

National Health Sciences Students' Association in Canada (NaHSSA)

Formed in January 2005, the National Health Sciences Students' Association (NaHSSA) is the first ever national interprofessional student association in the world. As a diverse network of university and college-based chapters, NaHSSA seeks to address the unmet need of actively involving Canada's health and human service students in interprofessional education while promoting the attitudes, skills, and behaviours necessary to provide collaborative patient-centred care. NaHSSA has great potential to positively influence the educational and professional development of Canada's next generation of health-care providers and will become a premier pan-Canadian student federation capable of achieving great success in this area. NaHSSA aims to:

* promote interprofessional education for collaborative patient-centred practice;
* facilitate and potentiate opportunities for interprofessional interaction;
* foster student champions to lead interprofessional efforts now and in the future.

NaHSSA is an "association of associations" that is currently composed of health sciences students from 18 university and college-based chapters (Dalhousie University; Memorial University of Newfoundland and Labrador; McGill University; McMaster University; Queen's University; Université de Montréal; Université de Sherbrooke; Université Laval; University of Alberta; University of British Columbia; University of Manitoba; University of New Brunswick at Saint John–New Brunswick Community College–Atlantic Health Sciences Corporation; University of Ottawa; University of Saskatchewan; University of Toronto; University of Waterloo; University of Western Ontario; and York University) and 4 additional schools (George Brown College; University of Calgary; University of Northern British Columbia; and University of Victoria) across Canada, including over 20 different health and human service professions.

51

The Network: Towards Unity for Health

The Network: TUFH is a global association of institutions for education of health professionals committed to contribute, through education, research and service, to the improvement and sustainability of health in the communities they serve.

The Network: TUFH member institutions seek collaboration with their health systems to adapt to each other the education of health personnel and the operation of the health-services in order to improve the health of the community. The Network: TUFH members also explore innovative educational approaches (e.g. community-based education, problem-based learning) to fulfill this mission. The Network: TUFH emphasizes educational research, research on priority health needs and on the efficacy of the health-services. In these endeavours The Network: TUFH invites the collaboration of like-minded organizations.

Nordic Interprofessional Network (NIPNet)

NIPNet is a learning network to foster interprofessional collaboration in education, practice and research and is primarily for Nordic educators, practitioners and researchers in the fields of health. The network's members represent interprofessional education inititatives in Denmark, Finland, Norway and Sweden.

NIPNet aims to:
* explore theories and evidence bases of interprofessional collaboration;
* develop approaches, methods and evaluations of interprofessional learning and practice;
* stimulate collaboration among Nordic countries and international collaboration in research and development of interprofessional education.

Framework for Action on Interprofessional Education and Collaborative Practice

52

Centre for the Advancement of Interprofessional Education (CAIPE)

CAIPE is an independent charity, founded in 1987. It is a membership body with some 300 members who form a network of mutual support and interest. They include organizations and individuals across the United Kingdom statutory, voluntary and independent sectors, and a growing international membership. It has expanded from its roots in primary care to include individual and organizational members in local government, higher education, professional associations, Royal Colleges, professional regulatory bodies and the voluntary and private sectors. CAIPE is a national and international resource for interprofessional education in both universities and the workplace across health-care.

CAIPE promotes and develops interprofessional education as a way of improving collaboration between practitioners and organizations, engaged in both statutory and non-statutory public services. It supports the integration of health-care in local communities. CAIPE's focus is on ways of enabling professions and occupations in the community, education institutions and the workplace to learn and work together, foster mutual respect, overcome barriers to collaboration and engender joint action. CAIPE promotes interprofessional learning that actively involves service users and local communities as essential partners. Closely associated with the work that has established the evidence base for interprofessional education through systematic review, CAIPE is concerned to ensure the quality of interprofessional education and disseminates findings from relevant research and best practice.

53

ANNEX 3 Methodology

The World Health Organization Programme on Interprofessional Education and Collaborative Practice was launched in May 2007 to help Member States strengthen their health systems and address the global health workforce challenge. In collaboration with the International Association of Interprofessional Education and Collaborative Practice (InterEd), the WHO Health Professions Networks Team formed a WHO Study Group on Interprofessional Education and Collaborative Practice consisting of 25 leading education, practice and policy experts from around the world who were divided into three working groups: 1) interprofessional education; 2) collaborative practice; and 3) system-level supportive structures. Building on the considerable progress achieved since WHO issued previous reports* related

to interprofessional education and collaborative practice, the WHO Study Group was tasked with the following:

*   review of the 1988 report of the WHO Study Group on Multiprofessional Education of Health Personnel and evaluate the positive outcomes of this report and the areas in which little or no progress has been made;

*   assess the current state of research evidence on interprofessional education and collaborative practice, synthesize it within an international context and identify the gaps that must still be addressed;

*   conduct an international environmental scan to determine the current uptake of interprofessional education and collaborative practice, identify examples of successes, barriers, enabling factors and the best practices currently known in this area;

*   develop a conceptual framework that would identify the key issues that must be considered and addressed by WHO and its partners when formulating a global operational plan for interprofessional education and collaborative practice;

*   identify, evaluate and synthesize evidence on the potential facilitators, incentives and levers for action that could be recommended as part of a global strategy for interprofessional education and collaborative practice;

---

* 1) World Health Organization. *Continuing education for physicians.* Geneva, World Health Organization, 1973 (WHO Technical Report Series, No. 534); 2) World Health Organization. *Working interrelationships in the provision of community health-care (medicine, nursing and medicosocial work): Report of a Working Group. Florence, 23-26 October 1978.*Copenhagen, World Health Organization Regional Office for Europe, 1978 (ICP/SPM 006); 3) World Health Organization. *Studies on communication and collaboration between health professionals (physicians and nurses: teamwork).* Copenhagen, World Health Organization Regional Office for Europe, 1978 (ICP/HMD 054); 4) World Health Organization. *Innovative tracks at established institutions for the education of health personnel: An experimental approach to change relevant health.* Geneva, World Health Organization, 1987 (WHO Offset. Publication No. 101); 5) World Health Organization. *Multiprofessional education of health personnel in the European region: Proceedings of a WHO meeting on study for analysing multiprofessional training programmes and defining strategies for team training. Copenhagen, 5-7 March 1986.* Copenhagen, World Health Organization Regional Office for Europe, 1988; 6) World Health Organization. *Learning together to work together for health: Report of a WHO Study Group on Multiprofessional Education for Health Personnel: The team approach.* Geneva, World Health Organization (WHO Technical Report Series, No. 769), 1988.

Framework
for Action on
Interprofessional
Education and
Collaborative
Practice

54

* evaluate the efforts and contributions of the WHO Study Group.

In order to meet these terms of reference, the WHO Study Group has prepared the *Framework for Action on Interprofessional Education and Collaborative Practice*, which is based on original and available research evidence and the principles of primary health-care. Meetings were held in Geneva, Switzerland, on 11 September 2007 (for the Central Leadership Team and Theme Leaders) and in Stockholm, Sweden, on 1 June 2008 (for the entire WHO Study Group), and were supplemented by several teleconferences for the three working groups. Partnerships were established with the following organizations to enhance the international relevance of the work and to engage as many people as possible throughout the interprofessional and global health communities:

1. Australasian Interprofessional Practice and Education Network
2. Canadian Interprofessional Health Collaborative
3. European Interprofessional Education Network
4. *Journal of Interprofessional Care*
5. Canada's National Health Sciences Students' Association
6. The Network: Towards Unity for Health
7. Nordic Interprofessional Network
8. Centre for the Advancement of Interprofessional Education

In addition to an extensive review of the research literature and consultation process, the WHO Study Group engaged in several activities that further informed this Framework and provided representative examples of innovative initiatives being undertaken throughout the world.

* An international environmental scan of interprofessional education practices was undertaken between February and May 2008. A custom-designed descriptive questionnaire was developed and targeted individuals who worked on the design, delivery or evaluation of interprofessional education at higher education institutions. Respondents were recruited via email using a wide range of distribution lists, including WHO Country Offices, WHO Collaborating Centres and the membership of 15 international professional associations.[†] Participants represented 42 countries and each of WHO's six regions.

* A targeted call was made throughout WHO's six regions for international case studies of collaborative practice and faculty development for interprofessional education.

---

† The following international organizations, their associated membership and e-mail distribution lists facilitated contact with prospective participants: Association for Prevention Teaching and Research, the United States; Australasian Interprofessional Practice and Education Network; Canadian Interprofessional Health Collaborative; Centre for the Advancement of Interprofessional Education, the United Kingdom; Council of Deans of Health, the United Kingdom; European Interprofessional Education Network; Higher Education Academy, the United Kingdom; International Association for Interprofessional Education and Collaborative Practice; International Pharmaceutical Federation; *Journal of Interprofessional Care*, Informa Healthcare; Linköping University, Sweden; Nordic Interprofessional Network; Secretariat of the All Together Better Health IV Conference (2–5 June 2008, Karolinska Institutet & Linköping University, Sweden); Secretariat of the North American Interprofessional Education Conference (24–26 October 2007, University of Minnesota, the United States); The Network: Towards Unity for Health.

55

* Relevant international policy documents, government publications and global health reports were comprehensively collected and reviewed.
* The wider interprofessional community of practice was engaged through several announcements, teleconferences and meetings, including a workshop and plenary presentation at the All Together Better Health IV Conference, held in Stockholm, Sweden, in June 2008.
* Definitions were developed using an iterative process involving research literature, input from members of the WHO Study Group and other key informants. For example, the definition of "collaborative practice" was based on a review of key publications, adaptations from an existing definition from the Ontario Interprofessional Care Steering Committee‡ and the inclusion of new elements through extensive discussion which ensured the representation of global perspectives. As a result, the term "health worker" was used to reflect internationally-accepted terminology, the importance of families, carers and communities in health-care delivery was recognized, and the reality that care is delivered across settings was incorporated. This working definition was presented to the

wider interprofessional community during a plenary presentation at the All Together Better Health IV Conference, in Stockholm, Sweden, in June 2008, and was further refined by the Collaborative Practice Working Group. Similarly, the definition of "interprofessional education" was adapted from that of the Centre for the Advancement of Interprofessional Education in the United Kingdom§ and Lesley Bainbridge's work¶ to better reflect the global health context.

* Several scoping literature reviews were conducted on key issues, such as staff development for interprofessional education and learning outcomes.

While this Framework addresses many of the major policy-relevant issues related to interprofessional education and collaborative practice, it is by no means exhaustive or all-encompassing. It is the hope of the World Health Organization Study Group on Interprofessional Education and Collaborative Practice that the work outlined in the Framework will be the beginning of lasting change and provide a catalyst for health systems around the world to begin implementing interprofessional education and collaborative practice within their local context.

---

‡ Ontario Interprofessional Care Steering Committee. *Interprofessional care: a blueprint for action in Ontario.* Toronto, HealthForceOntario, 2007 (http://www. healthforceontario.ca/upload/en/whatishfo/ ipc%20blueprint%20final.pdf, accessed 11 August 2008).

§ Centre for the Advancement of Interprofessional Education and Collaborative Practice, the United Kingdom, 2002.
¶ Bainbridge L. *The power of prepositions: learning with, from, and about in the context of interprofessional health education* [doctoral dissertation]. Vancouver, Canada, University of British Columbia, 2008.

Framework for Action on Interprofessional Education and Collaborative Practice

56

ANNEX 4   Public announcement on the creation of the WHO Study Group on Interprofessional Education and Collaborative Practice[**]

World Health Organization Study Group on Interprofessional Education and Collaborative Practice

JEAN YAN, RN, PHD[1], JOHN H. V. GILBERT, PHD[2], & STEVEN J. HOFFMAN, BHSC[3]

[1]Co-Chair, WHO Study Group on Interprofessional Education and Collaborative Practice and Chief Scientist for Nursing & Midwifery, Department of Human Resources for Health, World Health Organization, Geneva, Switzerland, [2]Co-Chair, WHO Study Group on Interprofessional Education and Collaborative Practice; Principal and Professor Emeritus, College of Health Disciplines, University of British Columbia, Vancouver, Canada; Project Lead, Canadian Interprofessional Health Collaborative, [3]Project Manager, WHO Study Group on Interprofessional Education and Collaborative Practice, Department of Human Resources for Health, World Health Organization, Geneva, Switzerland

The urgency for action to enhance human resources for health internationally was recently highlighted by the *World Health Report 2006: Working Together for Health* which revealed an estimated worldwide shortage of almost 4.3 million doctors, midwives, nurses and support workers.[1] The 59th World Health Assembly recognized this crisis and adopted a resolution in 2006 calling for a rapid scaling-up of health workforce production through various strategies including the use of "innovative approaches to teaching in industrialized and developing countries".[2]

  As one innovative strategy to help tackle the global health workforce challenge, we are pleased to announce the launch of the World Health Organization (WHO) Study Group on Interprofessional Education and Collaborative Practice. Working in collaboration with the International Association for Interprofessional Education and Collaborative Practice (InterEd), this initiative builds upon the considerable progress that has been achieved in this area since WHO first identified interprofessional education as an important component of primary health care in 1978[3] and issued its technical report on this subject in 1988.[4] Not only will the WHO Study Group conduct a much-needed international environment scan and an assessment of the current state of research in this area, but it will also identify, evaluate and synthesize the evidence on potential facilitators, incentives and levers for action that could be adopted as part of a global strategy for interprofessional education and collaborative practice (Exhibit 1). This work will form the basis for follow-up efforts and ensure that future activities are rooted in the best evidence possible.

  The WHO Study Group consists of 25 top education, practice and policy experts from across every region of the world; members have formed three separate teams on

[**] Yan J, Gilbert JHV, Hoffman SJ. World Health Organization Study Group on Interprofessional Education and Collaborative Practice. *Journal of Interprofessional Care*, 2007, 21:588–589.

Exhibit 1. Tasks of the WHO Study Group on Interprofessional Education and Collaborative Practice.

- Review the 1988 report of the WHO Study Group on Multiprofessional Education of Health Personnel (WHO, 1988)[4] and evaluate the positive outcomes of this report as well as the areas in which little or no progress has been made;
- Assess the current state of research evidence on interprofessional education and collaborative practice, synthesize it within an international context, and identify the gaps that must still be addressed;
- Conduct an international environmental scan to determine the current uptake of interprofessional education and collaborative practice, discover examples that illuminate successes, barriers, and enabling factors, and identify the best practices currently known in this area;
- Develop a conceptual framework that would identify the key issues that must be considered and addressed by WHO and its partners when formulating a global operational plan for interprofessional education and collaborative practice;
- Identify, evaluate and synthesize evidence on the potential facilitators, incentives and levers for action that could be recommended as part of a global strategy for interprofessional education and collaborative practice; and
- Evaluate the efforts and contributions of this WHO Study Group.

Exhibit 2. Partnering organizations.

1. Australasian Inter Professional Practice and Education Network (AIPPEN);
2. Canadian Interprofessional Health Collaboration (CIHC);
3. European Interprofessional Education Network (EIPEN);
4. *Journal of Interprofessional Care* (JIC);
5. National Health Sciences Students' Association in Canada (NaHSSA);
6. The Network: Towards Unity for Health;
7. Nordic Interprofessional Network (NIPNET); and
8. UK Centre for the Advancement of Interprofessional Education (CAIPE)

interprofessional education, collaborative practice, and system-level supportive structures that are led by Prof Peter G. Baker (University of Queensland, Australia), Prof Yuichi Ishikawa (Kobe University, Japan) and Prof Dame Jill Macleod Clark (University of Southampton, UK) respectively. The WHO Study Group has also established partnerships with several existing communities of experts and enthusiasts (Exhibit 2) to further engage the wider community in this historic initiative while maximizing the specialized knowledge and local experiences of individuals worldwide.

It is clear that now is an exciting time of progress for interprofessional education and collaborative practice. Working together for better health is more important than ever, and we look forward to updating you as the WHO Study Group and its partners move towards a greater understanding of this important issue.

References

[1] World Health Organization. *World Health Report 2006: Working Together for Health.* Geneva: World Health Organization; 2006.
[2] World Health Organization. WHA59.23: Rapid Scaling Up of Health Workforce Production. *Fifty-Ninth World Health Assembly. A59/23, 37–38.* Geneva: World Health Organization; 2006.
[3] World Health Organization (1978). Alma-Ata 1978: Primary Health Care. *Report of the International Conference on Primary Health Care.* 6–12 September 1978. Alma-Ata, USSR. Geneva: World Health Organization.
[4] World Health Organization (1988). Learning to Work Together for Health. Report of a WHO Study Group on Multiprofessional Education for Health Personnel: The Team Approach. *Technical Report Series 769:1–72.* Geneva: World Health Organization.

Framework
for Action on
Interprofessional
Education and
Collaborative
Practice

58

ANNEX 5   Key recommendations from the 1988 WHO Study Group on Multiprofessional Education for Health Personnel technical report

The following are the draft recommendations put forward in the technical report prepared by the WHO Study Group on Multiprofessional Education of Health Personnel in 1988.[††]

8. Promoting the concept of multiprofessional education

These draft recommendations refer to action at different levels and on the part of various bodies: institutional (universities and other schools for health personnel, other education institutions, organizations of health professionals, etc.), inter-institutional (joint action by different educational institutions), and national (ministries of health and education).

8.1 Institutional level

* Formal and informal links should be established between neighbouring institutions responsible for the education of different member of the health team, and between these and the non-health sectors that may have a substantial impact on health and are already involved in community development activities.
* The roles and responsibilities of each member of the health team should be redefined (service,

training, administration, community relations, etc.).
* Communication between health professionals at all levels should be encouraged and improved.
* Continuous joint in-service training should be provided for all member of the health team with a view to strengthening the team approach in the field.
* Ways of reducing any staff overload should be investigated, in order to allow better team functioning.
* Groups should be formed in educational institutions to review:
  - systems for selecting students and staff;
  - curricula and learning resources, laboratories, etc.;
  - systems for evaluating performance of students and teachers;
  - physical arrangements, office needs and use, field facilities, transport, etc.;
  - integration of programmes;
  - Iindividual staff roles and responsibilities.
* Workshops on the team approach should be organized for all teaching and administrative staff in educational institutions.
* It is important to recognize the particular organizational and logistic difficulties that arise in establishing and maintaining cooperative educational activities between different faculties or departments and to make

††   World Health Organization. *Learning together to work together for health: report of a WHO Study Group on Multiprofessional Education for Health Personnel: the team approach.* Geneva, World Health Organization (WHO Technical Report Series, No. 769), 1988.

59

allowance for them in funding arrangements.

* Integration of the community development services with the education sector should be strengthened.

* An incentive system to encourage the team approach should be introduced.

* The involvement of the community should be promoted.

* Research on the health-team approach by educational institutions and health-services should be launched or strengthened.

* Multiprofessional committees should be set up to follow up the utilization of the team approach.

* An international directory of multiprofessional education programmes would be useful for promoting the dissemination of information about multiprofessional education.

8.2 National (or provincial) level

* It is important to have a strong and enduring commitment to the team concept on the part of the ministries and educational institutions concerned.

* The resources of the ministries concerned should be developed and strengthened to enable them to put the health team concept into effect.

* The organizational structure of the health system should be reviewed with the object of making wider use of the primary health-care approach and applying the health team concept.

* Health manpower needs should be determined and the role of the educational institutions for health sciences in meeting those needs should be defined.

* The system for evaluation and supervision of all categories of health workers should be reviewed in the light of its suitability for a team approach.

* Job descriptions for all team members should be distributed to all health centres, and efforts made to develop a scheme for modifying job descriptions as necessary.

* It would be useful to publish descriptions of the role of each of the occupations represented in the health team. The descriptions should indicate how the skills and knowledge pertaining to each discipline can enhance team functioning. They should be made widely available throughout the health sector and the educational institutions.

Framework for Action on Interprofessional Education and Collaborative Practice

60

ANNEX 6   Summary chart of research evidence from systematic reviews on Interprofessional Education (IPE)

SYSTEMATIC REVIEW	STUDY OBJECTIVE(S)	STUDIES	RESULTS	AUTHOR'S CONCLUSIONS
Reeves S et al. Interprofessional education: effects on professional practice and health care outcomes. *Cochrane Database of Systematic Reviews*, 2008, Issue 1.	To assess the effectiveness of IPE interventions compared to education interventions in which the same health-care professionals learn separately from one another; and to assess the effectiveness of IPE interventions compared to no education intervention.	Six included (four RCTs and two CBA studies)	Four studies indicated that IPE produced positive outcomes in areas such as emergency department culture and patient satisfaction; collaborative team behaviour; and management of care delivered to domestic violence victims. Two studies reported mixed outcomes and two of the six studies reported that IPE had no impact on professional practice or patient care.	Although the studies reported some positive outcomes, it was not possible to draw general inferences about IPE and its effectiveness (due to small number of studies, heterogeneity of interventions and methodological limitations).
Hammick M et al. A best evidence systematic review of interprofessional education. *Medical Teacher*, 2007, 29:735–751.	To identify and review the strongest evaluations of IPE; to classify the outcomes of IPE and note the influence of context on particular outcomes; to develop a narrative about the mechanisms that underpin and inform positive and negative outcomes of IPE.	21 included	Staff development is a key influence on the effectiveness of IPE for learners who all have unique values about themselves and others. Authenticity and customization of IPE are important mechanisms for positive outcomes of IPE. Interprofessional education is generally well received, enabling knowledge and skills necessary for collaborative working to be learnt; it is less able to positively influence attitudes and perceptions towards others in the service-delivery team. In the context of quality improvement initiatives interprofessional education is frequently used as a mechanism to enhance the development of practice and improvement of services.	Measuring outcomes of IPE, and thus enabling informed judgements to be made about the impact of the many different IPE initiatives delivered internationally, continues to evolve towards a robust science. This review shows that such work leads to evidence informed interprofessional education, practice and policy-making, and thus learner satisfaction and ultimately enhanced patient/client care and care service delivery.
Barr H et al. *Effective interprofessional education: assumption, argument and evidence.* Oxford, Blackwell Publishing, 2005.	To review conventional wisdom about IPE in the light of evidence from more rigorous and better-presented evaluations.	884 identified, 353 reviewed, 107 high quality	Well planned pre-registration IPE can meet intermediate objectives (i.e. establish common knowledge bases and modify reciprocal attitudes). Well planned employment-led, post-registration IPE can meet ultimate objectives (i.e. improving services and patient experiences).	Improvements in evaluative rigour need to be sustained within both qualitative and quantitative paradigms. IPE needs to be developed as a continuum with progressive objectives.
Cooper H et al. Developing an evidence base for interdisciplinary learning: A systematic review. *Journal of Advanced Nursing*, 2001, 35:228–237.	To explore the feasibility of introducing interdisciplinary education within undergraduate health professional programmes. This paper reports on the first stage of the study in which a systematic review was conducted to summarize the evidence for interdisciplinary education of undergraduate health professional students.	141 identified, 30 included	Student health professionals were found to benefit from interdisciplinary education with outcome effects primarily relating to changes in knowledge, skills, attitudes and beliefs.	Effects upon professional practice were not discernible and educational and psychological theories were rarely used to guide the development of the educational interventions.
Reeves S. A systematic review of the effects of interprofessional education on staff involved in the care of adults with mental health problems. *Journal of Psychiatric Mental Health Nursing*, 2001, 8:533–542.	To assess the extent and quality of published evidence in relation to staff who care for adults with mental health problems.	173 identified, 67 reviewed, 19 included	All 19 papers report positive outcomes from the use of IPE with staff involved in the care of adults with mental health problems. However, after assessing these studies, it was found that they generally contained a number of shortfalls, including: lack of information relating to the methods employed and their associated limitations; little account of how IPE impacted on user care; uncertainty whether initial effects of IPE remained or diminished over time; poor descriptions of the evaluated IPE programmes; limited applicability due to cultural influences.	Although this study offers an initial effort at collecting and assessing the published evidence of IPE, further work would usefully extend and strengthen this study: further searching of other health-care databases; contacting experts in the field to search for grey literature; and scanning the reference sections of these papers to identify other potentially useful studies.
Barr H et al. *Evaluations of interprofessional education: a United Kingdom review for health and social care.* London, BERA/CAIPE, 2000.	To identify where and how IPE had been evaluated in the United Kingdom. To assist others in replicating and developing methods found.	40 reviewed, 19 included	Reviews reported that IPE was enjoyed and valued by learners with positive modification of reciprocal attitudes. Work-based IPE is capable of modifying practice and patient care. Most evaluations were conducted by the teachers themselves.	This small-scale qualitative review revealed the methodologies employed in IPE evaluations and confirmed classifications of types of IPE and learning methods.

61

ANNEX 7   Summary chart of research evidence from select systematic reviews related to collaborative practice

SYSTEMATIC REVIEW	STUDY OBJECTIVE(S)	STUDIES	RESULTS	AUTHOR'S CONCLUSIONS
Malone D et al. Community mental health teams (CMHTs) for people with severe mental illnesses and disordered personality. *Cochrane Database of Systematic Reviews*, 2007, Issue 2 (Art. No.: CD000270. DOI: 10.1002/14651858. CD000270.pub2).	To evaluate the effects of community mental health team (CMHT) treatment for anyone with serious mental illness compared with standard non-team management.	80 identified, three included	CMHT management did not reveal any statistically significant difference in death by suicide although overall, fewer deaths occurred in the CMHT group. Significantly fewer people in the CMHT group were not satisfied with services compared with those receiving standard care. Also, hospital admission rates were significantly lower in the CMHT group compared with standard care. Admittance to accident and emergency services, contact with primary care, and contact with social services did not reveal any statistical difference between comparison groups.	Community mental-health team management is not inferior to non-team standard care in any important respects and is superior in promoting greater acceptance of treatment. It may also be superior in reducing hospital admission and avoiding death by suicide. The evidence for CMHT-based care is insubstantial considering the massive impact the drive toward community care has on patients, carers, clinicians and the community at large.
Holland R et al. Systematic review of multidisciplinary interventions in heart failure. *Heart*, 2005, 91:899–906.	To determine the impact of multidisciplinary interventions on hospital admission and mortality in heart failure.	74 identified, 30 included	Multidisciplinary interventions reduced all-cause admission, all-cause mortality and heart failure admission. These results varied little with sensitivity analyses.	Multidisciplinary interventions for heart failure reduce both hospital admission and all-cause mortality. The most effective interventions were delivered at least partly in the home.
McAlister FA et al. Multidisciplinary strategies for the management of heart failure patients at high risk for admission. *Journal of the American College of Cardiology*, 2004, 44:810–819.	To determine whether multidisciplinary strategies improve outcomes for heart failure patients.	29 identified but were not pooled, because of considerable heterogeneity. A priori, the interventions were divided into homogeneous groups that were suitable for pooling.	Strategies that incorporated follow-up by a specialized multidisciplinary team (either in a clinic or a non-clinic setting) reduced mortality, heart failure hospitalizations and all-cause hospitalizations. In 15 of 18 trials that evaluated costs, multidisciplinary strategies were cost saving.	Multidisciplinary strategies for the management of patients with heart failure reduce heart failure hospitalizations. Those programmes that involve specialized follow-up by a multidisciplinary team also reduce mortality and all-cause hospitalizations.
Naylor CJ, Griffiths RD, Fernandez RS. Does a multidisciplinary total parenteral nutrition team improve outcomes? A systematic review. *Journal of Parenteral and Enteral Nutrition*, 2004, 28:251–258	To critically analyze the literature and present the best available evidence that investigated the effectiveness of multidisciplinary total parenteral nutrition (TPN) teams in the provision of TPN to adult hospitalized patients.	11 included	Results of the studies indicate that the incidence of total mechanical complications is reduced in patients managed by the TPN team. However, the benefit of the TPN team in the reduction of catheter-related sepsis remains inconclusive. Although only two studies (n=356) investigated total costs associated with management of patients by the TPN teams, there was evidence that a team approach is a cost-effective strategy.	Overall, the general effectiveness of the TPN team has not been conclusively demonstrated. There is evidence that patients managed by TPN teams have a reduced incidence of total mechanical complications. Furthermore, the available evidence, although limited, suggests financial benefits from the introduction of multidisciplinary TPN teams in the hospital setting.
Simmonds S et al. Community mental health team management in severe mental illness: a systematic review. *The British Journal of Psychiatry*, 2001, 178:497–502.	To assess the benefits of community mental health team management in severe mental illness.	1200 identified, 65 reviewed, five included	Community mental health team management is associated with fewer deaths by suicide and in suspicious circumstances, less dissatisfaction with care and fewer drop-outs. Duration of in-patient psychiatric treatment is shorter with community team management and costs of care are less, but there are no gains in clinical symptomatology or social functioning.	Community mental health team management is superior to standard care in promoting greater acceptance of treatment, and may also reduce hospital admission and avoid deaths by suicide. This model of care is effective and deserves encouragement.
Zwarenstein M, Bryant W. Interventions to promote collaboration between nurses and doctors. *Cochrane Database of Systematic Reviews*, 2000, Issue 1.	To assess the effects of interventions designed to improve nurse-doctor collaboration.	Five identified, two included	First trial noted shortened average length of stay and reduced hospital charges, with no statistically significant differences in mortality rates. Second trial noted no significant differences between the intervention and control wards in terms of total average length of stay for patient. No significant difference in mortality rates.	Increasing collaboration improved outcomes of importance to patients and to health-care managers. These gains were moderate and affected health-care processes rather than outcomes. Further research is needed to confirm these findings. Interventions other than nurse-doctor ward rounds and team meetings should also be tested.

62

ANNEX 8   Summary chart of select international collaborative practice case studies

COUNTRY	PRACTICE SETTING	WHO IS INVOLVED?	WHAT ARE THE CHALLENGES AND FACILITATORS?
Canada	A family practice teaching clinic located in an urban setting	Complex patients living with chronic and mental illnesses Family physicians, mental health workers, nurses, nurse practitioners, nutritionists, pharmacists, public health nurses, receptionists and social workers	Challenges: lack of an electronic health record; interpersonal conflicts; lack of structured protocols Facilitators: remuneration models; a governance model that shares responsibility between professionals; interprofessional rounds; committed leadership
Denmark	General practice clinics in Denmark, each serving between 1600 and 2500 patients, in urban and rural areas	All types of patients General practitioners, administrative staff, nurses and laboratory technicians	Challenges: unsuitable office and administrative space for all tasks; unclear division of responsibility and competency between different staff groups Facilitators: self registration of patients; joint discussion of patients by general practitioners and staff
India	A psychiatric hospital located in a semi-urban setting	Patients living with mental illnesses (children, adolescents and adults) Nurses, occupational therapists, psychiatrists, psychologists, social workers, special education teachers and supportive staff	Challenges: miscommunication Facilitators: open communication; approachability and adaptability of team members
Japan	All types of health-services located in an urban setting	Pregnant women and young children Clinical psychologists, dental hygienists, nutritionists, paediatricians, public health nurses and social workers	Challenges: none identified Facilitators: supportive legislation; structured protocols; team conferences
Nepal	A hospital and an educational institution located in an urban setting	Mothers and their newborn babies Nurses and physicians	Challenges: time constraints; traditional care delivery models Facilitators: evidence; government policies
Oman	Four community health centres located in urban areas	All types of patients Doctors, nurses, assistant pharmacists, laboratory technicians, X-ray technicians, dieticians, health educators and medical orderlies	Challenges: managing difficult personalities; staff turnover Facilitators: commitment from high-level policy-makers; ongoing staff training, including communication skills training; clear guidelines; meetings between health workers and system planners; spirit of teamwork
Slovenia	A community health centre	All types of patients Dentists, nurses, physicians, physiotherapists and social workers	Challenges: new members being introduced into teams Facilitators: supportive health legislation; same payment scheme for all professions; professional development programmes that focus on teamwork
Sweden	Four major hospitals located in an urban setting	All types of patients Medical, nursing, occupational therapy and physiotherapy students	Challenges: professional prejudices and attitudes Facilitators: standard protocols
Thailand	A community clinic located in a rural setting	All types of patients Nurses and physicians	Challenges: lack of time and resources Facilitators: supportive policies from universities, agencies and government; common goals; regulatory bodies; financial support; trusting relationships
United Kingdom	An outpatient clinic located in an urban setting	Patients living with incontinence Nurses, occupational therapists and physiotherapists	Challenges: discord between teams; time constraints; lack of managerial support Facilitators: regular face-to-face meetings; respect for other professions

WHO/HRH/HPN/10.3

Health Professions Networks
Nursing & Midwifery
Human Resources for Health

World Health Organization
Department of Human Resources for Health
20, avenue Appia
1211 Geneva 27
Switzerland

www.who.int/hrh/nursing_midwifery/en/

A priori Outcome predictions that are made before the measurement phase begins.

Absolute risk reduction The value that gives the reduction in risk in absolute terms. It is the difference between the observed risk in those who did and did not experience the event/disease.

Action Plan Is a written document developed by those leading implementation and other key stakeholders that outlines the objectives, actions, and responsibilities of individuals or groups necessary to implement the EBPs.

Active dissemination Real-time interaction with the intended audience to impart key messages or information. This type of dissemination is bidirectional communication, and multiple conversations are used to discuss EBPs and rationale for use.

After-only design This is a less frequently used and weaker design composed of two randomly assigned groups, but unlike the classic experimental design, neither group is pretested. The independent variable is manipulated for the experimental arm but not for the control group.

AGREE II tool A standardized tool and method for appraising clinical practice guidelines.

Altmetrics The nontraditional impact of a study, tracked by many publishers at the article level, may measure downloads, captures (bookmarks, favorites, watchers, and other indications a reader wants to return to an item), "mentions" in news outlets, blogs, tweets, and other social media.

Audit and feedback Ongoing auditing of performance indicators, aggregating data into reports, and discussing the findings with practitioners on a regular basis during the practice change.

Auditability Is a feature of establishing scientific rigor where the reader can follow the line of thinking used by the researcher in the development of thematic and the exhaustive description.

Background question Those questions that lead you to investigate information about a disease, a condition, or a treatment that is derived from a knowledge-focused trigger.

Benchmarking The process of comparing a practice's performance with an external standard.

Bias Any influencing factor that may affect a study's results.

Blinding Sometimes called masking, is the process of concealing from the researchers, recruiters, interventionists, and subjects and/or data collectors what treatment the subjects are receiving in the study.

Boolean connectors Search operators such as "AND", "OR", and "NOT" that define relationships among search terms to narrow or expand search results.

Case control study Study designed to assess the association between an exposure (independent variable) and an outcome (dependent variable).

Case series Study that collects data from a consecutive sample of patients treated in a similar manner without a control group.

Case study Research is rooted in sociology and focuses on describing elements of an individual case.

cause-and-effect diagrams Used to identify and treat the causes of performance problems.

Change champion Individual who takes a role in organizing and brokering change because of his or her advocacy and personal network relationships.

Citation management tools Tools, such as Endnote, Zotero, Mendeley, and Refworks, among others, that are platforms for downloading citations from library catalogs, article databases, and websites to build a personal data/article repository.

Climate for evidence-based practice implementation Staff's shared perceptions of the practices, policies, procedures, and clinical behaviors that are rewarded, supported, and expected to facilitate effective implementation of evidence-based practices.

Clinical decision support Tools often designed in the form of algorithms that can help illustrate the compatibility of a new practice in the context of the organization.

Clinical meaningfulness The degree to which the differences and relationships reported in a study are relevant to nursing practice.

Clinical Microsystems A quality improvement model developed specifically for health care. It is considered the building block of any health care system and is the smallest replicable unit in an organization.

Clinical practice guidelines Systematically developed statements or recommendations that link research and practice and provide an evidence-based best practice guide for clinicians.

Clinical question Forms the basis for searching the literature to identify supporting evidence from research to inform development or revision of clinical standards, protocols, and policies that guide professional nursing and interprofessional best practice.

Cohort study Study that collects data from the same group of subjects.

Common cause variation Occurs at random and is considered a characteristic of the system.

Concealment A method of protecting the randomization process to make sure the group assignment is not readily known by anyone before the subject is assigned to a group.

Conduct of research The systematic investigation of a phenomenon to answer research questions or hypotheses that generate new knowledge and advance the state of the science.

Confidence interval Represents a range of values within which a given population parameter (e.g., a mean, test statistic, or effect size) may be expected to fall.

Confirmability Refers to confirmation of the researcher influence in interpreting data and evidence of bracketing their biases through journal writing.

CONSORT Diagram The abbreviation used for the Consolidated Standards of Reporting Trials. A CONSORT diagram often is required to report the enrollment of participants in a trial.

Constancy Sameness in methods and procedures of data collection.

Context Characteristics of the physical setting of implementation and the dynamic practice factors in which implementation processes occur.

Contextual barriers Challenges in the environment, health care system, clinical workflow, administrative, and patient care context that make engagement more difficult to accomplish.

Continuous data A variable that measures a degree of change or a difference on a range.

Control Measures that the researcher uses to hold the conditions of the study consistent.

Control chart Is used to track system performance over time, but it is a more sophisticated data tool than a run chart.

Control group The group in a study that receives a different or no intervention or treatment.

Controlled vocabulary An online thesaurus of terms that disambiguate and facilitate more precise retrieval using search terms.

Cost/benefit ratio Mathematic representation of the relationship of the cost of an activity to the benefit of its outcome.

Credibility Refers to the conscious effort to establish confidence in an accurate interpretation of the meaning of the data.

Cross-sectional study Study design that assesses data at one point in time.

Crossover design A repeated measures design in which subjects serve as their own controls. Subjects are randomized to one of two groups; one group initially receives the intervention, and the other group serves as the control.

Data saturation Is determined by the researcher when no new information emerge from the informants.

Dependability Refers to whether the informants recognize the exhaustive description as their reality when the narrative is returned to them.

Dependent variable Outcome variable.

Descriptive statistics Statistics used to describe or summarize elements of the sample.

Diagnosis A diagnosis question focuses on the establishment of the power of a test to differentiate between those with the disease or problem and those who do not experience the problem.

Dichotomous data A type of nominal data with only two levels that typically have no hierarchy.

Diffusion of Innovation Broad framework explaining the adoption of many types of innovations by various groups or populations.

Dissemination The act of widely spreading information or ideas to many individuals. In health care, dissemination is the purposeful distribution of information and intervention materials to a specific public health or clinical practice audience.

DMAIC Model Control is achieved by applying an improvement model.

Double blind Means that neither the subject nor the researcher knows to which arm the subject is assigned, that is, the intervention or the control arm of the study.

Effect size A measure of the degree to which the null hypothesis is false, that is, the treatment makes a significant difference.

Effectiveness When a study is designed to test an intervention under "real-world" conditions.

Efficacy When a study is designed to test an intervention under well-controlled conditions.

Emic Is the insiders' view of a culture.

Environmental scan Assessment of internal strengths and challenges for implementation of evidence-based practices. Environmental scans include the structure and function of the organization.

Ethnography Is associated with anthropology, the work of describing culture and the people of a particular culture.

Etic Is the outsider's view of a culture.

Evaluation A structured approach to evaluating the impact of evidence-based practices (EBPs) when implemented in practice. It includes collection and analysis of data from the practice setting to determine whether the EBPs should be retained, modified, or eliminated.

Evidence summary A short summary of available evidence that may provide pre-synthesized data as well as recommendations for research and clinical practice.

Evidence-based practice The conscientious and judicious use of current best evidence in conjunction with clinical expertise, patient values, and circumstances to guide health care decisions.

Exclusion criteria Specific factors or characteristics of potential research participants that should not be present when someone enrolls in a research study (e.g., poor health, pregnancy, moving soon).

Experimental arm The part of a randomized trial in which participants receive the investigational treatment or the new intervention.

Experimental group The group that receives the experimental treatment.

Exposure A harmful or beneficial condition that can affect the outcome of illness or health.

Extent of adoption Number of evidence-based practice users after implementation compared with the number before implementation.

External validity The degree to which findings can be generalized to other populations or environments.

Extraneous variable Variables that interfere with study and cannot be manipulated or controlled. Also called mediating variables.

Fail-safe number Uses an odds ratio to calculate the number of studies reporting no treatment effect that would need to be included in the analysis to reduce the pooled odds ratio to a nonsignificant value.

Fiscal outcomes Estimated health care costs that may be affected by implementing evidence-based practices. Fiscal measures can address cost savings, cost reductions, and cost benefit.

Fishbone diagrams Can be used proactively to prevent quality defects including errors and retrospectively to identify factors that potentially contributed to a quality defect or error that already has occurred.

Flowchart Depicts how a QI process works, detailing the sequence of steps from the beginning to the end of a process.

Forest plot A visual reporting diagram of the individual study odds ratios (ORs) and confidence intervals (CIs) and the pooled OR and CI for the combined studies, which illustrates the magnitude of the effect of the intervention.

Funnel plot A graph based on odds ratios that detects small study treatment effects.

Generalizability The extent to which a study's findings can be applied to a different population.

GRADE A standardized system for grading evidence.

Gray literature Fugitive, ephemeral, invisible, or unpublished, is unevaluated and not peer-reviewed.

Grounded theory Research is used to generate theories about clinical practice and understanding about many different aspects of health care.

Harm A harm question focuses on the potential harm of a symptom or group of symptoms, disorder, treatment, or intervention.

Health literacy An individual's ability to access, interpret, and understand qualitative data about his or her health (i.e., delivered without numbers, typically as words or pictures).

Health numeracy An individual's ability to access, interpret, and understand quantitative data about his or her health (i.e., delivered with numbers or portraying numbers).

Heterophily Transfer of ideas between opposite or different groups where the individuals have different attributes (e.g., various levels of education or different organizational roles).

History Internal validity threat that refers to events outside the study that many affect the dependent variable.

Homogeneity Similarity of the sample's characteristics.

Homophily Transfer of ideas among groups of people who are similar (e.g., members of the same professional groups or specialty practices).

Hypothesis Is used in research studies to predict the outcome(s) of the study. A hypothesis is predictive in nature and typically used when significant knowledge already exists on the subject, which allows the prediction to be made.

Implementation Is the processes and strategies used to promote the uptake and use of EBPs by clinicians, consumers, and policy makers.

Implementation fidelity Measures the degree to which participants carry out the evidence-based practices as intended.

Implementation science Testing implementation interventions/strategies to improve uptake and use of evidence to improve patient outcomes and population health, as well as to clarify what implementation strategies work, for whom, in what settings, and why.

Independent variable The antecedent or variable that has the presumed effect on the dependent variable.

Inferential statistics Tests used to apply findings from a sample to a population

Instrumentation Changes in the measurement of a variable that may account for changes in the obtained measurement.

Integrative review Critical appraisal of the literature in an area of interest that does not include a statistical analysis due to the limitations of the study designs or the heterogeneity of the designs and sam-

ples. A systematic approach using explicit criteria is often used.

Intent-to-treat method The statistical process of analyzing data according to randomized groups, exactly as it exists upon randomization (even if participants receive no or minimal exposure to the intervention)

Internal validity The degree to which one can infer that the experimental treatment, rather than another condition or variable, resulted in the outcome or observed effects.

Interval data A type of data where the values are numeric, there is a hierarchy to the data, and the distances between categories have consistent, set values with the same interpretation.

Intervening variable A variable that occurs during a study that affects the dependent variable.

Intervention dose An important component of intervention fidelity, is the amount of the "something" that is given to the study participants to create a change in the dependent variable(s).

Intervention fidelity Also called treatment fidelity, implementation fidelity, adherence to protocol. Process used to ensure that the research intervention was delivered exactly as planned; typically involves collecting data on how research staff were trained and the consistency with which the intervention was delivered and received by the participants.

Intervention studies Often called randomized controlled (clinical) trials and abbreviated as RCT, reflect the strongest design type for an individual study, located at Level II on the Evidence Hierarchy.

Knowledge-focused triggers Ideas that are generated when clinical teams or quality improvement committees read research studies, listen to scientific papers presented at professional conferences, or encounter practice guidelines published by federal organizations.

Leadership behaviors for evidence-based practice (EBP) implementation Enactment of behaviors by leaders that reflect the extent to which they support and foster EBP implementation.

Lean A quality improvement framework focused on eliminating waste from the production system by designing the most efficient and effective system.

Likelihood ratio Expresses the magnitude by which the probability of disease in a specific patient is modified by the result of a test.

Longitudinal study Also known as cohort, repeated measures, or prospective study.

Manipulation Means using a different dose of "something" in one group (the intervention arm) and not the other group (the control group).

Maturation Developmental, biological, physiological, or psychological processes within an individual as a function of time that are external to a study's events.

Mean The average of all the data in a set.

Meaning A meaning question focuses on the situation or processes related to how people experience, cope, or adapt to conditions, illnesses, or circumstances.

Measurement effects Administration of a pretest that affects the generalizability of a study's findings to other populations.

Median The value in a set that is closest to the middle of a range.

Meta-analysis A type of systematic review, combines the results of multiple studies in a specific area, quantitatively analyzes the findings as an aggregate, and presents a quantitative conclusion about the strength of the evidence provided by the group of studies and makes a recommendation about the applicability of the findings.

Metaliteracy An "ongoing adaptation to emerging technologies and an understanding of the critical thinking and reflection required to engage in these spaces."

Metasynthesis Is a rigorous synthesis of a critical mass of qualitative research evidence that relates to answering a specific research question (sometimes call a metasummary).

Mode The value that occurs most frequently in a data set.

Model for improvement Focuses on the aims, identifies measures to assess change, and specifies changes that will result in improvement.

Mortality Loss of subject.

Narrative review Review of the literature that includes studies that support an author's perspective and provides a broad background discussion in a focused area of interest. A systematic approach to searching for and appraising papers is often not used.

Negative predictive value The proportion of those with negative test results who truly do not have disease.

Nominal data A type of data that is not numerical and has no established hierarchy between values.

Nonparametric statistics Distribution-free statistical method used to analyze nominal and ordinal level data.

Null hypothesis A hypothesis that assumes there is no relationship between two variables.

Null value The value of no effect; in experimental study design it often means there is no difference in the outcomes between the experimental and control groups.

Numbers needed to treat The number of patients who need to be treated to get the desired outcome in one patient who would not have benefited otherwise.

Observational study A category of non-experimental studies that constructs a picture of variables at one point or over a period of time. The variables are not manipulated or randomized as in a randomized clinical trial.

Odds ratio A numeric value that indicates the probability of an outcome occurring given exposure to a variable of interest. It compares the odds of the disease (or other phenomenon) occurring with those of the disease (or other phenomenon) not occurring when exposed to the variable of interest.

Opinion leader Individual who is able to informally influence others' ideas, attitudes, or overt behavior in a desired way.

Ordinal data A type of nonnumerical data that has an associated hierarchy but the distance between values may not be consistent and may have different interpretations.

Outcome The consequence of the exposure.

Outcome measures Measures projected to change as a result of evidence-based practice (EBP) implementation. They are used to evaluate whether implementation of the selected EBPs are resulting in improvements in health outcomes.

Outcomes The effect that the processes of care have on patients and populations.

Parametric statistics A method used to analyze data at the interval or ratio level. The parameters tested must be normally distributed in the population.

Passive dissemination A one-way communication or top-down process such as publishing or posting information with the expectation that the intended audience will access and use the information.

Patient activation The knowledge, confidence and skills that a patient possesses and is willing to use to make decisions about his or her health.

Patient portal A web-based platform that compiles various resources for patient engagement, such as decision making aids, educational materials and communication applications. It typically is connected to the Electronic Health Record used by providers to communicate health care data back to the patient.

Performance gap assessment The baseline practice performance that provides information about the state of current practices at the beginning of a practice change.

Phenomenology Is a science whose purpose is to describe particular phenomena, or the appearance of things, as lived experience.

PICO Provides an effective format for developing focused and searchable clinical questions. PICO is a tool to help you formulate the clinical question.

Pilot Trying an evidence-based practice for a period of time before full adoption

Pilot study A small sample study conducted as a prelude to a larger scale study, often called the "parent study."

Plan-Do-Study-Act (PSDA) Improvement Cycles The improvement changes identified in the planning phase of the quality improvement process are tested using the PDSA improvement cycle, the last step in the quality improvement process.

Point-of-care tool Designed to aid decision support for clinicians by synthesizing evidence for common clinical problems, diseases, drugs, and therapies.

Positive predictive value The proportion of those with positive test results who truly have disease.

Power analysis A method of determining statistical power, the probability of correctly rejecting a null hypothesis.

Pragmatic trials Trials that evaluate the effectiveness of an intervention previously tested for efficacy in traditional experimental designs.

Prevalence Epidemiological term used to describe the number of people with a disease in a specified time period.

Primary source A book or article that contains original evidence.

PRISMA flowchart A graphical depiction of the process of identifying, screening, determining eligibility, and applying exclusion criteria during the process of creating an integrative or systematic review that can be very useful as a graphical depiction of your search.

Probability value (P-value) A numeric value that helps determine whether the null hypothesis should be rejected or accepted

Problem-focused triggers Those identified by staff through quality improvement, risk surveillance, benchmarking, and financial data or recurrent clinical problems.

Process measures Methods to evaluate staff's use of the evidence-based practices (EBPs) as detailed in the local EBP standard. They measure whether the EBPs demonstrated to benefit patients are being followed.

Processes of care The services and treatments patients receive.

Prognosis A prognosis question focuses on a patient's likely course for a disease state or factors that may alter a prognosis.

Public reporting Systems that compare treatment results, costs, and patient experiences.

Publication bias Misleading results as the set of published data may not be a representative sample of the overall evidence.

Purposive sampling Indicates that a sample is homogeneous and reflects the population being studied.

Qualitative research Is explanatory, descriptive, and inductive in nature and comprises methods that help us formulate an understanding of phenomena and their context answered by discovery-oriented research questions.

Quality health care Care that is safe, effective, patient-centered, timely, efficient, and equitable.

Quality improvement Uses data to monitor the outcomes of care processes and improvement methods to design and test changes to continuously improve the quality and safety of health care systems.

Quasi-experimental design A design located at Level III on the Evidence Hierarchy. Quasi-experimental designs differ from RCTs in that they lack either a comparison group or randomization and, as such, have a higher risk of bias.

Quick reference guides Guides that provide targeted, concise information designed to help practitioners perform specific tasks.

Randomization A sampling procedure in which each person has an equal chance of being selected to either the experimental or control group.

Randomized clinical trial Research study having at least two arms where the decision as to which arm the subject is assigned to is made by chance (usually computer-generated).

Range The lowest and highest values reported in a data set

Rapid review Methodology that uses shorter time frames than for other evidence-based summaries. It provides a timely and valid view of evidence but sacrifices rigor. As such, RRs are both review and assessment and respond to urgent clinical and public health-related questions.

Rate of adoption Speed at which users begin to use new evidence-based practices

Ratio data A type of data where the values are numeric and contain absolute zero (the complete absence of the variable), there is a hierarchy to the data, and the distances between categories have consistent, set values with the same interpretation.

Reactivity Distortion created when those who are being observed change their behavior because they know they are being observed.

Realist review Provides explanatory analysis aimed at discerning what works for whom, in what circumstances, and how. Sources can include theoretical, policy, and research literature that combine theoretical understanding with empirical evidence and focus on the context in which an intervention is applied, the mechanisms by which it works, and the outcomes it produces.

Receiver Operating Characteristics (ROC) curve A plot of the true positive rate against the false-positive rate for the different possible cutpoints of a diagnostic test.

Recognition Formal or informal action that recognizes staff for their efforts in implementing evidence-based practices. Examples include highlighting work in organizational publications; personal thank-you notes from leaders; highlighting the work at system-level quality improvement meetings; and nominating individuals or teams for practice excellence awards offered by the health system or professional organization.

Relative risk A numeric value that describes the probability of developing a disease when exposed to risk factor(s) compared with the probability of developing the disease when not exposed to risk factor(s).

Repeated measures study A study design in which data are collected from the same subjects on multiple occasions.

Research The systematic investigation of a phenomenon to answer research questions or hypotheses that generate new knowledge and advance the state of the science.

Research question Addresses a gap or conflict in the literature. Tests a measureable relationship between the independent and dependent variable that is examined in the study.

Retrospective study A study that begins with an outcome (dependent variable) and examines its relationship to another variable (independent variable) that preceded it.

Review An evidence summary that synthesizes information from quantitative and qualitative research studies as well as theoretical and conceptual published and unpublished outputs.

Reward Form of monetary compensation such as a bonus payment, salary increase, or educational funds to be used at the discretion of the individual, team, or practice. For example, an individual or team who has been instrumental in implementing evidence-based practices may receive financial support to attend a regional or national conference to present their work.

Risk/benefit ratio Ratio of the risk of an action to its potential benefits. Risk–benefit analysis is analysis that seeks to quantify the risk and benefits.

Root cause analysis (RCA) Identify system design failures that caused errors.

Run chart A graphical data display that shows trends in a measure of interest; trends reveal what is occurring over time.

Scoping review A preliminary search and assessment of the potential size and scope of available research literature, including ongoing research. It aims to determine the value of undertaking a full systematic review.

Scoping search Identifies the existing evidence or a gap in research and informs the focus for developing a refined PICO question.

Search bias The skewed or insufficient retrieval of literature that results from a careless or incomplete search strategy or selection of the wrong database.

Secondary source Derived from or interpretation of primary sources.

Selection bias Internal validity threat that arises when pretreatment differences between the experimental and control group are present.

Sensitivity The ability of the instrument or test to predict a positive result when the phenomenon of interest is also positive or will occur.

Sensitivity analysis Used to examine the effect of studies that are "outliers."

Shared decision making A process by which patients and clinicians partner to make informed health decisions.

Shared decision making aids Evidence-based documents or tools that portray health care options; give information about risks, benefits, and outcomes for the options; assist patients in clarifying their values; and incorporate clinical judgment and counseling.

Single blind Occurs when the subject does not know which intervention he or she is receiving. Solomon four-group design – A design with four groups (two experimental and two control). Two groups are identical to those used in the classic experimental design described earlier, plus two additional groups including an experimental after-group and a control after-group. Subjects are randomly assigned to one of four groups before baseline data are collected. This design results in two groups that receive only a posttest rather than a pre- and posttest.

Six Sigma A quality improvement framework that emphasizes meeting customer requirements and eliminating errors or reworking with the goal of reducing process variation. Focuses on tightly controlling variations in production processes with the goal of reducing the number of defects using the DMAIC model.

Snowballing Following reference lists backward and following articles that cite an article following publication

Social system Context of a care delivery or practice setting where the evidence-based practices are being implemented.

Special cause variation Arises from a special situation that disrupts the causal system beyond what can be accounted for by random variation.

Specificity   The ability of the instrument or test to predict a negative result when the phenomenon of interest is also negative or will not occur.

SQUIRE Guidelines   Promote standardized guidelines for the publication and interpretation of applied research and used to evaluate QI projects.

Stakeholder   A key individual or group of individuals who will be directly or indirectly affected by the implementation of the EBP.

Standard deviation   A numeric measure of the variation or spread of values in a set of data.

Survey studies   Provide information in areas where little is known, often ask broad questions, and generally have large sample sizes. Survey studies are also classified as descriptive, exploratory, or comparative.

Sustainability   Occurs when a new practice becomes embedded into daily workflow.

Synthesis   Critical appraisal of the overall strengths and weaknesses of the studies as a group to establish the state of the science for answering your PICO question and provide an evidence-based foundation on which to base practice and standards of care.

Systematic review   A collection of research studies based on a clearly focused question that uses a clearly defined search strategy to locate and then assess relevant evidence for applicability to clinical practice.

Test for heterogeneity   Sometimes referred to as the test of homogeneity, calculated to determine that the hypothesis that each study is measuring is similar across studies and for the same population.

Testing   The effects of taking a pretest on a posttest that includes defining, measuring, analyzing, improving, and controlling processes.

Therapy   A therapy question focuses on determining the effect of an intervention(s) on patient outcomes.

Total Quality Management/Continuous Quality Improvement   A holistic management approach used to improve organizational performance. TQM/CQI tools and techniques are applied to specific performance problems in the form of improvement projects.

Transferability   Focuses on whether the findings are applicable outside the study situation.

Translating Research into Practice Model   Is a conceptual model to guide selection of implementation strategies for promoting adoption of EBPs. The model is derived from Roger's (2003) seminal work on diffusion of innovations.

Translation science   Focuses on testing the implementation of interventions to improve uptake and use of evidence to improve patient outcomes, population health, and to clarify what implementation strategies work for whom, in what settings, and why.

Triple blind   Occurs when the researcher, interventionist, and subjects do not know which arm is receiving the experimental treatment versus the placebo.

Trustworthiness   Refers to whether the participants recognize the experience as their own and whether adequate time has been allowed to fully understand the phenomenon.

Type I error   When an instrument or test incorrectly predicts that a phenomenon of interest will occur.

Type II error   When an instrument or test incorrectly predicts that a phenomenon of interest will not occur.

Users of EBPs   Members of a practice setting who will be using and implementing the evidence-based practices. This may include nurses, physicians, respiratory therapists, and professionals from other disciplines.

Note: Page numbers followed by "f" indicate figures, "t" indicate tables and "b" indicate boxes.